CORNEAL ASTIGMATISM
ETIOLOGY, PREVENTION, AND MANAGEMENT

Computed corneal topology of a series of corneas with astigmatic error in a classification system suggested by Waring.

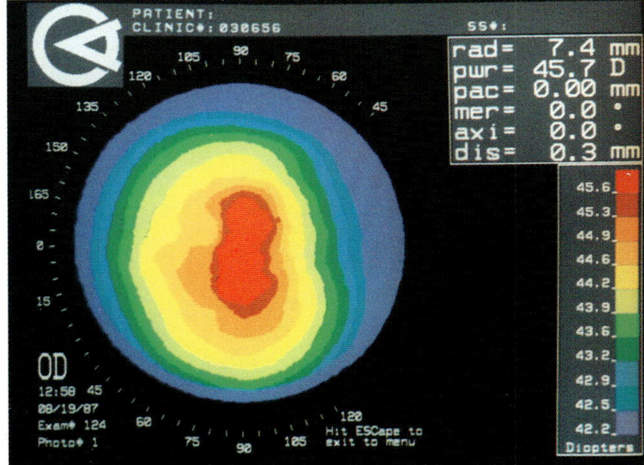

A. Oval.

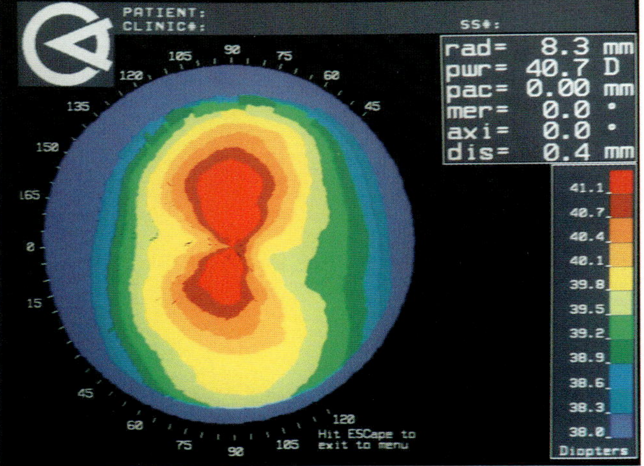

B. Hourglass.

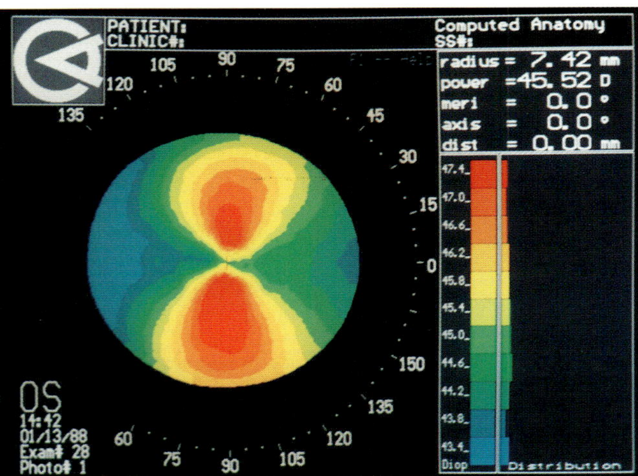

C. Equal bowtie.

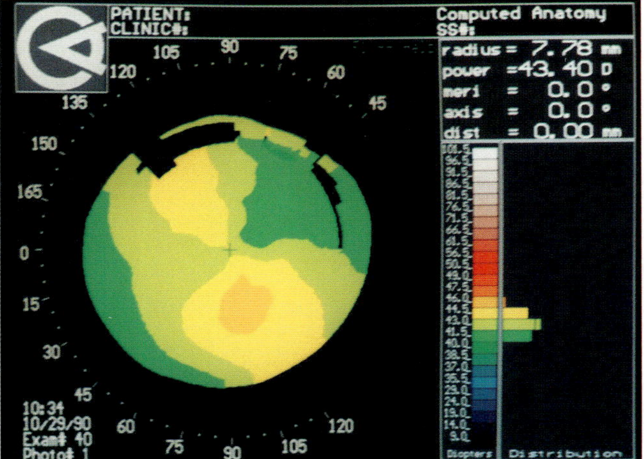

D. Unequal bowtie.

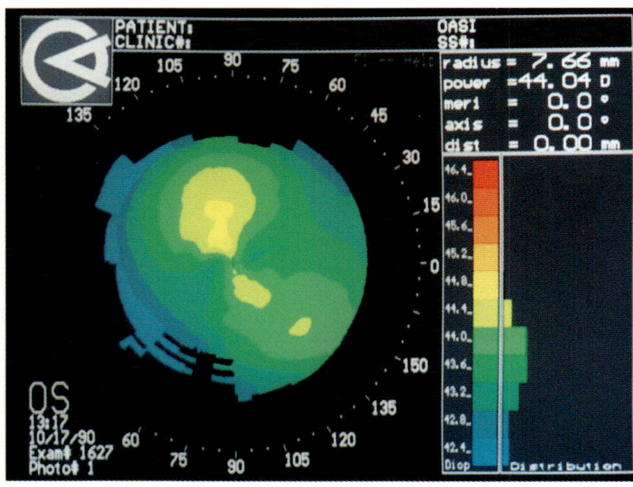

E. Tipped.

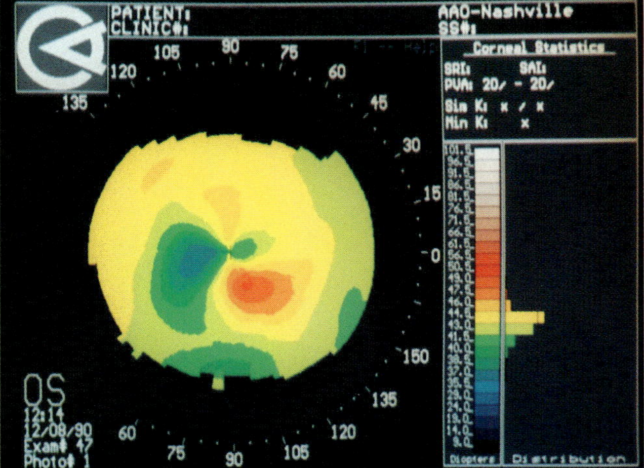

F. Irregular.

Corneal Astigmatism
Etiology, Prevention, and Management

RICHARD C. TROUTMAN, M.D., F.A.C.S., F.C.Oph.
Attending Surgeon and Director of Corneal and Refractive Surgery Clinics
Manhattan Eye, Ear, and Throat Hospital
Clinical Professor of Ophthalmology
The New York Hospital
Cornell Medical Center
New York, New York

KURT A. BUZARD, M.A.(Physics), M.D., F.A.C.S.
Assistant Clinical Professor of Ophthalmology
University of Nevada
Las Vegas, Nevada

450 illustrations by:
VIRGINA HOYT CANTARELLA, A.M.I.

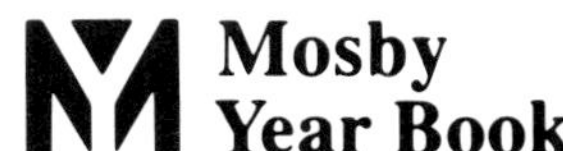

St. Louis   Baltimore   Boston   Chicago   London   Philadelphia   Sydney   Toronto

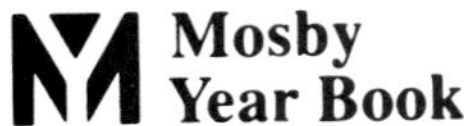 **Mosby
Year Book**

Dedicated to Publishing Excellence

Sponsoring Editor: Kim Kist
Assistant Editor: Penny Rudolph
Assistant Managing Editor, Text and Reference: George Mary Gardner
Production Supervisor: Carol A. Reynolds
Proofroom Manager: Barbara Kelly

1   2   3   4   5   6   7   8   9   0   CL MB   96   95   94   93   92

Library of Congress Cataloging-in-Publication Data

Troutman, Richard C. (Richard Charles), 1922-
    Corneal astigmatism : etiology, prevention, and management /
Richard C. Troutman, Kurt A. Buzard.
        p.   cm.
    Includes bibliographical references and index.
    ISBN 0-8016-5531-5
    1. Astigmatism.   2. Astigmatism—Surgery.   3. Cornea—Surgery.
4. Microsurgery.   I. Buzard, Kurt A.   II. Title.
    [DNLM: 1. Astigmatism—etiology.   2. Astigmatism—prevention &
control.   3. Astigmatism—surgery.   4. Cornea—physiopathology.
5. Cornea—surgery.   WW 310 T861c]
RE932.T76   1991
617.7′55—dc20
DNLM/DLC   91-30023
for Library of Congress   CIP

DEDICATION

We dedicate this volume to our spouses
  Suzanne Véronneau-Troutman
    and
  Carol Buzard
without whose encouragement, help, and participation this work never could have been realized, and to our patients, who have contributed with us in the advancement of our understanding of the management of congenital and surgically induced astigmatism.

FOREWORD

Corneal astigmatism is a complex problem. Every anterior segment surgeon searches for its solution: how to end up with minimum astigmatism when performing a cataract operation and how to obtain an "acceptable" astigmatism when doing a corneal transplant.

There are other types of astigmatism that make the question more difficult: congenital, traumatic, following corneal surface disease, and keratoconus, among others.

What to do about this condition is a dilemma. No one has yet come up with generally acceptable solutions. Most techniques to correct it are controversial.

Of all the learned surgeons on this subject, I can think of no one more apt to discuss this subject in depth and to give us solutions that work than Richard Troutman, M.D. I am therefore delighted to write a Foreword for this excellent book, *Corneal Astigmatism: Etiology, Prevention, and Management*.

When we intend acquiring a book, we naturally want to know as much as possible about the senior author and why he or she is deserving of our trust in what is said and recommended in that book.

Richard Troutman is a superb ophthalmic surgeon, a world-recognized authority on the cornea. In 1954 he pioneered use in the United States of the surgical microscope for ocular surgery. In that same year Troutman began to use edge-to-edge sutures for penetrating keratoplasty with Grieshaber needles. He was also the one to advocate the seated position for ophthalmic microsurgery. At that time, ophthalmic surgeons operated standing so that they could approach the eye readily from different directions.

In 1966, to stimulate development in the infant microsurgery of the eye, Mackensen, Harms, and Troutman formed the International Microsurgery Study Group, which still serves as an international forum for exchange of ideas on the subject.

In 1967 Troutman performed the first corneal wedge resection in the flatter corneal meridian, which is still considered the procedure of choice in high astigmatism following penetrating grafts. This was the first attempt at secondary correction of postkeratoplasty astigmatism. Until that time the only surgical treatment, suggested by Castroviejo and others, was to regraft with a larger graft.

In 1976 Troutman proposed relaxing incisions as an alternative procedure performed in the steeper meridian. He discusses in depth both corneal wedge resection and relaxing incisions in this masterful volume.

Troutman has dedicated his entire professional life to microsurgery, particularly of the cornea. To the many and significant contributions he has made to Ophthalmology, he now culminates his career with this magnificient volume in which he shares with us the great value of experience, acute powers of observation, great surgical skill, and the search for the truth.

Benjamin F. Boyd, M.D., F.A.C.S.
Editor-in-Chief
Highlights of Ophthalmology
Panama City, Panama

PREFACE

As we complete this volume, I am mindful of the privilege I have enjoyed to have practiced our specialty during a time of remarkable achievement. It has been almost half a century since, in 1945, inspired by my father, Erwin Webster Troutman, an eye, ear, nose, and throat specialist, I began my training in ophthalmology under John McLean at The New York Hospital, Cornell Medical Center.

At that time astigmatism was a refractive anomaly managed primarily by spectacles. Although the scleral supported contact lenses of the era could sometimes neutralize severe astigmatic anomalies, they were so uncomfortable that patients often could function with them for only a few hours. Nevertheless, they were a welcome alternative to the problematic results of corneal surgery practiced in those years using overlying silk sutures. Surgeons were only just beginning to use edge-to-edge closure for cataract incisions. Postoperative astigmatism was accepted without question, and patients often functioned less than adequately with compound high-powered aphakic spectacles. Anterior segment surgery was done without magnification. When I used the 2× loop, with which we then customarily removed corneal foreign bodies, for a cataract procedure, I encountered considerable skepticism from my mentors and peers alike. This was nothing compared with their reaction when, in 1954, I began to use an otologic surgical microscope I had modified for both cataract and corneal surgery. In 1957 my interest in the prevention of astigmatism resulting from cataract surgery and keratoplasty began. This was stimulated by my introduction to anterior chamber intraocular lenses, 8-0 virgin silk sutures, and sharper corneal needles by Joaquin Barraquer. In addition to the anatomic benefits derived from the more accurate cataract and corneal wound closure afforded by the better needles and finer sutures, I noted a decrease in corneal astigmatism.

However, my patients still rarely enjoyed astigmatism-free pseudophakia, because we still continued to experience against the rule astigmatism from slippage of the wound as the silk threads lost their tensile strength a few weeks after surgery. With penetrating keratoplasty too, although we now achieved more accurate edge-to-edge wound closure, the relatively short-term apposition did not result in firm circumferential healing. High astigmatic bands following penetrating keratoplasty were still the rule rather than the exception. In 1962, at the behest of Günter von Norden, I visited Günter Mackensen and Heinrich Harms in Tubingen, Germany. They introduced me to elastic monofilament nylon suture material, which permitted not only secure primary approximation of the wound but

"

also maintained it optimally closed until secure first intention healing could take place. This made a remarkable difference in the optical consequences of the healed cataract incision, virtually eliminating the sometimes severe, progressive against the rule astigmatism endured and accepted by ophthalmologists for more than a century.

For keratoplasty, the secure suturing eliminated the majority of my previous anatomic wound problems, and I began almost routinely to obtain clear grafts with firm, level postoperative scars. Nevertheless I continued to see cases of severe astigmatism, and rapidly it became my most annoying postoperative optical complication. Repeating the corneal graft, the only operation recommended at the time, did not solve the problem. Looking for another solution, in 1967, to convert the oblate cornea to a sphere, I applied the theories of spherical physics. I excised a wedge of tissue from a sector of the healed graft scar across the flatter corneal meridian in a highly astigmatic post-keratoplasty cornea. The nylon sutured wound healed firmly, and when the sutures were removed the reduced corneal radius was retained, correcting the high astigmatic error in that and five additional eyes on which I reported in 1970.

In 1976, for smaller degrees of post-keratoplasty astigmatism I began to apply a principle I discovered later that Snellen had suggested in 1869 for cataract incision–induced astigmatism. Rather than incise the peripheral cornea in full thickness, as he had done, I made two curved deep lamellar relaxing incisions in the keratoplasty scar in the opposing sectors crossing the steeper astigmatic meridian. The unsutured, partially penetrating wounds spread and filled with scar tissue and the corneal radius lengthened, the astigmatic correction being assisted by steepening of the flatter opposing meridian, in a ratio of 2:1. This phenomenon of spherical psychics, now referred to as coupling, I had also reported with corneal wedge resection.

I mention these historic facts to enable the reader to understand the evolution toward the current surgical approaches to the correction of corneal astigmatism. Time is too short to include all of the concomitant advances and events of these decades that have contributed to the present state of the art. Surgically induced astigmatism, like many other surgical concerns, has always been present to a greater or lesser degree. Its correction has become of contemporary interest because of the solution of more pressing surgical problems.

In cataract surgery, for example, the intraocular lens has become widely used only after microsurgery, phacoemulsification, and the refinement of extracapsular extraction made possible the secure positioning of the lens implant in the capsule, as originally proposed but unsuccessfully practiced by Ridley. Contemporary small incision techniques, by avoiding the optical corneal ring, cause minimal to no alteration of preoperative corneal curvatures. In this volume, management of astigmatism with cataract surgery will deal less with prevention than with the management of preexisting and the now minimal residual astigmatic errors.

Preventive measures at wound level have not solved the problem of postoperative astigmatism following penetrating keratoplasty, because of the many disparate anatomic, pathologic, and optical anomalies of the donor and recipient tissues. Though there is little probability that astigmatism from these causes will ever be eliminated, we should not abandon our attempts at its prevention; rather we must continue to apply them as we evolve better secondary corrective procedures. For the same reasons, we will need to be able to correct astigmatism from trauma and from other anterior segment conditions that involve healed corneal incisions.

As we reach for the cornea and refractive surgeon's utopia of eliminating the need for glasses or contact lenses, congenital and developmental astigmatism will continue to demand our surgical attention, especially as they accompany spherical ametropia. Appropriately, this volume will deal in some detail with astigmatism as it relates to refractive surgery for myopia, and in particular to radial keratotomy. We shall only briefly discuss excimer laser photoablation and its possibilities for the correction of corneal refractive anomalies, because it still is investigational.

This volume would not have been started had it not been for the encouragement of my spouse, Dr. Suzanne Véronneau-Troutman, who has on more than one occasion rescued this effort from oblivion. It would not have been completed had it not been for the coauthorship of Dr. Kurt Buzard, my former fellow, whose background in physics and whose creative intelligence, in addition to his not inconsiderable surgical skills, were ideally suited to this task. In particular, we enjoyed his state-of-the-art computer facility presided over by his accomplished spouse, Carol, as well as her staff, who not only relieved us of the details of production but whose perfectly run household gave us the time and intellectual leisure to pursue this goal. Our artist, Virginia Cantarella, who has worked with me on *Microsurgery of the Anterior Segment of the Eye,* volumes 1 and 2, has with her superb illustrations perfectly complemented the text. In truth, her pictures speak louder than our words.

I have asked Dr. Benjamin Boyd to write the foreword to this volume, not only because he is a close personal friend but because, as editor of the multilingual, global *International Highlights of Ophthalmology,* he is the most lucid and objective ophthalmologic chronicler of our time.

Above all, our work is designed to be practical, readable, and translatable to everyday practice. Where appropriate, we have added more detailed discussions of theory as they relate to these practical aspects. We will have succeeded if you, the reader, on finishing this volume, accept that the prevention and correction of astigmatism should be a part of your everyday anterior segment surgical practice.

Finally, I would like to dedicate this volume to my patients, my former residents and fellows, and my colleagues, without whom my work and life would have been incomplete.

Richard C. Troutman, M.D., F.A.C.S., F.C. Oph.

PREFACE

Within this book we have attempted to portray corneal astigmatism in the patho-physiologic setting in which it occurs. We wish not only to present the medical and surgical intervention used to identify and treat the problem but to approach the subject in a more global fashion. By presenting the etiology of astigmatism, the structure of the cornea, the mechanics of wound healing, and the particulars of sutures, needles, and instruments, we hope to impart the excitement of corneal surgery as we have known it. With this perspective, readers of this volume should bring their imagination and creativity to explore what we have written here and to use this knowledge to expand on these concepts and surgical techniques. Thus we present this book not as a compilation of what is known but as a starting point for future exploration and experience.

There are many people I would like to thank for their help and dedication over the years contributing to my training as a research scientist and clinical ophthalmologist. Dr. John Ketterson and Dr. Bernard Abraham taught me experimental physics and have given me advice ever since. The late Dr. David Shoch influenced me to choose ophthalmology, and his assistance made it possible for me to enter this field. Dr. Bradley Straatsma, Dr. Tom Pettit, Dr. Allan Kreiger, and Dr. Bartly Mondino made my residency at the Jules Stein Eye Institute the rich educational experience that it was and influenced me to enter cornea as a subspecialty. Dr. Richard Elander, Dr. Donald Dickerson, and Dr. Sam Masket each contributed extra personal and clinical experiences that continue to influence my clinical judgment even today. My coauthor, Dr. Richard Troutman, has been not only my mentor as a corneal surgeon but a personal friend as well. The opportunity to write this book combining Dr. Troutman's expertise in corneal grafting and astigmatism with some of my own techniques in refractive and corneal surgery has been both a pleasure and in many ways a fellowship of its own. This book would not have been possible without the forebearance of my associate, Dr. Steven Shearing, who encouraged me and taught me many of the subtleties of cataract surgery.

The elegant, artistic, and accurate illustrations accompanying this text are the result of the skilled efforts of Virginia Cantarella. Toni Thorn, Carol Shepherd, and Carolyn Makaena provided the hours of patient translation and typing that made this book a reality. I would like to thank Tara Bussey for all of her efforts on our behalf. This list of acknowledgements could not be complete without thanking my wife, Carol, who spent many hours encouraging and organizing to allow the smooth integration of everyone involved. Throughout a sometimes trying and difficult period she maintained her support even when completion seemed farthest away.

All of us hope that our efforts will please and stimulate you, the reader, to use these techniques and ideas in your practice of ophthalmology.

Kurt A. Buzard, M.A.(Physics), M.D., F.A.C.S.

CONTENTS

Introduction to Microsurgery for Astigmatism

Astigmatism, like most ophthalmic terminology, is of Greek origin (*alpha,* privitive; *stigma,* a point). It is described as that condition of refraction wherein a point focus of light cannot be formed on the retina. In theory, no eye is stigmatic (spherical), and as a result, in practice we include under this form of ametropia only those anomalies that induce an appreciable optical error by the unequal refraction of light in different meridians.

Sir Isaac Newton, who himself appears to have been astigmatic, first considered the question of astigmatism in 1727. This optical error received its first detailed investigation in 1801 from the renowned scientist Thomas Young. He had 1.7 D of astigmatism, and because it remained when he immersed his head in water, thus eliminating the influence of corneal refraction, he attributed the defect to the lens. The Cambridge astronomer Airy (1827) was the first to correct the defect with a cylindrical lens, but it was the invention of the keratometer by Helmholtz (1856) and the treatise of Donders (1864), "Astigmatism and Cylindrical Lenses," that impressed the ophthalmologic world with the prevalence and importance of this anomaly. Early attempts at its surgical prevention and correction were made by Snellen (1869) in cataract incisions. His theories and those of others (e.g., Bates, 1891; Luciola, 1893; Dogonoff, 1895) were confirmed experimentally in animal eyes by the Dutch ophthalmology student Lans in 1897. Several attempts were made to correct congenital astigmatism, notably by Sato and José Barraquer.

Secondary correction of astigmatism following otherwise successful penetrating keratoplasty was not performed until 1967, by Troutman. Only recently, with the more successful correction of spherical ametropias by cataract implant surgery, refractive surgery, and penetrating keratoplasty, has there been a sustained interest in the prevention and correction of surgically induced or preexisting astigmatism. The causes, prevention, and surgical management of corneal astigmatism, in particular that induced by corneal and cataract surgery or by trauma, has been a career-long interest of the authors. Congenital astigmatism, although relatively rare, also has occupied our attention, as have the axial- and corneal-induced spherical ametropias that often accompany astigmatism.

Astigmatism may be induced by an error of curvature or of centering, a change of refractive index, and by tilting. Curvature astigmatism is of primary interest to corneal and refractive surgeons. Curvature astigmatism in small degrees is present in just about everyone. In youth, the cornea is typically more curved in the vertical meridian, flattening slightly with age, presumably from pressure of the upper lid. When the steeper, more curved meridian is vertical, it is termed *with the rule* astigmatism. Conversely, when the steeper meridian is horizontal, the vertical meridian having the lesser curvature, it is termed *against the rule* astigmatism. When tilted to the right or left, it is called oblique astigmatism. Whether alone or combined with axial errors, when it occurs to greater degrees, it can interfere significantly with clear vision even when corrected.

In this volume, the emphasis in cataract surgery is primarily on prevention of surgically induced astigmatism and secondarily on its correction. In corneal surgery, it is the secondary correction of residual astigmatic errors that is given greater emphasis. Astigmatism of a degree unacceptable after cataract surgery still occurs frequently after the most meticulously performed penetrating keratoplasty. Nevertheless, the corneal surgeon must use every possible technical aid at the primary procedure to assure accurate apposition and in-depth healing to restore the optical integrity of the cornea so as to reduce to a minimum the necessity for secondary correction. Topographic analysis of the corneal curvatures before, during, and after any surgical procedure involving the cornea is one of the essentials in the prevention of astigmatism, and when indicated, delineates the surgical parameters for a secondary corrective procedure. The development of noninvasive monitoring of wound healing by topographic analysis, as discussed by Buzard, represents a new dimension in the precise and appropriate correction of wound healing abnormalities. This is being reinforced by new pharmaceutical developments to accelerate and enhance wound healing.

Edge-to-edge suturing, as first applied to cataract wounds, gave the ophthalmic surgeon the opportunity not only to better control wound apposition and healing but also significantly reduced optical distortions of the previously unsutured wounds, in particular, excessive corneal astigmatism. In keratoplasty, however, the pathologic, often optically distorted recipient cornea as well as the unknown optical status of the donor buttons have continued to hinder our best efforts at primary control. As a result, an acceptable level of postsurgical astigmatism approaching that

   Introduction to Microsurgery for Astigmatism

which is now almost routinely enjoyed by cataract surgeons has eluded the corneal surgeon. However, any surgical or traumatic wound of the cornea, especially with less than meticulous wound closure, can induce significant astigmatic distortion.

Macroscopic edge-to-edge suturing of corneal wounds, performed initially with 5-0 absorbable and silk threads, was facilitated by finer nonabsorbable suture materials such as 7-0 and 8-0 silk. Microsurgery has made possible the use of even finer 9-0 to 11-0 synthetic elastic monofilament suture materials. Combined with more precise instrumentation, the improved visualization afforded by the surgical microscope allows more accurate and stable wound apposition. Improved local and general anesthetic agents and technique have given the surgeon the additional time required to perform the more meticulous surgical techniques.

Furthermore, exacting in-depth apposition of precisely cut wound edges is a prerequisite for predictable correction of any excessive astigmatic band resulting from cataract and keratoplasty incisions. Surgical correction of an astigmatic band resulting from a poorly apposed and healed wound has a significantly different prognosis than a numerically identical one in which the wound is healed accurately in depth. Notwithstanding, because of individual tissue variability, there can be no routine procedure to assure predictable correction of a postoperative corneal astigmatism.

To minimize astigmatism in keratoplasty, it is the first obligation of the corneal surgeon to substitute an optically clear donor disc of normal thickness and of identical diameter to the excised pathologic disc and then to fix it as accurately as possible in depth as well as circumferentially to the recipient corneal margin. This process begins with a careful examination and accurate diagnosis of the presenting corneal anomaly or disease, followed by detailed topographic analysis. A recipient cornea with an irregularly thinned periphery can be expected to influence significantly the postoperative astigmatic result, a prime example being keratoconus. The more advanced the keratoconus, the greater the probability of a significant residual error. The patient must be informed that postkeratoplasty astigmatism requiring secondary correction can occur just as the patient is advised of the possibility of a graft rejection. At the same time, assurances should be given that with an otherwise successful graft, such a problem, should it occur, can be readily corrected.

Postoperatively, during the period that the sutures remain in place ("sutures in" period), through selective removal of interrupted sutures, early suture adjustment of a continuous suture, or suture addition to correct microdehiscences, astigmatism often can be compensated and reduced to an optically acceptable and functional level.

When all sutures are removed, even several years after the primary procedure, secondary correction of the then uncompensated astigmatism may be required. Both secondary astigmatism and its correction are promoted by and complicated by less than optimal full-thickness wound apposition at the primary procedure.

To avoid a prolonged postoperative course, we use deeply placed, opposing continuous sutures. These permit earlier suture removal, from 6 months to 1 year after the primary surgery, depending on the peripheral pathology. Then any excessive astigmatism can be fully corrected and the patient rehabilitated significantly earlier, often within the first postoperative year.

The purpose of this volume is to bring together for the reader not only the current state of the art in the management of excessive corneal astigmatism but also a look to the promise of the future. At present, it appears that astigmatism, particularly that following penetrating keratoplasty, may always be with us. In penetrating keratoplasty, even using the most precise surgical instrumentation and techniques at the primary surgery, the individual variability of the pathologic recipient and the unknown optical properties of the donor make it virtually impossible to control every astigmatism-inducing contingency. Although excessive astigmatism is much less prevalent after cataract surgery, because of the large numbers of cases performed and the greater visual expectations of the patients since the introduction of posterior chamber intraocular lenses, an even larger number of postcataract eyes may require surgical correction of residual astigmatism. The goal of this volume is to provide readers with essential information to enable them to detect, evaluate, and correct iatrogenic and natural astigmatism. Combining these corrective techniques with the equally important preventive techniques should result in an essentially astigmatism-free postoperative patient population. Combining these techniques with the surgical techniques for ametropias by thickness volume, incision, laser, or all three, may result ultimately in the utopia of a spectacle- and contact lens–free society.

Chapter 1

Terminology and Definitions, Optical and Surgical Principles, Tenets of Refractive Surgery

To understand the principles and to practice refractive surgery for astigmatism, it is first necessary to be familiar with its associated terminology. Astigmatism, as with other ophthalmic entities, has its *key words*. First, there is the word astigmatism, itself, which is defined and its origins outlined in the Introduction to this volume. In this chapter we discuss in greater detail the eye with astigmatism.

The astigmatic eye, instead of focusing rays of light on a single point, refracts two focal lines separated from each other by a focal interval (the conoid of Sturm). The length of this focal interval is a measure of the degree of astigmatism. The correction of a refractive error thus induced can be accomplished only by reducing these two foci into one.

WHY CORRECT ASTIGMATISM?

Why are we concerned with correction of astigmatism, and in particular, why do we advocate surgical correction of uncompensated errors? The higher degrees of astigmatism alone or in combination with axial errors have long been recognized as a principal cause of asthenopia and eye strain. When the eye attempts to focus the disparate meridians, especially in hyperopia, severe symptoms can occur. The patient often compensates by tilting the head or making a stenopeic slit by half closing the lids to modify the ray path in one meridian so that the viewed object may appear more distinct. This compensatory posturing is particularly noticeable in patients with higher degrees of oblique astigmatism and in irregular astigmatism, for example, in keratoconus.

Initially, optical correction of such errors may be more disturbing to patients than no correction at all. When their distorted world is normalized optically, it becomes wider or taller or obliquely displaced. When correction of such errors by spectacles or a spherical, rigid contact lens becomes intermittent or poorly tolerated, surgical correction is the only means to optical rehabilitation. This is true in the patient who has a residual astigmatic error following otherwise successful penetrating keratoplasty or cataract surgery. It is this group, in particular, on which we focus in this volume. Moderate to high degrees of congenital astigmatism and traumatically induced astigmatism, although rarer, cause similar problems and respond to similar management.

REGULAR ASTIGMATISM: VARIABLE AXIAL LENGTH

When astigmatism can be fully corrected by a spectacle lens, it is termed *regular*. Moderate degrees of regular astigmatism are corrected by a spherocylindrical lens that refracts rays of light in one plane and leaves unaltered rays in the plane perpendicular to this, that is, in the plane of its axis. A properly oriented lens of a cylindrical power equal to the astigmatic error of the cornea changes the refraction so that the rays from all meridians are brought to a focus at the same distance, the visualized spherical image being focused on a single plane at the retina. Correction of astigmatic errors can be accomplished also by a rigid spherical-surfaced contact lens that becomes a new spherical front refractive surface separated from the astigmatic cornea by a spherocylindrical layer of fluid.

Regular refractive astigmatism in eyes with the same astigmatism and variable axial length is classified into *simple astigmatism, compound astigmatism,* and *mixed astigmatism* (Plate 1–1). In *simple astigmatism,* the focus of one meridian falls on the retina, the other behind the retina in a short eye (hyperopic astigmatism) (Plate 1–1,A) or in front of the retina in a long eye (myopic astigmatism) (Plate 1–1,C). *Mixed astigmatism* (Plate 1–1,B) occurs when the focus of one meridian is in front of the retina and the second is behind it so that the refraction is hypertropic in one direction and myopic in the other. In *compound astigmatism,* both foci fall either behind or in front of the retina. In the former case, the astigmatism is called *compound hypertropic* in a still shorter eye (Plate 1–1,D) and in the latter, *compound myopic* in a still longer eye (Plate 1–1,E) astigmatism. When there are such irregularities in the curvature of the meridians that no geometric foci are adhered to, the condition is called *irregular* astigmatism.

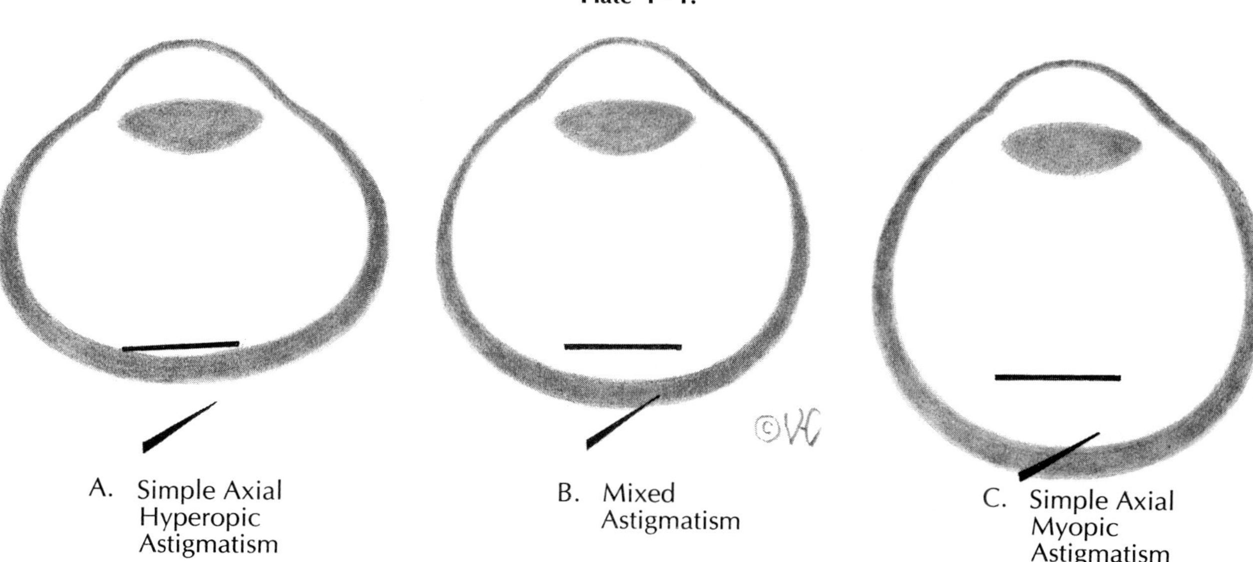

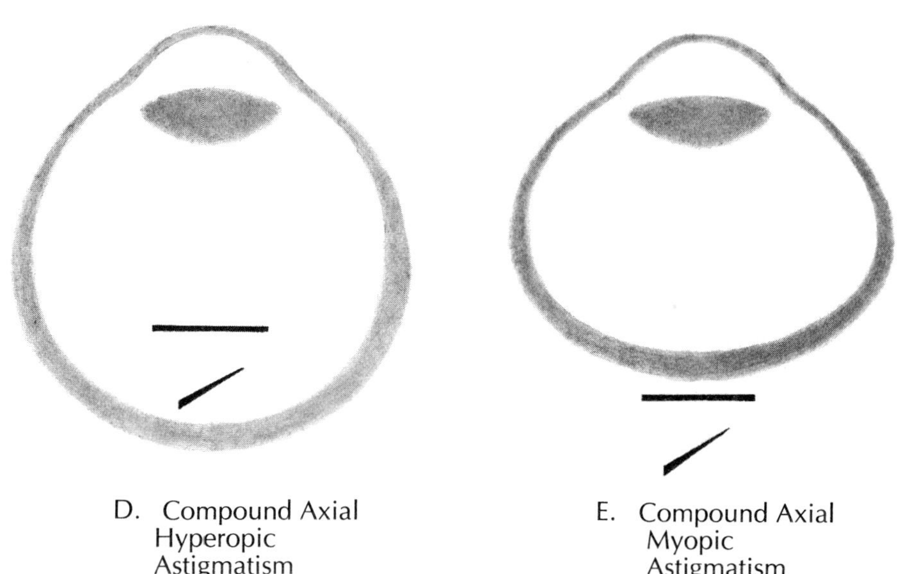

A, simple hyperopic astigmatism, short eye. **B,** mixed astigmatism, normal axial length. **C,** simple myopic astigmatism, long eye. **D,** compound hyperopic astigmatism, shorter eye. **E,** compound myopic astigmatism, longer eye.

ASTIGMATIC ORIENTATION IN SPACE

For the purpose of spatial orientation of an astigmatic band, the terms *axis* and *meridian* are commonly and interchangeably used. Their description in texts on physiologic optics can sometimes be confusing to the corneal surgeon because the terminology in these texts refers primarily to cylindrical corrective lenses. Nevertheless, it is simpler, as well as more logical, to describe the cornea in physiologic optic terms because they are more familiar to us. We can then more readily orient ourselves to the astigmatic cornea.

Axis

The concept of axis is simplified if one remembers that the principal axis of the corneal clock is an absolute, always at the 12-o'clock position, 90 degrees in relation to the cornea circumference, just as a compass needle always points north. The axis notations on the corneal clock begin at the 3-o'clock position, zero degrees, and proceed to the left, counterclockwise, to 90 degrees at the principal meridian, then continue counterclockwise to the 9-o'clock position, 180 degrees. The inferior cornea clock repeats, continuing counterclockwise, each point on the clock corresponding numerically to the degree notation directly opposite it (Plate 1-2,A).

Meridian

The meridians (Plate 1–2,B) are variable, their individual positions being identified by their relationship to the principal axis and the corneal clock. The meridians are further identified as vertical at 90 degrees, horizontal at 180 degrees, and oblique if a meridian falls anywhere between the two principal axes. In relation to each other, the meridians are steeper (myopic) or flatter (hyperopic).

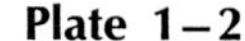

Plate 1–2.

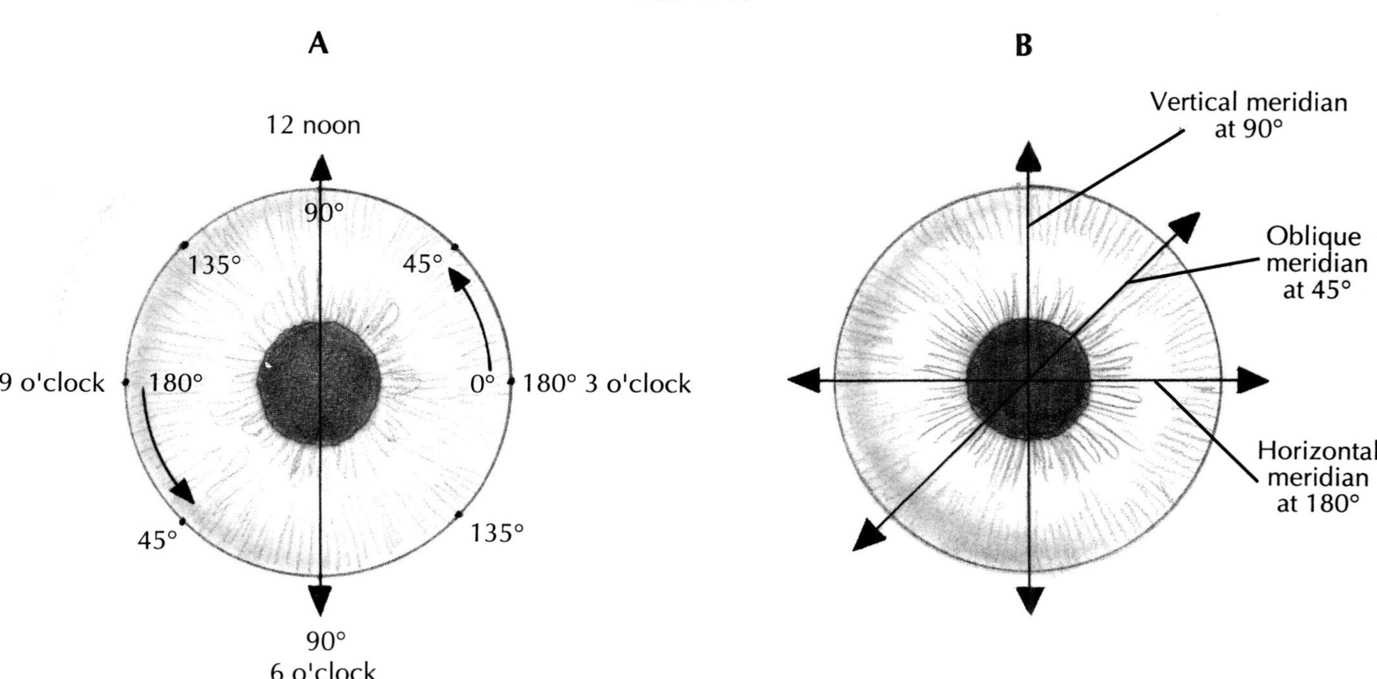

A, axis. Corneal clock as related to the principal axis. Axis notations proceed counterclockwise from zero degree or 180-degree meridian. **B,** meridian. Variable in relation to corneal clock.

Cylinder Axis: Spectacle Lens

A simple cylindrical spectacle lens correcting a simple regular astigmatism (Plate 1–1,A and C) has two axes, one powered, the other neutral (unpowered) at 90 degrees to each other. The neutral axis is always the cylinder axis of a correcting spectacle lens. In a simple myopic astigmatism (Plate 1–1,C), in reference to the cornea, the more curved corneal meridian, at 90 degrees, is myopic and will be corrected by a minus cylinder spectacle lens with its neutral axis at 180 degrees (Plate 1–2,C). In a simple hyperopic astigmatism (Plate 1–1,A), the steeper vertical corneal meridian is neutral, and will be corrected by a plus cylinder spectacle lens with its powered meridian at 180 degrees (Plate 1–2,D). In both instances the astigmatic lens neutralizes the ametropic, myopic, or hyperopic corneal meridian to focus at a single point on the retina. When the cornea is steeper at axis 45 degrees and correspondingly flatter at axis 135 degrees, a minus cylinder at axis 135 or a plus cylinder at axis 45 provides correction in an eye with a simple myopic or hyperopic astigmatism.

Therefore, to characterize underlying corneal curvature differences in relation to their meridians and axes, *one need only to imagine the astigmatism in a cornea as a mirror image of the back surface of the corresponding correcting spectacle cylinder* where the astigmatism-correcting spectacle lens has always a neutral unpowered axis and a powered meridian at 90 degrees. On the other hand, the astigmatic cornea has no neutral axis, being more or less curved in opposing meridians, and has power (greater or lesser) in both axes and meridians at right angles. In refractive surgery, corneal meridian power is always measured objectively, with the keratometer, the keratoscope, a computer-aided topology system, or preferably with all three, to avoid the errors inherent in retinoscopy and subjective spectacle refraction. *It is important to remember that the surgeon operates on the cornea and not on the refraction. The results of refractive surgery should never be measured only by retinoscopy or subjective refraction. Only direct measurements of the cornea can provide an objective assessment of the corneal refractive error to be corrected and the results of corneal refractive surgery.*

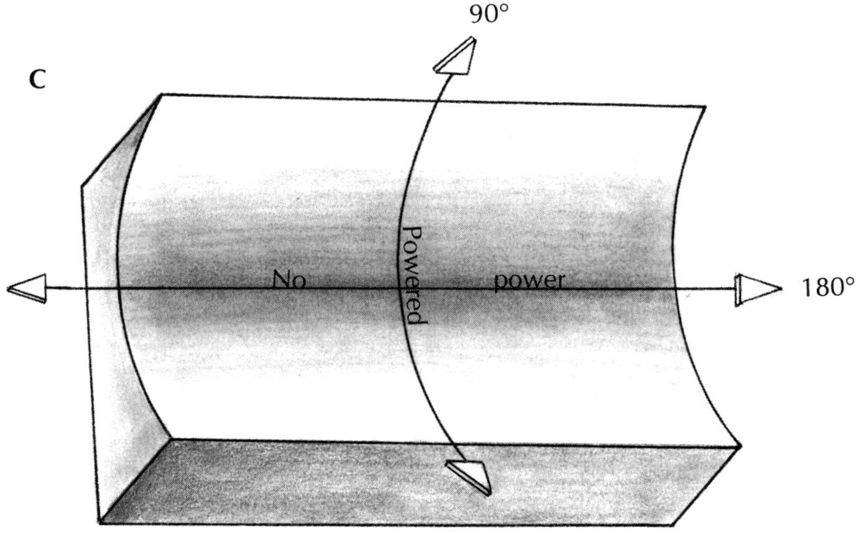

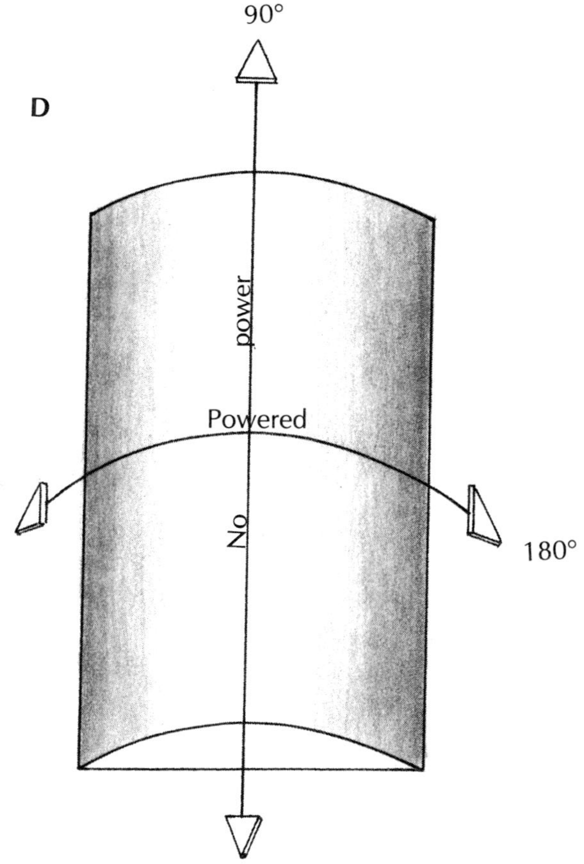

C, minus cylinder lens. To correct a cornea steeper at 90 degrees the neutral, unpowered axis is placed across the horizontal meridian at 180 degrees. D, plus cylinder lens. To correct a cornea steeper at 180 degrees the neutral, unpowered axis is placed across the vertical meridian.

With the rule and *against the rule* are confusing as they apply to axis and meridian. *With the rule* means that the cornea is more curved, more myopic, in its vertical meridian, the meridian at 90 degrees being less curved (not neutral as in a simple cylindrical spectacle lens; Plate 1–3,A). When the cornea is less curved in the vertical meridian it is termed *against the rule* (Plate 1–3,B). The expression *with the rule* was coined because of the observation that during one's early life, physiologic astigmatism is characterized by a steeper (more myopic) vertical corneal meridian and a corresponding flatter (more hyperopic) horizontal meridian. The term *against the rule* indicates the opposite condition, the reversal from steeper vertical to steeper horizontal, which occurs later in life, presumably from the continuous pressure of the upper lid on the originally steeper vertical corneal meridian. One can readily observe this phenomenon with a keratometer. As one observes the keratometer projection with the upper lid in its normal position and then lifts the lid from the cornea, the vertical meridian flattens slightly (Plate 1–3,C). When the upper lid is distorted by trauma or disease, the corneal curvature may change because of excessive or unequal pressure. Oblique astigmatism can be induced when pressure is applied obliquely to the 90-degree axis or vertical meridian. A teardrop (steeper vertical meridian) shape of the keratoconic cornea also is caused by the pressure of the upper lid on the pathologic elastic corneal tissue.

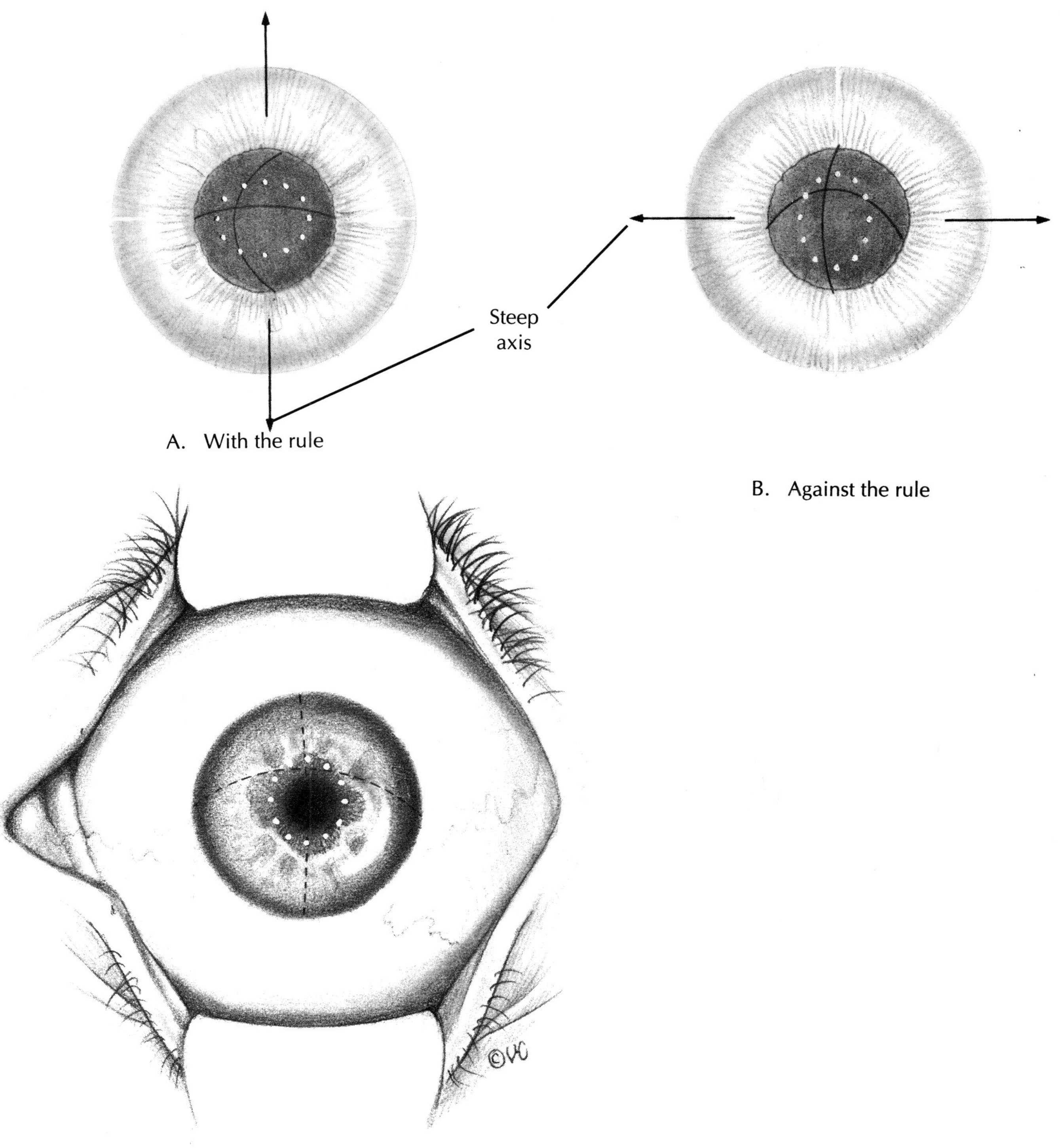

A, with the rule astigmatism. The cornea is more curved, more myopic in the vertical meridian, and flatter in the horizontal meridian. **B,** against the rule astigmatism. The cornea is less curved, more hyperopic in the vertical meridian, and steeper in the horizontal meridian. **C,** The corneal vertical meridian flattens, inducing against the rule astigmatism on release of upper lid pressure.

SYMMETRY AND ASYMMETRY OF ASTIGMATISM

Astigmatism usually is *symmetric* (Plate 1–4,A), the steeper and flatter meridians crossing at approximately 90 degrees. If the axes of the corneal meridians of an eye are not at right angles to each other (scissored), they are *asymmetric* (Plate 1–4,B). With the new computed topology instruments, which allow us to see the periphery of the cornea in more detail, it is increasingly evident that absolute symmetry is the exception rather than the rule, particularly when astigmatism is present. For practical purposes, we need to assume symmetry in the diagnosis and treatment of most corneal astigmatism.

When considering paired (fellow) eyes, corneal astigmatism is described also as *symmetric* (Plate 1–4,C) or *asymmetric* (Plate 1–4,D). Usually it is symmetric, even in paired pathologic corneas (e.g., keratoconus). Symmetry exists when the axis of the astigmatism is at 135 degrees in the right eye and at 45 degrees in the left eye, or in corresponding oblique axes (e.g., 120 and 60 degrees) up to axis 90 or 180 degrees (Plate 1–4,B). Conversely, asymmetric astigmatism exists when the axes do not geometrically coincide (e.g., right eye 60 degrees, left eye 45 degrees). An extreme example would be when a meridian is steeper at 90 degrees in one eye and flatter at 90 degrees in the fellow eye.

ISOMETROPIC AND ANISOMETROPIC ASTIGMATISM

When the astigmatism has the same power in the two eyes, it is *isometropic*. It becomes *anisometropic* when the power of the affected meridians is different in each eye whether or not they are symmetrical (e.g., +2.00 C × 80 = OD +5.00 C × 100 = OS).

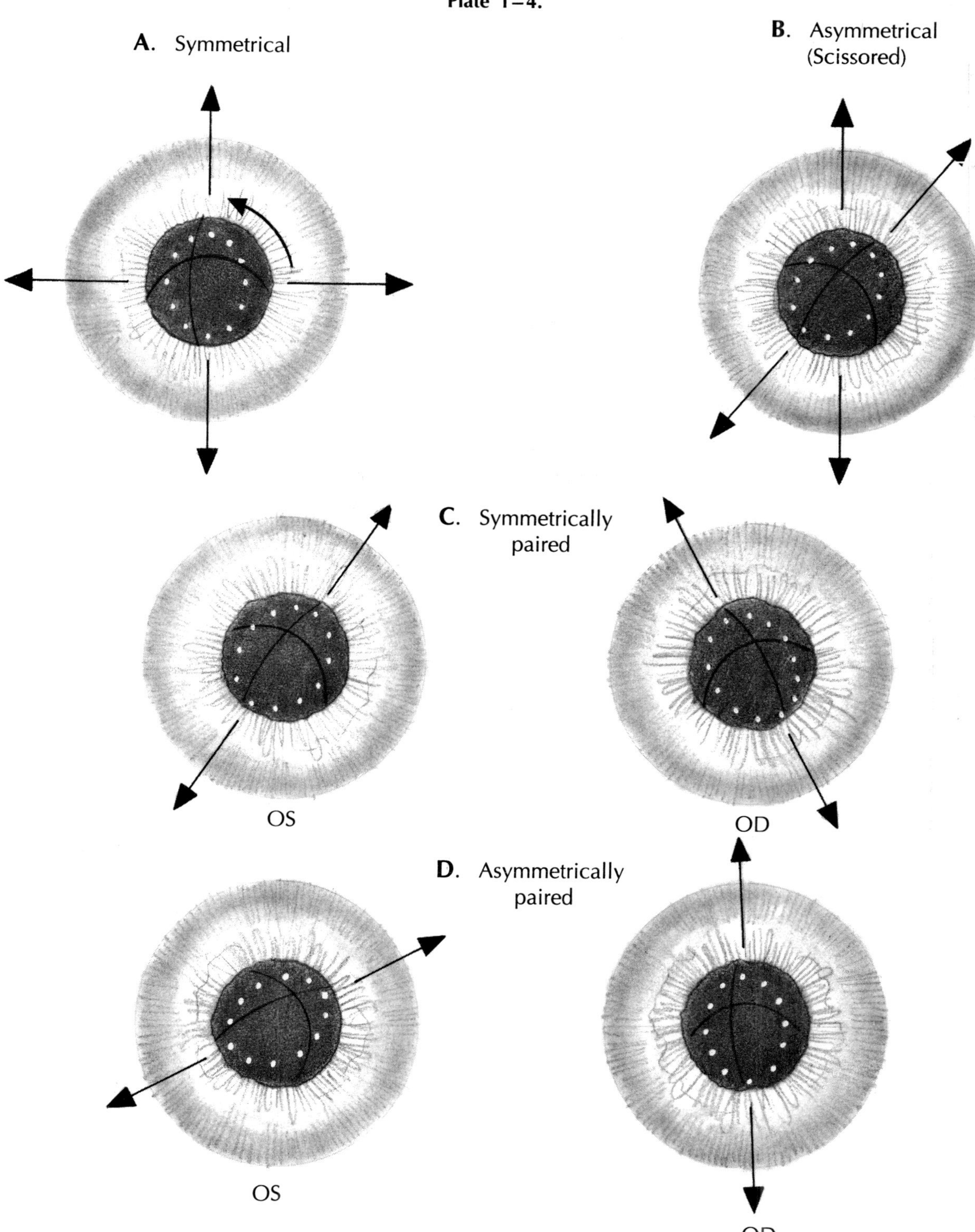

A, symmetric astigmatism. Meridians cross at 90 degrees. **B,** asymmetric astigmatism. Meridians cross obliquely (scissored). **C,** symmetric paired eyes. Meridian and axis correspond geometrically. **D,** asymmetric paired eyes. Meridian and axis do not coincide geometrically.

CORNEAL ASTIGMATISM: VARIABLE POWER, FIXED AXIAL LENGTH

Astigmatism can be characterized also in relation to the refractive power of steeper or flatter than average corneal meridians as they influence total eye power at a given axial length. If both corneal meridians focus on and anterior to the retina, the corneal astigmatism is simple *myopic* (Plate 1–5,A). When the image refracted by the two corneal meridians focuses on and posterior to the retina, the astigmatism is termed simple *hyperopic* (Plate 1–5,C). If one corneal meridian is hyperopic and the other myopic, in relation to retinal imaging, the astigmatism is *mixed* (Plate 1–5,B). When a concomitant spherical error is present, the astigmatism becomes *compound myopic* or *compound hyperopic* (Plate 1–5,D–E).

REGULAR ASTIGMATISM

Corneal astigmatism is described also in relation to its surface topography as regular or irregular. If the surface topography of the cornea is perfectly smooth and light is refracted regularly by the meridians crossing at right angles, the astigmatism is termed *regular*.

Regular astigmatism is most responsive to primary refractive surgery corrective procedures.

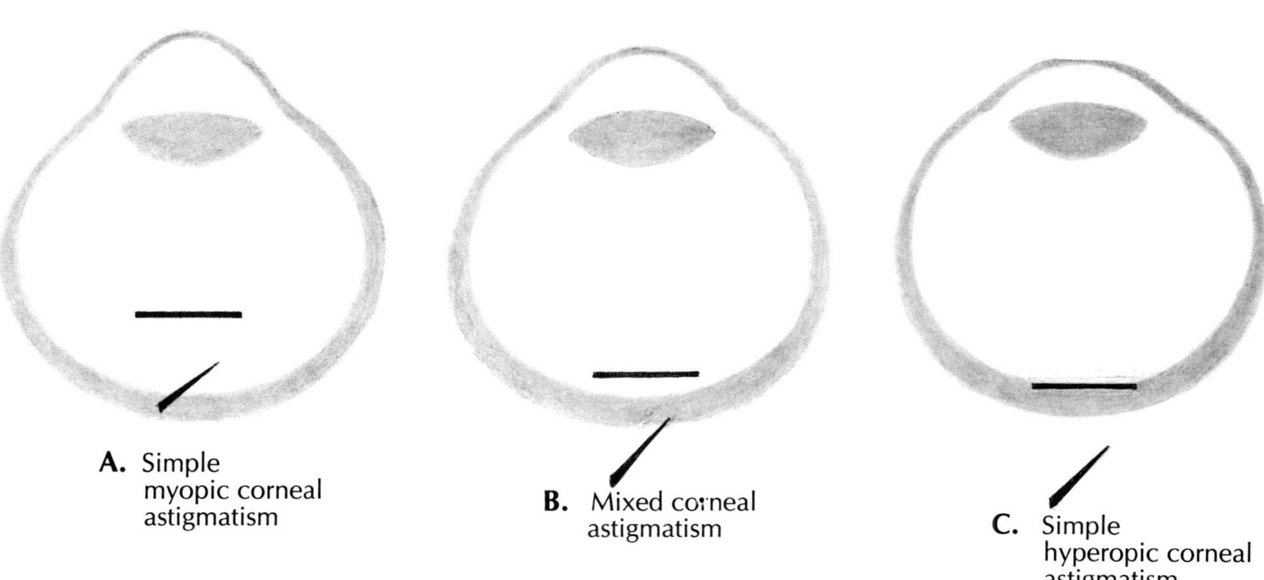

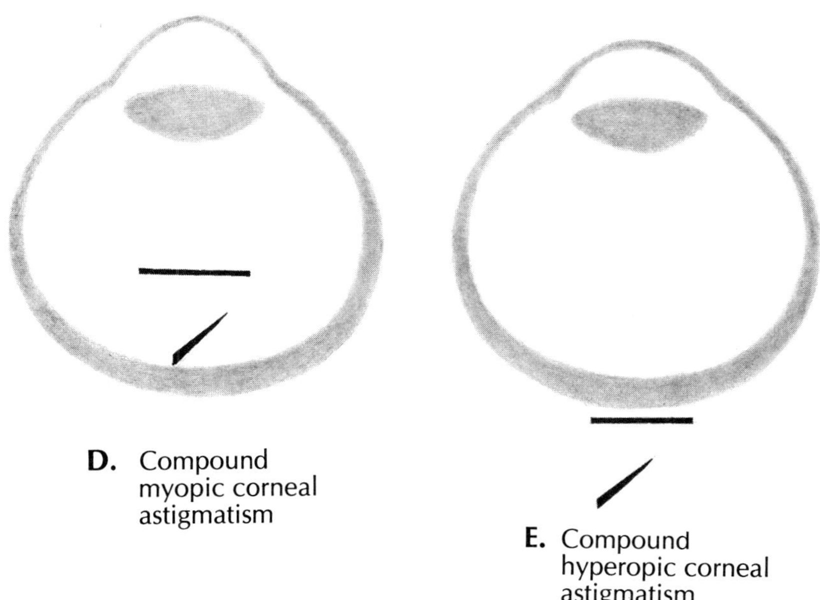

A, simple myopic corneal astigmatism, fixed axial length. Steeper corneal meridians at right angles focus on and anterior to the retina. **B,** mixed corneal astigmatism, fixed axial length. Corneal meridians at right angles focus anterior and posterior, respectively, to the retina. **C,** simple hyperopic corneal astigmatism, fixed axial length. Flatter corneal meridians at right angles focus on and posterior to the retina. **D,** compound myopic corneal astigmatism, fixed axial length. Both meridians focus anterior to the retina. **E,** compound hyperopic corneal astigmatism, fixed axial length. Both meridians focus posterior to the retina.

Astigmatism is termed *irregular* when refraction is interrupted by any variation of the refractive corneal surface and may be present to a different degree as characterized by the following terms.

Regular-irregular refers to astigmatism, such as in early keratoconus, where the surface is smooth enough to regularly refract light but is of variable curvature or scissored, or both, so that correction with spectacles is less accurate and contact lenses or keratoplasty is required for normalization.

Irregular-regular refers to corneas, such as seen in the later stages of keratoconus or keratoglobus, where the surface is so irregular or scarred that spectacle correction is impossible and *only* contact lenses or keratoplasty can correct.

True irregular astigmatism (Plate 1–6) refers to a corneal surface so irregular that it cannot be refracted with any optical corrective device and requires surface smoothing by excimer laser photoablation, surface regeneration by lamellar keratoplasty, or a full-thickness corneal replacement, depending on the extent and depth of the pathologic condition.

The use of accurate descriptive terminology allows the surgeon to better understand and apply refractive surgery to a given astigmatic cornea. For refractive surgery, ideally the cornea should be both physiologically and optically intact, of normal thickness and clarity centrally, and have a regular peripheral support zone ending at a normally configured optical ring (see Chapter 2). Only such a cornea may be predictably altered optically by incision, excision, suture compression, thickness alteration, or selective addition or removal of corneal tissue to correct astigmatism.

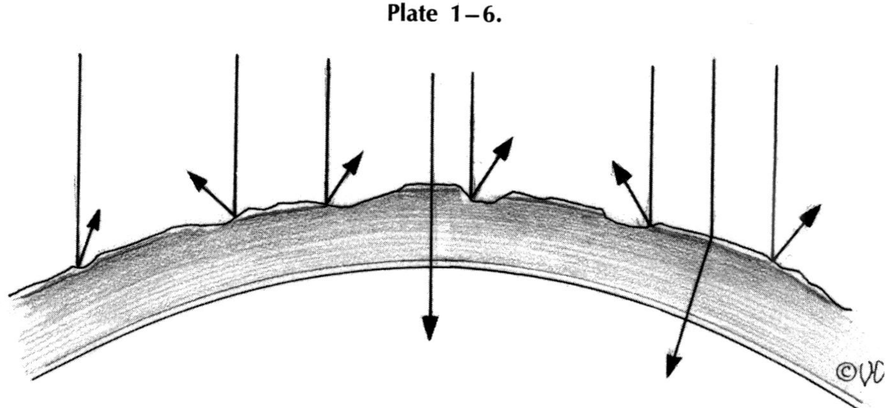

True irregular astigmatism.

Over the years many investigators, beginning with Snellen (1869), have proposed useful fundamental principles that continue to guide the understanding and application of incisions, excisions, and sutures to the practice of refractive surgery. These principles, as they apply to the surgery of astigmatism, are summarized below.

1. Any incision(s) in corneal tissue that interrupts Bowman's layer will induce a permanent change in corneal curvature. The more numerous, longer, or deeper the incisions, the greater the curvature change induced.

2. The more peripheral the incision(s), the less effect on the central corneal curvature. Conversely, the closer the incision(s) to the central optical zone, the greater the effect that will be achieved (Bates, 1891). An exception to this tenet occurs with transverse incisions, which have a maximal effect in the mid-cornea and a lesser effect as they progress either more centrally or more peripherally.

3. The effect in the area immediately anterior to an incision is localized steepening (tenting) of the cornea. Central and peripheral to the incision, the cornea abruptly flattens. Either radial or transverse (linear or arcuate) incisions, or a combination, will induce flattening of the central optical zone in the incisional meridian.

4. Suturing an incision will inverse the tenting, inducing flattening at the suture line and steepening peripheral and central to it. After normal wound healing and removal of the sutures the cornea should return to its preincision curvature.

5. Sector (meridional) transverse incisions, for example, curvilinear Troutman relaxing incisions or T-cuts, have a negligible and variable effect on total corneal power. Such linear or arcuate transverse incisions made across a steeper meridian cause a corresponding steepening of the formerly flatter meridian at 90 degrees, in a ratio of approximately 2D of flattening to 1D of steepening, recently termed "coupling" (Plate 1–7). This phenomenon tends to maintain the preincisional spherical equivalent power of the cornea.

6. Radial incisions have a coupling effect opposite that of transverse incisions. Radial incisions flatten in the meridian parallel to the incision and *flatten* 90 degrees away. When used in conjunction with transverse incisions the coupling effect cancels 90 degrees away. Radial incisions do not block coupling; rather, they act in opposition to transverse incisions and nullify the combined coupling.

7. A partial penetrating circumferential incision will cause the cornea central to the incision to steepen and the peripheral cornea to flatten as Bowman's layer retracts. With a penetrating circumferential incision, both peripheral and central cornea retract and steepen. When sutured and

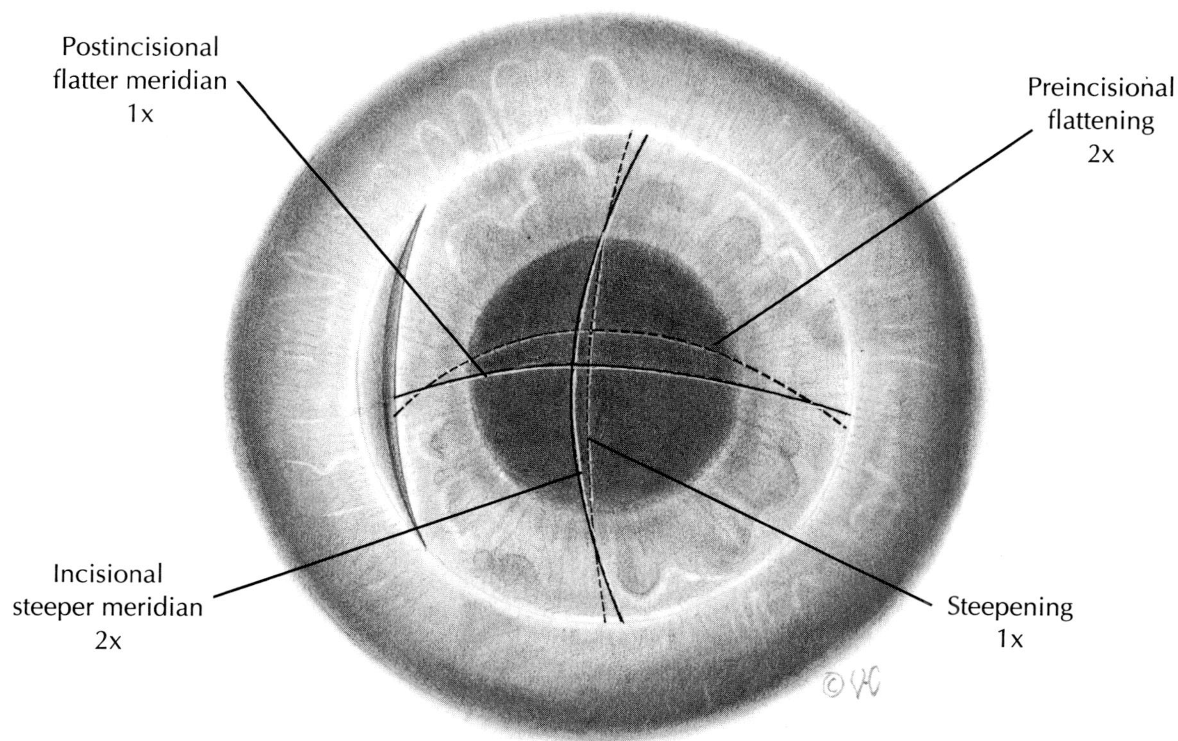

Coupling

Coupling. Troutman relaxing incision induces flattening of the incisional meridian, with corresponding steepening of the meridian at 90 degrees, in 2:1 ratio. "Coupling."

healed, the circumferential scar forms an internal corneal *pseudo-optical ring* that serves to isolate the central optical zone from the peripheral support zone. This pseudo-optical ring assumes the mechanical functions of the limbal *corneal optical ring*. Any corrective procedure for *central optical zone* astigmatism must then be done at or within the confines of this pseudo-optical ring (see Chapter 2).

8. Displacement of the pseudo-optical ring, relative to the visual axis, induces astigmatism. In corneal transplantation, the visual axis must coincide with the center of the graft regardless of peripheral support zone pathology.

9. An unsutured corneal incision creates flattening of the adjacent corneal surface by addition of a wedge of scar tissue, or in the case of a poorly healed incision by an epithelial plug. As a corollary, addition of tissue in any meridian flattens the cornea.

10. Removal of tissue and edge-to-edge suturing in a single meridian (e.g., Troutman corneal wedge [block] resection) causes flattening immediately over the excised and sutured area and steepening central and peripheral to it in the 2:1 ratio noted previously. Permanent correction results on removal of the closing sutures from the healed wound.

11. Compression sutures placed in unincised cornea induce reversible steepening of the cornea central to the compressing suture loops and flattening in the meridian at 90 degrees, *coupling*. They can be used to enhance the effect of Troutman relaxing incisions in the meridian at 90 degrees. Similarly, this coupling effect can be used to reduce the temporary overcorrection induced by sutured excisions (e.g., Troutman corneal wedge [block] resection.)

12. A toric interlamellar or epicorneal homograft or alloplastic lens selectively increases curvature in a meridian to correct hyperopic astigmatism. Conversely, a selective decrease in the thickness (curvature) of a meridian by intralamellar or surface tissue removal induces a toric flattening to correct a myopic astigmatic error.

The curvature of the posterior cornea is maintained as the curvature of the anterior cornea is altered by selective tissue addition or removal to effect the refractive change. In contradistinction, the deep focal disruption of the cornea from the various incisional techniques, tenets 1 through 11, induces the refractive effect by effective posterior as well as anterior curvature changes (see Chapter 2).

Such corneal thickness-volume modification techniques, as originally described by José Barraquer, have been used relatively infrequently for correction of astigmatic refractive errors, because of limited accuracy. However, new techniques, such as photoablation with the excimer laser, may make such meridional thickness modification techniques sufficiently accurate to be feasible.

Anatomy and Physiology

In contrast to most other body organs, the cornea is unique in that for its optimal function as an optical organ it depends on an absence of vascular tissue. Its physiology and clarity are compromised by the close proximity to or invasion by blood vessels. It is privileged immunologically by this avascular physiology. In the absence of secondary vascularization it can, in most instances, be replaced successfully by randomly supplied, unmatched donor tissue. This circumstance, however, confines such surgical interventions, for example, penetrating keratoplasty, to a closely circumscribed area of limited dimensions. In the surgical cornea, these restricted anatomic parameters are so precise that they must be duplicated almost exactly or revised only minimally to preserve or to restore optical function after any surgical incision or excision. In the prevention or correction of astigmatism in cataract, and especially in corneal surgery, the surgeon often must deal simultaneously with sometimes opposing anatomic and optical functions.

LIDS AND OCULAR ADNEXA

The physiologic, anatomic, and optical functions of the cornea depend on the integrity of the structures surrounding or covering it. The lids, the extraocular muscles, the sclera and conjunctiva and their sensory and motor nerve supplies, as well as the tear mechanism must be intact for the cornea to survive and function optimally. Even normally functioning lids and extraocular muscles provide only partial protection for the cornea should the sensory nerves to the cornea be compromised, for example, in herpes zoster ophthalmicus. If tears are deficient, conjunctival and corneal epithelium is more readily dehisced and not consistently replaced, which can result in irregularity of the corneal surface.

Therefore, at the initial examination of the patient who is to undergo surgery that involves the cornea, the prudent surgeon verifies that the cornea is adequately covered by the lid excursions, that the conjunctiva and extraocular muscles are unrestricted and allow full movement of the globe, and that a normal Bell's phenomenon is present. Tear function is assessed for both quantity and quality, using Schirmer testing and tear breakup time, to mention only two evaluations. The sensory response of the cornea to a graded stimulus is determined. If it is anesthetic, healing and regularity can be significantly compromised. Only when all of the cornea's direct or indirect protective physiologic mechanisms are intact, or have been repaired or substituted, should a surgical intervention be undertaken.

The lids have an important interaction with the cornea in terms of astigmatism. Both axis and scalar amount of astigmatic error are affected by lid tension (Plate 2–1,A). In children younger than 3 years a high incidence of *against the rule* astigmatism is appreciated. In these young children eyelid tension is poor, allowing the cornea to assume an *against the rule* astigmatism. As the children become older, lid tension increases, resulting in little astigmatism or slight *with the rule* astigmatism for most of adulthood. Buzard (1988) has shown increasing *against the rule* astigmatism in patients in their sixties and older, again related to easing of lid tension. Both the axis and the degree of astigmatism are thus influenced by lid tension.

This balance can be disturbed by many external factors, such as trauma, inflammation, and scarring. It is well known that patients with corneal abrasion often report diminished visual acuity for several weeks after the eye injury, even when the cornea and adjacent structures have returned to a normal appearance. Refraction in these eyes often reveals a slight increase in *with the rule* astigmatism related to increased lid tension due to ocular irritation. This astigmatism diminishes as photophobia and injection clear from the eye.

Wilson (1982) found that retraction of the eyelids of young adults for at least 10 seconds produced less *with the rule* astigmatism measured by keratometry in corneas that had at least 1D *with the rule* astigmatism (Plate 2–1,B). Robb (1977) found that patients with lid hemangiomas had increased astigmatism at a later age, related to the position of the hemangioma (Plate 2–1,C). We examined a patient with acid burns to the face that produced severe scarring of the lids (Plate 2–1,D). High *with the rule* astigmatism developed. Transverse relaxing incisions had little effect; in fact, the astigmatism increased slightly. Recognizing the contribution of the extremely tight eyelids to astigmatic error, the lids were loosened by oculoplasty. The incisions were reopened, and a hard contact lens was used to isolate lid tension from the cornea, allowing the cornea to heal with minimal astigmatism. Each of these examples emphasizes the bal-

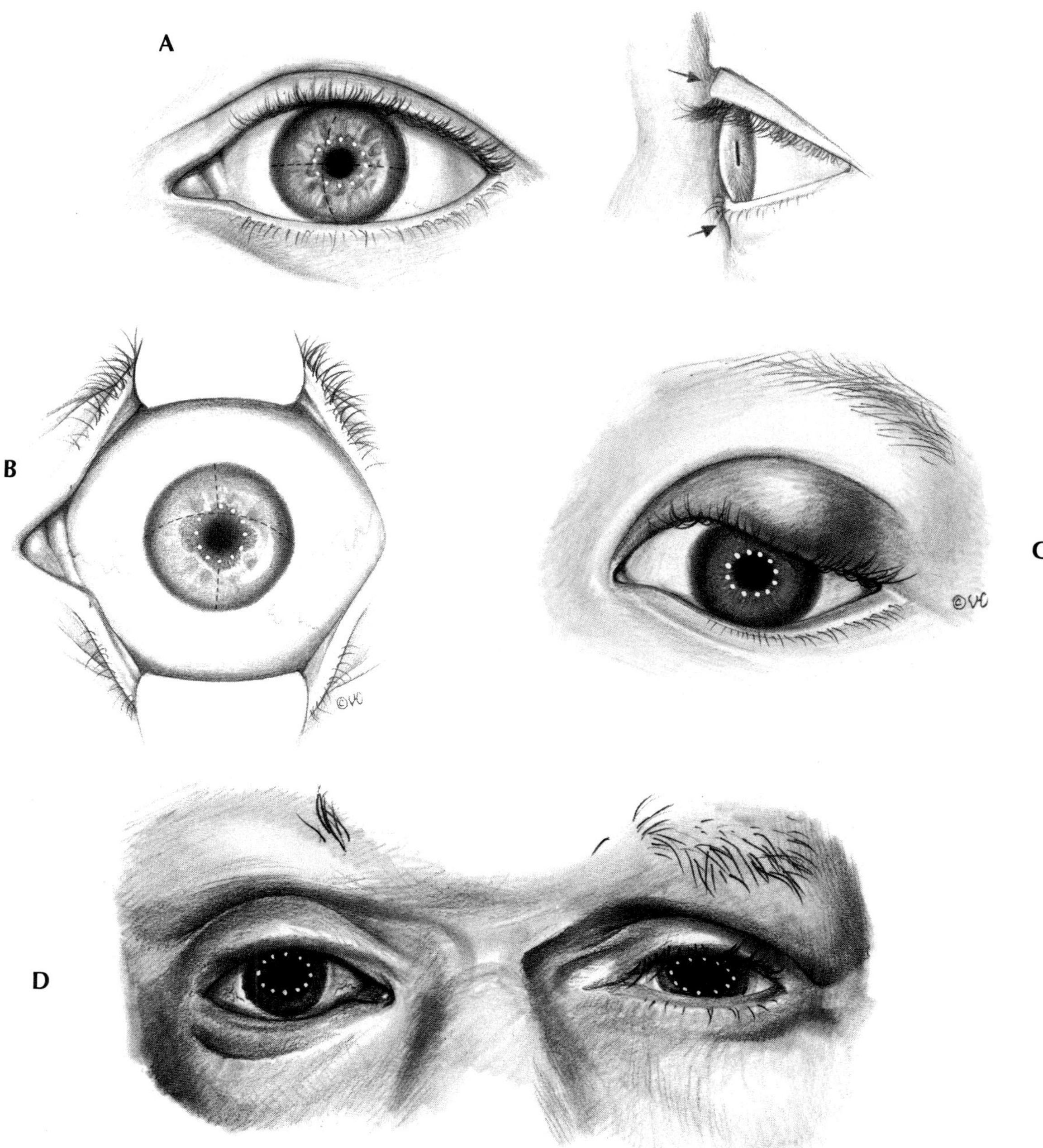

A, effect of lid tension on corneal astigmatism. **B,** against the rule astigmatism with retraction of the lids in a young adult, (exaggerated for emphasis). **C,** with the rule corneal astigmatism induced by a lid hemangioma. **D,** severe with the rule astigmatism due to tight lids in a patient with acid burn.

ance between eyelid tension and central corneal astigmatism that must be considered in treatment of corneal astigmatism.

TEAR FILM

The tear film is the most anterior layer of the cornea and represents the true anterior refractive surface of the eye. It is often overlooked in this role because of its dynamic nature, despite its well-defined structure. The tear film is composed of three layers. The superficial oily layer is derived from the meibomian glands and the accessory sebaceous glands of Zeis. This layer prevents the evaporation of fluid from the tear film and is affected by diseases of the meibomian glands, such as blepharitis. Potential corneal surgical patients with blepharitis should therefore be treated both from the standpoint of infection and to improve the tear film.

The middle aqueous layer is secreted by the lacrimal glands and the accessory glands of Krause and Wolfring. This layer is the largest and represents the real water content of the tears. The third mucoid layer is produced by goblet cells of the conjunctiva and coats the hydrophobic microvilli of the epithelium to prevent tear breakup. When a patient with dry eye has a diminished aqueous layer, the superficial oily layer and mucoid layer meet and mix, which causes the cornea to become hydrophobic and increases tear breakup time. Preservatives in drops, such as artificial tears, also can adversely affect these three layers, indicating the importance of preservative-free tear substitutes for patients who require frequent administration of these drops. The stability and regularity of the tear film is fundamentally important to good vision, and this goal often can be attained with a basic understanding of its anatomy.

EPITHELIUM

Histologically, exclusive of the tear film, the cornea consists of five distinct layers. Each layer has a particular importance to corneal surgery, and each must be restored or preserved intact for an functional result (Plate 2–2). The epithelial layer, normally seven to nine cells thick, serves to stabilize the tear film as the primary refractive surface by means of microvilli on the most anterior surface of the epithelium. If these microvilli are deficient due to lack of vitamin A or to trauma, such as over a scar, the tear film will adhere poorly and will break up, exhibiting diminished tear breakup time. Physiologically, the epithelium contributes less than the endothelium to the fluid balance of the cornea through active transport. The basement membrane of the epithelium and the interlocking of its cells provides the anterior water barrier of the cornea.

The cornea does not heal readily unless its most anterior layer, the epithelium, is intact. When the epithelial layer is incised or dehisced during

Plate 2–2.

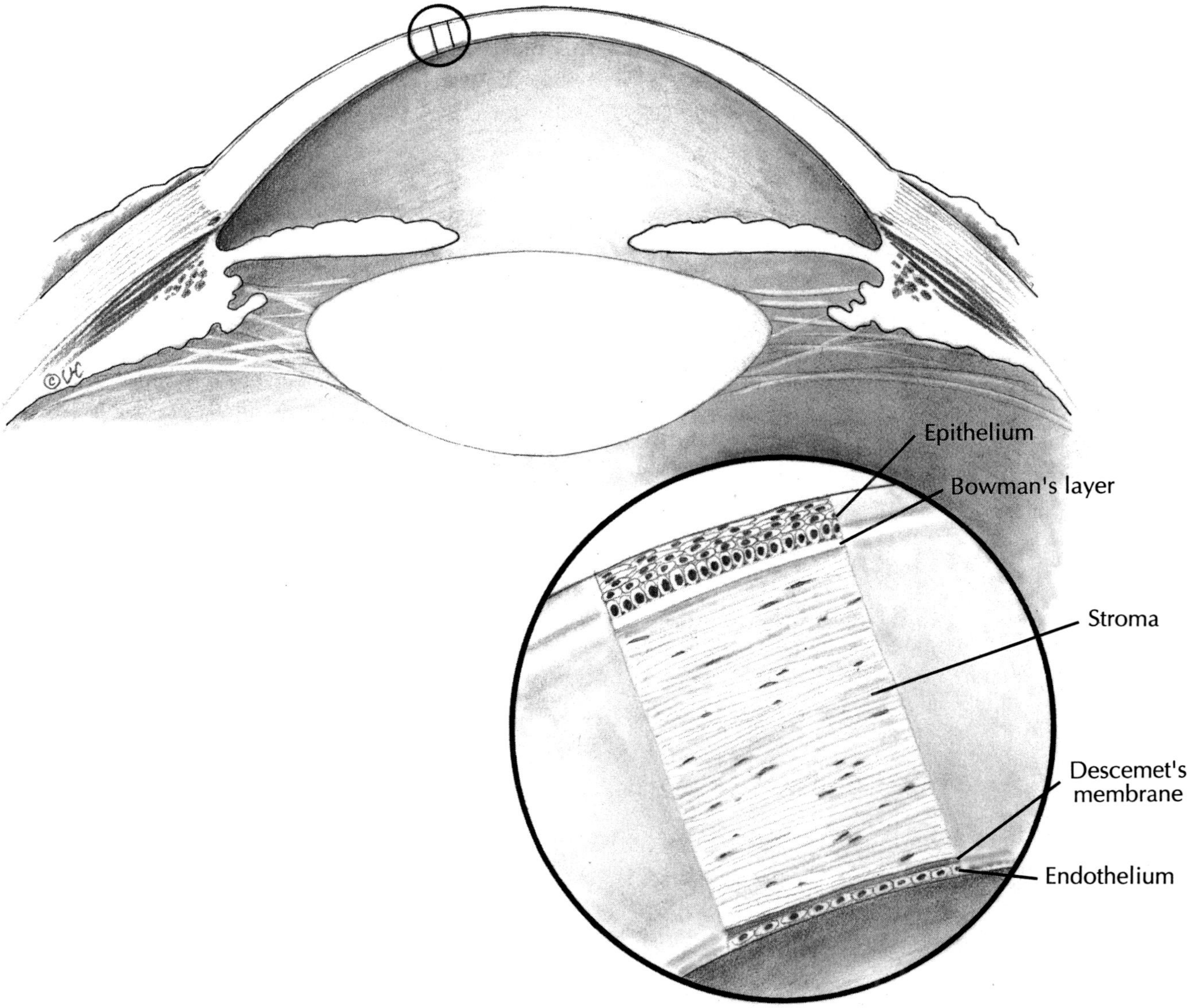

Anatomy and the five layers of the cornea.

either cataract or corneal surgery, when it is removed in whole or in part from a donor or from the recipient corneal periphery, new epithelium must slide in from peripherally to fill the defect. New epithelial cells are created at the limbus by transdifferentiation from conjunctival epithelial cells. A second important maturing movement of the epithelium occurs from the posterior cuboidal epithelial cells to mature anterior wing cells. The regenerated epithelium must be smooth and regular for an optimal optical result. Various medications, for example, chlorpromazine (Thorazine) can interfere with the normal maturation of epithelial cells, as can the presence of sutures in the cornea, which can result in *vortex epitheliopathy,* disturbing the smooth nature of the anterior surface of the epithelium.

The epithelium must adhere firmly to the underlying Bowman's layer. This is accomplished by the basement membrane, which is secreted by the epithelium and acts as a "glue" to stick the epithelium to the underlying Bowman's layer. Because this disturbs the anterior water barrier diminished visual acuity due to mild corneal edema can result. Defects in the basement membrane, such as that seen in map-dot-fingerprint dystrophy, allow recurrent corneal erosions that not only delay healing but invite infection and compromise vision by their irregularity. With extensive loss of Bowman's layer and anterior stromal defects, the epithelial cell layer tends to increase irregularly in thickness in an attempt to restore a more regular anterior contour to the damaged cornea. Excimer laser area photoablation can stimulate changes in the thickness of the epithelial layer, and may reverse in part the effect of ablations for large refractive errors. Parel (1991) has demonstrated that variations in the radial thickness of the normal epithelium contribute to overall corneal power. The epithelium has been shown to induce as much as 1.5 D myopic effect by means of this thickness variation.

BOWMAN'S LAYER

Bowman's layer, which is unique to humans and some mammals, provides a tough, elastic, acellular, smoothly regular, external envelope for the cornea. The absence of Bowman's layer in some laboratory animals, such as rabbits, has important consequences in terms of the measurement of intraocular pressure. Animals without Bowman's layer have markedly less rigid corneas, and thus applanation pressures in these animals differ significantly from measurements calibrated for humans. This stiffening of the cornea by Bowman's layer is an important difference between the eyes of humans and the eyes of animals without this structure. This is seen clearly in the markedly diminished effectiveness of lamellar refractive techniques of Barraquer if Bowman's layer is not incised circumferentially.

Bowman's layer is the only layer of the cornea that does not regenerate or migrate. Dehiscences of Bowman's layer not only alter the anatomy but also, when irregular, significantly compromise the optics of the cornea. Because Bowman's layer is the permanent corneal anterior refractive surface, dehiscence results in reduction of visual acuity to the extent that the overlying epithelium mimics the underlying irregularity of the stroma. Only recently in photoablative optical surgery have we begun to question the necessity for its preservation. Carefully controlled micrometric excimer laser surface ablation can change corneal surface curvature to induce power changes. It remains to be seen whether, when Bowman's layer and the anterior stroma are removed by laser energy, the epithelium will regenerate regularly enough over the ultrastructurally altered substrata so as not to significantly degrade acuity and whether the anterior cornea will permanently retain its new curvature. Although visible scarring usually is minimal in areas that have undergone area excimer laser ablation, micrometric irregularities may compromise vision function.

A linear, tangential, or radial incision through an intact Bowman's layer releases the surface tension of the cornea within its limbal physiologic *optical ring* and permanently alters corneal optics, not only in the incised meridian but also in the meridian approximately perpendicular to it, so-called coupling. The fact that sutures or incisions in a given meridian may alter the curvature of the meridian 90 degrees away is the basis for many of the refractive techniques discussed in this book. Similarly, these techniques clearly have an effect on the spherical equivalent power of the cornea, and these effects must be considered before performing astigmatic refractive procedures.

The third, or middle, layer of the cornea, the stroma, comprises 99% of its thickness and rigidity. Its semirigid structure supports the primarily optical anterior surface and the primarily nutritional (by active transport) posterior surface. Corneal fibrils are organized in regular layers with a 64 to 66 nm periodicity of collagen with the fibrils extending from limbus to limbus. The regular arrangement of these fibers allows the transmission of light, and disruption of this regular arrangement by corneal edema degrades the transmission of light (Plate 2–3,A). In the interfibrillar space, glycosaminoglycans (GAGs) or mucopolysaccharides are present and play a large role in the attraction of water into the cornea. When abnormal concentrations of these substances are present, as in Hurler and Scheie syndromes, corneal haziness occurs due to an imbalance between the attraction of water by GAGs and the ability of the endothelium to remove this water. The cellular component of the cornea, the keratocyte, represents a relatively small fraction of the corneal volume, and when keratocytes are completely killed, as in a keratomileusis lenticle, the stroma remains clear, although keratocytes may migrate back into the acellular tissue after 1 to 2 years. These cells play an important role in healing and regeneration of the cornea by differentiation into fibroblasts.

Corneal clarity is attributed to the regular arrangement of collagen fibrils and GAGs and is maintained by the water balance established between the tendency of the stroma to attract water and the active transport of water away from the stroma by endothelial cells (Plate 2–3,B). The balance of water in the cornea is a complex process that begins with the osmotic flow of fluid into the cornea due to the attraction of the GAGs. This process is retarded by water-tight barriers at both the epithelial and endothelial surfaces. This water is removed by the sodium-potassium pump, which requires adenosine triphosphate (ATP), located primarily in the endothelial cells, although some water transport is also performed at the epithelial surface. The production of ATP is performed under aerobic conditions through the Krebs cycle using oxygen and glucose in the mitochondria of the endothelial and epithelial cells. If the flow of oxygen from the surface of the eye is diminished by patching or contact lenses, the corneal cells must switch to the anaerobic pathway for the production of ATP, which is less efficient and produces lactate. This in turn causes corneal edema, which is reversible if oxygen flow returns. The flow of glucose, primarily from the anterior chamber, is the second important component of the Krebs cycle and is rarely a problem for the endothelial cells in close proximity. However, if this flow is interrupted by an impermeable, intracorneal lens placement, such as that introduced by Choyce, the overlying stroma becomes weakened, and can necrotize.

Centrally, the optical quality of the cornea is dependent on the paral-

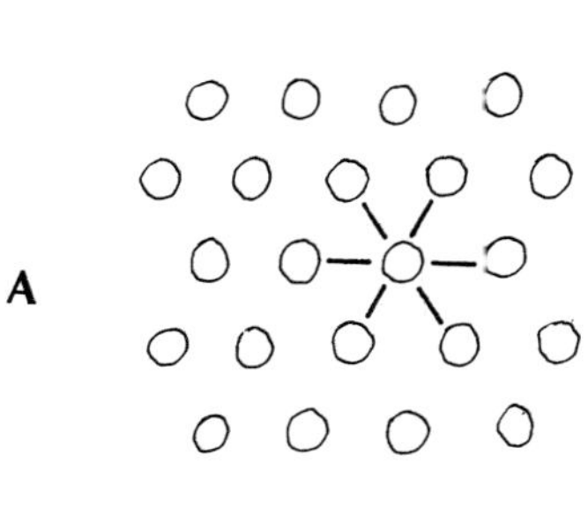

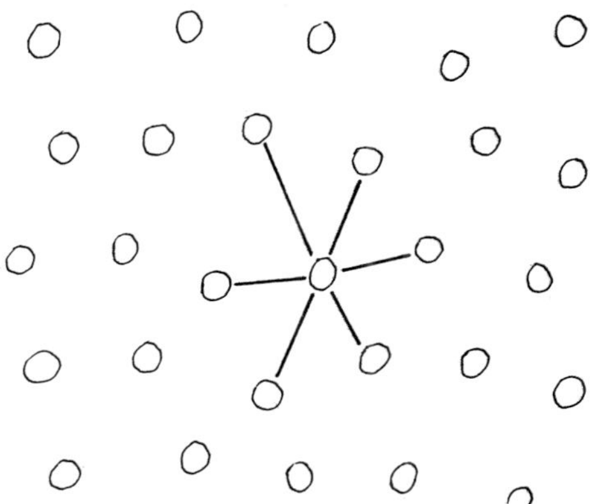

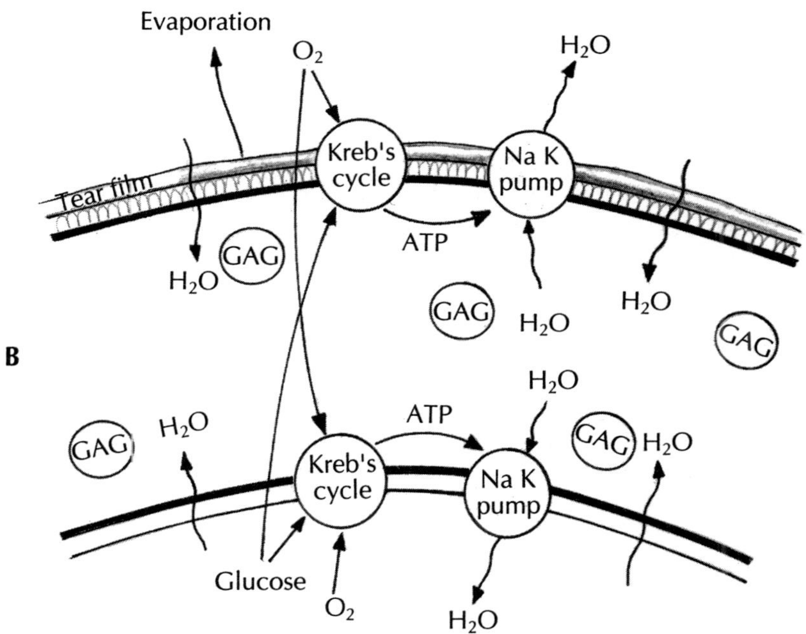

Osmotic Balance
of the Cornea

A, regular arrangement of collagen fibrils allows transmission of light; irregular arrangement of collagen fibrils with corneal edema limits transmission of light. **B,** physiology of corneal water balance.

lelism of its internal and external faces. Any accidental or deliberate alteration of its uniform central thickness will flatten or steepen the curvature of the anterior refractive surface, changing the corneal refraction. To maintain its physiologic optical function, the surgeon must therefore preserve or restore the thickness and regularity of the central optical zone. Incisional wound edges must be held to heal in full thickness, because any in-depth irregularity in apposition will compromise optical function. Precise segmental excisions of such healed, full-thickness scars, when accurately closed with sutures, more predictably steepen the cornea in the excised sutured meridian to correct an excessive astigmatic band.

When surgically modifying corneal refraction the surgeon must consider the corneal stroma from two dimensions, anatomy and optics, and when a corneal graft is involved, from the third dimension of implant physiology, for an optimal visual result.

DESCEMET'S MEMBRANE AND ENDOTHELIUM

Descemet's membrane forms the posterior limiting membrane of the cornea. It is a smooth, optically regular surface contiguous posteriorly with the stroma and lined by a single layer of endothelial cells that provide the physiologic function on which normal corneal thickness and optical clarity depend. Unlike Bowman's layer, Descemet's membrane is regenerated by a normal intact endothelium and consists of type IV collagen with a tight interfibrillar structure. Descemet's membrane is similar to basement membranes in other tissues, such as kidney glomeruli and blood vessels, and is relatively more resistant to collagenase than corneal stromal collagen. Thus in corneal ulcers Descemet's membrane provides a relative barrier to the melting of the cornea into the anterior chamber.

Not only is Descemet's membrane compromised by loss of its underlying complement of endothelial cells, but the remaining cells do not mitose or regenerate but respond by enlarging to cover depleted areas. The enlarged cells do not reconstitute a damaged Descemet's membrane to the same thickness or regularity as do normal cells; therefore, to retain physiologic and optical corneal function, it is essential to replace by graft a severely compromised Descemet's membrane and its underlying endothelium. The cellular integrity of the corneal endothelium should be verified in vivo with specular microscopy and pachymetry before any surgery involving an apparently optically clear cornea is attempted.

Following incision and closure, the cornea heals from posteriorly (back to front) once the epithelial integrity has been reestablished. When the depth of the suture closure of the wound is less than full thickness, an irregular gaping of the posterior wound edges will occur *(lambda-shaped wound profile)*. The gap is covered by enlargement and sliding of adjacent endothelial cells, which prevent posterior wound apposition and healing, resulting in a thinned elastic wound profile. Not only is wound healing compromised, but removal of sutures must be delayed, causing unpredictable alteration of corneal curvature. After suture removal the weak wound stretches and the corneal curvature excessively flattens, often forming an unstable astigmatic band. When meridional distortion results from such a thinned defective wound, its repair not only is more difficult and unpredictable than in a deeply sutured wound, but endothelial function is more likely to be compromised.

LIMBUS

The limbus is a complex structure at the periphery of the cornea representing the transition between sclera and cornea (Plate 2–4). Many important physiologic and optical activities occur in this region. First, the curvature changes in this location from that of the cornea to the sclera. Collagen fibers become much more tightly packed, illustrated by lack of lacunar spaces on histologic preparation. A healthy limbus allows active transdifferentiation of conjunctival epithelial cells to corneal epithelial cells, and the absence of this activity results in a rough anterior surface with diminished vision and healing activity across the entire cornea. The filtration of aqueous humor leaving the eye is accomplished by the trabecular meshwork and Schwalbe's canal, which is directly under the surgical limbus. Incisions in this area can easily affect this delicate process, leading to glaucoma and diminished vision. The coalescence of uveal tissue, including the iris and ciliary body, add additional structural support to the region. The combination of change of curvature, collagen compaction, and uveal thickening creates an effective barrier to the transmission of forces from the cornea to the sclera, and likewise in the opposite direction. From the standpoint of astigmatism, the limbus is pivotal to the understanding of a wide range of corneal behavior, including coupling and central corneal astigmatism related to the cataract incision. Loss of structural integrity in this structure can result in long-term instability in corneal power and astigmatic error, and such problems can be difficult to repair.

SUMMARY

The dual functions of the cornea, optical transmission of light and mechanical support of the globe, result in a structure with properties that are unique compared with any other human organ. Physiology and function combine in the cornea to provide admirably for both responsibilities. However, even minor structural or physiologic alterations can result in unintended distortion of vision. For corneal surgeons, appreciation of these many interactions is essential to successful manipulation and repair of the human cornea.

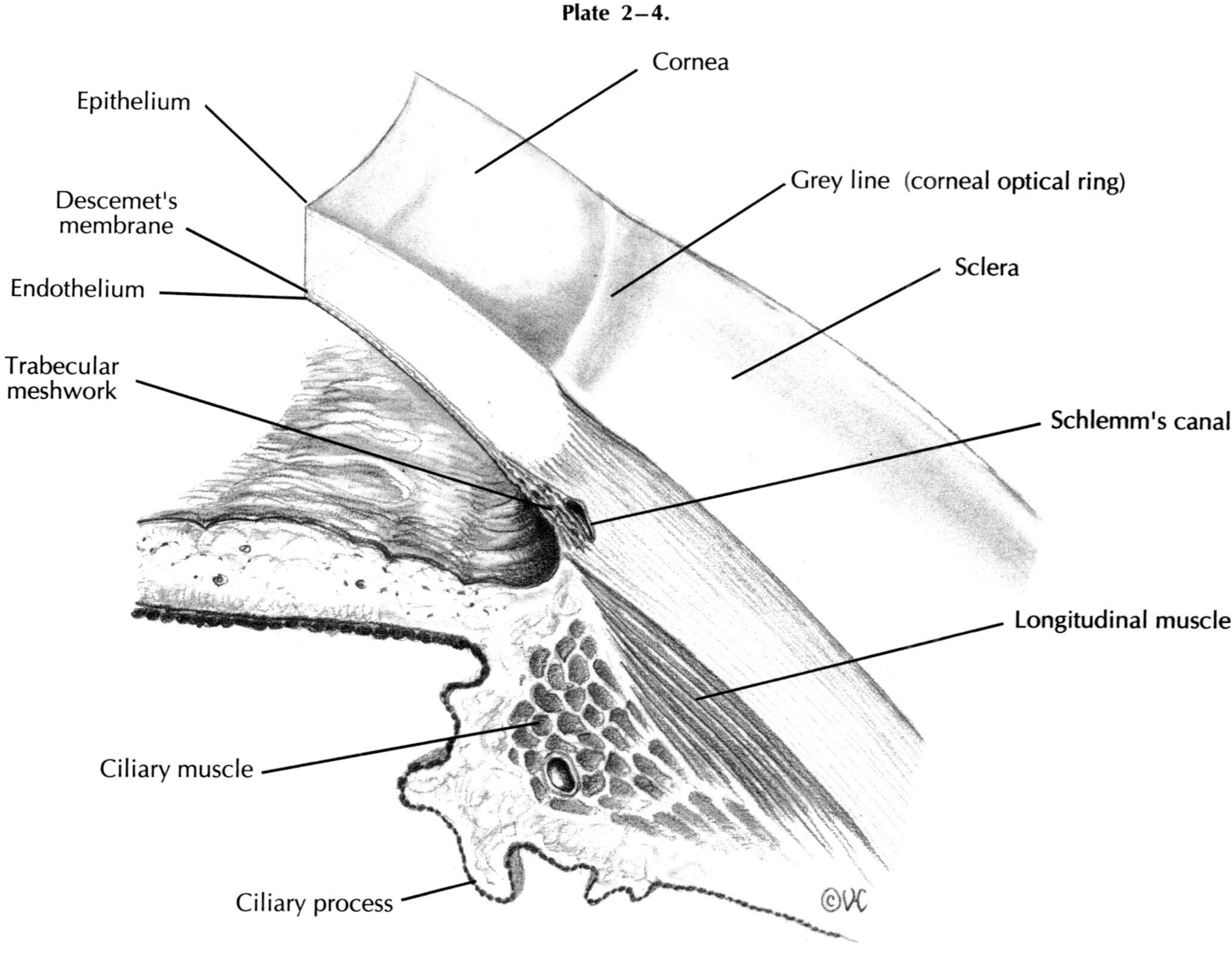

Anatomy of the limbus.

The Cornea: Optical Considerations

The ultimate goal of corneal and refractive surgery is to achieve a regular, spherical emmetropic optical result. To accomplish this, an in-depth understanding of corneal optics as it relates to anatomic structure is essential to the final surgical result. In the human eye the cornea comprises approximately one sixth of the external surface of the eye and is responsible for two thirds of its refractive power. The ability of the cornea to refract light accurately depends not only on its clarity but on the regularity and parallelism of its refractive surfaces. For this discussion, it is assumed that the cornea is of normal physiology and transparency.

CENTRAL OPTICAL ZONE

The central optical zone of the average cornea has an anterior curvature approximately +48.83 diopters (radius 7.70 mm) and a posterior curvature approximately −5.88 D (6.80 mm) (Plate 3–1). This central zone is 4 mm in diameter and approximately 0.55 mm thick, and its anterior and posterior surfaces are parallel.

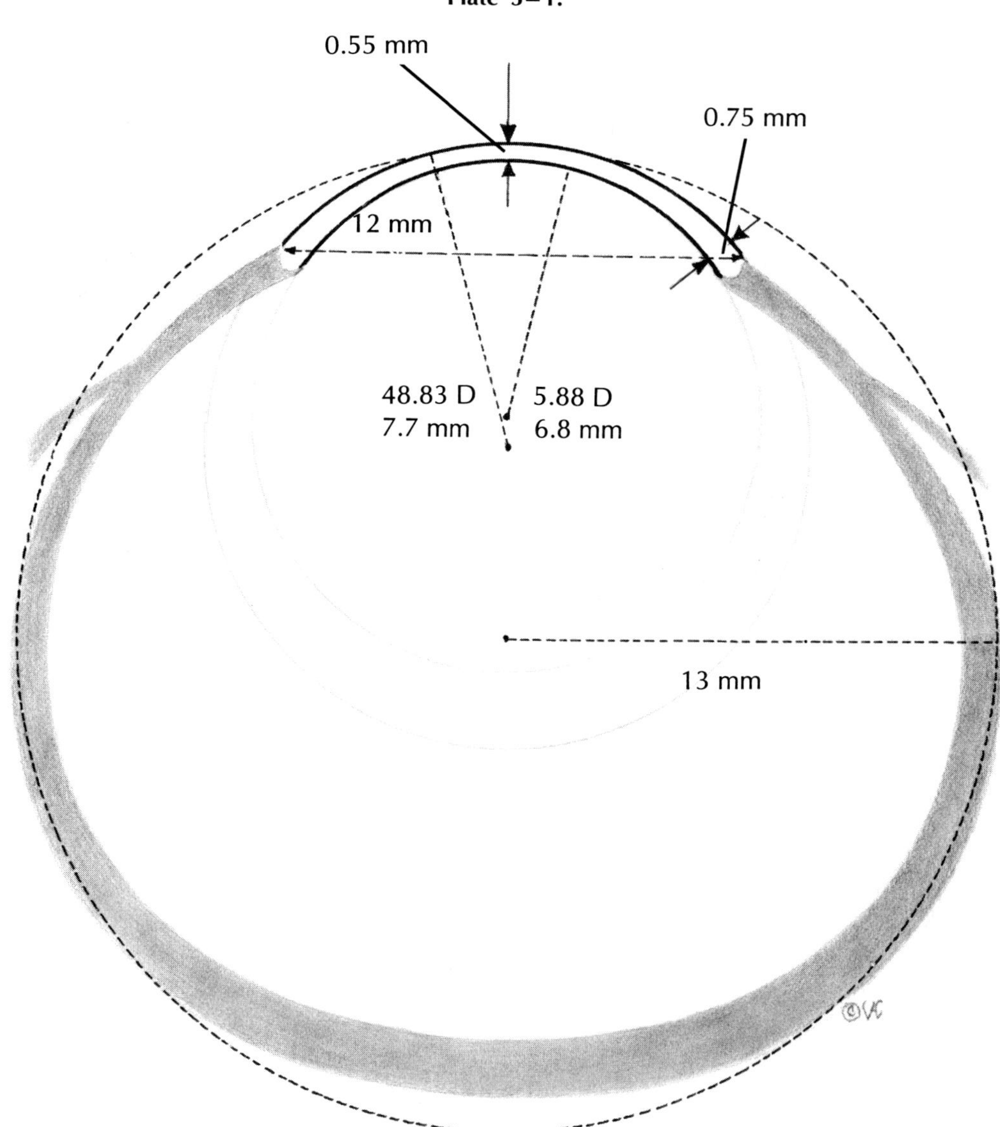

Schematic eye, optical dimensions.

The main power of the cornea is derived predominately from its anterior surface (Plate 3–2,A). The bending of light is greatest when the change in index of refraction is greatest. The change from air to cornea is greater than that of the posterior surface of the cornea in contact with aqueous humor. The anterior surface of the cornea therefore is the most important refractive surface of the human eye.

For the purpose of this discussion, the cornea is represented with regular surfaces of a fixed optical power. At each level of the cornea, the artist's drawing includes a *guy wire,* either circular, representing the fixed circumference of the cornea, or linear, representing the variable diameters (Plate 3–2,B). These are altered in their dimensions as they affect corneal curvature. A given disease or corneal refractive procedure induces or corrects astigmatism by altering the diameter in a meridian, in turn inducing a change in the shape of the corneal ring while maintaining the circumference. Careful attention should be paid to these alterations of diameter and shape.

Quantitative clinical and surgical keratometers measure only the front surfaces of the central cornea and are calibrated to read the average power of the anterior and posterior curvatures (e.g., 48.83 D minus 5.88 D equals 42.95 D; see Chapter 5). This fact is most important in the calculation of absolute refractive power. The variation of the curvatures of these two surfaces as they relate to each other produces the final refractive result, whether the radius and refractive change are affected by a change in corneal thickness, in volume, or a change in its surface area, or all three.

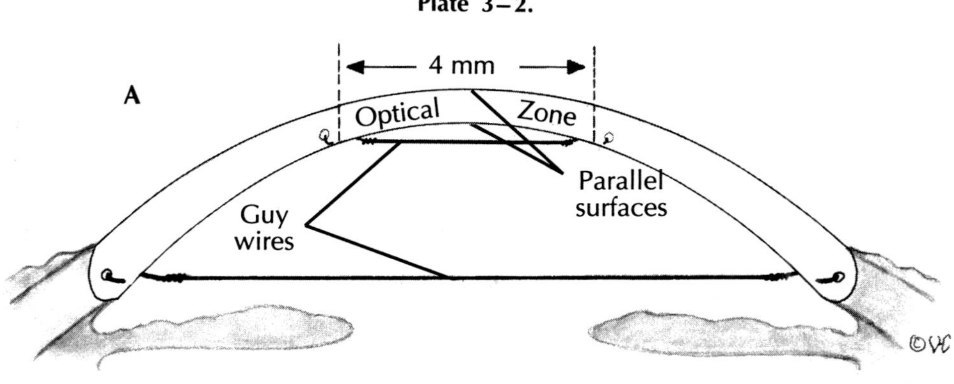

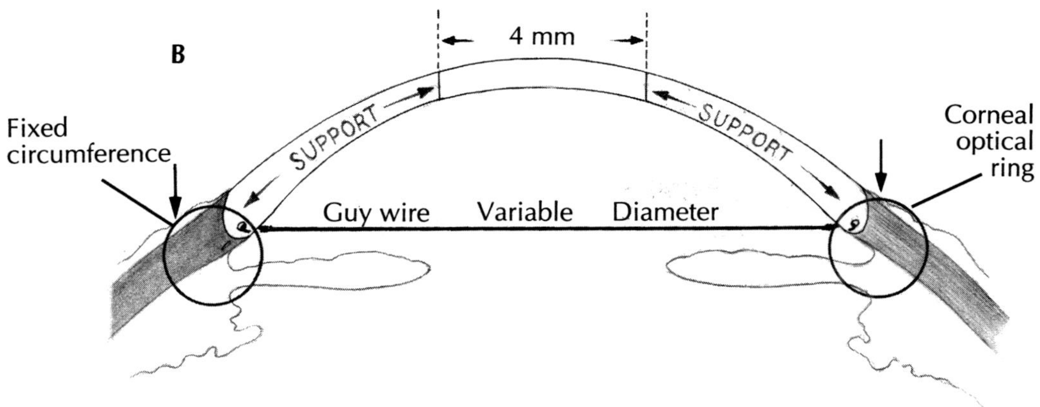

A, four-millimeter central optical zone with parallel surfaces. **B,** peripheral support zone ending in corneal optical ring (of fixed circumference).

As one proceeds peripherally from the optical zone, the cornea, although retaining its clarity, progressively increases in thickness from 0.55 mm at the optical zone to about 0.75 mm at the limbus, *the corneal optical ring* (see Plates 2–4 and 3–3). This intermediate zone functions primarily as a semirigid aplanatic *support zone* ending at the limbus (Plate 3–3). Any disease or surgical modification of this peripheral support zone, delimited by the fixed circumference of the corneal optical ring, will directly affect the curvature of the central optical zone (see Plate 3–3).

Until recently, peripheral support zone curvatures could not be measured quantitatively. Now this peripheral area can be measured accurately and reproducibly by one of several computerized topographic corneal mapping systems, for example, the Corneal Modeling System (CMS) and the Topographic Modeling System (TMS), developed by Computed Anatomy of New York, and the EyeSys System (see Chapter 5). These instruments project a series of equidistant concentric alternating black and white circles on the cornea that can be imaged by a high-resolution television monitor. These lines are digitized from the center to the periphery, converting the subjective data of reflections from the corneal surface into objective data points. These data points are analyzed by the computer and are displayed as a color-coded topographic map (see frontispiece).

Klyce has developed a useful representational system for mapping the cornea with these and other instruments. In this system, red represents the steeper cornea, and blue the flatter cornea, with intermediate zones in spectral progression. From this display, one can quantitatively measure the corneal periphery as it affects the curvature of the central optical zone. Spherical or meridional differences, as well as in the axis of astigmatic bands, ±5 degrees, are demonstrated graphically in absolute (0.5–5.0 D) and normalized (0.2 D) stepped scales. These systems enable the refractive surgeon treating abnormal refraction to compare presurgical and postsurgical measurements for treatment groups or for individual patients, providing more precise information on the interaction between the peripheral support zone and the central optical zone.

CONCEPT OF CORNEAL OPTICAL RING

To enlarge on our understanding of corneal optics, it is necessary to review the entire globe anatomy and the effect of alterations distal to the cornea and limbus. Why does a muscle shortening or lengthening procedure or an extensive scleral buckling procedure not have a significant or lasting effect on corneal curvature? Close scrutiny of the anatomy and topography of the cornea in relation to the globe reveals that the cornea and its optics are isolated from the posterior segment by a circumferential

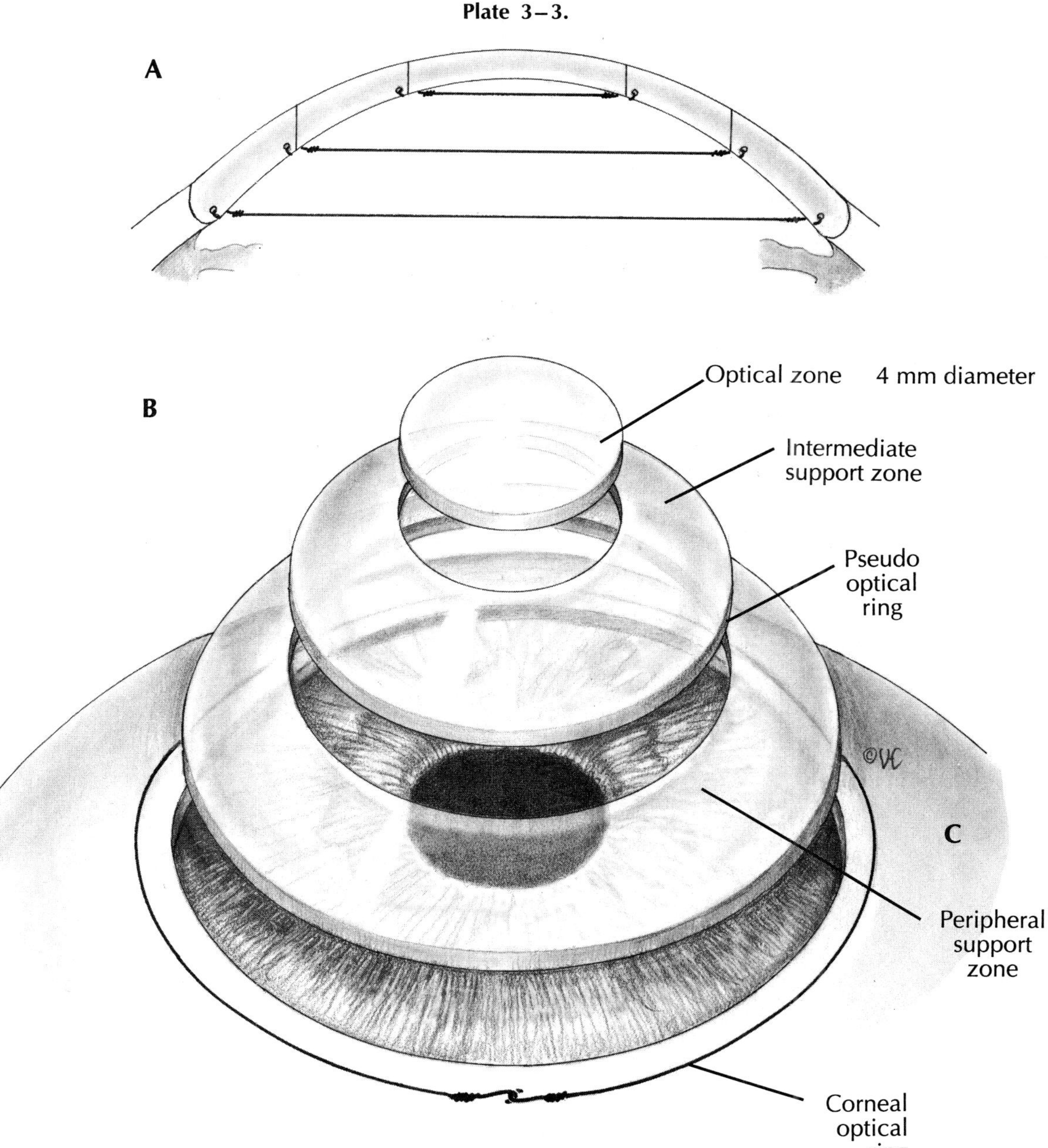

Exploded three-quarter view. **A,** central optical zone. **B,** intermediate support zone ending at pseudo-optical ring. **C,** peripheral support zone ending at corneal optical ring of fixed circumference, variable diameter.

transition zone (Plate 3–3). We have termed this zone, characterized by curvature and tissue differences both distal and proximal to it, the *corneal optical ring.* This ring corresponds roughly to the so-called *surgical limbus,* where the greater curvature of the cornea is continuous with the lesser scleral curvature. Here the regular transparent lamellae of the cornea interlock with the multidirectional, fibrous, opaque scleral tissue to form, in cross section, a pyramid-shaped transition zone, the scleral spur (see Chapter 2). This roughly circular anatomic landmark forms a delimiting ring separating the cornea from the sclera (see Plate 3–2,B).

Surgical or pathologic alteration of the scleral dimensions or elasticity peripheral to this zone (e.g., scleral buckling, myopic staphyloma, scleromalacia) will not induce significant changes in corneal curvature. Conversely, dimensional changes induced within the cornea do not appreciably affect scleral curvature. A cataract incision entering the anterior chamber by tunneling from 3 to 4 mm peripheral to this corneal ring will have minimal effect on the corneal curvature. In contrast, an incision made into or including the corneal optical ring (surgical limbus) in any of its extent will tend to induce a sometimes severe, always unstable, residual corneal astigmatism. A cataract incision inside the ring in clear cornea can induce astigmatism. However, if it is accurately closed in its vertical dimension, its effect on corneal curvature is more predictable and more stable than a limbal incision. In addition, it can be more readily modified when it is necessary to correct a preexisting astigmatic band, than can a scleral tunnel incision (see Chapter 12).

The healed circumferential scar of a lamellar or penetrating corneal graft in effect creates a second, internal *corneal pseudo-optical ring* (see Plate 3–3) at the graft-host junction, due to the extensive crosslinking of layers that occurs during normal healing. Because of its close proximity to the central optical zone, such an incision has a greater potential for inducing excessive spherical or astigmatic errors. In theory, if the graft scar could be made homogeneous circumferentially, corresponding to the circular symmetry of the eye, residual meridional defects should be minimal, or at worst, more readily correctable by a secondary surgical procedure.

Correction of a residual optical defect after either a cataract or a corneal graft procedure always should be done in or inside its respective optical ring. Corrective incisions or excisions for excessive astigmatism after keratoplasty, performed in clear cornea external to a graft scar, will have a minimal or temporary effect on the central optical zone. Also, surgery to correct postcataract astigmatism that is performed external to the limbal optical ring will have a minimal effect on the central zone. Within the respective rings, the closer an incision or excision is made to the optical zone the greater its dioptric effect, with the exception of transverse or arcuate incisions (see Tenets, Chapter 1).

When a corrective incision or excision is placed too close to the apex of the central corneal optical zone, it can induce irregularity and glare. For this reason, corrective (relaxing) incisions within the graft scar or an excision (corneal wedge resection) of the graft scar induces less irregularity and glare than do more internal T-cuts or trapezoidal configurations that more closely approach the apex.

SCHEMATIC EYE

Let us now examine further the influence of the corneal optical ring on the optical parameters of the cornea as represented in a schematic eye (see Plates 3–1 through 3–3). The schematic eye illustrated is assumed to be axially emmetropic and the cornea anastigmatic with a total power of 43 D. The delimiting corneal optical ring is represented by a circular inextensible hooking wire (see Plate 3–3). The variable diameter of the cornea is represented by an elastic band in the cross-sectional two-dimensional view (Plate 3–2,B). We will study the schematic eye for the effects of variation of one or both of these dimensions with pathologic and surgical entities as they relate to corneal curvatures. The *corneal optical ring* is assumed to be inelastic but flexible, permitting meridional variations within its fixed circumference. To maintain these relationships, it is assumed that the globe of the schematic eye is filled with an incompressible fluid.

If we excise an 8 mm circular button from the center of the schematic cornea and replace it, there should be no resulting difference in curvature (or power) (Plate 3–4,A). In this instance, the rigidly supported limbus maintains its radius and the excised button its radius, so that when replaced, no change in central corneal curvature is induced. *In vivo this would not be necessarily the case, because cutting of the anterior limiting (Bowman's) layer induces an increase in curvature of the excised button, a flattening when it is sutured in place, and a return to a steeper configuration when the sutures are removed.*

If an 8.5 mm corneal button from a donor is placed in the same opening (Plate 3–4,B), initially it will overlap until its diameter is reduced by forcing it into the recipient opening, steepening its curvature (increasing its power) in relation to the peripheral cornea. This occurs because the area of the donor button is excessive for the size of the opening. Because of the elastic nature of the cornea, when such a cornea is healed in position, the curvatures blend at the periphery of the donor button. This forms the internal *pseudo-optical ring,* and an overall steepening of the central cornea occurs. The optical ring remains round, because the forces exerted are equal in all directions.

If a 7.5 mm corneal button is placed in the 8.0 mm recipient opening, no change will occur in the curvature of either tissue (Plate 3–4,C). However, when the smaller button is sutured so as to heal to the larger recipient opening, an overall flattening of the central cornea (decreasing its power) will occur as a result of the reduced tissue within the limbal optical ring. It maintains its round configuration, again because the forces are equal in all directions, this time pulling instead of pushing.

In each instance it will be noted that the diameters of the corneal optical ring and the new pseudo-optical ring remain constant. The variation occurs in curvature of the oversized or undersized button taking place within these circumferences.

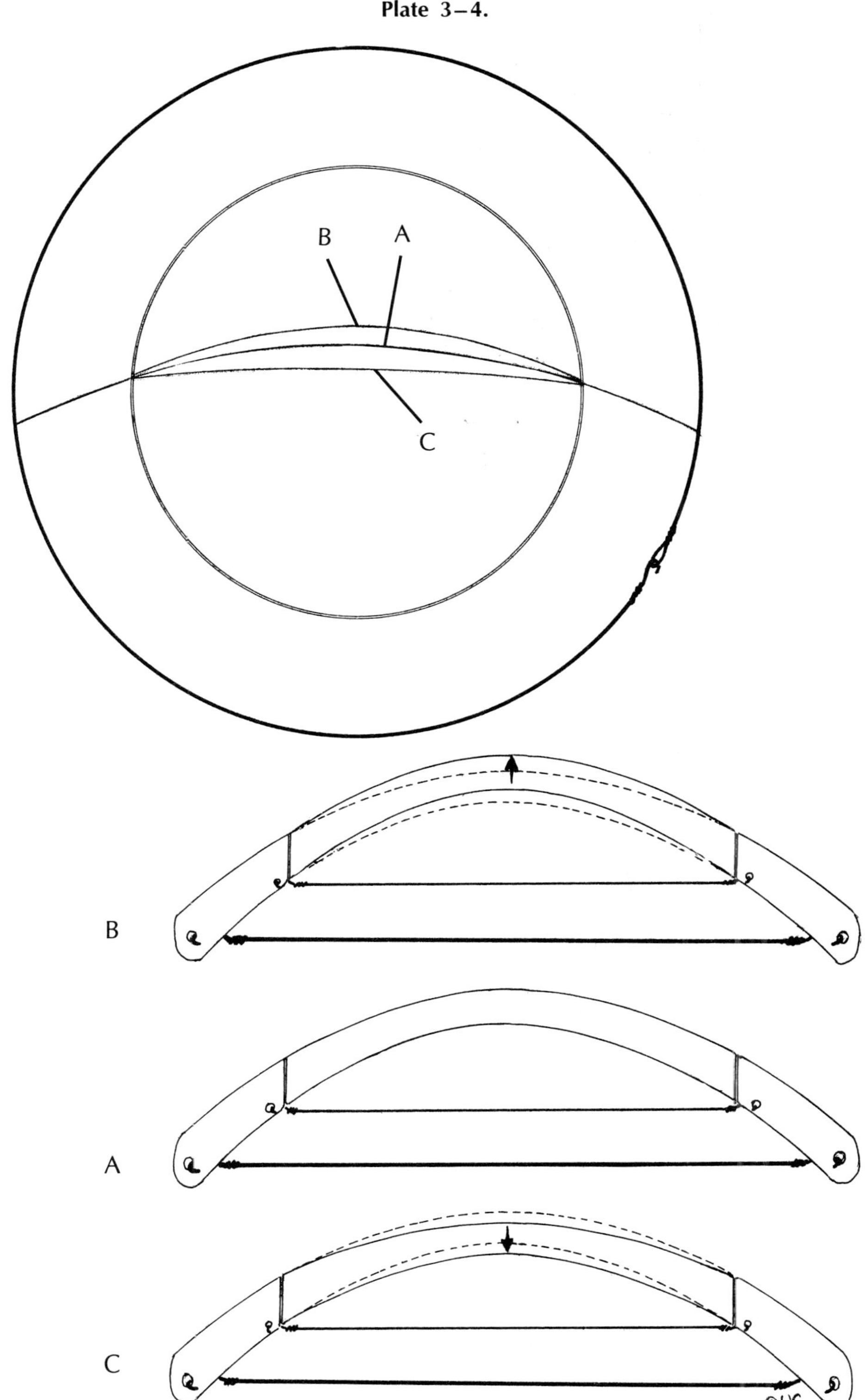

Effects of disparate-diameter graft in fixed-diameter recipient. **A,** 8.0 mm graft in 8.0 mm recipient; no change in curvature. **B,** 8.5 mm graft in 8.0 mm recipient; steepening induced. **C,** 7.5 mm graft in 8.0 mm recipient; flattening induced.

Variation of the shape but not the area of the donor button, or the recipient opening, or both, will have a neutral effect on average curvature while inducing astigmatism by the difference in diameter of the opposing meridians. When an oval graft is inserted in a round recipient bed the cornea becomes flatter in the meridian of the greater donor diameter (Plate 3–5,A). When a round recipient is placed in an oval recipient opening the cornea becomes steeper in the meridian of the greater recipient diameter (Plate 3–5,C). The effects are similar when the graft and recipient are ovaled in opposite dimensions, but depending on their respective dimensions, tending more or less to compensate each other (Plate 3–5,B).

In these instances, although the circumference of the optical corneal ring remains constant, it becomes oval. The narrowed dimension of the oval corresponds to the steeper meridian, whereas the widened dimension of the oval corresponds to the flatter meridian.

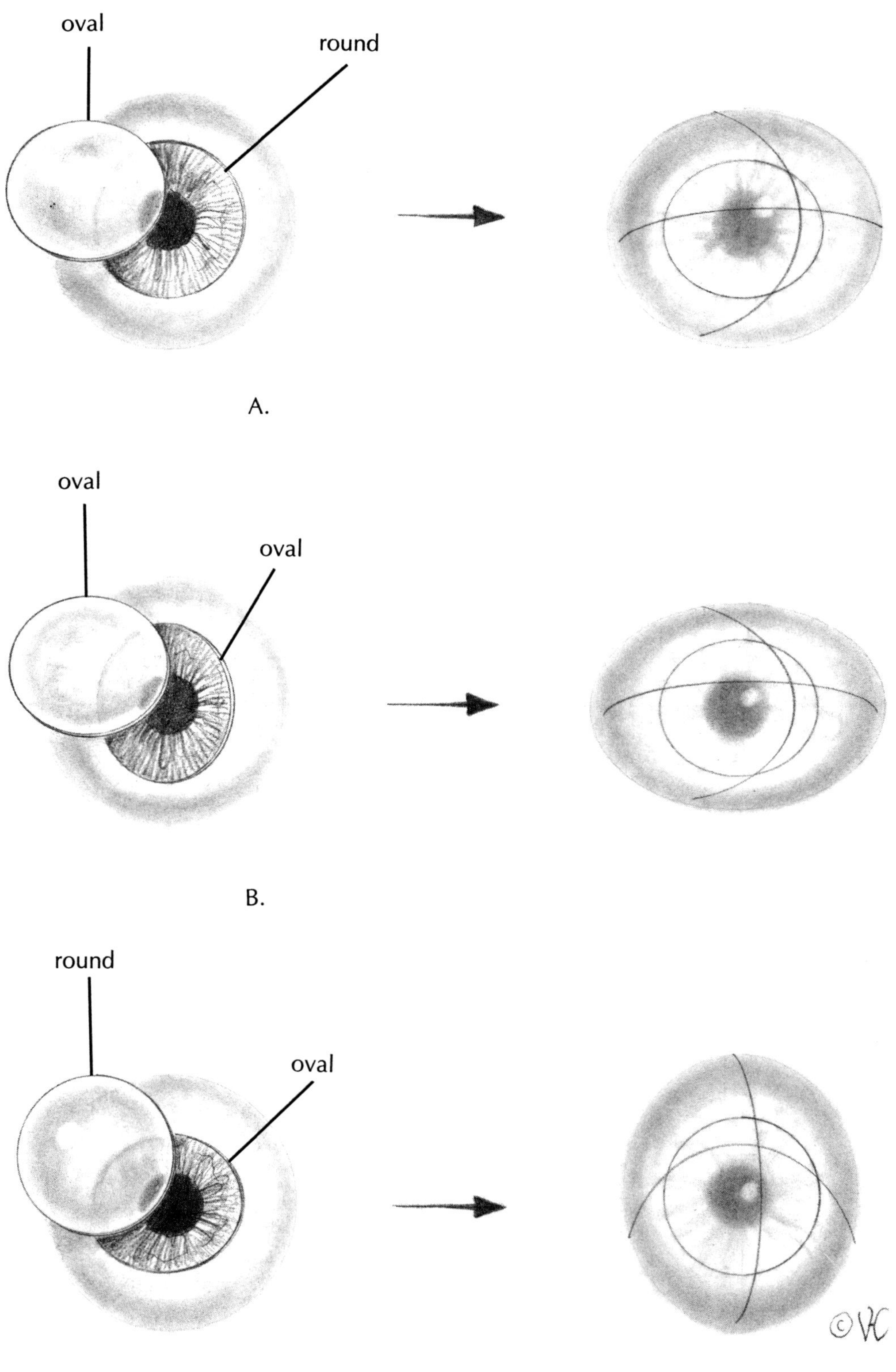

Effect of ovaling of graft or recipient or both. **A,** effect of oval graft in round recipient. **B,** effect of oval graft in oval recipient. **C,** effect of round graft in oval recipient.

When a round donor button is placed in a round recipient opening in an abnormally curved astigmatic cornea (e.g., in a keratoconus where an irregularly thinned elastic inferior recipient bed is present), similar meridional dioptric distortions are induced in the donor (Plate 3–6,A and B). When the normally thick, consistently firm edge of the donor cornea is apposed to the pathologically thin, soft, inferior recipient edge and to the more normal thickness of recipient cornea superiorly, the differences in apposition tension around the healed circumference will induce astigmatism.

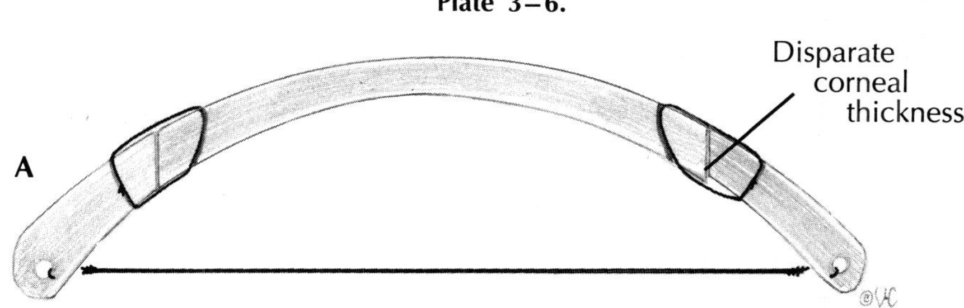

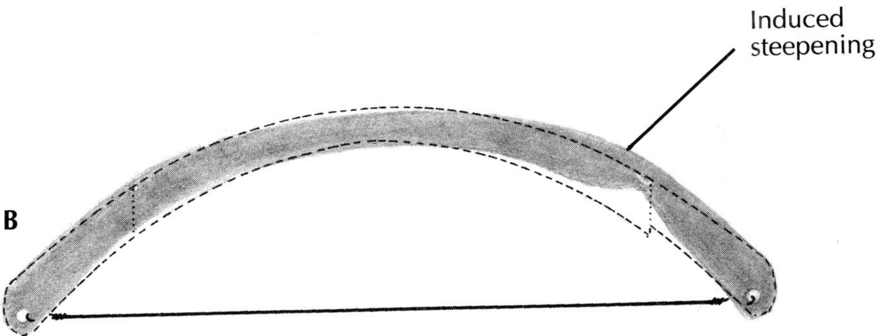

Effect of round graft sutured into round recipient opening with thinned sector (e.g., keratoconus). **A,** disparate thickness sutured. **B,** disparate thickness healed. Cornea steepens within fixed-circumference corneal optical ring.

Coupling

It was noted as early as 1891 by Bates that when an incision was made that flattened one meridian of the cornea, corresponding, but not equal, steepening of the meridian occurred at 90 degrees away. The engineering term for this effect, *coupling,* recently has been applied to this long-recognized phenomenon. Coupling, as we have learned from computerized topographic mapping systems, is usually asymmetric, but for purposes of illustration, and even for practical purposes in most instances, can be assumed to be symmetric.

If the circumference of the limbal corneal optical or pseudo-optical ring is compromised by an incision across or along its length, the cornea will become flattened in the meridian of the disrupted ring sector and steepened at approximately 90 degrees. In contradistinction to incisions made within the intact rings, when a ring is violated the overall corneal curvature tends to flatten and the eye becomes more hyperopic. This occurs because the circumference of the ring increases while the area of the cornea internal to it remains the same (e.g., the limbal cataract incision or corneal relaxing incisions).

This phenomenon can be duplicated schematically (Plate 3–7). In this instance, in the meridian of a partial penetrating incision made into the pseudo-optical ring, as the incisional edges retract the ring stretches, increasing its circumference and diameter, inducing flattening of the central cornea in the incisional meridian. At 90 degrees the pseudo-optical ring proportionally reduces in diameter and the central cornea steepens in a ratio of approximately 1 D of steepening to each 2 D of flattening (see Poisson's ratio and Gauss' law, below). Within the constant circumference of the corneal optical ring, these effects combine, tending to maintain average curvature and power.

When an excision and suture of a graft scar is made in a quadrant, the cornea central to the resected meridian steepens as the pseudo-optical ring is reduced in diameter and circumference. The meridian at 90 degrees flattens in a 1 D flattening to a 2 D steepening ratio, tending to maintain total corneal curvature and power within the fixed circumference of the corneal optical ring.

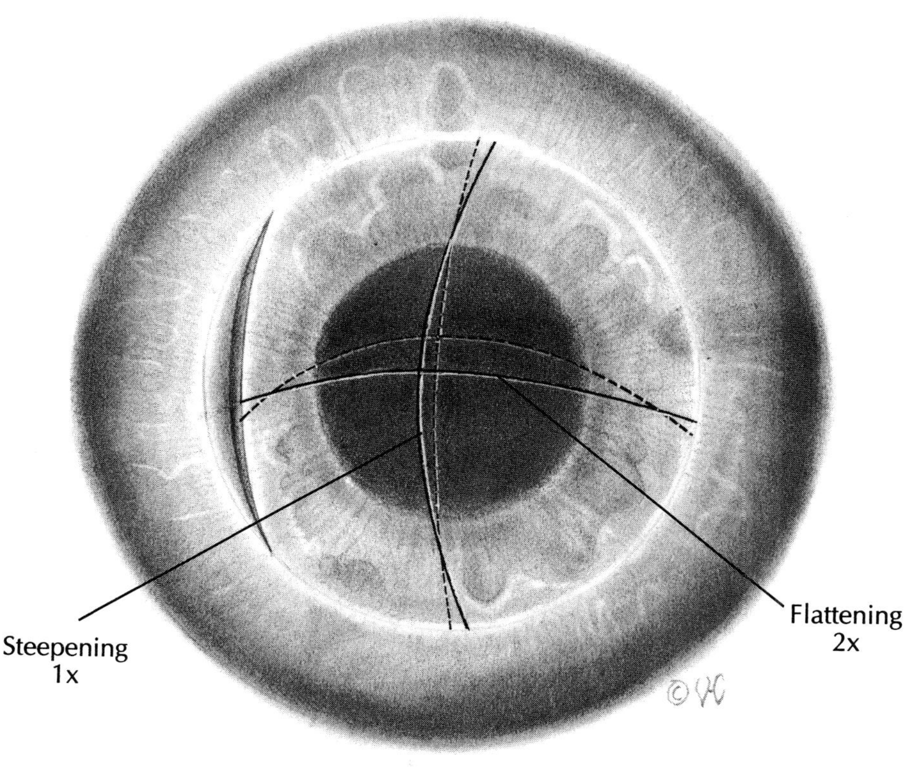

Coupling

Coupling. A relaxing incision in a graft scar (pseudo-optical ring) across the steeper corneal meridian flattens the incisional meridian, inducing steepening of the meridian at 90 degrees in a 2:1 ratio.

When radial incisions are made from the optical zone to but not including the optical corneal ring, flattening of the central optical zone will occur, due to an increase in corneal diameter and circumference of the midperipheral support zone while the cornea is being held in its constant circumference at the corneal optical ring (Plate 3–8). The effect can be meridional when the incisions are placed in a sector, or circumferential, as in radial keratotomy, when placed equidistant around the entire corneal circumference.

In combination, the effects of radial and meridional transverse incisions, whether the latter are curvilinear or linear, have a unique effect to reduce coupling ratio and effect the curvature change only in the incisional meridian. In this instance, the effect of coupling being neutralized, decrease in total corneal power is induced.

The above phenomena depend on the *physics of incompressible fluids*. Incompressible fluids, such as those found inside the eye, have the property that their volume is constant at all times. Thus a sphere filled with fluid, when compressed, will expand to half the amount in the direction 90 degrees away. This coupling of perpendicular forces is described in mechanical terms by *Green's tensor,* and in a simple isotropic incompressible fluid by a single value called *Poisson's ratio* (ratio of movements 90 degrees apart), which is 0.5 in this situation.

A second means of understanding coupling can be gained from consulting *Gauss' law* of total curvature of a toric surface, which states: *If a perfectly flexible and inextensible surface is bent in a given meridian, the total curvature remains constant as the second main radius changes in the opposite way. The total curvature is defined as the product of the inverse of the radius of each meridian.*

These properties are not perfectly proportional clinically, as they would appear to be in the schematic eye, because of the variable physical properties of the cornea.

Clinical Application of Theoretic Phenomena

Why are we so concerned with variations of corneal curvature? To answer that question, we need only query any corneal or cataract surgeon as to the most common optically debilitating problem following an otherwise successful surgical intervention. Most will indite excessive astigmatism. After cataract surgery, differences in meridional curvature are regular and minimal and are readily correctable by spectacles or by contact lenses. After corneal surgery, however, moderate to severe astigmatism is the rule. Spectacle correction may be inadequate, and contact lenses may be uncomfortable or contraindicated. The patient who has worn contact lenses for years, particularly to correct keratoconus, may object to their wear.

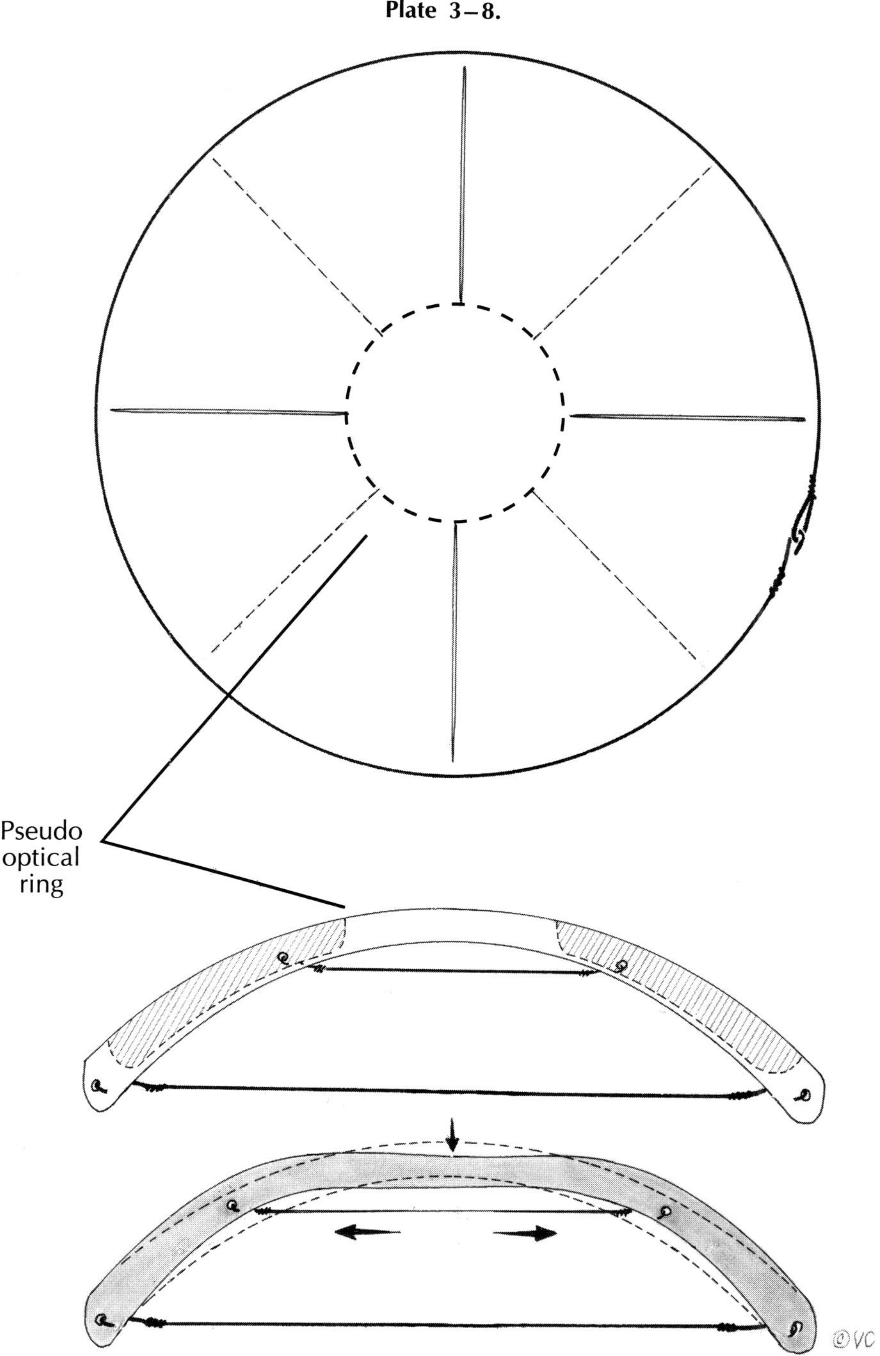

Effect of radial incisions. Flattening induced in optical zone central to incision-induced ectasia in peripheral support zone.

A second, less well-recognized optical problem following penetrating keratoplasty, often seen combined with astigmatism, spherical ametropia, can be more difficult to manage effectively. The postoperative donor cornea can become flatter (more hyperopic) or steeper (more myopic) than the average seen in a normal cornea or the cornea of the fellow eye. Where the length of the recipient eye is normal, an excessively flat or steep donor cornea may induce a *6-D Surprise* akin to cataract or implant surgery.

The potential for such compound refractive problems after otherwise successful penetrating grafts, both unilateral and bilateral, requires the development of new measuring techniques for both donor and recipient as well as improved surgical techniques with which we can anticipate and compensate or correct both astigmatism and ametropia simultaneously.

At minimum, preoperative keratometry should be performed with an office keratometer supplemented by a photokeratoscope, and when possible with a computerized topographic mapping instrument. Detailed preoperative measurements obtained with these instruments have the potential to improve the predictability of postoperative ametropic errors. Technical steps, based on these measurements, then can be taken at the primary procedure to compensate for anticipated astigmatic distortions.

Intraoperative keratometry should be routinely used during each surgical step to identify and to monitor such compensating or correcting procedures. Detailed quantitative evaluation during the postoperative course completes the trilogy to identify the parameters for necessary intermediate or definitive secondary corrective procedures.

If one could reliably predict preoperatively the amount and axis of such an anticipated curvature change, then a graded ovaling of the donor button or of the recipient opening, or both, should primarily compensate the anticipated distortion. However, when such compensatory ovaling of the recipient opening was attempted clinically with the Lieberman trephine (Troutman, 1976), no consistent results were obtained. However, with computerized corneal topography and mechanical modeling of the cornea and the potential for infinite alteration of graft or recipient shape using the excimer laser it soon may be possible to design the compensating operative procedure primarily. The digitized results can then be used to control automated instrumentation to guide a precise cutting device, such as the excimer laser, to perform the definitive procedure and to correct any optical residuals. In another dimension, a laser might be developed that might actually weld corneal tissue, making sutures unnecessary, and at the conclusion of the procedure corneal topology might identify minor surface optical alterations that can be corrected with area photoablation.

At present, correction of an induced meridional defect, whatever the cause, is more predictably performed at a secondary procedure. Current corrective procedures are performed within or inside the graft incision or cataract scar at or within the corneal optical or pseudo-optical ring. They are positioned selectively across either the flatter (corneal wedge resection) or the steeper (corneal relaxing incisions) corneal meridian or across both by a combination of the two procedures. In a cornea with a residual astigmatic band and a myopic (excessively steep) spherical equivalent power, a circumferential resection of the scar (circumferential wedge resection) in the graft-host junction or of a cataract incision scar across the flatter corneal meridian will tend to reduce overall corneal myopia in addition to the astigmatic correction. Conversely, when the spherical equivalent power of the cornea is hyperopic (excessively flat), a circumferential incision placed at or just internal to the graft-host junction that connects the steeper (myopic) meridians paradoxically increases overall corneal curvature (power), reducing the corneal hyperopia. Combining these procedures can better compensate more complex (CMS delineated) errors, and in theory has a more neutral effect on corneal spherical equivalent power.

KERATOPLASTY AND CORNEAL AMETROPIA

We have used keratoconus as a model to study the optical effects of several penetrating keratoplasty incision and closure techniques, because of the uniformity of its pathologic features and the consistency of the anatomic and physiologic results. Further, and as important, because of the variable circumferential recipient consistency and thickness, it shows a greater than average tendency for the development of significant post-keratoplasty spherical equivalent ametropia and excessive astigmatism. More often than not, the keratoconic eye would be axially emmetropic, if it had on average 43 D corneal curvature. Because the characteristic compound myopic ametropia is corneally induced, a dioptric surprise can occur when the grafted cornea is too flat, less than 43 D (hyperopic), or conversely too steep, greater than 43 D (myopic). It follows that when the recipient eye is axially myopic or hyperopic, (by A-scan) the ametropia can be predictably compensated by deliberately inducing flattening or steepening of the donor. It is always important to tell the patient preoperatively not only of the virtual certainty of some astigmatism but also of the probability of a less readily correctable residual myopia or hyperopia.

Disparate diameter graft to recipient opening (Troutman, 1976) has been suggested as a means to correct such axially induced myopia or hyperopia. With the Krumeich trephine system, when a donor cornea button is cut from anteriorly with an 8 mm diameter trephine blade and an 8 mm diameter recipient opening is cut with the same blade (see Chapter 7), an approximately 43 D average keratometry results. When a donor corneal button is punch cut with an 8 mm blade from its endothelial side

(Amsler technique), a slightly smaller (0.2 mm) anterior diameter is obtained. When healed in an 8 mm diameter recipient opening, a flatter (±40 D) average cornea power will result. However, when a 0.2 mm larger diameter trephine blade is used to punch the donor button (8.2 mm), the average 43 D is obtained. Varying diameter combinations have been used to vary the postoperative corneal curvature from the average (43 D) to compensate axial ametropias. In aphakic keratoplasty, before the use of intraocular implants, a larger donor diameter difference (0.5 to 1.0 mm) was used in aphakic eyes to induce a steeper than average cornea to compensate partially the aphakic hypermetropia. Currently, larger donor diameters may be used to compensate an anticipated (A-scan) axial hypermetropia. However, when a 1.0 mm or greater difference is used, an excessive, sometimes irregular astigmatism can be induced. Occasionally a smaller donor diameter (e.g., 7.7 or 7.5 mm diameter in an 8.0 mm diameter recipient) is used to compensate a higher axial myopia or to flatten a severely stretched steep cornea, such as encountered following trauma or in congenital glaucoma. Here, too, more than average induced astigmatism can result. After the graft is healed, a circumferential wedge resection, as described by Buzard (1990), can induce the same effect. This tendency to irregularity has limited the application of this technique to the correction of smaller degrees of axial ametropia ±5–10 D. Above that level, until the potential of excimer laser photoablation is fully realized, there has been no possibility for accurate surgical compensation of residual ametropias.

It is interesting that a wedge resection (removing area) along a given meridian causes steepening, yet a wedge resection performed in two meridians or circumferentially causes central cornea flattening. Similarly, a relaxing incision (adding area) along a given meridian causes flattening, yet relaxing incisions circumferentially (for instance in hexagonal keratotomy) cause central corneal steepening.

REFRACTIVE KERATOPLASTY SURGICAL PRINCIPLES

Having reviewed the basis of refractive surgery, stating its tenets, and demonstrating it in principle on the schematic eye, we now have the understanding to approach its clinical application. First we will consider the principles involved in the performance of the various refractive keratoplasty procedures. These are considered in the order of their evolution rather than frequency of performance. Thus the techniques of José Barraquer, who has been characterized as the "father of refractive keratoplasty," although currently less frequently performed, qualify to be described first. His principles are seminal to the development of the specialty of refractive keratoplasty and thus essential to understanding of any subsequent procedures for the prevention, limitation, and correction of corneal ametropias, in particular, astigmatism.

Refractive surgery includes several distinctly different underlying principles, described according to the surgical method used to effect the corneal refractive change. In the first group, the change in curvature of the anterior cornea is effected by graded surgical removal of or addition to the corneal stroma without posterior radius change: *thickness-volume* techniques. In the second group, refractive change is induced by addition to or subtraction of tissue from the anterior corneal surface to induce a combined posterior and anterior radius change: *surface modification* technique. When such surgical corrections are applied equally circumferentially, axial ametropias can be corrected; when the corrective procedure is confined to a corneal meridian, it can compensate corneal astigmatism.

Barraquer not only developed but defined the terminology for the thickness-volume techniques.

Keratomileusis (corneal carving) induces an anterior curvature and power change by optical modification of the posterior stromal surface of a resected anterior corneal cap. For correction of myopia, the central area of the resected corneal cap is thinned to flatten the cornea when healed in place (Plate 3–9,A). To effect a refractive change to correct hyperopia, the corneal cap is thinned in its periphery so as to steepen the central refractive zone (Plate 3–9,B). Here, too, posterior corneal radius and circumference do not change. Because all of the surgery is done on the cornea, the volume of the cornea is reduced to effect the thickness change. Ruiz induces the same optical effect for correction of myopic by graded removal of the corneal tissue from the posterior lamella with a second pass of the microkeratome using a nonfreeze technique.

Keratophakia (cornea-lens) effects an anterior curvature change by increasing both corneal thickness and volume by insertion of a concavoconvex lenticle of donor cornea of predetermined plus power between the layers of a lamellarized normal cornea (Plate 3–9,C). The corneal radius and circumference remain constant. This technique is used to correct higher degrees of hyperopia, particularly that of aphakia.

Epikeratoplasty. In this instance a planolamellar homograft is used to replace the lamellarized anterior surface of an irregular cornea. The epikeratoplasty lenticle may be modified optically to correct an anticipated refractive error.

The term *epikeratophakia* has been substituted for the term *epikeratomileusis,* originally coined by Werblin and Kaufman. In this case, an optically modified lamellar homograft is placed on the deepithelized Bowman's layer of a normal cornea (Plate 3–9,D). The corneal radius and circumference remain constant. Although this technique initially was thought applicable to correct adult myopia and hyperopia, it is currently being used only in aphakic hyperopia in children.

In all of these techniques, the change in refraction is effected primarily by a change in anterior corneal curvature *without changing the posterior corneal radius* (Plate 3–9, guy wire), except in the case of epikeratophakia for keratoconus in which simultaneous radius change occurs as a result of the compression of the underlying pathologic condition.

The Barraquer procedures and epikeratophakia originally were performed by freezing the corneal tissue and modifying it optically in the frozen state. More recently, Barraquer and colleagues have devised the BKS (Barraquer, Krumeich, and Swinger) system to prepare keratophakia, keratomileusis, and epikeratophakia lenticles by a nonfreeze technique. Using metal optical dies, the excised corneal cap is cut with the

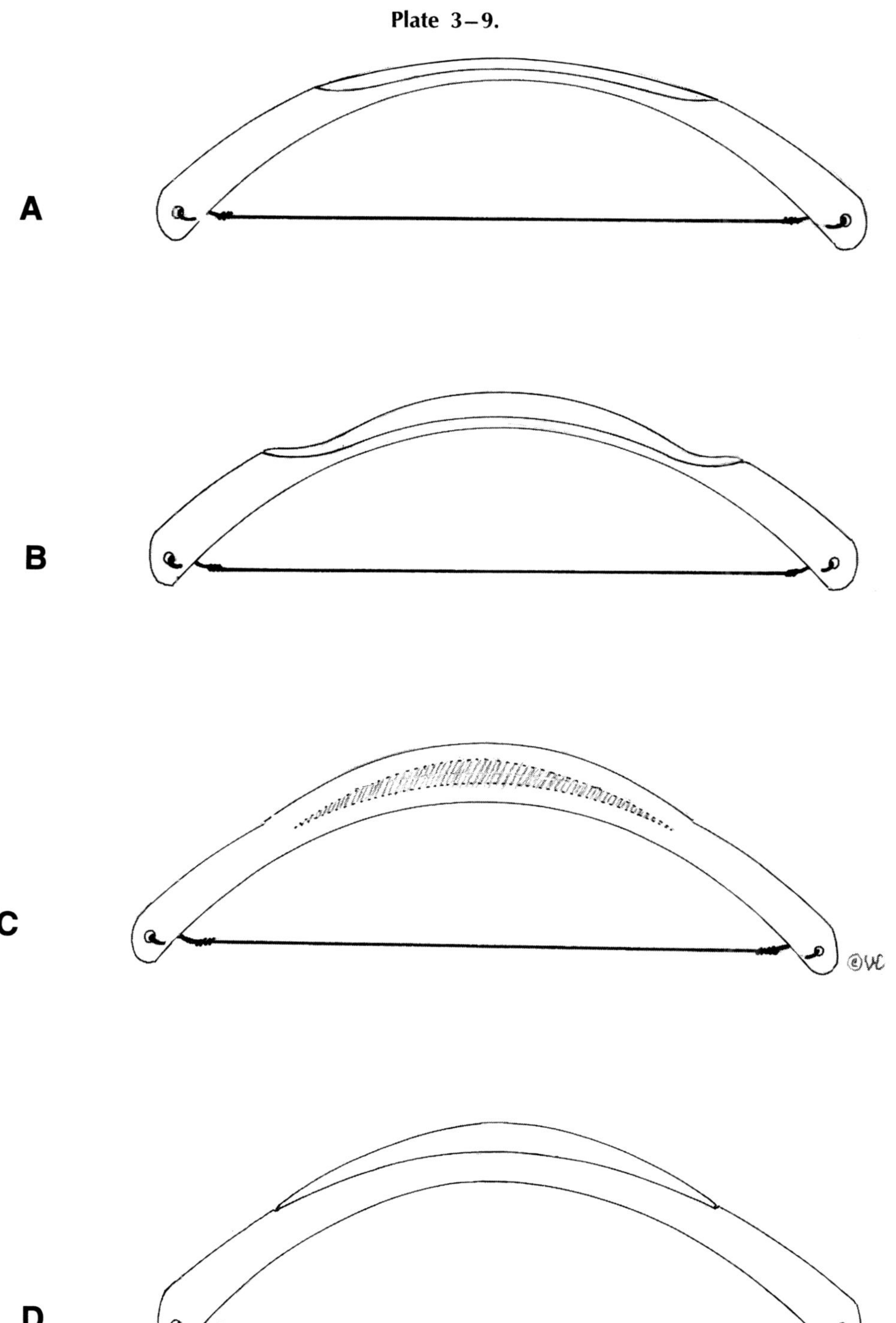

Thickness-volume techniques of Barraquer. **A,** myopic keratomileusis. Flattening of the optical zone is induced by central thinning of the corneal cap. **B,** hyperopic keratomileusis. Steepening of the optical zone is induced by peripheral thinning of the corneal cap. **C,** keratophakia. Steepening of the central optical zone is induced by interposition of a corneal tissue lenticle in lamellarized stroma. **D,** epikeratophakia. Steepening of the central optical zone by overlay of lamellarized lenticle on intact Bowman's layer.

microkeratome to a predetermined power in its natural state. The major problem with the Barraquer techniques and epikeratophakia has been accuracy. Both the freeze-thaw cycle of the cryotechnique and the non-freeze techniques can induce significant deviation from the planned power. The excimer laser may solve the problem of accuracy and make possible higher power corrections and retention of Bowman's layer, now sacrificed with photorefractive keratectomy (PRK).

SURFACE AREA MODIFICATION TECHNIQUES

The second group of refractive keratoplasty procedures effect a change in refraction primarily by increasing or decreasing posterior and anterior corneal radii by surface area modification. This principle originally was applied by Sato, who made multiple radial cuts, sparing the center of the cornea, from the internal or external corneal surface. He, in effect, created a peripheral keratoconus that secondarily caused central flattening. Because of severe corneal complications, almost 30 years passed before Fyodorov (1978) revived and popularized this technique for correction of myopia and minor degrees of astigmatism.

Troutman (1970) was the first to describe curvilinear keratectomy (corneal wedge resection) across the flatter corneal meridian for correction of excessive astigmatism following keratoplasty. He also applied the principle of Snellen (1869) to keratoplasty (Troutman, 1975), using curvilinear keratotomies (corneal relaxing incisions) across the steeper corneal meridian for correction of lesser degrees of post-keratoplasty astigmatism.

Fyodorov and others used sector radial keratotomy to correct for small degrees of astigmatism, and later transverse keratotomies (T-cuts) were added to their primary myopic procedure for the correction of astigmatism.

Surgical procedures for the correction of refractive errors by surface modification are divided into two groups: surface modification by excision and suture, and surface modification by unsutured incisions.

Troutman Corneal Wedge (Block) Resection

In this technique for correction of excessive astigmatism after penetrating keratoplasty, as originally described by Troutman (1970), an in-depth wedge of corneal tissue, arcuate shaped to include the graft scar, was resected across the flatter meridian. The resulting defect was sutured and allowed to heal. The cornea was steepened to correct the excessively flat meridian. A corresponding flattening at 90 degrees (coupling) was noted (see Gauss' law).

In 1980 the wedge technique was modified to effect the change in corneal curvature by resection of a block rather than a wedge of tissue. Not only was less width of resection required for the same dioptric effect, but less irregular astigmatism was induced.

These techniques are unique because they are the only astigmatism correcting techniques to use a reduction in area to effect surface curvature modification. The result, in addition to meridional correction, is a slight tendency toward overall steepening of the cornea (increasing corneal power). Paradoxically, circumferential block resection has been used to effect overall corneal flattening (Buzard, 1991).

Troutman Corneal Relaxing Incisions

These curvilinear (arcuate) relaxing incisions are done in pairs in or within the graft and scar across the steeper meridian. Single full-thickness incisions were used by Snellen (1869) for correction of high astigmatic bands following the unsutured cataract incisions of the late 19th century. Troutman (1976) applied this principle using partial penetrating keratotomies to correct postpenetrating keratoplasty astigmatism. Paired relaxing (arcuate) incisions have been used by Merlin (1987) for correction of congenital astigmatism. Compression sutures were added (1980) to enhance the effect and predictability of relaxing incisions.

Combined Procedures

A combination of relaxing incisions and corneal wedge resection, giving more accurate stable results in higher degrees of astigmatism, has been advocated by Troutman (1989) based on computerized topographic data analysis to further enhance and permanently maintain the compression effect along the flatter meridian.

Bowtie Procedure

The bowtie procedure (Tchah, 1986) combines two incisional modalities, paired sector curvilinear relaxing incisions connecting peripherally to a four-incision radial keratotomy to flatten a steeper meridian. It has been largely abandoned because of poor healing and instability at the crossing of incisions.

Corneal Relaxing Incisions (Linear)

These T-cuts and variations originally were used by Hoffman, Thornton, and others to correct small degrees of astigmatism concomitant with the correction of myopia by radial keratotomy. They continue to be used for correction of small degrees ($\leq$3 D) of astigmatism occurring after cataract surgery or radial keratotomy.

Trapezoidal Keratotomies

Several combinations of radial and transverse incisions have been applied meridionally for the correction of astigmatism (Ruiz, personal communication, 1982). Because they are inherently unstable, their use, including several modifications of the procedure, has been largely abandoned.

Astigmatic Radial Keratotomy

Paired multiple radial incisions (Fyodorov L=procedure) were applied meridionally in this technique for combined correction of small degrees of astigmatism and myopia.

This technique corrects astigmatism by inducing a flattening central to and peripheral to the incisional zone. The surface area was modified by the width of the scars of the cuts in the corneal surface to induce a combined radius and central corneal curvature change, but was inherently unstable.

REFRACTIVE INDEX MODIFICATION

Interlamellar inlay of alloplastic material with a higher refractive index, such as polysulfone, increases the power when either a plus or minus lenticle is inserted in the cornea between its layers. The primary refractive change, in this case, is effected by the greater refractive index of the material. The technique has been abandoned because of the tendency for corneal melting over the implant in favor of a lower refractive index material, such as Hydrogel, which still shows some promise primarily as a volume technique (similar to keratophakia).

EXCIMER LASER SURFACE MODIFICATION

A second evolving investigational group are those techniques effecting anterior curvature change by excimer laser area photoablation. In this technique, the anterior corneal surface is shaped to effect a concentric anterior curvature change of central corneal thickness without changing internal radius. Because Bowman's layer is removed, this technique might better be termed epikeratomileusis. The long-term effect of removal of Bowman's layer is unknown, and may limit the final effectiveness of this technique. The excimer laser also is applicable to keratomileusis or keratophakia techniques to optically carve the lenticle or lamellarized stroma, which will effect correction while preserving Bowman's layer.

PENETRATING KERATOPLASTY AS A REFRACTIVE PROCEDURE

Penetrating keratoplasty also can be considered as an inherently secondary refractive keratoplasty technique, because some control or modification of postoperative corneal curvatures is necessary to achieve an optimal final refractive result. Significant ametropia can be induced by penetrating keratoplasty combined with cataract implant surgery. A knowledge of corneal optical changes that can be induced by using different diameters of corneal buttons and variable suture tension, as they are related to the corneal recipient, is essential to the result. A dioptric surprise can occur should the calculation of intraocular lens power, based in part on the curvature of the cornea, be altered by a significantly steeper or flatter curvature of the healed corneal graft.

In keratoconus, in particular, it is our opinion that this procedure represents the ultimate refractive technique in penetrating keratoplasty. A penetrating keratoplasty in a keratoconic eye converts irregular astigmatism to regular astigmatism and significantly reduces corneal myopia in a single procedure. The management of keratoconus becomes primarily surgical as soon as the diagnosis can be established and uncorrectable irregular astigmatism and myopia can be attributed primarily to the cornea.

INTRAOCULAR LENS AS REFRACTIVE SURGICAL TECHNIQUE

The intraocular lens must be considered as dependent on refractive surgery. Although it does not directly involve the cornea, its calculation depends on corneal power. A knowledge of corneal optics is essential to the selection of lens power even when the cornea is not involved directly and particularly when keratoplasty is combined with intraocular lens surgery. In addition, it is the only current practical means for the correction of very high degrees of spherical ametropia.

INTRACORNEAL ANNULAR RING

An innovative approach to the control of spherical ametropia and astigmatism has been the introduction of a polymethylmethacrylate ring inserted peripherally near the limbus in corneal tissue. This ring may be expanded to flatten the cornea or contracted to steepen the cornea, and its presence reduces regular astigmatism. Parel and others have used this ring in laboratory animals, but human trials have not yet been performed.

Wound Healing

Never before have the number and variety of surgical procedures performed on the cornea been so numerous. With its unique avascular system of metabolic supply, it is not unreasonable that healing of this tissue also should be a unique and special process. As refractive and corneal surgeons, we bear a special responsibility to ensure that the procedures that we perform on these corneas heal as well as the tissue allows. To ensure this, we must understand the clinical and pathologic appearance of normal corneal wound healing and the variance that represents delayed wound healing. A remarkable array of surgical and pharmacologic agents are available to modify the progress of wound healing. To achieve the fine refractive results, which we and our patients desire, we must not only master the surgical technique but recognize the nuances of the postsurgical period.

HISTOPATHOLOGY OF WOUND HEALING

Healing of normal corneal anatomy after injury with a sharp instrument, such as a knife, can be best understood by reviewing healing of the various layers of the cornea.

Epithelium

Repair of the epithelium begins on a microscopic level within 1 to 2 hours of corneal injury (Plate 4–1), moving into the wound in 3 to 5 hours

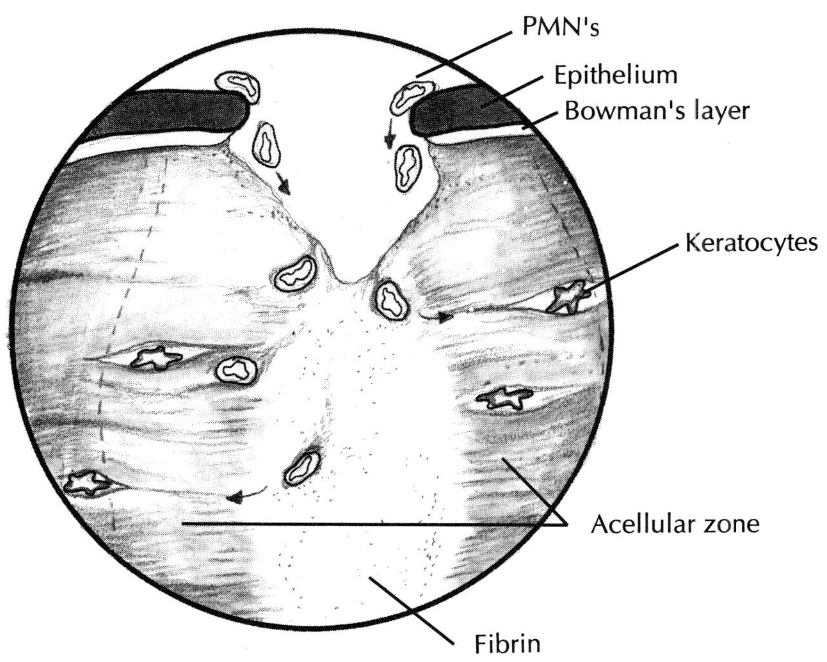

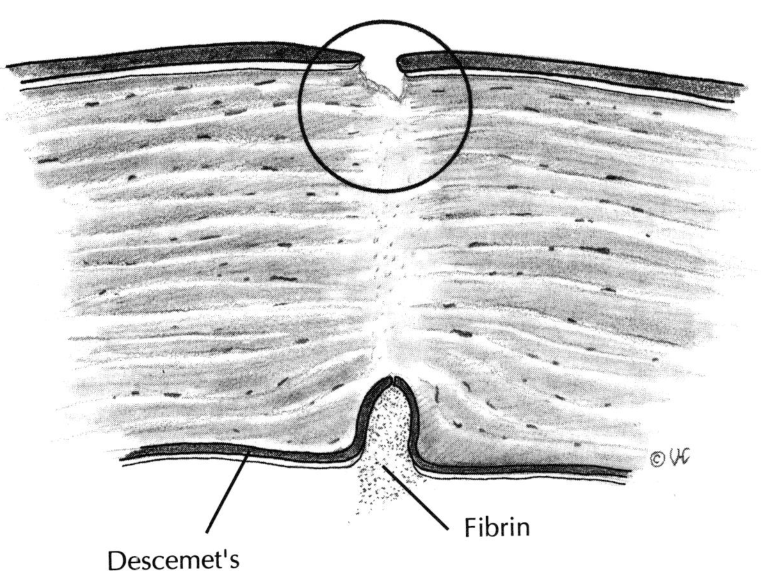

Corneal wound healing 1 to 3 hours after perforating injury.

(Plate 4–2). On a more macroscopic level, a clean corneal wound usually is bridged by epithelium within 6 to 8 hours after injury (Plate 4–3). This process begins by the sliding of adjacent cells, followed by mitosis of the deepest layers of the epithelium, thickening of the epithelium, creation of an epithelial plug in the depths of the corneal wound, and finally secretion of basement membrane substance to adhere the epithelium to the underlying cornea. This secretion of basement membrane substance is delayed under optimal circumstances as long as 24 hours, and can be delayed indefinitely under more adverse circumstances, leading to map-dot-fingerprint dystrophy. The energy for sliding is provided by glycogen in the basal epithelial cells. A denuded corneal epithelium can regenerate, under optimal conditions, within 3 to 4 days, although these conditions rarely exist.

In large abrasions, the glycogen stored in the epithelial cells under total anoxia lasts only 4 to 6 hours. The anoxic use of glucose, resulting in production of lactic acid in cellular metabolism creates only 5% of the energy of the aerobic pathway, producing large amounts of lactic acid leading to corneal swelling. The use of patching to heal corneal abrasions rests on the foundation of diminished trauma to the healing edge of the epithelium, whereas it is clear that oxygen available for aerobic conversion of glucose is decreased by this technique. Thus, in the presence of a denuded epithelium after penetrating keratoplasty, many surgeons prefer to leave the eye open, using lubricants to decrease mechanical trauma and to improve oxygen availability. Friedlander and Zinny have shown that therapeutic contact lenses of varying oxygen permeability enhance corneal wound healing with high oxygen permeability and similarly inhibit corneal wound healing if the thickness of the lens or the oxygen transmissibility is low. This emphasizes the importance of oxygen in epithelial sliding. The availability of inexpensive, disposable contact lenses has made a significant impact on the treatment of epithelial damage after trauma, and on corneal surgery in general. Aside from enhanced epithelial closure, the use of disposable contact lenses allows better apposition of wound edges through anterior support, and diminished pain through the reduction of trauma secondary to blinking. This control of pain and the maintenance of vision has made the use of disposable contact lenses in our practice almost routine in simple abrasions, and has contributed significantly to patient acceptance of refractive surgical procedures.

The healing of epithelial scrape wounds is a complex sequence of events that is influenced by several factors. First, corneal innervation plays an important role in proper regeneration of epithelial cells through the release of neuropeptides. These neuropeptides of the tachykinin family induce neurogenic inflammation, which aids stromal wound healing and stimulates proliferation of both epithelial and mesenchymal cells. Suppression of these neurons, either by naturally occurring processes re-

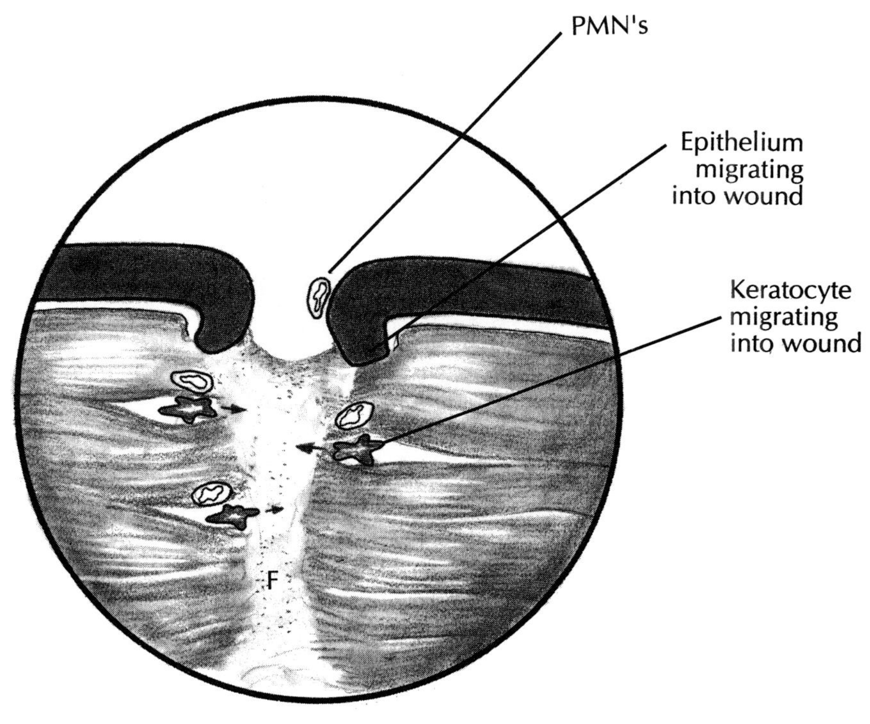

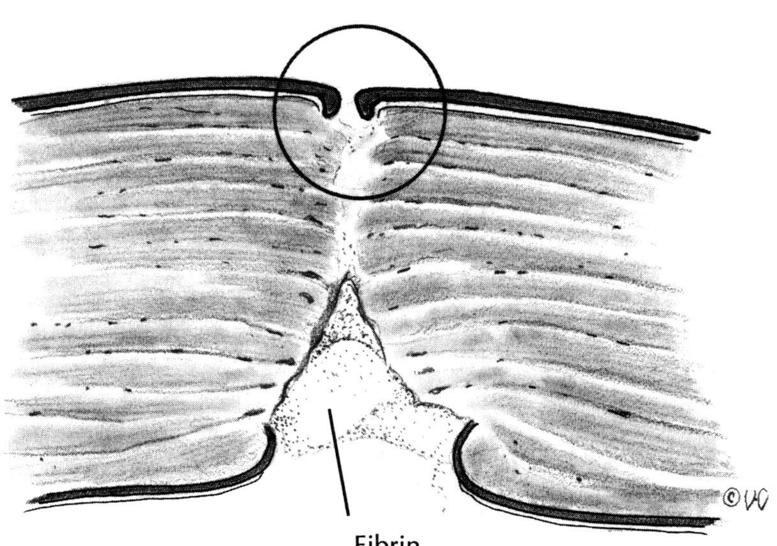

Corneal wound healing 3 to 5 hours after perforating injury.

sulting in corneal anesthesia or by capsaicin, a neurotoxin, causes significant delays in epithelial closure, as shown by Gallar and coworkers. The role of proper innervation for epithelial closure and subsequent stromal healing cannot be overemphasized.

In normal epithelial healing, spreading and adhesion of the cells is mediated by fibronectin, which is a large glycoprotein that has binding activities to collagen, fibrin, and extracellular matrix. There are two types of fibronectin in the body; one is present as a soluble substance in the blood plasma, and the other is elaborated by cells, such as normal epithelium. When epithelial cells are damaged, as after chemical or thermal burns or in the presence of herpetic infection, the secretion of this substance is decreased, resulting in diminished epithelial healing, as shown by Phan and coworkers. In addition to fibronectin, a host of epithelial growth factors have been identified that together with fibronectin may provide the additional stimulus necessary to heal damaged epithelial cells.

Stroma

The corneal stroma, which accounts for most of the mechanical strength of the cornea, heals less rapidly than the epithelium. Much of our information on corneal wound healing comes from studies performed in rabbit corneas, and much of the material presented here has been developed from the studies of rabbit corneal healing, particularly the excellent work of Matsuda and Smelsen. Within 3 to 5 hours after injury, a fibrin clot fills the incision, proceeding in the rabbit from the posterior surface to the anterior surface (see Plate 4–2). The epithelium, which had begun sliding toward the wound (see Plate 4–3), fills the wound as an epithelial plug, reaching a maximum in the rabbit at about 48 hours and displacing the fibrin clot anteriorly (see Plate 4–3). The extent of the epithelial plug depends in great measure on the gaping of the wound.

Polymorphonuclear leukocytes (PMNs) appear within the first 5 hours (see Plate 4–2) and become more numerous, spreading into the superficial stroma. Cells that have been damaged by the surgery are lysed by proteolytic enzymes derived from the PMNs. Relatively inactive stellate fibroblasts in the nearby corneal stroma become active and transform into fibroblasts that migrate across the wound at about 12 hours, and enter the anterior wound in large numbers in 24 to 48 hours. In rabbits, the posterior fibrin clot persists at 48 hours, with little infiltration of fibroblasts (see Plate 4–3).

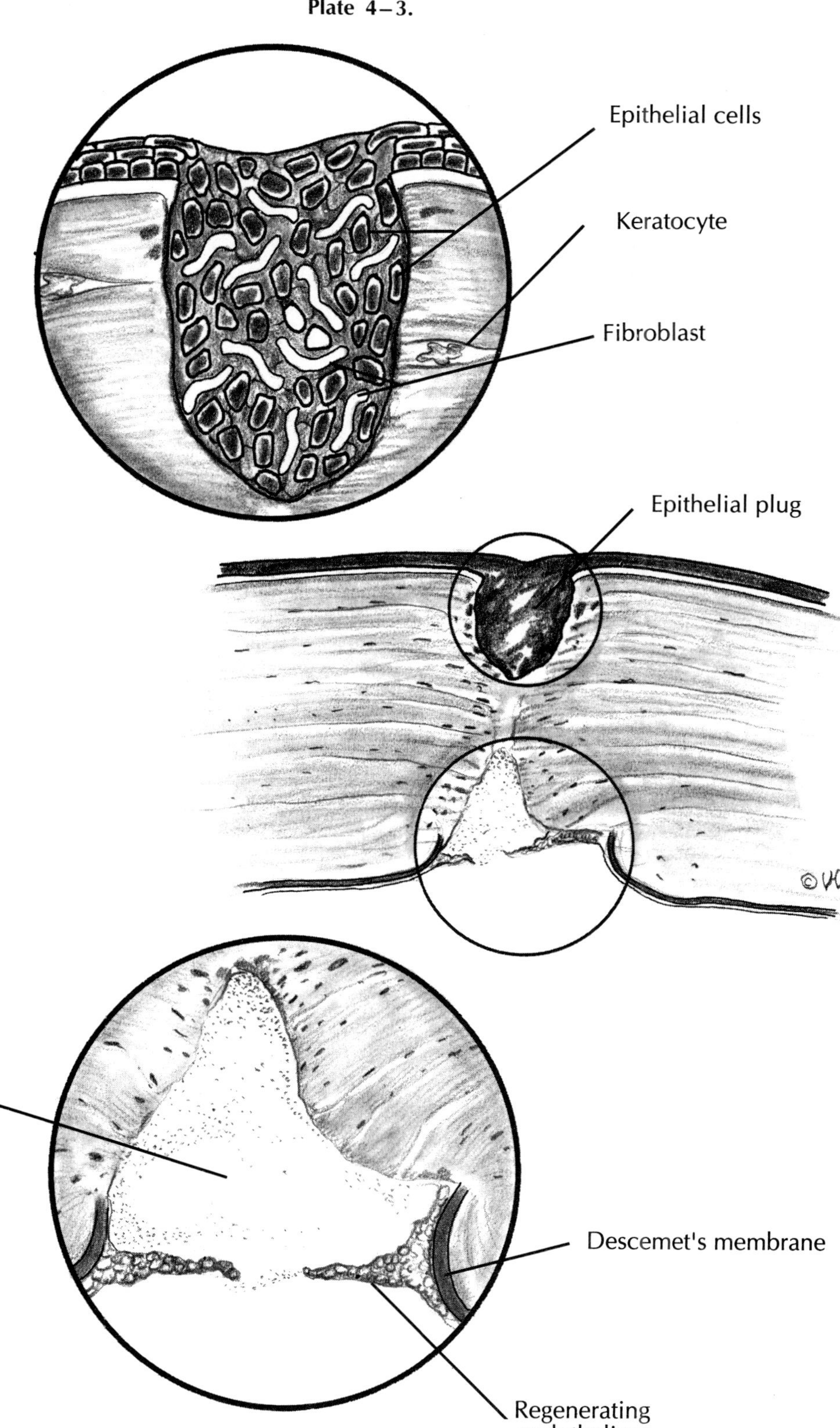

Corneal wound healing 2 to 4 days after perforating injury.

The fate of the epithelial plug is of some importance because it is at this stage that we often see a halt to corneal wound healing in the unstable cornea or poorly closed corneal wound. By 3 to 4 days in the rabbit, we see regression of the epithelial plug with the filling of this space by fibroblasts and immature collagen fibrils. In the posterior portion of the cornea, the fibrin plug persists with little activity in this area. Many organelles, such as rough-sided endoplasmic reticula, mitochondria, ribosomes, Golgi complexes, and vesicles are observed in the fibroblasts. This indicates a high level of metabolic activity in the production of collagen and proteoglycans. The epithelial plug is extruded for the most part at about 5 to 8 days, whereas the posterior fibrin clot remains in place during this time period (Plate 4–4).

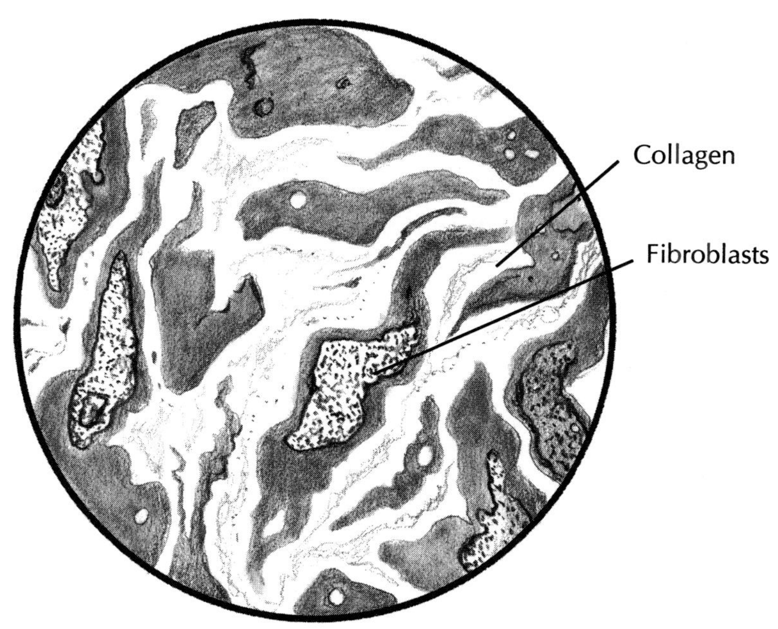

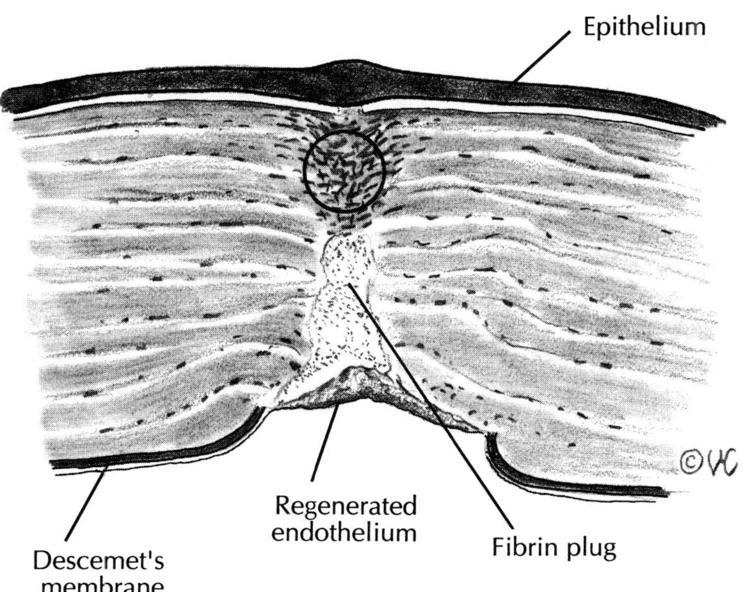

Corneal wound healing 8 days after perforating injury.

Significant differences in the healing of anterior and posterior stroma are observed in the rabbit model, and clinical correlation can be seen in penetrating keratoplasty in which partial-thickness sutures are used to close the wound. In the rabbit posterior stromal healing progresses much more slowly, with significant fibroblastic activity in the posterior cornea occurring only in the 2- to 4-week period (Plate 4–5). This area represents an unsupported penetrating incision in the model of an unsutured penetrating incision and shows the importance of secure posterior closure in penetrating corneal wounds. With secure through-and-through closure, the penetrating wound is converted to a wound in which anterior and posterior wound healing can progress at more equal rates. In addition, we may appreciate the fact that radial keratotomy incisions, which by their nature are securely closed posteriorly if not penetrating, require no suturing and heal relatively quickly due to the vigorous nature of anterior wound healing.

The normal corneal stroma is comprised predominantly of collagen fibrils interspersed in a mixture of glycosaminoglycans (GAGs) consisting of three major fractions: keratan sulfate (50%), chondroitin (25%), and chondroitin sulfate (25%). These proteoglycans are responsible for the tendency of corneal tissue to swell, and disruptions of these molecules during corneal wound healing account for much of the opacity of the corneal scar. The activated fibroblasts secrete GAGs and collagen, and by the fourth week of normal healing GAG levels have returned to three-fourths normal concentrations.

Collagen fibrils are produced that initially are randomly oriented (see Plate 4–4) but gradually line up perpendicular to the wound (see Plate 4–5) and approach the concentration found in normal stroma by approximately the ninth week. The new fibers are coarser than normal corneal collagen bundles, but gradually achieve strength comparable to the normal cornea as crosslinking occurs involving hydroxylysine. After a corneal wound, the normal corneal remodeling process can extend for many months, although clinical resolution of corneal healing is thought to be relatively complete at 6 to 12 months (Plate 4–6).

It is well known that the defects in Bowman's layer do not regenerate; however, close approximation of Bowman's layer allows a smooth epithelial surface to regenerate (see Plate 4–6). Without proper approximation

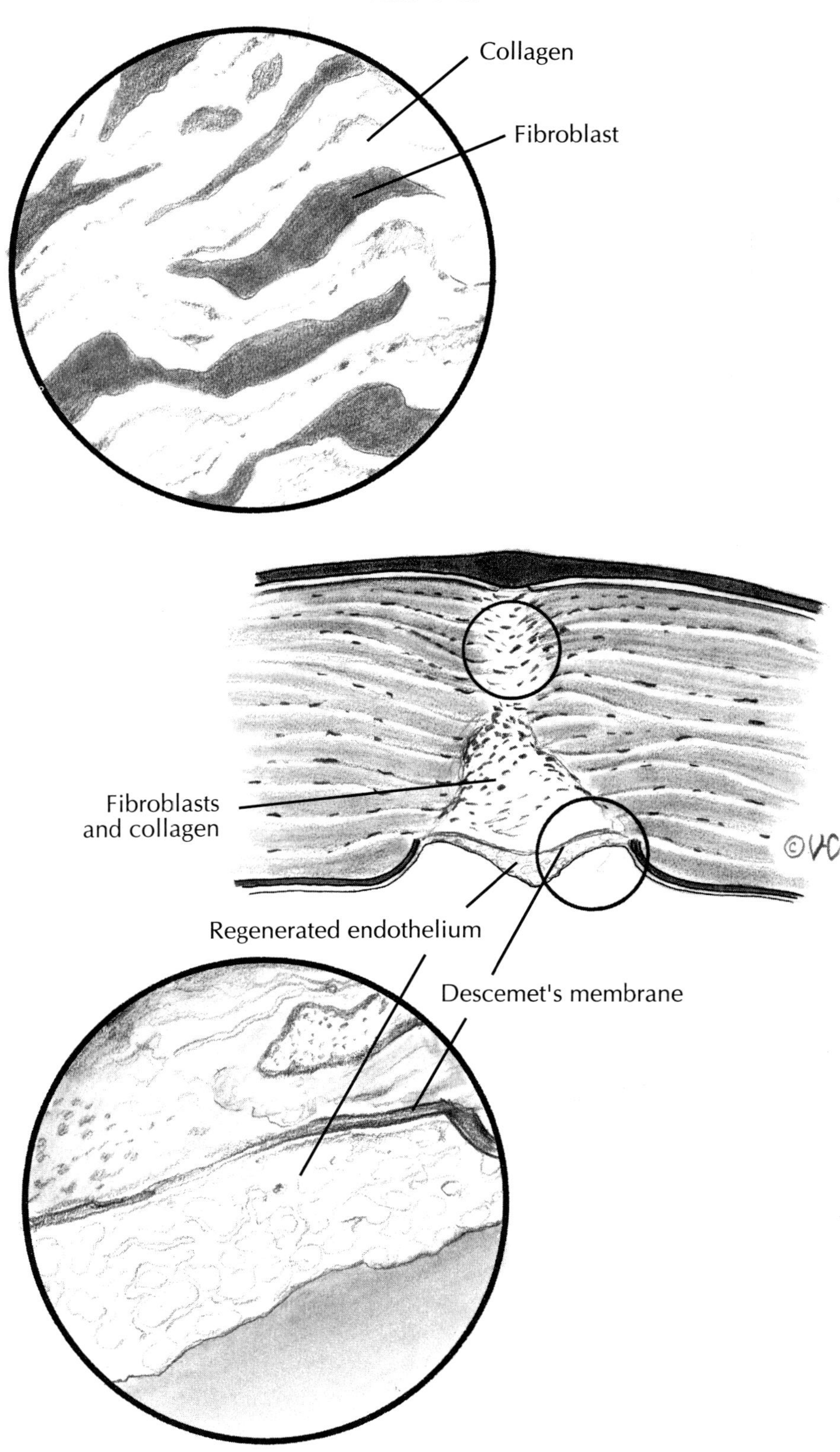

Corneal wound healing 2 weeks after perforating injury.

of Bowman's layer, the water-tight nature of the epithelium and the associated basement membrane can become incompetent, allowing fluid to enter the wound and accounting for significant diurnal variation of corneal thickness. Moreover, failure to mate the edges of Bowman's layer can result in epithelial hyperplasia with a persistent epithelial plug and possible weakness of the resulting wound.

Descemet's membrane is much firmer than the underlying stroma and can easily be stripped away during surgery. In a small defect, if good approximation of the underlying tissues is obtained, a new Descemet's membrane will reappear microscopically several weeks after surgery (see Plate 4–5), becoming more normal in thickness several months after surgery (see Plate 4–6). The larger the posterior defect, with respect to Descemet's membrane, the longer this process will take. If Descemet's membrane is dislodged and incarcerated into the wound, it can create long-term posterior corneal instability. In addition, large posterior defects of Descemet's membrane can encourage a persistent fibrin clot, with subsequent proliferation of fibrous tissue projecting into the anterior chamber. Certainly all of these possibilities are undesirable, and for optimal wound strength, close approximation of Descemet's membrane is mandatory.

Endothelium

The corneal endothelium is a monolayer of polygonal cells resting on Descemet's membrane, and generally is considered relatively amitotic. Restoration of a continuous endothelium after penetrating corneal incision is accomplished by the sliding and spreading of adjacent endothelial cells, beginning approximately 24 hours after surgery. With good posterior wound apposition, this process is almost complete by the fifth day (see Plate 4–3). With poor posterior apposition, the endothelium is hard pressed to cover the defect. In some cases, a retrocorneal membrane can occur in which fibrous tissue with fibroblast-like cells covered with endothelial cells extends beyond the posterior aspect of the wound (see Plate 4–8,D). The origin of these fibroblast-like cells is controversial, and may represent fibroblasts derived from keratocytes, circulating mononucleocytes, or even endothelial cells undergoing metaplasia into fibrocytes. Such membranes are undesirable from the standpoint of corneal clarity, because the osmotic balance of the overlying cornea is likely to be affected because the membrane is not covered by endothelium along its growing edges. In addition, the mechanical strength of the wound is impaired. If wound apposition is even more abnormal, epithelial cells may extend entirely through the cornea, resulting in an epithelial downgrowth and possible loss of the eye. The importance of precise posterior corneal closure cannot be overestimated, and provides the rational for through-and-through closure of penetrating incisions.

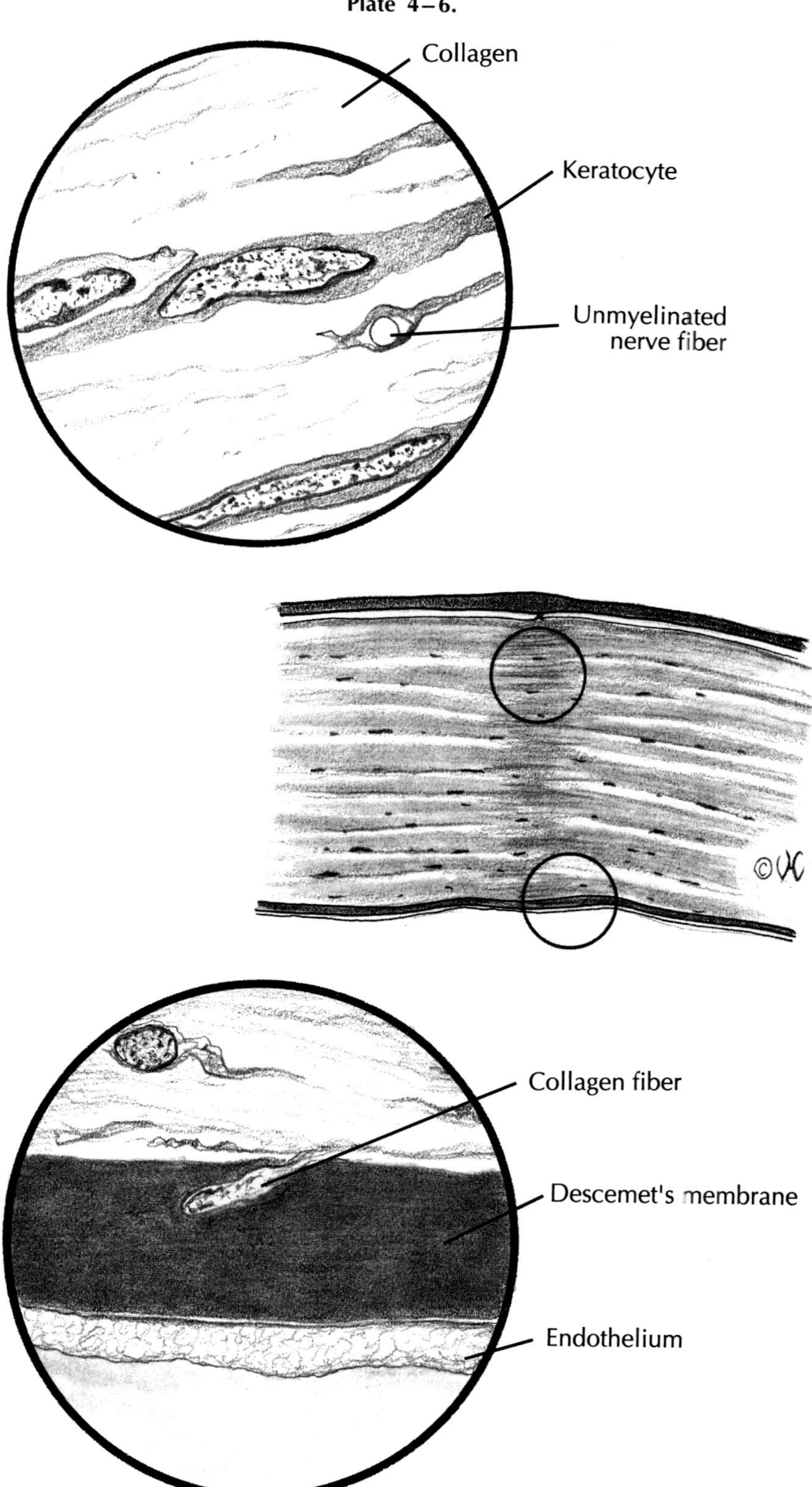

Corneal wound healing 7 months after perforating injury.

Precise apposition of wound surfaces is essential to normal corneal wound healing, and a wide variety of circumstances can lead to a halt in the healing process. It is essential that the clinician be able to identify the signs and symptoms of delayed wound healing so that appropriate action may be undertaken. Abnormalities in corneal wound healing can manifest themselves in a variety of ways, but in general can be identified by observing disruption in the normal functioning of the cornea. One such disruption that occurs with incomplete wound healing is in electrolyte-water balance in the cornea. Corneal abrasions, incisions, and trauma all disrupt the barriers created by the cornea to prevent unrestricted entry of water into the cornea. Immediately after a radial keratotomy, the stroma will imbibe fluid, creating a slight elevation around each incision. This is evident on corneal topology as *breaking of the mires* over the incisions, because small elevations will appear in these areas. Similarly, after corneal transplantation the stroma adjacent to the trephination will swell, causing elevation of the wound margin. The use of the slitlamp and the photokeratometer to observe these elevations will give evidence of the progression of wound healing, because with incomplete wound healing the ability of the cornea to maintain water balance around the incisions may be compromised (Plate 4–7,A).

Clinical variables, such as visual acuity, also can be compromised by fluid balance in the cornea. The diurnal variation of vision seen immediately after radial keratotomy results from the differences in fluid balance between the nighttime sleeping hours and the daylight hours, during which the eyes are kept open, allowing for more dehydration. Hydration of the cornea gives a radial keratotomy slightly more effect, so that a patient with undercorrected vision sees better in the morning and worse as the day progresses, and a patient with overcorrected vision sees worse in the morning and better as the day progresses. Even in a technically perfect radial keratotomy, slight diurnal variation of vision occurs for 6 to 10 weeks. Similarly in penetrating keratoplasty, corneal swelling under the sutures enhances the effective tightness of the sutures, thus flattening the cornea. With resolution of this edema the cornea will steepen slightly over 1 to 2 months as wound healing progresses.

The use of fluorescein can enhance subtle features of the wound that may not be visible otherwise. Certainly delayed wound healing will result in slight elevations of the stroma on each side of the incision, pooling the dye in the incision (Plate 4–7,A). The pooling of dye late in the postoperative course is an indication of localized corneal edema and wound healing abnormality. Likewise, delayed wound healing may result in areas of actual staining of the incisions. If this condition is allowed to continue and staining of the incisions persists for a long time, eventual wound healing

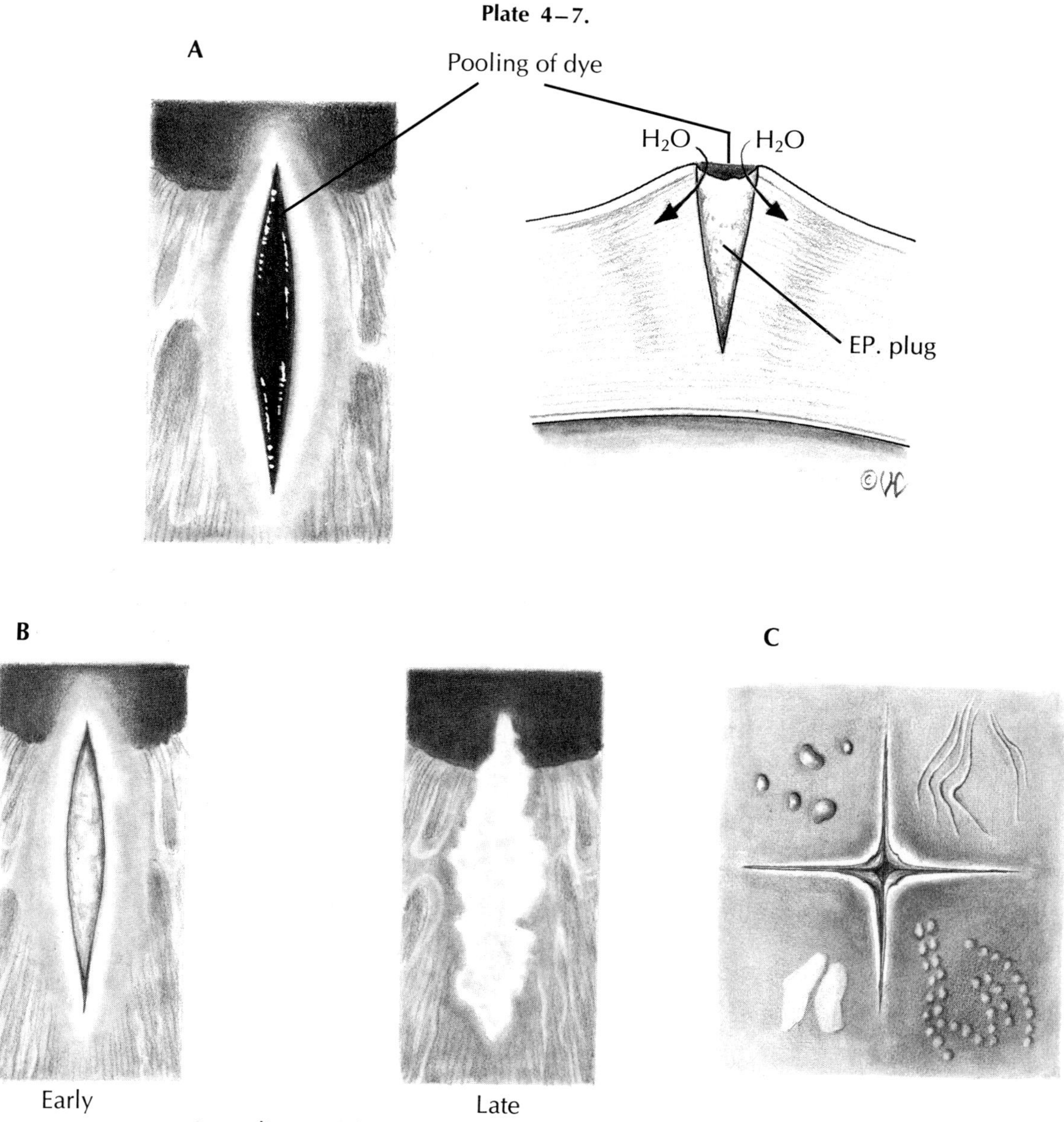

A, swelling around incision indicates incompetent corneal water balance and incomplete corneal healing. **B,** gaping incision with early appearance of swelling around the incision and staining, followed by late appearance of a wide, irregular corneal scar. **C,** crossed corneal incisions show gaping and swelling around the incision site. Map dot–fingerprint dystrophy is an additional sign of wound healing abnormality.

will be disordered, appearing clinically as a wide irregular scar (Plate 4–7,B). If corneal incisions cross, a particularly prominent form of this problem occurs. Marked corneal swelling occurs in the area, resulting in poor wound apposition and the development of a calcified area at the intersection of the two incisions. In addition map-dot-fingerprint dystrophy may appear in the surrounding epithelium, indicating the abnormal wound healing in this area (Plate 4–7,C).

If the wound closure problem is severe enough, subepithelial fibrosis may occur (Plate 4–8,A). Similar in nature to the retrocorneal membrane, subepithelial fibrosis is relatively common after penetrating keratoplasty (Plate 4–8,B), and accounts for at least a portion of the haze seen along the donor-host wound after this procedure. There are two possible origins of the subepithelial fibrosis. The first is growth from the suture tract, which is more pronounced if large needles are used or if the sutures are left in for an extended period. This fibrosis usually can be peeled away, and does not attach itself significantly to the wound. The other type of subepithelial fibrosis emanates from the wound itself, is usually thicker, and often results from incomplete wound closure at the affected area. Mechanical strength of the wound is impaired in the second form of this disorder. Often the subepithelial fibrosis can cause traction on the cornea that results in flattening (Plate 4–8,C). This problem can be reversed if the subepithelial fibrosis is peeled away when possible before closing sutures are removed, thus releasing the traction on the cornea.

The retrocorneal membrane, associated with the posterior lambda effect, is a more serious abnormality (Plate 4–8,D). Abnormal anterior wound healing weakens the wound, resulting in a cosmetically objectionable scar. Abnormal posterior wound healing creates a lambda-shaped wound that mechanically will tend to split open when suture support is removed, due to the direction of intraocular pressure into the wound. In addition, endothelial cells can be lost in the attempt to bridge the wound with epithelium, and a retrocorneal membrane can prevent this bridging. This can result in a permanently weak wound, which can be difficult to repair.

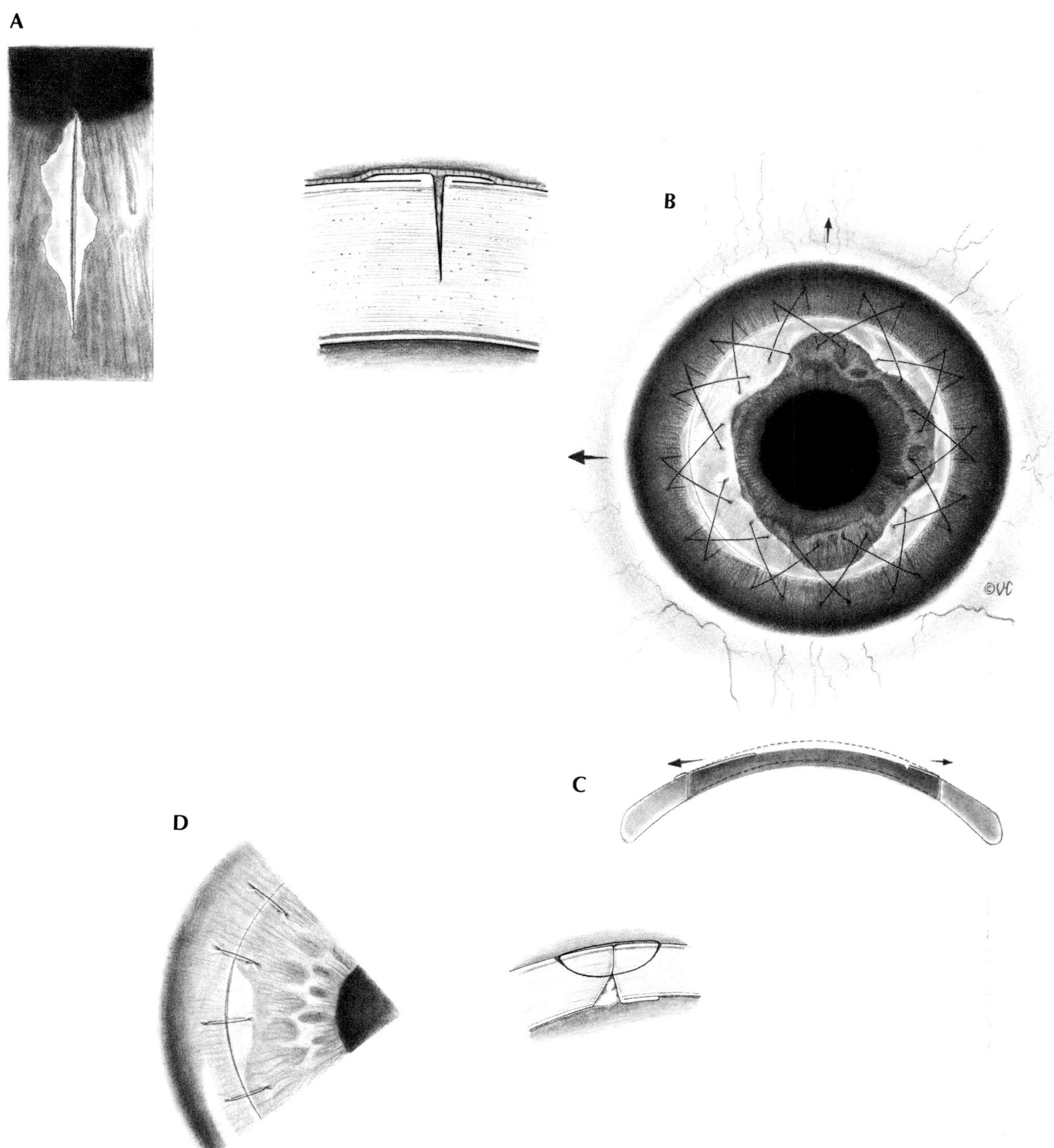

A, subepithelial fibrosis, stimulated by poor wound healing and persistent epithelial plug formation. **B,** subepithelial fibrosis after penetrating keratoplasty shows broad membrane extending from
the wound to suture tracts. **C,** surface tension induced by subepithelial fibrosis shows flattening of
the cornea. **D,** retrocorneal membrane formation stimulated by poor posterior corneal wound closure.

In radial keratotomy, we also see subepithelial fibrosis in patients with severe wound-healing abnormalities (Plate 4–9,A). This problem is seen almost exclusively in patients with 16- and 32-incision radial keratotomy. The many radial incisions in a restricted area of the cornea create *block lifts* of corneal tissue that disrupt the contiguous anterior corneal surface (Plate 4–9,B). Because the incision does not close appropriately, stromal keratocytes transform into fibroblasts that migrate over Bowman's layer and under the epithelium. This migration can create localized corneal surface tension, resulting in irregular astigmatism and disruption of the normal water balance of the cornea. In extreme cases, subepithelial fibrosis can extend over the visual axis and cause diminished best corrected vision. Peeling away this fibrosis does not solve the problem of mismatched incision edges, and the fibrosis will recur. Penetrating keratoplasty seems to be the only permanent correction currently available for this form of subepithelial fibrosis.

Although this problem has been discussed with respect to radial keratotomy, any incisional keratotomy procedure that places many incisions in a limited area of the cornea can result in subepithelial fibrosis. For example, the Ruiz procedure exhibits this and other wound-healing abnormalities.

A

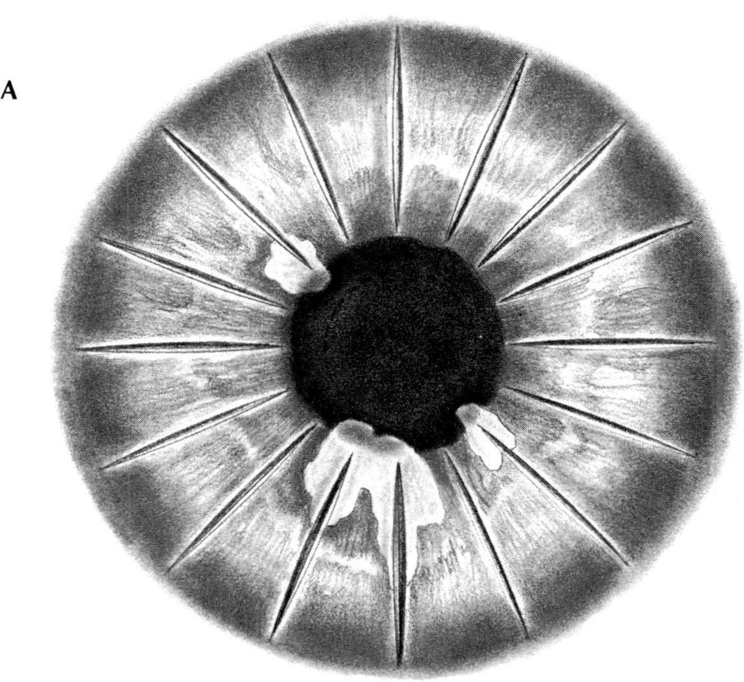

B

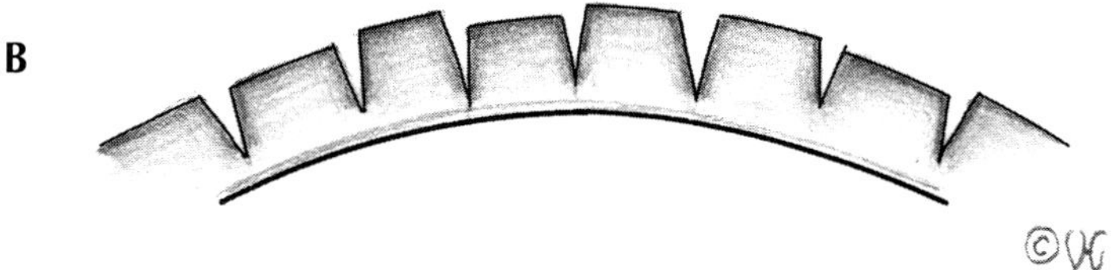

A, subepithelial fibrosis after 16-incision radial keratotomy shows poorly healed radial incisions and subepithelial fibrosis emanating from the incisions. **B,** block lifting of corneal tissue with closely spaced radial incisions.

A significant finding of wound instability in transverse and arcuate incisions, such as in penetrating keratoplasty and cataract surgery, can be seen on corneal topology in the form of the *microdehiscence* (Plate 4–10,A). The characteristic photokeratometric finding of a triangle-shaped abnormality pointing to an area of wound weakness is seen in a variety of clinical situations. In penetrating keratoplasty, recognition of this abnormality allows a noninvasive appreciation of delays in wound healing. Appreciation of delayed wound healing in a given area allows the surgeon to take corrective action before the condition leads to central astigmatism. Because wound healing is most frequently delayed by inadequate apposition of corneal tissue, the addition of a suture across the involved area improves wound apposition and can lead to permanent resolution of the problem, even when sutures are removed. Using this approach, *sutures in* astigmatism can be monitored and controlled, with resulting diminished long-term astigmatism and stabilization of spherical equivalent. Removal of sutures based on photokeratometric evidence reduces tensile strength across the wound and can lead to wound instability with increased long-term variability of astigmatism and spherical equivalent. Manipulation of the corneal graft wound requires not only photokeratometry or computed corneal topology but a careful interpretation based on a clear understanding of corneal wound healing.

The microdehiscence can be seen in corneal relaxing incisions, which are generally left unsutured. If a microdehiscence persists into the late postoperative period, it represents evidence of delayed wound healing and usually means that the incision is gaping, resulting in delayed extrusion of the epithelial plug, with refractive overcorrection. Again, this condition is repaired by increasing the tensile strength across the wound, with the addition of sutures to allow both normal extrusion of the epithelial plug and normal corneal wound healing. This approach of recognition of delayed wound healing and subsequent action by improving wound apposition is the basis for correction of a wide variety of wound-healing abnormalities.

Although radial incisions will not show a pattern of microdehiscence, the sign of breaking of the mires (Plate 4–10,B) over incisions, diurnal variation, and staining of incisions all indicate poor wound healing. Generally in such patients refraction is overcorrected, although the patient may not show signs of overcorrection at the time of examination. The same approach is used in this problem; that is, tensile force across the wound is increased through the use of pilocarpine, which seems to draw the incisions together early in the postoperative course, and/or the use of a circular suture to mechanically draw the incisions together later in the surgical course. Signs of wound-healing abnormality should generally be treated, because overcorrection no doubt will occur later if the incisions

A

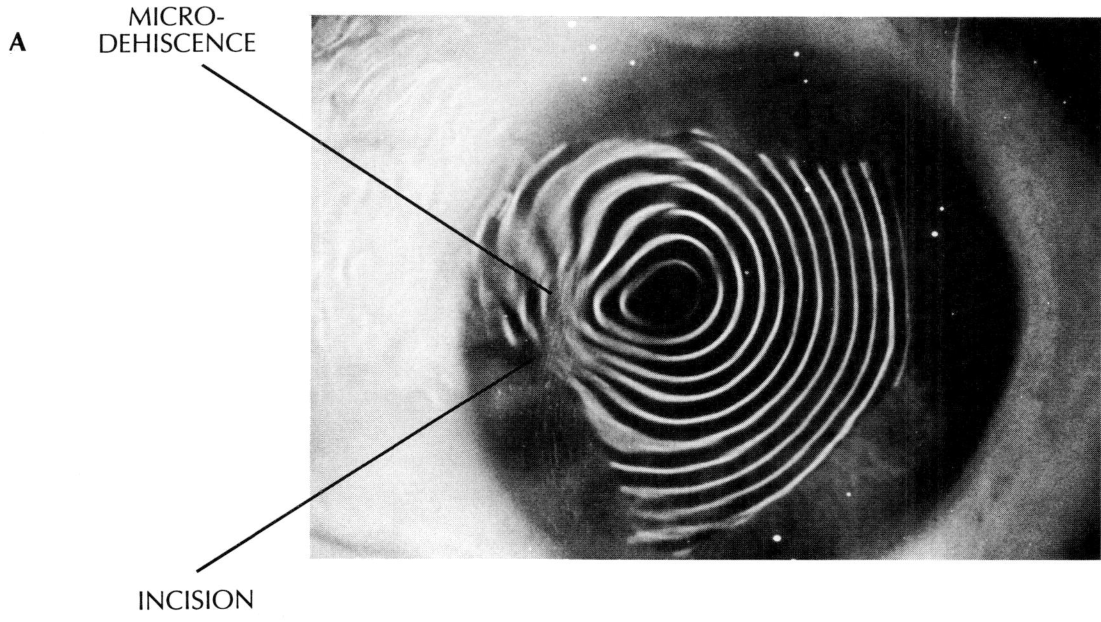

B

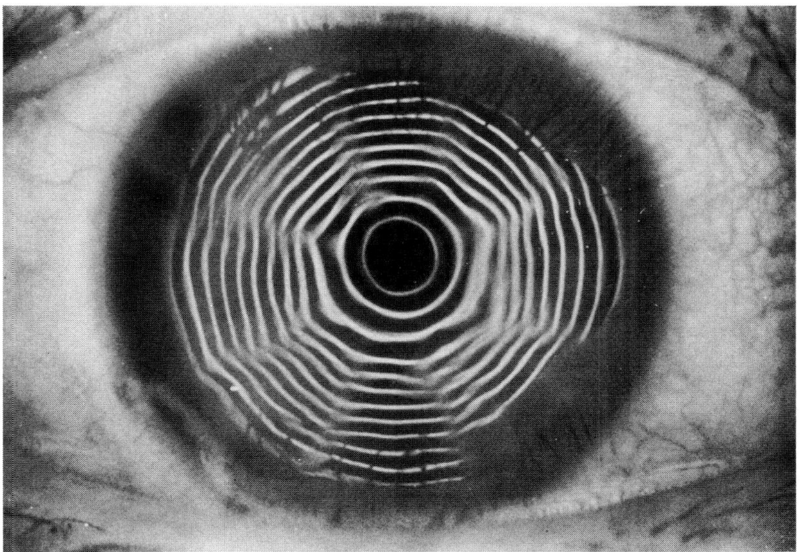

A, photokeratograph shows a microdehiscence representing abnormal corneal wound healing. **B,** photokeratograph shows breaking of mires over swollen incisions in radial keratotomy.

are allowed to continue in an unhealed state. The wise surgeon will appreciate the consequences of poorly healed incisions despite the appearance of a good clinical result and will take steps to prevent this condition from continuing. Often, the utility of "cleaning" the incisions is discussed as a prelude to suturing. Although this practice does not seem to cause long-term harm, it certainly delays eventual healing, and in our opinion is unnecessary. Simply improving the tensile strength across the wound will promote the reengagement of normal corneal wound healing, with eventual extrusion of the epithelial plug. Careful slitlamp examination, photokeratometry, and computed corneal topology can be invaluable in identifying the exact location of the abnormality so that precise and effective action can be taken.

In more extreme problems of corneal wound healing, the wound edges can become displaced relative to one another, as is sometimes seen in corneal transplant surgery when sutures are removed prematurely. This can result in a microdehiscence on photokeratometry and represents a potential finding on slitlamp examination. By confining the beam of the slitlamp to a thin area, one can appreciate discontinuities across the surface (Plate 4–11) that represent a corneal edge lift. Proper treatment involves incising the area that has become displaced, and resuturing to allow proper wound apposition to occur. It is important to identify this abnormality on slitlamp examination, because the appearance on photokeratometry is identical to that of delayed wound healing. The treatment for the two disorders is quite different, as discussed previously.

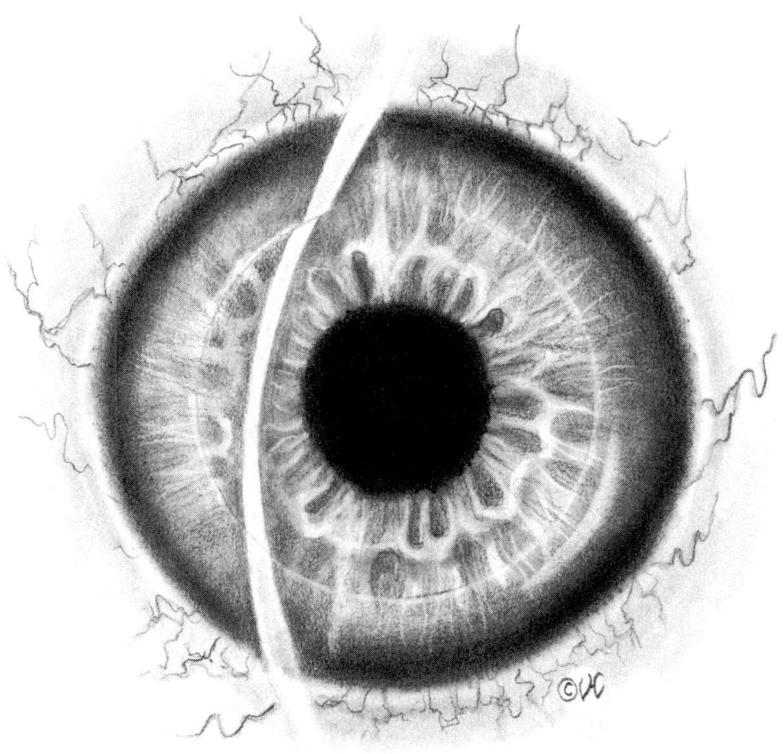

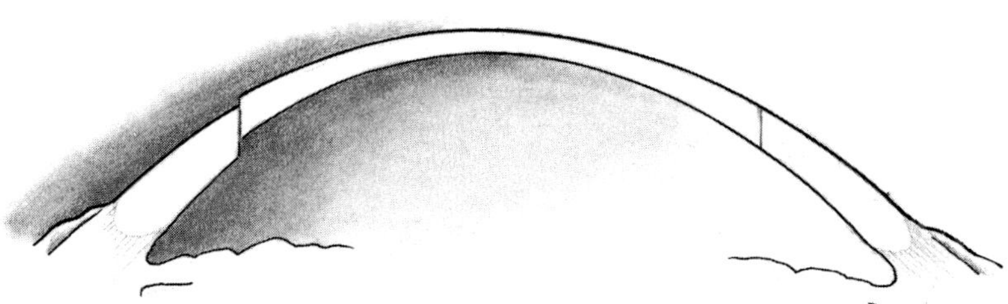

Corneal edge lift demonstrates one cause of flattening in a given meridian.

A final important consideration in delayed wound healing, although less common, involves the balance in stromal wound healing between collagen and proteoglycan synthesis by the fibroblasts and collagen and proteoglycan degradation by enzymatic activity. Particularly in connective tissue disease, the balance may shift toward increased enzymatic activity, with subsequent delayed wound healing due to the inability of the fibroblasts to keep up with enzymatic destruction. The appearance of the microdehiscence on photokeratometry or computed corneal topology may be quite similar to other circumstances, but clinical examination of the wound will reveal a softening of the tissue adjacent to the wound, with displacement of the sutures through the tissue and superficial punctate keratopathy in the surrounding area (Plate 4–12,A).

In this circumstance, additional sutures will serve no purpose, and an approach other than increased tension across the wound is needed. Topical and systemic steroids may be helpful; however, steroids in the presence of corneal melting tend to exacerbate the problem. Buzard has found that cytoxic medications have been extremely helpful under these circumstances, particularly the use of low-dose pulsed methotrexate. Although a discussion of cytoxic medication is beyond the scope of this discussion, low-dose pulsed methotrexate has been extremely helpful in the treatment of systemic disorders, such as arthritis, as they relate to eye disorders, such as scleritis, episcleritis, iritis, and corneal melting. These agents reestablish the proper balance between creation and destruction of collagen and proteoglycans and can often return the wound to relatively normal wound healing, although additional sutures may be required to restore tensile strength after this balance has been achieved. We have observed wound-healing abnormalities in well-sutured cataract and corneal transplant wounds that return to a photokeratometric appearance of wound dehiscence even after additional suturing. The addition of cytotoxic agents in these patients resolved the problem in many cases and reinforces our observation that collagen vascular-related healing disorders are more common in the elderly population.

One such patient with scleroderma and rheumatoid arthritis had evidence of corneal melting 3 months after penetrating keratoplasty, and a microdehiscence on photokeratometry with best corrected visual acuity of 20/200 (Plate 4–12,B). Treatment with low-dose pulsed methotrexate for 6 weeks completely resolved the corneal melting and microdehiscence (Plate 4–12,C), improving the visual acuity to 20/30 uncorrected. Treatment for 6 months resolved the problem, and the medication was tapered without recurrence.

Certainly epithelial integrity is necessary for normal wound healing, and if epithelial denudement remains a problem in the presence of an inflamed eye, the addition of steroid or other agents to quiet the eye may certainly encourage epithelialization and restore normal corneal wound

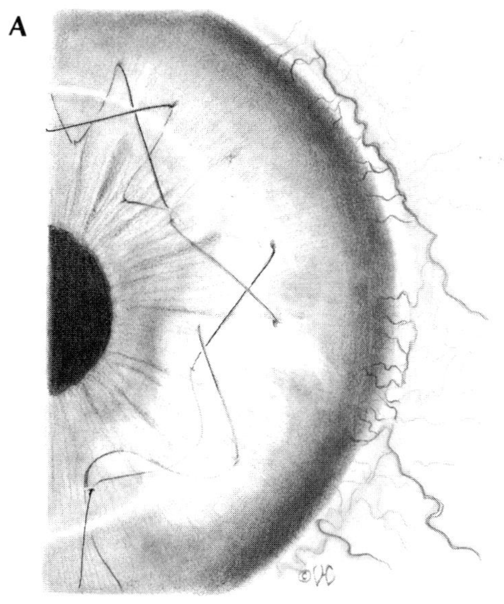

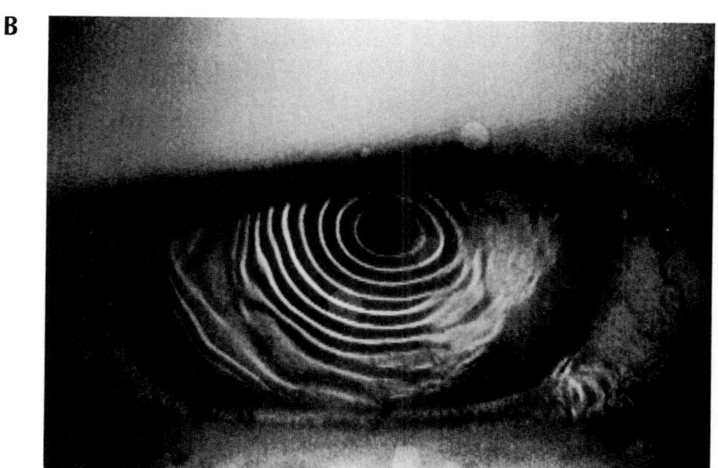

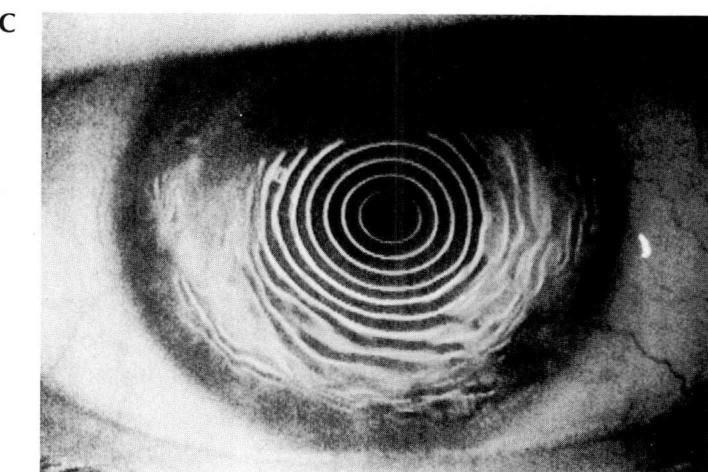

A, abnormal wound healing, seen with corneal melting, shows sutures displaced through softened tissue. **B,** photokeratograph shows microdehiscence in area of corneal melting. **C,** photokeratograph shows resolution of microdehiscence 6 weeks after treatment with methotrexate.

healing. Kenyon has demonstrated that polymorphonuclear neutrophils and extracts from them will delay epithelial migration and are one cause of failure to reepithelize.

The upshot of this discussion is that corneal wound healing is a complex and multifaceted process, and many difficulties are possible. A comprehensive understanding of the basic process and careful clinical examination are required to properly diagnose and treat abnormalities of corneal wound healing. A single routine approach does not exist that is adequate to always achieve the goal of optimal corneal wound healing.

THERAPEUTIC MEASURES TO SLOW WOUND HEALING

Wound healing is an important factor in the overall effect of refractive surgical procedures, and in a certain sense, all corneal interventions can be considered refractive surgical operations. In the presence of sutured wounds, pharmacologic agents have a much less noticeable effect than in unsutured wounds, such as radial and astigmatic keratotomy. To increase refractive effect, it is desirable sometimes to slow corneal wound healing.

Topical steroid preparations have been used traditionally as the primary pharmacologic means to slow wound healing. Certainly these agents have a dual effect. First, they increase intraocular pressure in a sizable number of patients, thus creating more gape in the wound, and enhance the effect of an unsutured keratotomy incision. Long-term changes in wound tensile strength are accomplished by a direct action of corticosteroids on fibroblasts, although ultimately if the wound is stable, healing strength remains approximately the same. By diminishing the number of PMNs, the early stages of wound healing can be slowed, which can lead to a greater refractive effect. Generally the effect of steroids in a stable incisional keratotomy is not large and should not be counted on to drastically increase the refractive effect. Other agents that have been tried as means to enhance the effect of incisional keratotomy include cyclosporin A, mitomycin C, and other cytotoxic medications that when used topically seem to have a minimal refractive effect. Capsaicin, which is a neurotoxin, slows epithelial wound healing in rabbits through blockage of the neurologic supply to the cornea. It is not entirely clear that it is beneficial, either to the refractive effect or to the long-term interests of the patient, to slow wound healing with these drugs. Usually refractive undercorrection is a result of miscalculation of the proper optical zone or evidence of shallow incisions. The possibility of long-term corneal instability from excessive use of either steroids or other medications affecting long-term corneal wound strength should be a major consideration in their use.

Mechanical factors that encourage gaping of the incision can be used as a means to enhance refractive effect and slow wound healing. Certainly the use of compression sutures in the Troutman relaxing incision gapes the arcuate incisions and leads to a larger refractive effect. Similarly, nighttime patching for 1 month has been suggested by Neumann as a means to increase the effect of radial keratotomy. Gas-permeable contact lenses that purposely fit flat, in a manner similar to that seen in orthokeratology, have been used in our practice on one or two occasions to create a greater refractive effect. We believe that orthokeratology-style molding after radial keratotomy may hold promise, but the contact lens fitting is exceedingly difficult, and most attempts in this direction have met with failure in our practice. One factor that has been beneficial in astigmatic keratotomy is the use of spherical contact lenses to mold the cornea into a spherical shape, particularly in patients with very tight lids. One such patient had acid burns to the face with a large amount of *with the rule* astigmatism (see Plate 2–10). Keratotomy incisions failed to correct the problem, but the temporary addition of a gas-permeable contact lens protected the cornea from the stiff, burned upper lids, allowing the cornea to heal, and ultimately aided in correction of the astigmatism.

Certainly in the undercorrected incisional keratotomy patient, attention should flow to the position, orientation, and depth of the incisions. Pharmacologic agents alone will not appreciably aid a poorly planned or poorly executed operation. In the event that the operation is believed suitable, the mechanical opening of incisions with a blunt hook, dubbed the *tickle* operation, may be an appropriate maneuver for increasing the wedge of corneal scar tissue and thus the refractive effect. If this fails to achieve the correction, the incisions may be deepened with a diamond knife. In astigmatic keratotomy, opening the incision and adding compression sutures may be another practical approach to reduce undercorrection. (These topics are discussed in greater detail in later chapters.)

THERAPEUTIC MEASURES TO ENHANCE WOUND HEALING

Pharmacologic approaches to enhancing wound healing after keratotomy include agents that reduce intraocular pressure and thus increase apposition of corneal tissue, for example, timolol (Timoptic), acetazolamide (Diamox), and pilocarpine. Pilocarpine has the additional effect of compressing the tissues by virtue of the miosis that it creates, and is the standard medication for overcorrections in radial keratotomy, although its use in astigmatic keratotomy may be more limited. For overcorrected astigmatic keratotomy, acetazolamide, which directly reduces intraocular pressure, may be more useful. When instituted, these medications should be continued for a minimum of 6 to 10 weeks, because the increased apposition that they induce needs to be maintained over this time to allow corneal strength to improve to the point that they are not needed.

Certainly sutures apply an order of magnitude of greater force across the wound, and crossed corneal incisions or widely gaping incisions should be closed with sutures. Therapeutic contact lenses may provide a slight additional stabilizing effect on the anterior cornea, and in some circumstances the combination of pressure-lowering medication and therapeutic lenses, either disposable or nondisposable, may provide the crucial extra stability to allow corneal wound healing. Epithelial defects will lead to abnormal wound healing, and the liberal use of artificial tears, ointments, and therapeutic contact lenses often stabilizes both the sutured and the unsutured wound and leads to better healing.

The use of growth factors has recently received much attention. The early optimism concerning a "magic bullet" to enhance both epithelial and stromal wound healing has gradually given way to more realistic expectations that a combination of these agents may indeed be clinically significant. A brief review of some of the more pertinent factors is indicated; however, it should be noted that much of this work remains in progress. The initial investigation was performed in vitro or in animal models, and frequently results of these studies do not agree. The ultimate test of any of these agents will be human trials, which thus far have been limited almost entirely to epidermal growth factor (EGF).

In 1962, Cohen isolated EGF from mouse submaxillary glands. EGF stimulates the growth of epidermal cells and enhances keratinization. Urogastrone is a polypeptide found in human urine, and has been designated as human EGF. Daniele found that EGF stimulated the regeneration of human epithelial scrape wounds and was effective in herpes lesions within 48 hours if the virus affected area was first scraped. In penetrating keratoplasty, randomized double-blind studies showed no increase in the healing rate, possibly because the cells are already proliferating maximally. A clinical trial of EGF by Chiron in a variety of epithelial defects was discontinued because the agent seemed to lack clear effectiveness and because of patient complaints of pain during administration. Current research in terms of epithelial defects has focused attention on a combination of fibronectin and EGF, possibly with other growth factors, that may be effective in more clinical situations. At least at this time, it seems clear that corneal epithelial regeneration is a complex issue requiring more than a single agent to effect the clinical situation. Attention also has been focused on the use of EGF in the preservative solutions for corneal tissue. Wound-healing studies by Serdarevic and Troutman demonstrated slightly increased wound strength with the addition of EGF, and growth factors may become an important addition to the solutions used in penetrating keratoplasty.

Fibronectin is not strictly a growth factor, but represents a plasma and cellular glycoprotein that mediates fibroblast adhesion to collagen matrixes and fibrin substrata. Foster has demonstrated in rabbit epithelial scrape wounds that fibronectin has little additional effect in accelerating wound healing. He theorized that the surrounding epithelial cells were basically normal and secreted fibronectin along the leading edge of healing. However, in corneas in which a significant metabolic abnormality occurs with inflammation or other endogenous or exogenous factors contributing to delayed epithelial coverage, the surface matrix provided by fibronectin might provide a more significant effect. In particular, alkali burns might represent a situation in which such a metabolic defect exists, and fibronectin has been shown to be effective in a rabbit model of alkali burns.

Mesodermal growth factor (MGF) accelerates the healing of rabbit and human corneal endothelium in organ culture and activates wound healing responses in rat corneas. Rich has demonstrated significant mitogenic activity for rabbit keratocytes after a single dose of either 2.5 or 5.0 μm MGF applied immediately after the incision is made. In a controlled study, expulsion of the epithelial plug was complete by the seventh day in rabbits treated with MGF, whereas untreated animals showed continued epithelial plugs. Human trials have not been reported, but it is clear that this may be a significant factor in improving the healing of stromal wounds.

A large number of other growth factors, including fibroblast growth factor (FGF), angiogenic growth factor, epithelial neurotrophic growth factor (ENF), insulin-like growth factor (IGF-I), and even insulin itself, have been found to induce mitogenic response in corneal cells. With genetic engineering, the long-term potential of these pharmaceutical agents should be bright indeed.

SUMMARY

Corneal healing is a complex process that, even today, remains incompletely understood. The importance of the epithelium and good wound apposition are prerequisites for the advance of normal corneal wound healing. In this chapter, we have attempted to focus on areas in corneal surgery in which this process goes awry. By careful observation with the slitlamp and corneal topology, many aspects of incomplete corneal wound healing can be identified and corrected. It is well to appreciate the limitations of corneal wound healing and prepare for them, both before and during surgery, so that postoperative correction does not become necessary. Attention to these principles will reduce the variability of the refractive error in corneal surgical patients and improve the stability in the years after surgery.

Chapter 5

Detection and Measurement of Astigmatism: Instruments and Techniques

Troutman keratometer
Quantitative keratometer
Javal-Schiotz (Haag-Streit) keratometer
Bausch & Lomb keratometer
Photokeratoscope

Computed corneal topology
Raster stereography
Holographic interferometry
Time-of-flight ranging methods
Summary

The detection of astigmatism can be considered the opposite of the problem of determining how far the optics of the human visual system deviate from perfectly spherical lenses. If we assume for the moment that most, if not all, of the astigmatism resides in the cornea and that the cornea is reasonably symmetric in thickness around the visual axis, we come to the most common instruments used to measure corneal astigmatism, the class of instruments known as keratometers. These instruments all share the common characteristic of depending on specular reflection from the surface of the cornea, or in actuality the tear film, to determine deviations from a perfectly spherical reflecting surface.

These assumptions are reasonable, and in practice correlate closely with clinical parameters of refraction but in fact are only assumptions, and in the wide diversity of naturally and iatrogenically occurring pathophysiology may frequently lead to inaccurate determinations of the true astigmatic error of the human optical system.

A second approach to the measurement of astigmatic error might be a determination through diffraction or the actual passage of light through the various media that comprise the optical pathway for the eye. Examples of this approach are retinoscopy and its newer relatives, the automated refraction devices. The assumptions inherent in this approach depend on the precise alignment of the eye relative to the observer, and misalignment can cause significant error. Moreover, the end point of such determination is often in question, and this method of quantifying astigmatic error when used as an objective procedure is less reliable than the keratometer in its many forms.

Finally, we might use the diffuse rather than the specular reflection of light to determine astigmatic error. This approach is the most difficult, because some computer-related analysis is required to determine irregularities in the diffusion of light from the corneal surface. Two such approaches have been described; the first relies on a technique known as photostereoscopy, and the other relies on laser interference holography. Both techniques are essentially new methods to quantify the corneal surface in detail, and are discussed later in this chapter.

The goal of this chapter is to explore the principles and techniques of the prevailing methods that claim to measure astigmatism and to illuminate and dissect the assumptions that underlie each technique. By understanding the limitations inherent in different approaches, we can more reasonably apply individualized techniques for particular problems and combinations of these techniques, to arrive at a better understanding of the true astigmatic error.

TROUTMAN KERATOMETER

The subjective Troutman keratometer, developed in 1972 and reported in 1974, is a device useful to consider before delving into the inner workings of more complex quantitative keratometers. If we shine a large circle of light on a convex shiny surface, such as the cornea, the image will be reflected back but appear much smaller than the original object. We can see that the image that we view on reflection from the cornea is a virtual image located some small distance behind the cornea. Thus the observation by the surgeon using the Troutman keratometer that if the operating microscope truly is focused on the surface of the cornea where sutures are being placed or manipulated, the image of the Troutman keratometer is slightly out of focus. Similarly, if the operating microscope is focused to bring the image of the operating keratometer into perfect focus, the corneal surface is seen to be slightly blurred. The relationship between the size of the operating keratometer (object) and the size of the virtual image can be described in a mathematical relationship as the magnification (M):

$$M = \frac{\text{Image size}}{\text{Object size}} = \frac{\text{Distance from image to corneal surface}}{\text{Distance from keratometer to corneal surface}} \qquad \text{(Eq 1)}$$

and

$$\frac{1}{\begin{array}{c}\text{Distance from}\\\text{image to corneal}\\\text{surface}\end{array}} + \frac{1}{\begin{array}{c}\text{Distance from}\\\text{keratometer to}\\\text{corneal surface}\end{array}} = \frac{2}{\begin{array}{c}\text{Radius of}\\\text{curvature of}\\\text{cornea}\end{array}} \qquad \text{(Eq 2)}$$

Because we have already stated that the object, in this case the keratometer, is larger than the image reflected from the surface of the cornea, we can conclude that the magnification factor of the cornea is less than 1, or that the reflected image is smaller than the object or operating keratometer. The actual surface from which the image is reflected is not really the anterior surface of the cornea. In reality, the image is reflected from the top of the tear film and not from the corneal surface. Because we assume the tear film has a constant thickness across the cornea, we can assume that it does not add power or astigmatism to the resulting image. However, the tear film is essential to obtaining a clear reflex from the Troutman operating keratometer and all other optical keratometers, and frequent use of balanced saline solution in the operating room or artificial tears in the clinic will aid the specular reflection from the surface of the cornea. An interesting new observation by Parel indicates that the epithelium contributes up to 1.5 D to the power of the human cornea, and if it is removed, this must be taken into account.

It follows from equations 1 and 2 that the size of the reflection of the operating keratometer will be proportional to the radius of curvature of the cornea, because the power of the cornea will increase as the radius decreases. Thus, compared with the reflection from a normal cornea (Plate 5–1,A), the reflection of the mires from the operative keratometer from a steep cornea (Plate 5–1,B) or keratoconus (Plate 5–1,C) will be smaller. Similarly, the reflection of the mires from the operative keratometer from a flat cornea (Plate 5–1,D) or Mooren's ulcer (Plate 5–1,E) will be larger. A device has been developed for the eyepiece of the microscope, to allow comparison to standard-size circles to determine relative steepness of the cornea.

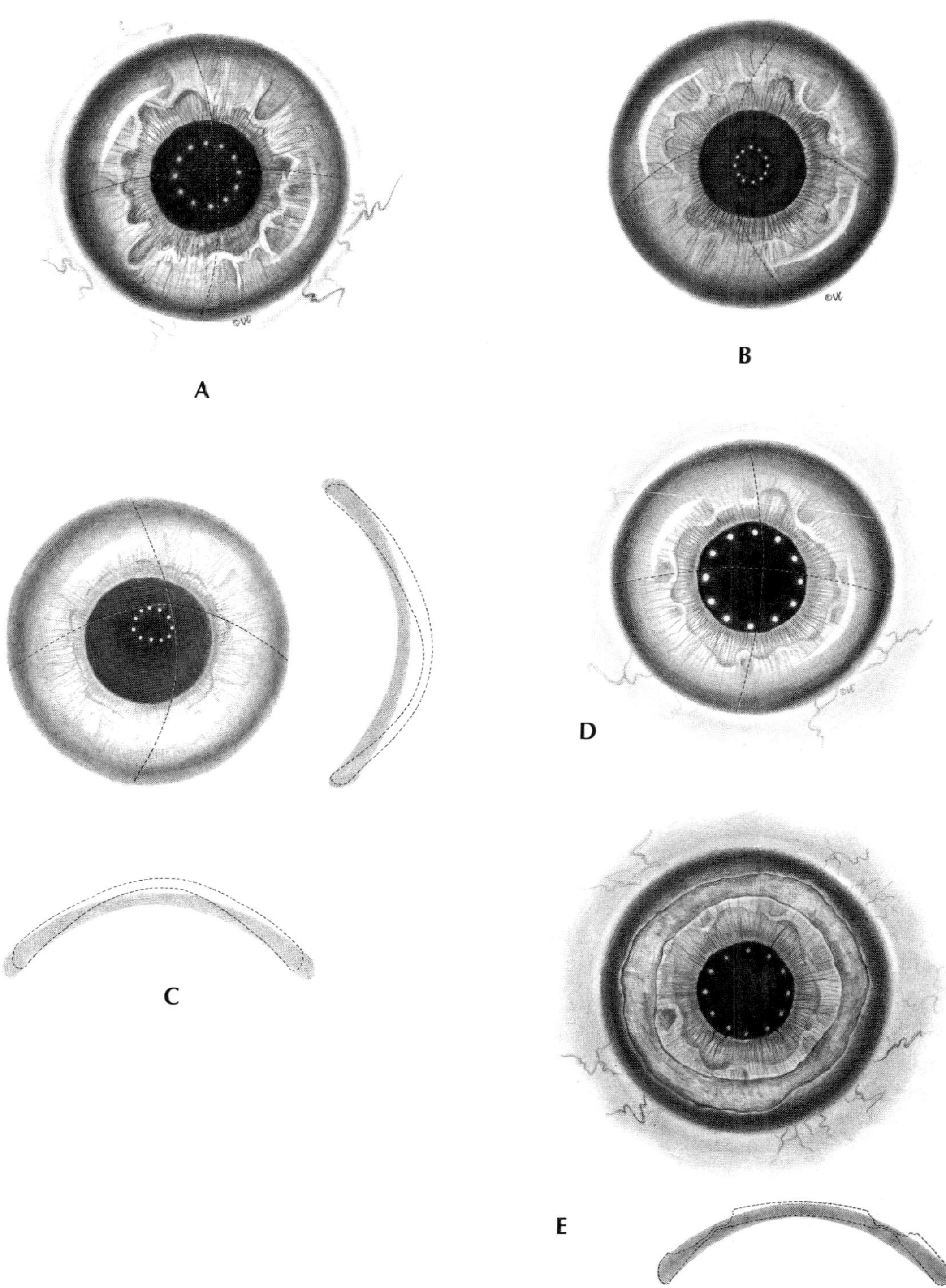

A, reflection of mires from normal cornea with Troutman operative keratometer. **B,** reflection of mires from steep cornea with Troutman operative keratometer. **C,** reflection of mires in keratoconus with Troutman operative keratometer. **D,** reflection of mires from flat cornea with Troutman operative keratometer. **E,** reflection of mires in Mooren's ulcer with Troutman operative keratometer.

The great usefulness of the subjective Troutman keratometer is that it gives a graphic but simple representation of astigmatism from the corneal surface in real time. Regular corneal astigmatism is represented by an ellipse reflected from the corneal surface with a long and short axis (Plate 5–2). As noted above, the minification is increased as the corneal radius decreases, so that the smaller of the two axes represents the steeper radius of curvature, whereas the larger of the two axes represents the flatter radius of curvature. This close relationship between radius of curvature and distortion of the round reflex of the simple Troutman subjective keratometer can be used to great effect in corneal surgery. Both steep and flat axes can be quickly and easily recognized, and adjustments can be made with immediate feedback from the keratometer.

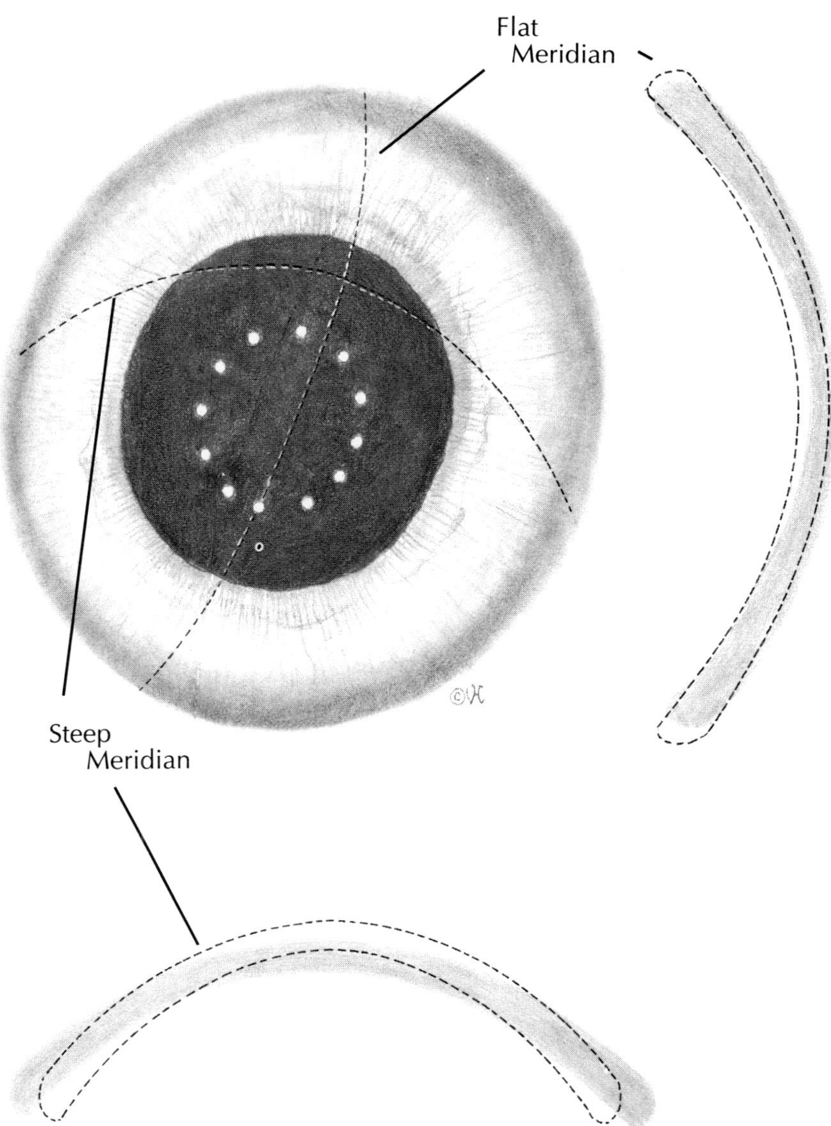

Appearance of cornea with astigmatic error showing oval appearance of mires from Troutman operative keratometer.

QUANTITATIVE KERATOMETER

The credit for the first keratometer, or ophthalmometer, as it was initially called, is given to Hermann von Helmholtz, who lived from 1821 to 1894. Building on this basic principle, but refining it for clinical use, Javal, Schiotz, and others made further contributions during the late 19th century. In all quantitative measurements using keratometry or specular reflection, we must keep in mind that the corneal radius is being measured on its anterior surface, and the power of this anterior corneal surface is obtained through a series of approximations.

The bending of light through an interface with different indices of refraction can be described in an exact mathematical formula by Snell's law. When light is bent by a curved surface, such as a sphere, the equation becomes considerably more complex and can only be approximated by a simple formula. A first approximation of the bending of light by a sphere is given by Littman's formula:

$$\text{Power (D)} = \frac{\text{Index of refraction of cornea} - \text{Index of refraction of air}}{\text{Radius of corneal curvature (m)}} \qquad \text{(Eq 3)}$$

where the index of refraction is a quantity that, based on measurement, is assumed by each manufacturer of keratometers. Both the Bausch and Lomb and the Javal-Schiotz (Haag-Streit) assume a value of 1.3375 for the index of refraction of the cornea, whereas the index of refraction of air is known to be 1.00. This equation can be transposed to provide a relationship between radius in millimeters and anterior corneal surface power in diopters:

$$\text{Power (D)} = \frac{337.5}{\text{Anterior corneal curvature (mL)}} \qquad \text{(Eq 4)}$$

This relationship is usually inscribed on the dials of the keratometer so that the corneal curvature can be recorded either in diopters or millimeters. It is important, however, to realize that this relationship between radius of curvature and dioptric power is based on several assumptions, which may vary from keratometer to keratometer. First, this index of refraction is adjusted to represent the total refractive contribution of the cornea, including the anterior and posterior surfaces. If we consider the cornea, we will immediately realize that the anterior surface is a converging lens, whereas the posterior surface is a diverging lens; thus the overall power of the cornea depends on both surfaces. Average parameters for the normal eye have been assembled by Gullstrand:

Gullstrand Data for Normal Eye

Radius of anterior corneal surface (mm)	7.70
Radius of posterior corneal surface (mm)	6.80
Thickness of cornea (mm)	0.48
Index of refraction of air	1.000
Index of refraction of cornea	1.376
Index of refraction of aqueous	1.336

We can see immediately that Gullstrand gives a different index of refraction for the cornea than the value noted earlier and used by the makers of the keratometer. If we use this data and apply Littman's formula to the anterior and posterior surfaces of the cornea, we find a convergence of 48.83 D at the anterior surface and a divergence of 5.882 D at the posterior surface. If we neglect the thickness of the cornea (an error in this case of <0.10 D) and apply thin-lens optical theory, we have a total corneal refraction of 42.95 = 48.83 − 5.882 D. Thus we see there is a far greater convergence at the anterior surface of the cornea than at the posterior surface, because of the great difference between the refractive indices of air and cornea as opposed to the much smaller difference between the refractive indices between cornea and aqueous humor. This illustrates the importance of the anterior surface of the cornea in refractive surgical procedures. A relatively small change in the anterior surface of the cornea can create large changes in refractive error, whereas the same change along the posterior surface of the cornea makes a much smaller refractive effect.

The makers of keratometers have hidden these details by assuming an average corneal index of refraction that accounts for the divergence of light on the posterior surface of the cornea. For most purposes these assumptions hold true, and the relationship between radius in millimeters and dioptric power of the cornea in diopters can be assumed to be the values noted on the dials of the keratometer. In some instances, however, particularly in the calculations required for the Barraquer procedures and other refractive procedures that modify the anterior surface of the cornea, the true index of refraction of the cornea must be used to obtain appropriate calculations. We will now explore the mechanical characteristics of two major clinical keratometers, the Javal-Schiotz (Haag-Streit) and the Bausch and Lomb.

JAVAL-SCHIOTZ (HAAG-STREIT) KERATOMETER

The Javal-Schiotz keratometer is based on the concept of varying the size of the object while maintaining a constant-sized image (Plate 5–3,A). Two mires illuminated by lamps are placed on a curved track that allows the two mires to be moved simultaneously relative to the center of the instrument by a mechanism beneath the housing. When the knob is turned in one direction the mires move together; when the knob is turned in the opposite direction the mires move apart. The essence of the keratometer is the use of a doubling prism, which was the original invention of Helmholtz. One might imagine that if the two lighted mires were set at a fixed distance, we might simply measure the distance between the two mires and thus determine the curvature of the anterior cornea using equations 1 through 4. Today such measurements form the basis of the new computed topology systems. However, in the early part of this century computers were not available, and using a simple ruler would have introduced inaccuracy into the measurement of the distance between the two mires. Instead, a doubling prism was used. The mires were moved to such location that the fixed distance, which the doubling prism produced, could be matched by the appearance of the mires in the eyepiece. Hence this keratometer produces a constant image size by virtue of the lens, which doubles the image and varies the object size by varying the distance between the two mires.

In practice, operation of the Javal-Schiotz keratometer is simple. The mires are observed and moved until they touch (Plate 5–3,B). At this point the dark line through the center of each mire is observed, and if the lines running through the right and left mire do not coincide, the entire housing is turned until the lines do coincide (Plate 5–3,C). The axis and corneal power are then recorded (Plate 5–3,D). The housing is then rotated 90 degrees and the mires are observed again. If the lines running through the center of each mire do not coincide, the housing is rotated until they do. The mires are then moved together or apart until they touch. The numbers are recorded again. The stepped appearance of the mire can be used to give a rough approximation of the degree of astigmatism present in the cornea, because each step corresponds to 1 D, and overlapping of the mires can then be used to estimate the corneal astigmatism to check the calibration of the instrument.

The Javal-Schiotz keratometer has the virtue of simplicity, and the configuration of the mires means that the cornea can be fairly irregular and yet still be adequate for objective keratometry. It is clear that two steps are required to obtain the full keratometry reading; in addition, this reading represents four points on the cornea, taken from the circumference of an optical zone approximately 3 mm in diameter. In general, we believe this keratometer is an excellent choice for the corneal surgeon, because of its simplicity and the ability to "read" relatively distorted corneas.

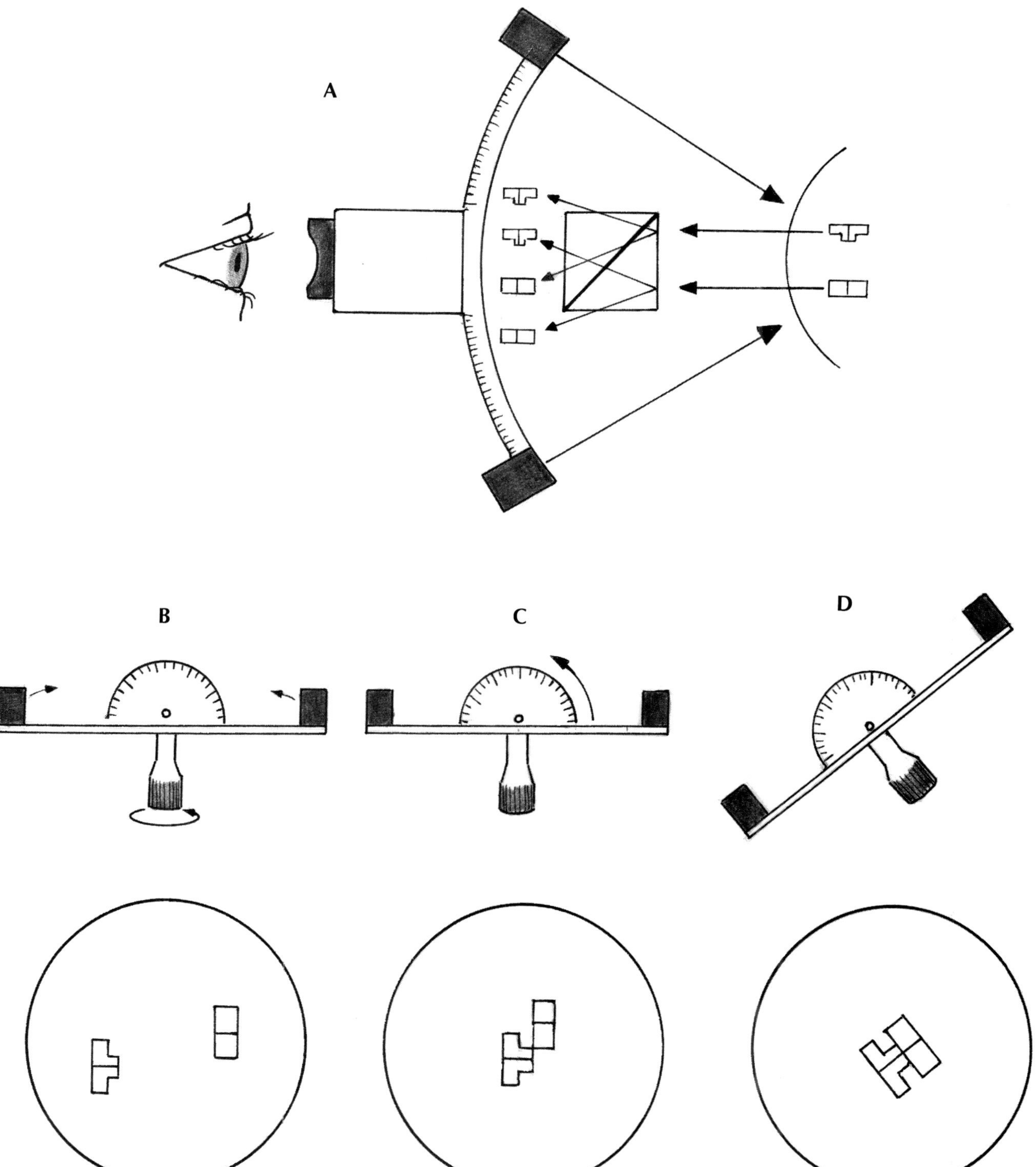

A, Javal-Schiotz (Haag-Streit) keratometer showing constant image size. B, initial configuration of mires, apart and misaligned. C, configuration after bringing mires together, but misaligned. D, alignment and juxtaposition of mires by rotation of keratometer.

BAUSCH & LOMB KERATOMETER

The Bausch & Lomb keratometer works on the opposite principle of constant object size and variable image size. This keratometer has the advantage that the measurement of both astigmatic axes can be accomplished at the same time without turning the instrument. The object or mire can be seen on the front plate of the instrument as a round circle with a cross at the 3-o'clock position and a minus at the 12 o'clock position. Internally, this mire is projected on the cornea, and an image is created behind the cornea. This image is then directed by converging lenses within the instrument to a diaphragm with four openings, one above, one below, and one on each side. The light emerging from each opening is directed through two prisms that can be moved independently parallel to the central axis of the instrument. Light passing through the left opening of the diaphragm is deviated by the base-up prism to place an image above the central axis. Light passing through the right opening is deviated by the base-out prism, placing an image to the right of the central axis. Light that passes through the lower and upper openings of the diaphragm does not pass through either prism, and an image is produced in the middle of the axis that is the same brightness as the other images, because the upper and lower openings are smaller.

In practice, this instrument is focused until the central image changes from double (Plate 5–4,A) to single. The horizontal and vertical dials are turned to bring the mires closer together (Plate 5–4,B). The housing is then turned until the crosses and minuses on the central image line up with the crosses and minuses on the secondary images (Plate 5–4,C). At this point, the horizontal and vertical dials are turned until the crosses and minuses coincide (Plate 5–4,D), and the readings are recorded from each drum (Plate 5–4,E). The horizontal meridian indicator is recorded with the horizontal dial, and the vertical meridian indicator is recorded with the vertical dial. One assumption of this instrument is that the astigmatic axes are always 90 degrees apart. As we will see later, this assumption is not always true, and in practice the instrument sometimes must be turned slightly after recording the plus cylinder axis to properly record the minus cylinder axis. In addition, the complexity of the pattern of mires can be a problem in distorted corneas, because the entire image sometimes may be obscured by various abnormalities.

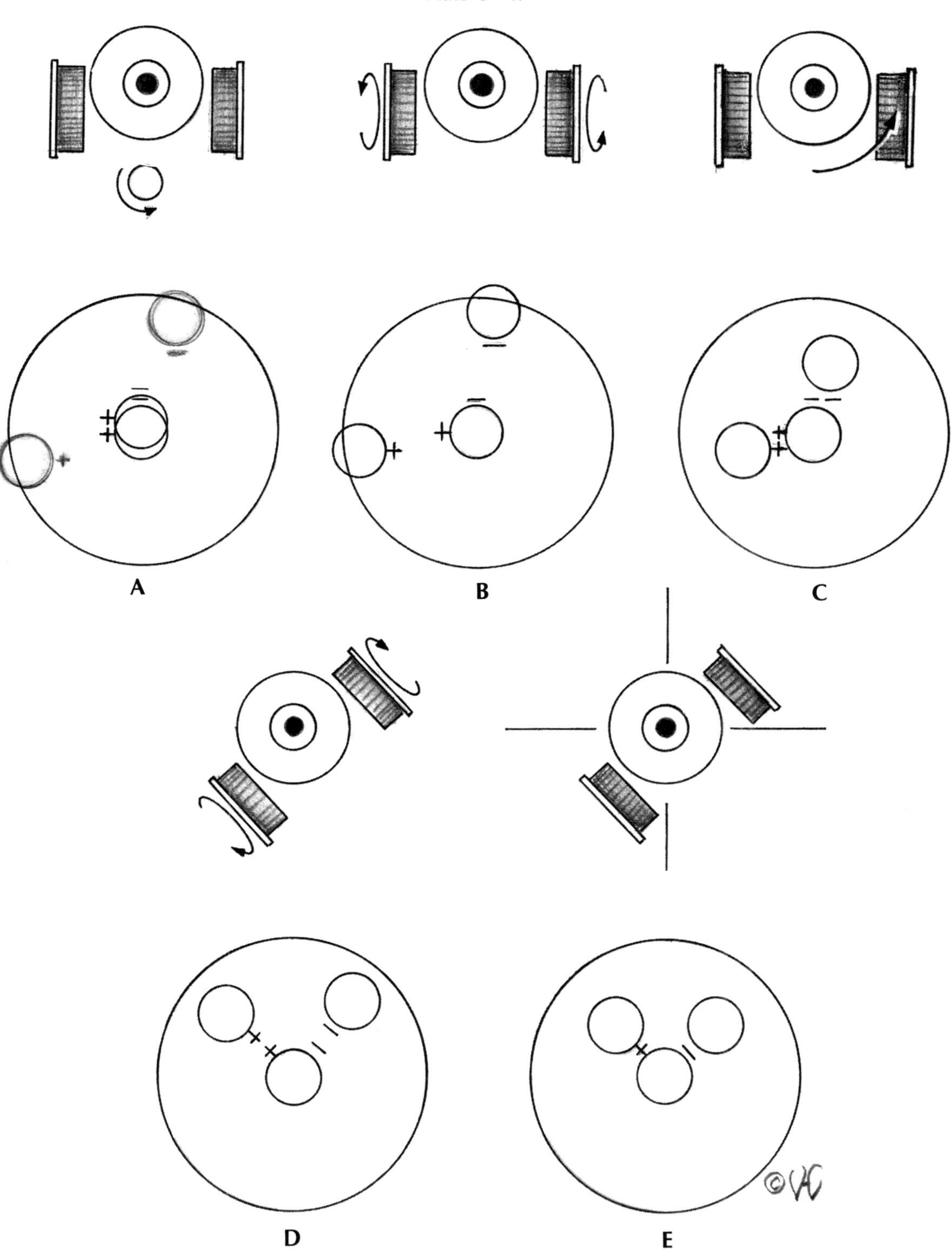

A, initial appearance of mires from Bausch & Lomb keratometer. Doubling of central mire indicates need for focusing. **B,** appearance of mires after focusing, showing misalignment and separation. **C,** appearance of mires after reduction of separation, but still misaligned. **D,** alignment of mires by rotation of keratometer, but separated. **E,** final alignment of mires; + and − coincide.

An advantage of the instrument is that it records a variable image size that is proportional to the corneal curvature, and it behaves much like a Troutman keratometer. Subjective observation of the mires of both the Bausch & Lomb and the Javal-Schiotz keratometers can be helpful in making the diagnosis of keratoconus and other irregular astigmatism. In this situation, an inability to properly align the mires or angulation in which the mires demonstrate an angled appearance relative to one another may indicate irregular astigmatism of the kind seen with keratoconus (Plate 5–5,A). Jumping of the mires also can be seen in keratoconus and other conditions in which the cornea is not smoothly continuous (Plate 5–5,B). Blurred mires usually indicate a deficiency in the tear film or a rough surface (Plate 5–5,C). If the mires are minified, there may be a steep cornea, as seen in keratoconus (Plate 5–5,D). Finally, distortion of the mires often is a reflection of distortion of the corneal surface, as seen in keratoconus and other conditions with irregular astigmatism (Plate 5–5,E). Careful observation of the mires during keratometry often reveals the presence of irregular astigmatism, and prompt clinical action is appropriate.

In addition, observation of the elliptical nature of the mires in the Bausch & Lomb keratometer in a patient with regular astigmatism can give a subjective estimate of the flat and steep axes and the general amount of astigmatism. The choice of a manual keratometer may be a matter of individual preference, although the clinician certainly should use the available choices in actual measurement before making a final choice.

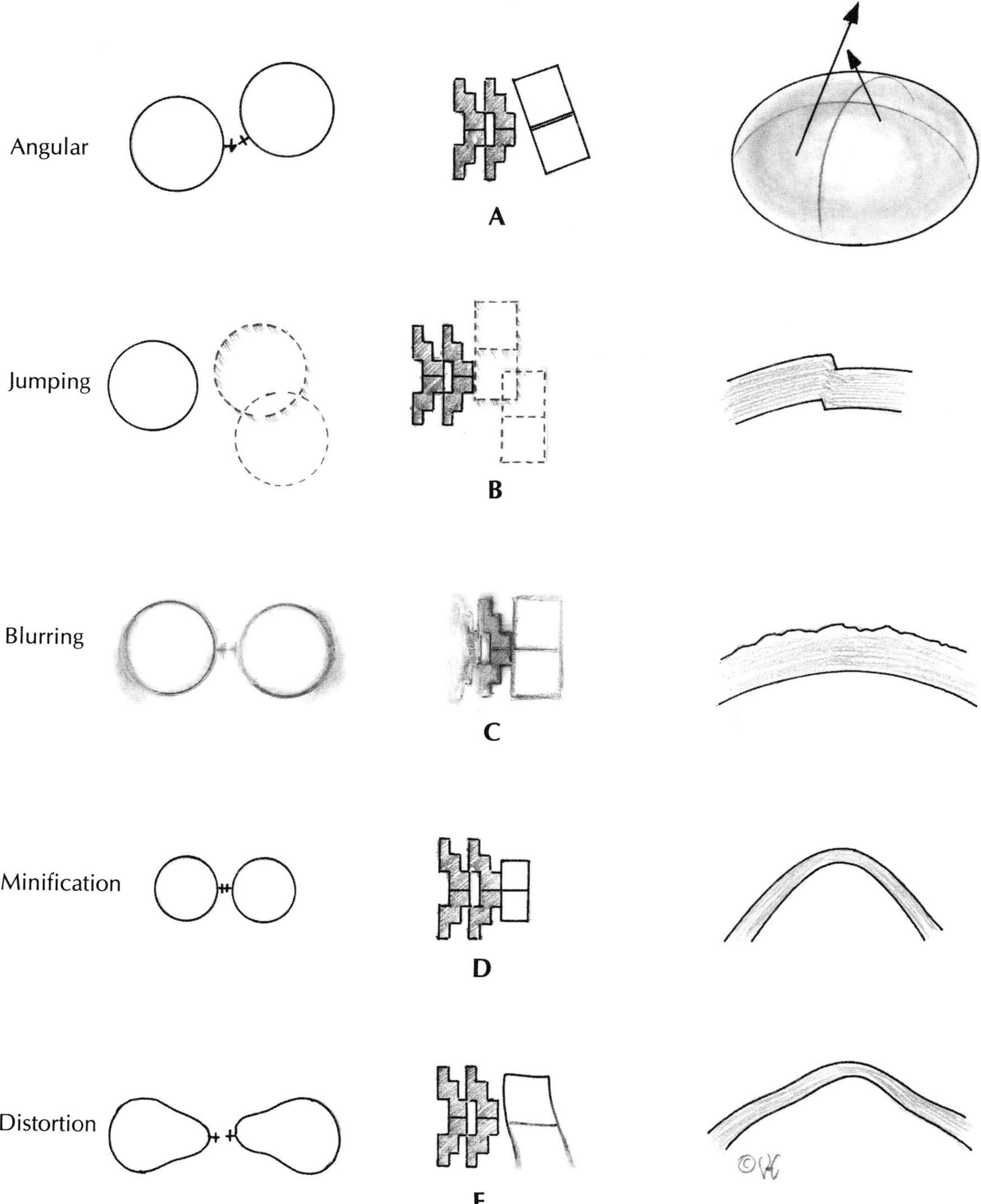

A, appearance of mires from Bausch & Lomb and Javal-Schiotz keratometers, with angulation. **B,** appearance of mires with jumping. **C,** appearance of mires with blurring. **D,** appearance of mires with minification. Both mires are minified with Bausch & Lomb keratometer; only one mire is minified with the Haag-Streit instrument. **E,** appearance of mires with distortion.

PHOTOKERATOSCOPE

The Placido disc was invented by Antonio Placido, and was popularized by Allvar Gullstrand. Today the limitations of orientation relative to the eye and coverage of the eye with reflected rings have been overcome with two instruments, one available from Nidek (Palo Alto, Calif.) and the other available from Kera Corporation (Japan). Photokeratometry, as demonstrated by these instruments, is a subjective evaluation of corneal topology (Plate 5–6,A). The pattern of rings can illuminate surface irregularities, such as incisions and sutures, and demonstrate both regular and irregular astigmatism. The instrument is reasonably easy to use, and in conjunction with the quantitative keratometer, a great deal of useful information can be obtained concerning the astigmatic characteristics of a given cornea. In practice, the rings are projected onto the cornea and a virtual image is created slightly behind the cornea, as with the Troutman keratometer. In general, the instrument is focused on the central rings, although it may be focused on the outer rings if this area is of particular interest. A button is depressed that activates a flash lamp, and a Polaroid photograph is taken. An advantage of the Nidek photokeratometer is the ability to take two images on a single photograph, although these images are smaller and more difficult to read than the single large image of the Kera unit.

Interpretation of keratoscopic patterns depends on the same basic principles as those used for interpretation of the subjective Troutman keratometer. Regular astigmatism is demonstrated by oval mires (Plate 5–6,B), and steep corneas will show smaller rings (Plate 5–6,E) than flat corneas. The distance between rings indicates the relative steepness of a particular cornea. Thus a steep area of the cornea will demonstrate rings that are very close together, and a flat area of the cornea will show rings that are farther apart and wider. In general, unsutured transverse incisions on the corneal surface (Plate 5–6,C) or sutured transverse or arcuate incisions, such as penetrating keratoplasty with wound dehiscence, demonstrate flattening of the cornea anterior to the area of interest, which we have named the microdehiscence. Similarly, excessively tight sutures or wounds in which very tight sutures are used, such as the Troutman wedge resection, show steepening of the cornea anterior to the area of interest, and the rings are closer together (Plate 5–6,D).

Irregular astigmatism, such as keratoconus, shows a characteristic pattern of steepening in the inferotemporal cornea, with flattening along the same meridian in the superior nasal cornea (Plate 5–6,E). Surface irregularities, such as those demonstrated by herpetic scars, will show blurring of the rings and often can demonstrate a cause of decreased visual acuity (Plate 5–6,F).

Plate 5–6.

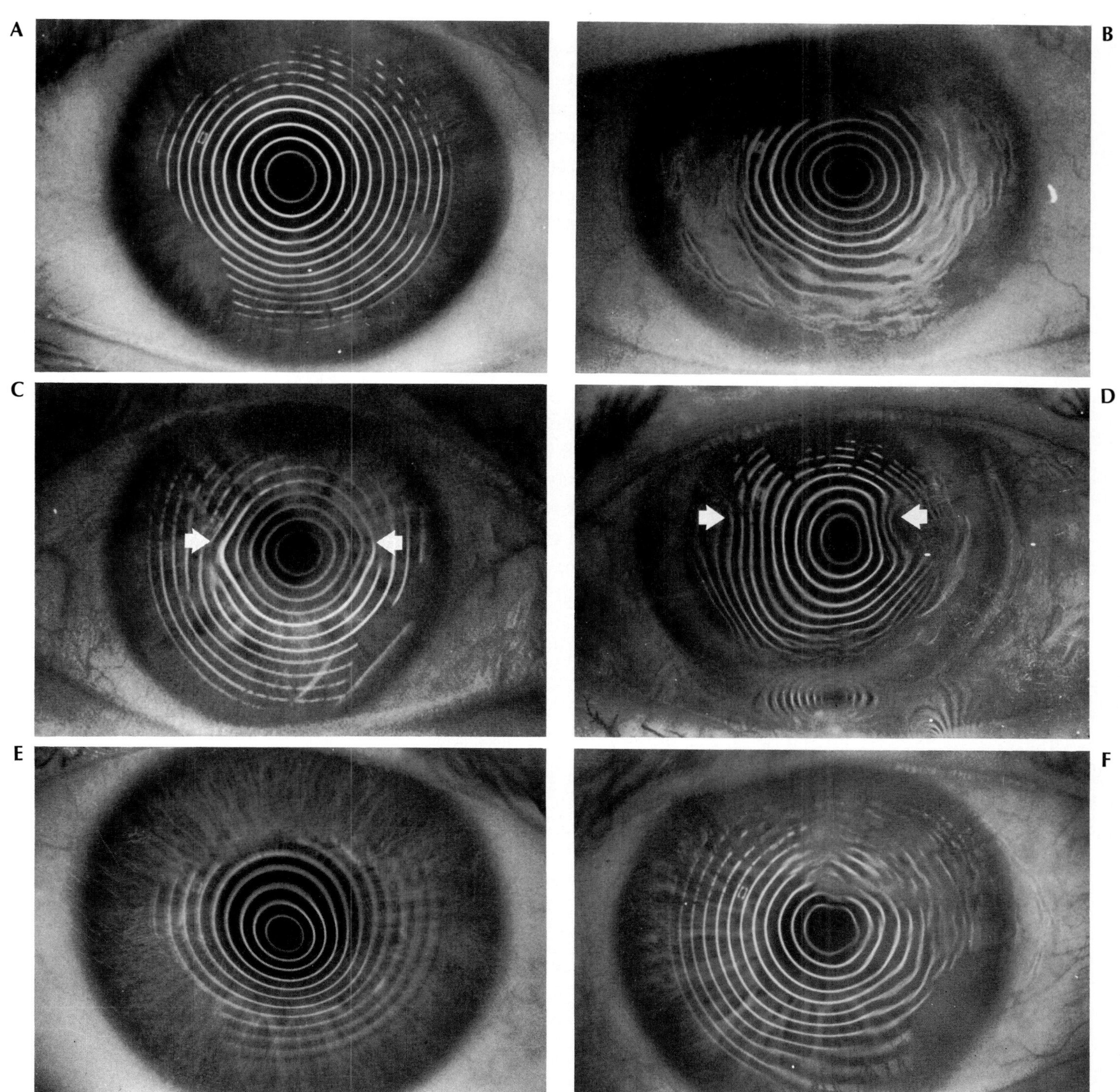

A, photokeratometry (Kera) of cornea without astigmatic error. **B,** photokeratometry (Kera) of cornea, with the rule astigmatic error. **C,** photokeratometry (Kera) of cornea with two transverse relaxing incisions shows microdehiscence *(arrows)*. **D,** photokeratometry (Kera) of cornea with two tight sutures *(arrows)*. **E,** Photokeratometry (Kera) of cornea with keratoconus shows irregular astigmatism and steepening. **F,** photokeratometry (Kera) of cornea with surface scarring due to herpes simplex keratitis shows blurring of mires.

Detection and Measurement of Astigmatism   107

By using the keratometer and photokeratometer together, areas of mid-peripheral corneal distortion often can be identified that may contribute to erroneous objective keratometric readings, and used together, the photokeratoscope and keratometer can provide a more accurate means of determining corneal astigmatism. In corneal transplantation, mid-peripheral distortion around the sutured incision is the rule, and it is our practice to combine keratometry and photokeratometry on every preoperative and postoperative visit. As the practitioner becomes more adept at interpretation of the photokeratometric image as it relates to objective keratometric readings, the combination becomes invaluable.

COMPUTED CORNEAL TOPOLOGY

With the advent of the computer, images that which once served as only subjective representations of corneal topology can now be quantified and represented in a variety of objective formats. The early precursors of this technique used large photographs and hand digitization, giving a map of the cornea with keratometer readings at various points. This technique was developed by Rowsey, and further development by Klyce converted these numerical values into color-coded maps of the corneal surface. The numerical interpretation of corneoscopic rings may at first seem complicated, but in fact is based on very simple principles, which are reviewed here.

To use the computer to assist our analysis of corneoscopic rings, we must first program the graphic representation of the rings into the computer in some manner. Devices are available that plug into any standard computer and allow input of a video-camera signal into the computer, resulting in the formation of the same image on the computer screen. The computer screen may be thought of as a piece of graph paper, divided into many small squares or pixels. A common standard is to convert the picture into a screen with 500×500 pixels. We can now accurately determine the location of the lines relative to the pixels, and by using the formulas discussed earlier in this chapter, can determine the corneal curvature that would correspond to rings in every location. Thus we obtain a detailed map of the cornea, with values of the corneal curvature at each location at which a ring appears. It is clear that providing more rings will give a more detailed mapping of the corneal surface, and for this reason, devices such as the Topographic Modeling System (Computed Anatomy, New York) provide many more rings than the older photokeratometer Kera. These numerical values can be presented in a variety of formats, but Klyce has demonstrated the usefulness of color-coded maps of the corneal surface, in which the cooler colors, such as blue, represent flatter areas of the cornea and the warmer colors, such as red, represent steeper areas.

Perhaps the most unexpected observations using this new technique have come in the area of astigmatism. By observation of rings of both the Troutman keratometer and photokeratoscopic images, clinicians were aware of a certain amount of irregular astigmatism, even in patients with good vision with normal astigmatic correction. Our observation of these rings over the years led us to consider astigmatism as an oval-appearing cornea with flat and steep axes 90 degrees apart. In fact, the surfaces demonstrated by the computed topology systems show us that only a minority of corneas truly satisfy the criteria of orthogonal flat and steep axes. In fact, a progression of astigmatic conditions, many of which have nonorthogonal astigmatic meridians, have been proposed by Waring as a classification scheme, based on the computed topographic appearance of the cornea after penetrating keratoplasty, (Plate 5–7). Cohen has taken this subjective classification by appearance and has created a computer-based analytical system, the Corneal Visualization Tool, which automatically classifies the cornea into the appropriate category. Using the same computer system, these authors hope eventually to create an artificial intelligence system that indicates surgical approaches to the astigmatic problem. This close interaction between the results of computed topology and real solutions to problems can be seen in another solution that has been proposed, that is, contact lens fitting. Using the results of the corneal topology system as a guide, a computer-controlled contact lens lathe can be used to create customized contact lenses for individual corneas. The variety and scope of applications for these new technologies are virtually limitless.

Plate 5–7.

Computed corneal topology of a series of corneas with astigmatic error in a classification system suggested by Waring.

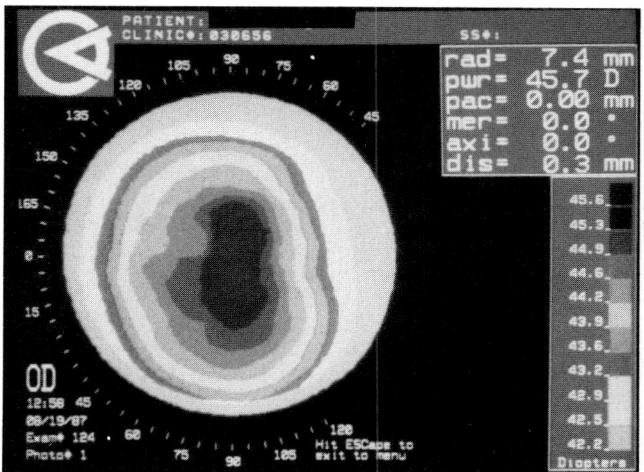

A. Oval.

B. Hourglass.

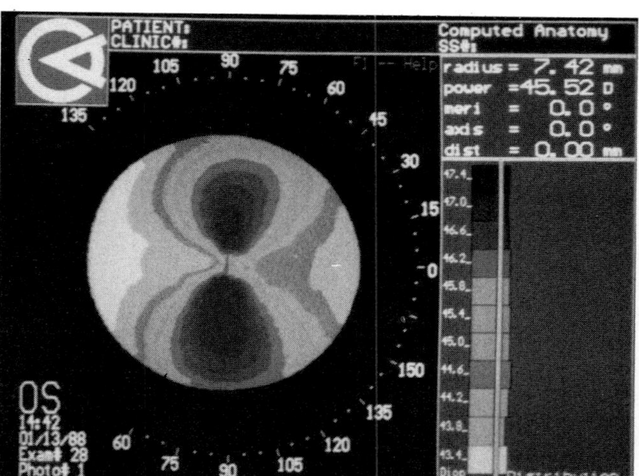

C. Equal bowtie.

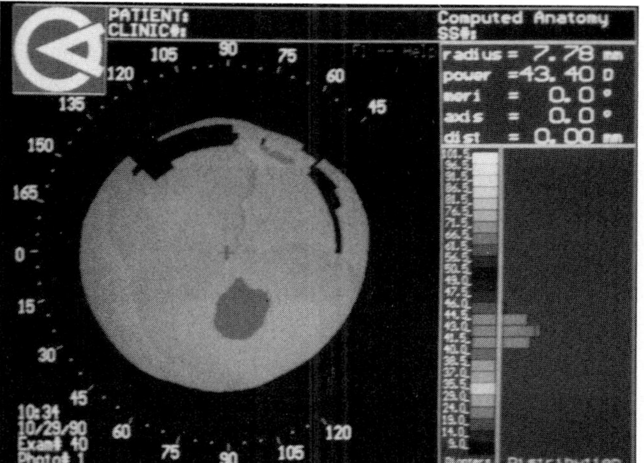

D. Unequal bowtie.

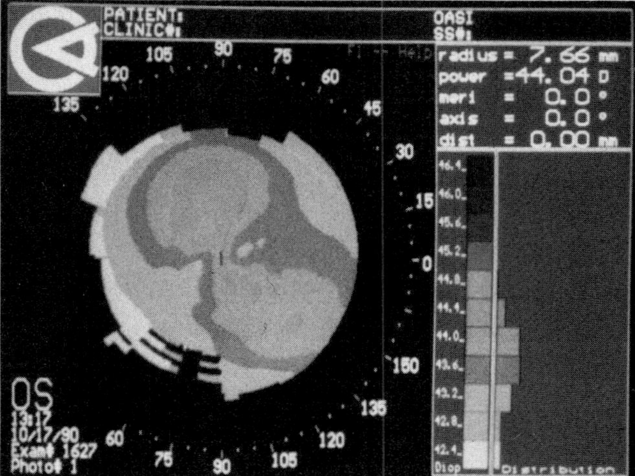

E. Tipped.

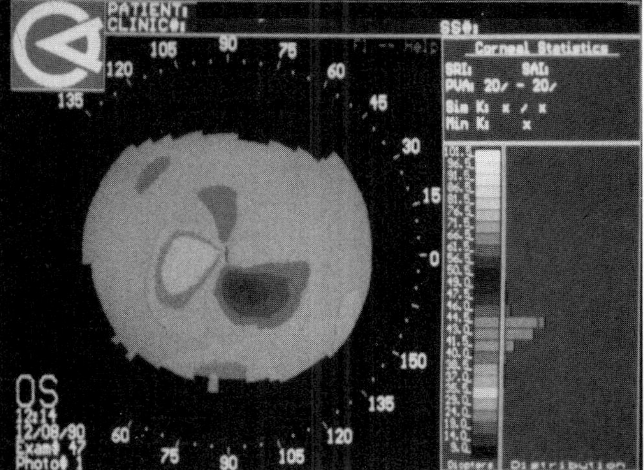

F. Irregular.

RASTER STEREOGRAPHY

One of the problems of photokeratometry is the necessity for an optically smooth surface to reflect the image of the photokeratoscope. In addition, the photokeratoscope measures changes in corneal curvature rather than elevations above a given baseline. Raster stereography represents a technique used in industry in which a pattern, in this case a grid, is projected onto the cornea and records distortions when viewed from a defined oblique angle. This technique was originally adopted for corneal topography by Warnicki and Rehkopf, and has been investigated as a clinical instrument in the form of the PAR Technology Corneal Topography System (PAR CTS) by Belin and associates.

This unit has been adapted to fit on a Topcon slitlamp. A pattern is projected onto the cornea by means of this device, completely covering the cornea (Plate 5–8,A). The pattern is not centered on the optical axis, and computational errors arising from inaccurate determination of the visual axis are not translated into errors of corneal topology. An important difference between this instrument and the computed photokeratometry devices is that this instrument reads elevations and not curvature. The PAR CTS is capable of both an elevation map (Plate 5–8,B) and a spherical subtraction map (Plate 5–8,C) in which a best-fit sphere is subtracted from the previous elevation map. In this example, an apparently spherical cornea (Plate 5–8,B) is shown to have a small amount of with the rule astigmatism (Plate 5–8,C). Approximately 5 D of with the rule astigmatism in spherical subtraction mode demonstrates a higher astigmatic error (Plate 5–8,D). The accuracy is calculated to be approximately ±0.015 mm, or between 0.15 D and 0.23 D over the normal range of curvature for the human cornea.

Because true elevations are measured, the unit is helpful in keratoconus (Plate 5–8,E) and in refractive procedures such as radial keratotomy (Plate 5–8,F). Because the PAR CTS does not depend on a smooth corneal surface, it is possible that it might be used in conjunction with excimer laser photoablation to monitor the effects of the procedure while it is being performed.

In observing these images, we are again reminded that a cylindrical lens has power 90 degrees away from the axis of the cylinder. Thus elevation mapping of the cornea for with the rule astigmatism shows elevations depicted as warm or reddish colors in a horizontal band or configuration as seen with the PAR unit. The same cornea demonstrating with the rule astigmatism as seen on a curvature plot of the cornea, for example, created with a Topographic Modeling System, will show warm or reddish colors, indicating the steep axis in a vertical band or configuration. Thus the basic principles remain the same despite the sophistication of the instruments used, and care should be taken in defining exactly what is being depicted on topologic plots of the cornea.

Plate 5–8.

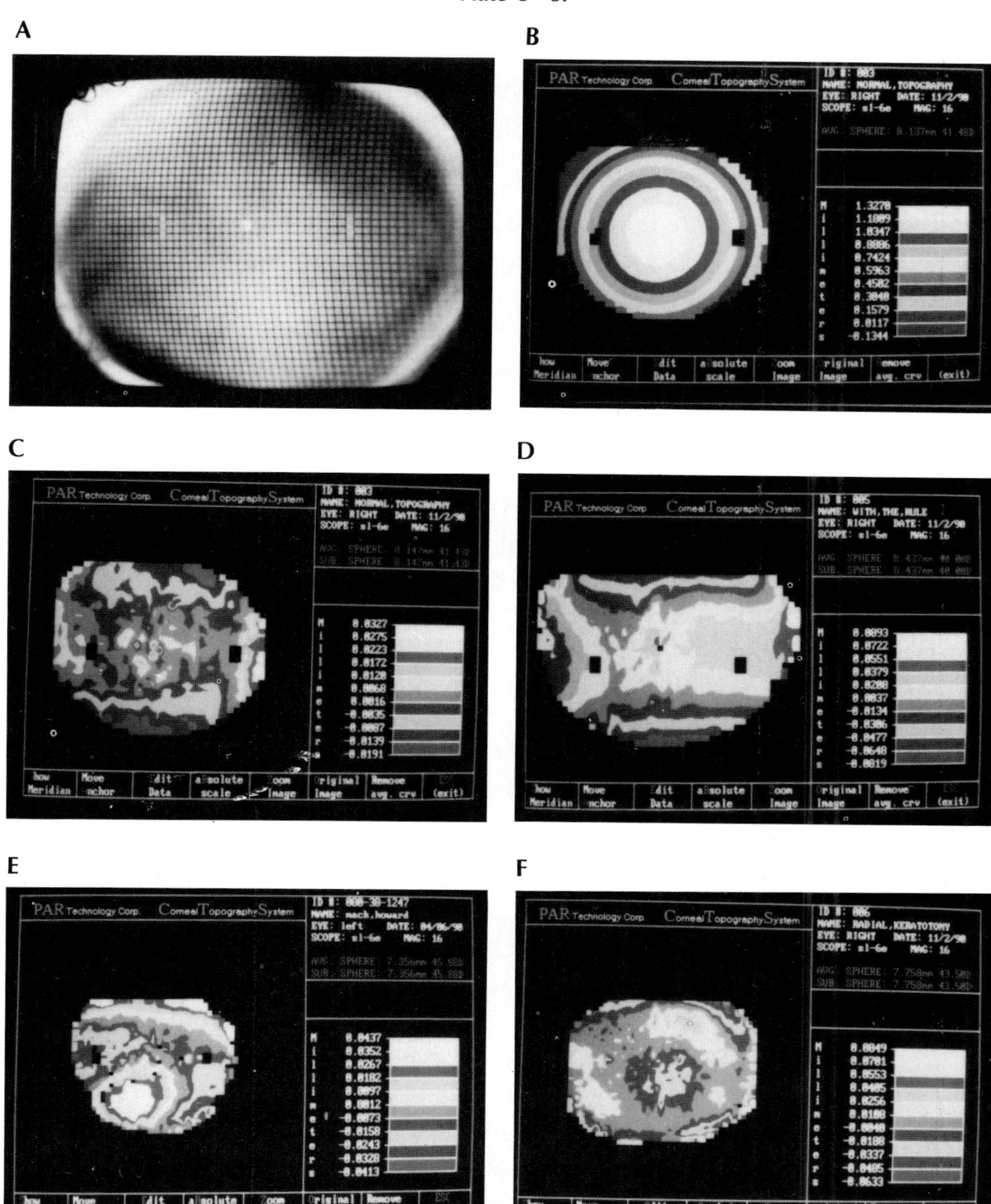

A, projection of grid on cornea by PAR corneal topology unit. **B,** appearance of a cornea with a small amount of with the rule astigmatism seen with the normal predetermined elevation scale, showing no astigmatic error. **C,** appearance of the same cornea as in **B,** in the subtraction mode demonstrates a small amount of with the rule astigmatism. **D,** appearance of a cornea with 5 D of with the rule astigmatism, seen in the subtraction mode. **E,** appearance of a cornea with keratoconus, in the subtraction mode. **F,** appearance of a cornea after radial keratotomy, in the subtraction mode. Fig 5–8,A–F courtesy of Michael W. Belin, M.D.

HOLOGRAPHIC INTERFEROMETRY

One of the newer approaches to analyzing the corneal surface is the application of laser holographic interferometry, which is simply a form of standard interferometry extended to an area measurement. This approach has been in development by Phil Baker in conjunction with DGH (San Diego), and the clinical work presented here was performed by Miles Friedlander. In standard interferometry used to measure one-dimensional length, we have a reference path and a path that is to be varied. The principle of this instrument depends on the interference of light from the fixed path as compared with light from the variable path. When the light is in phase, the wave fronts from the laser coincide and the light presented to the photodetector is twice as bright as the original beam. When the light is out of phase, the wave fronts cancel and the photodetector sees no light. By counting wave fronts as the variable path is moved, the instrument can measure linear displacements as small as a few nanometers. Holographic interferometry works on a similar principle, comparing the light emerging from a holographic reference object with a real object, in this case the cornea. The hologram is familiar to many as a means of creating a true three-dimensional image from a recording on film using laser light. Using the fringes of light and dark, which are created by interference from light coming from the holographic image and the cornea, computer analysis can re-create the surface of the cornea relative to the reference holographic object. In an astigmatic cornea, more fringes are observed in one direction (Plate 5–9,A) than in the direction 90 degrees away (Plate 5–9,B). By combining the information from these two orthogonal holographic views of the cornea, we can re-create the surface from which these views were taken. Of even more interest are the holographic interference fringes created by radial keratotomy (Plate 5–9,C) and penetrating keratoplasty (Plate 5–9,D). Here we see an indication of the remarkable level of sensitivity that we might expect from such an instrument. The capability to obtain very high-resolution modeling of corneal topology combined with the ability to view rough surfaces, such as those encountered during and after excimer laser area ablation (Plate 5–9,E) that might not have adequate specular reflection to allow photokeratometry, gives us a preview of things to come in the quantitative evaluation of corneal topology. Computer-generated mapping of the corneal surface (Plate 5–9,F) from these images is a complex task, but may offer details of the corneal surface that are not available from other modalities.

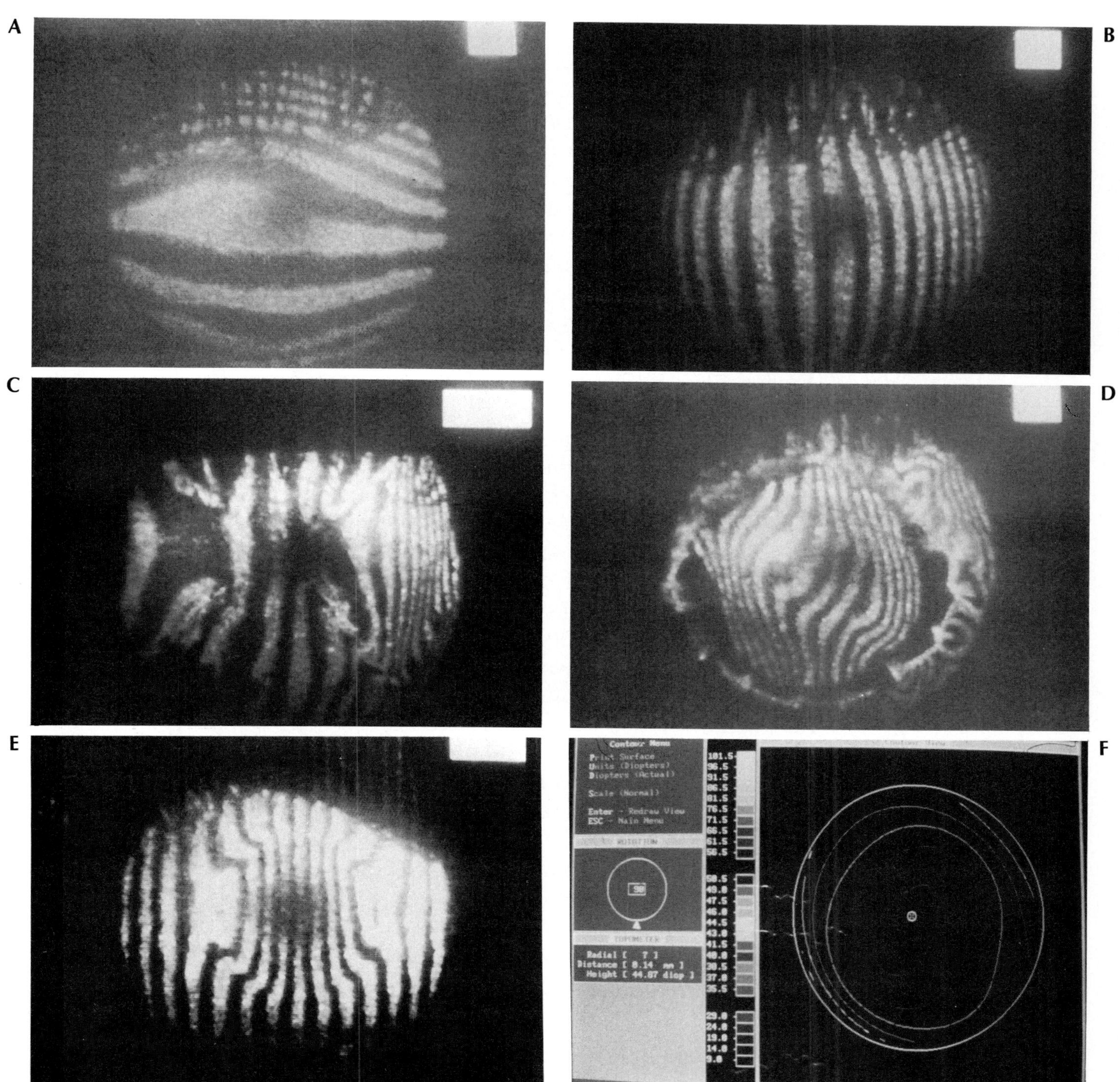

A, holographic interferometry of a cornea with 4 D of corneal astigmatism. **B,** holographic interferometry of the same cornea as in **A,** meridian 90 degrees away. **C,** holographic interferometry of cornea after four-incision radial keratotomy. **D,** holographic interferometry of cornea after penetrating keratoplasty. **E,** holographic interferometry of cornea 1 week after area excimer laser ablation. **F,** computer-generated elevation topology of keratoconus. Fig 5–9,A–F courtesy of Miles Friedlander, M.D.

TIME-OF-FLIGHT RANGING METHODS

Time-of-flight measurements of distance have been an established technique since the development of radar and sonar in World War II. Such techniques depend on the principle of pulses of energy flying outward from a central location and sending back an echo. If the velocity of the energy pulse in the media is known (speed of light for radar and speed of sound in water for sonar), the distance to the object can be calculated by determining the amount of time the round trip took for this pulse of energy. This is the principle used in ultrasound evaluation of corneal thickness. In this technique, a hand-held probe both creates a pulse of sound energy and receives it back, allowing electronics in the instrument to measure the transit time. Obvious sources of error relate to orientation of the probe relative to the surface, because a tipped probe will encounter more of the corneal thickness and thus give an abnormally high reading. Similarly, excessive pressure may distort the cornea and give abnormal readings. Attempts to obtain ultrasonic evaluation of corneal topology have thus far been unsuccessful, because of the necessity to include a fluid bath, which is messy and inhibits application of the technology. Moreover, the level of accuracy with the present generation of instrumentation is not considered adequate to obtain clinically useful information.

Femtosecond optical ranging, a new technique described by Puliafito and associates, involves the use of extremely short pulses of light. This technique has been used to determine the time of flight of these ultrashort laser pulses between the anterior corneal surface and the bottom of a keratotomy incision. Resolution is estimated to be 5 to 10 μm. Application of this instrumentation to photoablative excimer keratectomy has been discussed. The possibility of real-time monitoring of the very small changes occurring during this procedure might significantly improve the predictability and value of the procedure. Of particular interest, this technique does not require specular reflection, and may be used on rough surfaces such as those encountered during photoablative excimer keratectomy.

SUMMARY

The qualitative and quantitative determination of corneal position and curvature is an exciting frontier of corneal surgery. We are fortunate to live in a time when such instruments are available to us. Likewise, we are obligated to explore the basic principles of operation and to understand the appropriate limitations and strengths of each instrument so that we may gain the most information from their use. As in radiology, in which a similar proliferation of imaging devices recently has become available, it may be that a combination of measurements may yield the most accurate picture of a given cornea. For example, in our practice the combination of keratometry and photokeratometry provides excellent overall assessment of the preoperative and postoperative cornea. For assessment of optical zone, corneal curvature precisely at the corneal apex, and preoperative planning for corneal relaxing incisions, computed topology provides valuable additional information.

For the operating room, the Troutman keratometer is invaluable in both the real-time evaluation and performance of astigmatic and corneal surgery. In our minds, it is virtually impossible to accurately perform such surgery without a surgical keratometer. Although quantitative surgical keratometers have provided quantitative measurements in the operating room, their routine use must be qualified by somewhat clumsy mechanical operation and results that often do not correlate with measurements taken in the clinic. Nonetheless, continuing work in this area no doubt will provide us with accurate and easily obtained quantitative measurements. Should real-time computed topology someday become available in the operating room, it will be the challenge of the future to translate this development into better results for our patients.

Chapter 6

Special Refraction Techniques in Astigmatism

Among refractive disorders, astigmatism may be the least understood and the most undertreated, perhaps because of its relatively recent introduction into clinical practice. The early work of Helmholtz made detection of astigmatism an objective reality, and this was quickly incorporated as the major means for determining the astigmatic portion of the refraction. The early keratometers were clumsy to use, and fogging, retinoscopy, cross-cylinders, and astigmatic dials, to mention only a few, were developed as an alternative to the use of the keratometer. By the time Javal and Schiotz developed a more convenient instrument, these techniques were well established, and the keratometer for many ophthalmologists became of secondary importance. It was not until astigmatism could be corrected surgically that the interest of corneal and refractive surgeons in the keratometer as a primary refractive tool for the detection and correction of corneal astigmatism was rejuvenated.

SPHERICAL REFRACTION

A regular spherical surface (Plate 6–1,A) permits parallel light rays to focus at a single point. Because the distance between the lens and the focal point is unique for each lens, the power is defined as the inverse of the focal length. Spherical optics have been explored for hundreds of years, and form the basis of our understanding of the inner workings of the human eye. We realize that in the optimal circumstance of emmetropia, the eye acts as a lens system to focus light on the retina (Plate 6–1,B).

If the light is focused slightly forward of the retina, a spherical blur pervades the image, and we refer to the condition as myopia (Plate 6–1,C). If the light focuses slightly beyond the retina, we experience a

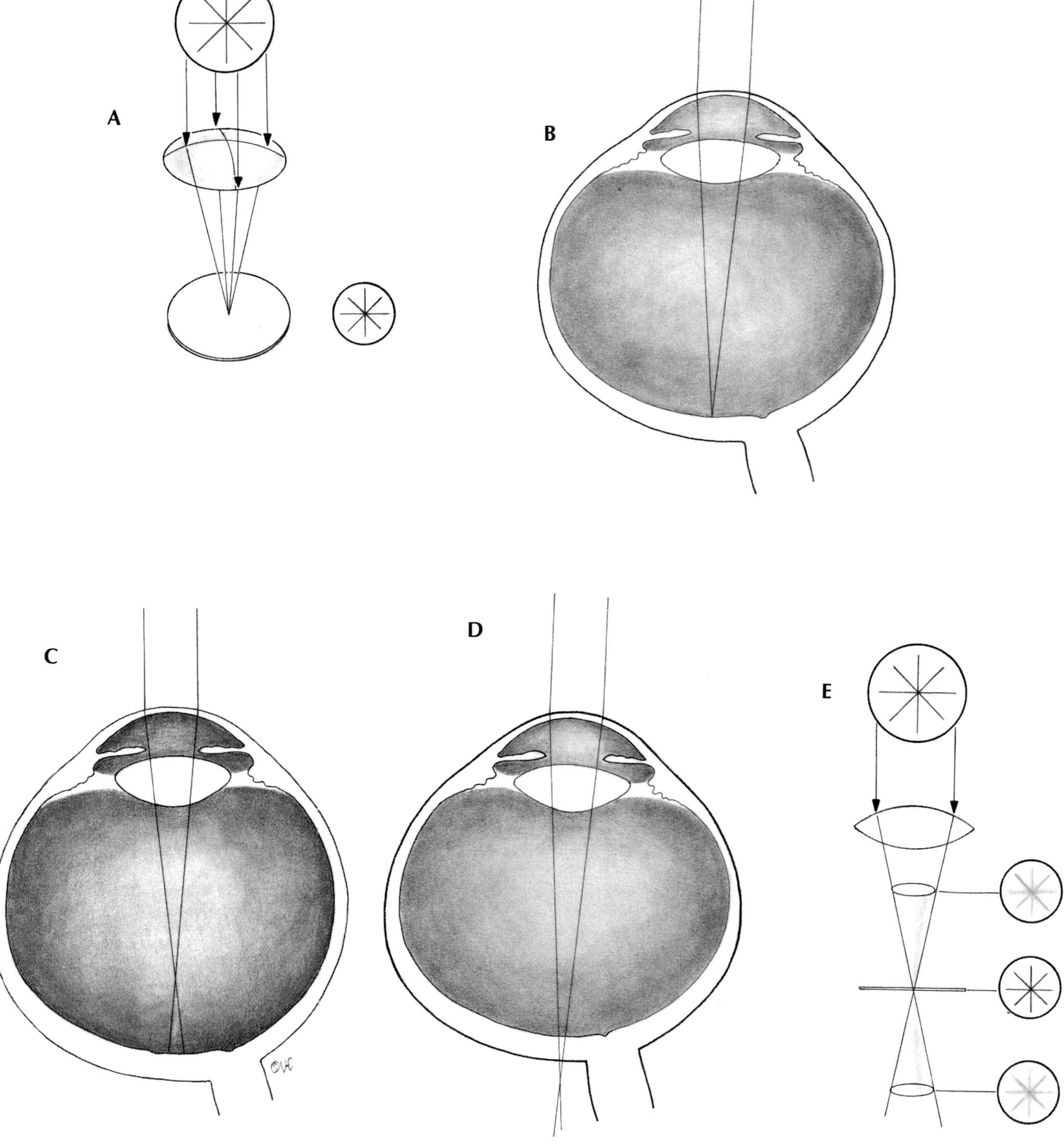

A, light impinging on a spherical lens focusing to a single point. **B,** emmetropic eye showing convergence of light rays on the macula. **C,** myopic eye showing convergence of light rays before reaching the macula. **D,** hyperopic eye showing convergence of light rays beyond the macula. **E,** light rays showing symmetric blur anterior and posterior to the focal point.

Special Refraction Techniques in Astigmatism **119**

symmetrical blur, or hyperopia (Plate 6–1,D). Reflection will quickly convince the reader that relative to the focal point of the lens or lens system, conditions are symmetric, both along the line bisecting the center of the lens and the focal point and angularly sweeping around this axis (Plate 6–1,E). The high degree of symmetry surrounding the focal point thus leads to the singularly successful nature of spherical manifest refraction.

CYLINDRICAL LENS

This discussion highlights the degree of three-dimensional thinking that is required to fully understand relatively simple concepts such as hyperopia and myopia. The ability to picture elements situated in three dimensions does not come naturally; it is far more common to think in two dimensions, as in lines on a piece of paper. Hyperopia and myopia can easily be represented in two dimensions (i.e., on a piece of paper) because of the high degree of symmetry. Astigmatism cannot be so easily represented. Light impinging on a cylindrical surface focuses on a line instead of a point (Plate 6–2,A). Light impinging on a true cylindrical surface focuses symmetrically on a line at a fixed distance from the cylindrical surface, defined as the focal length of the lens. In a lens with both spherical and cylindrical surfaces, the situation is analogous to that seen in the human eye (Plate 6–2,B). In this condition, astigmatism is most easily considered as light focusing on two specific planes, with the lines of focus 90 degrees apart. The well-known conoid of Sturm is actually not a cone coming to a single point, as in myopia and hyperopia, but instead represents an area of extreme complexity in which no true focus exists. The area at which the many rays of light come closest together is called the *circle of least confusion*, but in fact the light rays do not form a circle in this area, and this can result in a double image at this location. Blurring in the area of least confusion is reasonably symmetric, allowing a gross, spherical equivalent determination of a compound error.

Cylindrical lenses to correct astigmatic errors are available in both plus and minus cylinders. Minus cylinder astigmatic lenses have the desirable property of a minus spherical equivalent (Plate 6–2,C). Because most patients are slightly nearsighted, this lens can simplify refraction and is used in fogging. The cylindrical axis is oriented along the flatter meridian, which can be confusing for refractive surgeons. Plus cylinder lenses have a plus spherical equivalent that must be balanced by minus sphere. The steep meridian in which a tight suture (or sutures) is located conveniently corresponds to the axis of the plus cylinder, and is less confusing. (Plate 6–2,D).

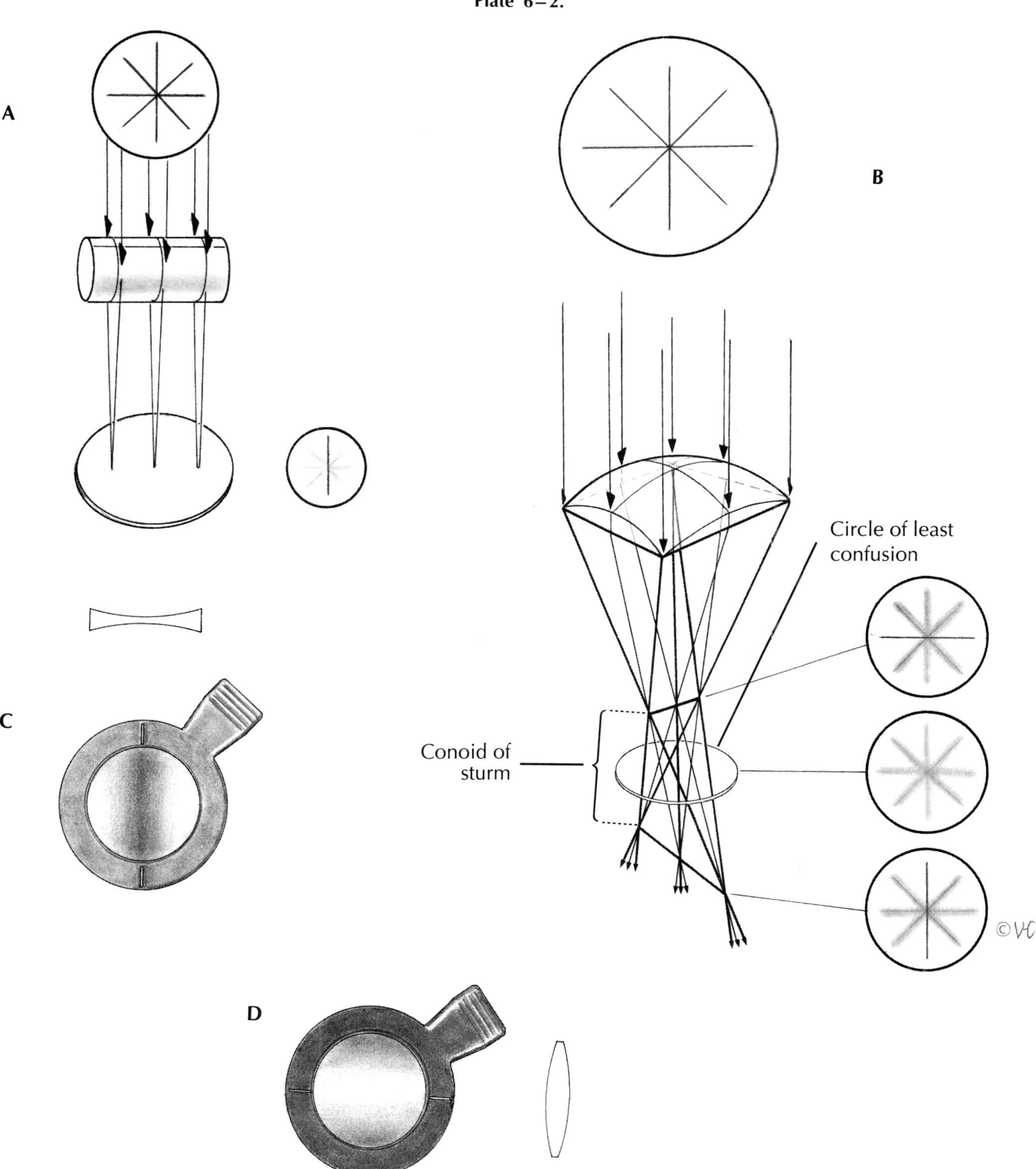

A, light impinging on a cylindrical lens focusing to a line. **B,** light impinging on a spherocylindrical lens, showing asymmetric blur around the circle of least confusion. **C,** minus cylindrical lens. **D,** plus cylindrical lens.

Because astigmatism is a vector problem, two values need to be determined during the manifest refraction, as opposed to the single value determined during a spherical refraction: the axis of the astigmatism in the plane of the cornea and the amount of astigmatism. That a single number can represent the spherical error is a reflection of the high degree of symmetry that exists for this problem; that is, the value is the same in all directions. That astigmatism must be represented by two numbers means that this element is not so symmetric and in fact is represented in mathematics by the term *vector quantity*. Vector quantities have special rules for addition and subtraction that are not the same as the conventional rules used in common mathematics. When we refract the cornea in a patient with astigmatism and place spherocylindrical lenses before the eye or when we perform refractive surgery on this eye, we are using the principals of vector mathematics.

Vector mathematics are not encountered often in everyday life, and a few relevant points should be mentioned. A vector is an object that can only be described by two separate quantities, such as direction and length, or in a different nomenclature by the projection on the X axis and on the Y axis (Plate 6–3,A). If two vectors are added together, we may add the X values together to determine the final projection of the resultant vector on the X axis, and similarly we may add the Y values together to determine the final projection of the resultant vector on the Y axis. Geometrically we may construct a rhomboid, with the initial vectors serving as the four sides. The result of adding these two vectors will be the diagonal of this rhomboid (Plate 6–3,B). It is clear that when vectors are added both the direction and the length of a vector change. When refracting a patient with astigmatism, these principles can be used to our advantage to determine both the axis and the amount of the astigmatic vector.

Two vectors of equal magnitude pointed exactly apart are equal to zero, whereas two equal vectors pointed in the same direction add together to give twice the length of the original vectors (Plate 6–3,C). If the two vectors are not pointed exactly apart but instead are aligned 10 degrees from one another, an interesting property emerges. A new vector is created that, in terms of degrees, is far from the direction of either of the two original vectors (Plate 6–3,D). If the vector is displaced 10 degrees farther, the size of the resultant vector is larger but only slightly displaced compared with the previous displacement of the second vector. If we create a collection of such displacements and resultant vectors, we can begin to see a pattern developing that will help us in determining the proper axis of astigmatism. If the patient is presented with an astigmatic correction at a given axis and the axis of correction is not consistent with the patient's own meridian of astigmatic error, a resultant vector will be created,

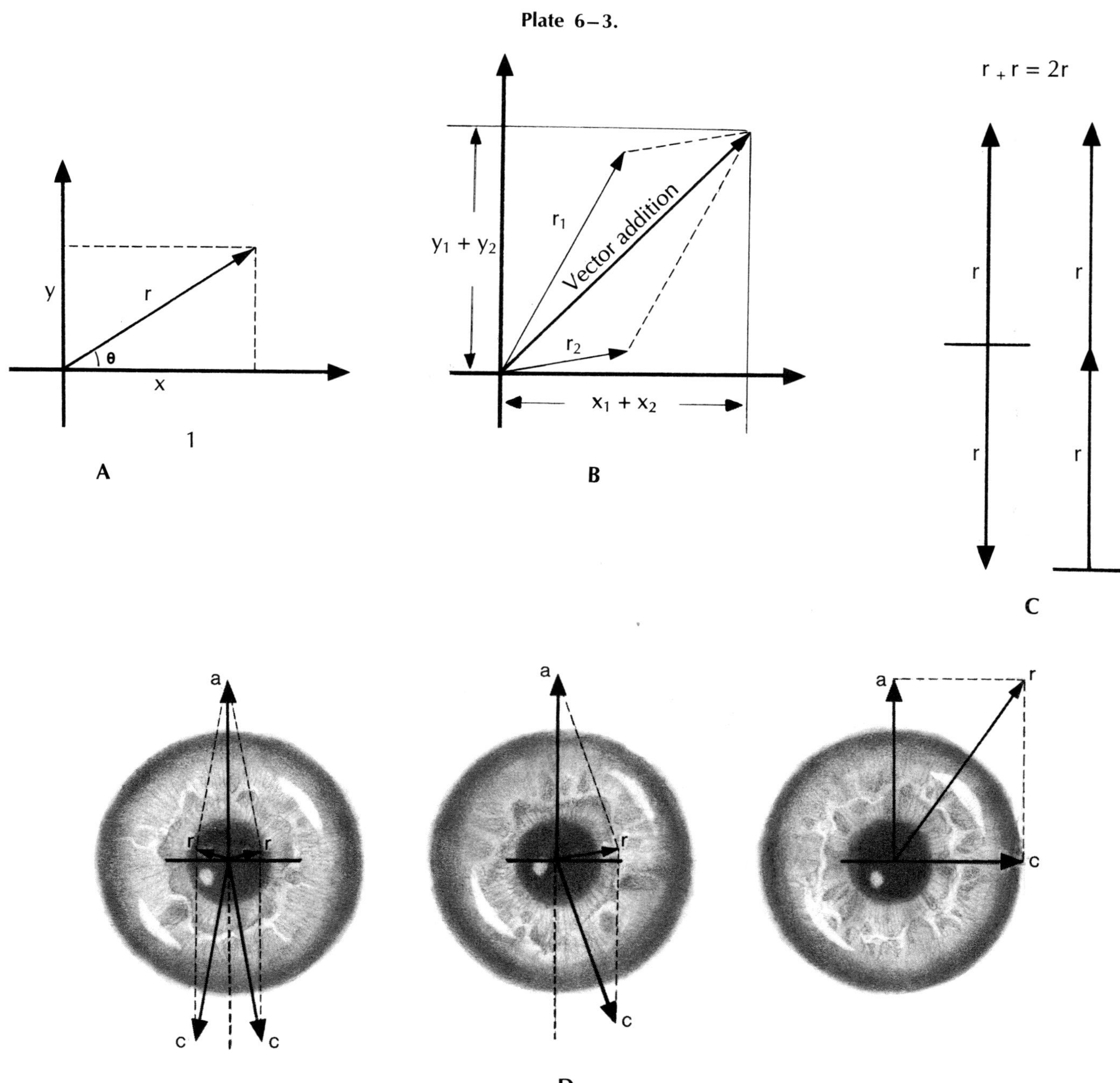

A, representation of a vector quantity by two values, axis and length (θ, r) or X and Y coordinates. **B,** addition of two vectors obtained by adding X values and separately adding Y values, resulting in the diagonal of a rhomboid. **C,** addition of two vectors of the same size in opposite directions, yielding zero, and in the same direction, yielding twice the length of the original vectors. **D,** vector diagram shows the effect of adding astigmatic lenses at different axes, showing diminished resultant vector as null point is approached.

as described. Because the patient when presented with a choice will always choose the smaller vector, this provides a way of guiding the refraction toward the proper axis to produce a null value for the astigmatic error. As the patient is gradually presented with choices closer and closer to the true astigmatic meridian, the resultant vectors will become smaller and smaller, until the patient is inevitably shown choices that straddle the astigmatic meridian, at which point the patient will report that the choices are the same.

JACKSON CROSS-CYLINDER

The first cross-cylinder was introduced in 1849 and named the Stokes lens. This lens consisted of two cylindrical lenses, one convex cylinder and one concave cylinder, that could be rotated relative to each other. If the cylinders were made parallel to one another the power was zero; if they were placed perpendicular to one another they formed a sphere, the power of which was determined by the cylinders being used (e.g., 2 D, 4 D, . . .). The lens was ungainly to operate and was not widely used. In 1885 W.S. Dennett improved the mounting, and Edward Jackson reported his results in 1887. The modern device with fixed lenses at axes perpendicular to each another has come to be known as the Jackson cross-cylinder (Plate 6–4). The significant attention that this instrument gained did not come from Jackson's original papers, but from W.H. Crisp, who popularized the instrument.

In practice, the Jackson cross-cylinder is available in powers ranging from 0.12 to 1.00 D. The eye is refracted with spherical power to a best-corrected refraction, thus placing the interval of Sturm astride the macula. An arbitrary cylindrical correction is placed before the eye, and a gross determination of cylindrical axis is determined by presenting the patient with various choices as the proposed astigmatic correction is rotated in front of the eye. Once an astigmatic axis is grossly determined, the Jackson cross-cylinder is introduced, straddling the axis of the cylinder in place before the patient's eye. The Jackson cross-cylinder is then twirled, reversing the positions of the plus and minus cross-cylinders. The patient is questioned as to the preferable location of the Jackson cross-cylinder. If the two locations are the same, the position of the axis is deemed appropriate. If the patient prefers one position of the cross-cylinder, the cylindrical correction is rotated, toward the white dot if the "plus" cylinder is being used, and toward the red dot if the "minus" cylinder correction is being used. This procedure is performed in a recursive manner until the cylindrical axis is defined. This portion of the procedure utilizes the vector properties, using the small astigmatic power of the Jackson cross-cylinder to add to the correcting astigmatic power, resulting in a vector addition that is closer or farther from the null correction. Although this is an ele-

Plate 6–4.

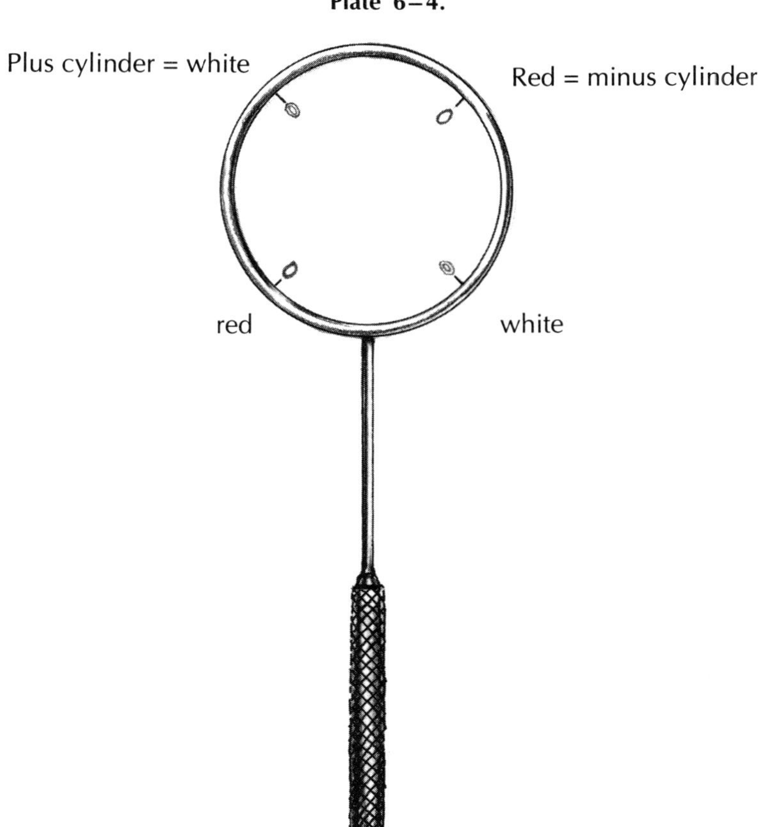

Jackson cross-cylinder.

gant approach, one might well ask why the refractionist does not simply rotate the correcting axis in a stepwise fashion and question the patient as to clarity of vision. This is discussed further in a later section.

The power of the cylindrical correction can be determined by aligning the dots on the Jackson cross-cylinder with the axis of correction or by rotating the handle 45 degrees. The patient is then presented with an alternative of the red dots or, by twisting the handle, the white dots along the astigmatic corneal meridian. If the patient finds both alternatives the same, the astigmatic correction in place is correct. If the patient prefers the white dots and one is working in plus cylinder correction, additional plus cylinder is added along that axis. As plus cylinder is added, minus sphere also must be added to the correction to keep the interval of Sturm balanced across the retina, or in other terms, to maintain the spherical equivalent. For example, if plus 0.50 D astigmatic correction is added, minus 0.25 D sphere must be inserted into the correction to maintain the spherical equivalent. This procedure is then repeated recursively until the proper astigmatic correction is obtained.

Again, this portion of the procedure uses the vector addition and subtraction of parallel vectors. One might well ask why simply changing the power of the astigmatic correction is not comparable to or perhaps better than use of the Jackson cross-cylinder. One answer might be that this instrument was introduced for use in conjunction with trial frames, which made the exchange of lenses somewhat clumsy. With a phorometer, changing astigmatic power is simple and probably obviates the use of the Jackson cross-cylinder for the determination of cylindrical power.

As we have seen, the Jackson cross-cylinder can be an effective means of refining both the power and the axis of the astigmatic correction. However, its limitation is that a reasonable approximation of the correction should be in place before use of this instrument. If the patient has a large astigmatic error and the Jackson cross-cylinder is used to find that correction, starting with an astigmatic correction that is significantly different from the final correction, the patient will be subjected to many recursive steps and may tire during this process. As a result, an incorrect astigmatic correction may be prescribed. The importance of the starting point is crucial to the successful outcome of this procedure.

One way to view the process of correction of astigmatism is to consider it a means of collapsing the interval of Sturm, thus converting the astigmatic refraction into a simple spherical refraction. One means to accomplish this end is to use the concept of hyperopic fogging (Plate 6–5,A). The concept involves use of the plus sphere to move both astigmatic focal points within the eye, thus creating a compound myopic astigmatism (Plate 6–5,B). The patient is asked to observe an astigmatic clock in which the lines parallel to the plus cylinder axis or perpendicular to the minus cylinder axis are seen as sharper than the rest. Minus cylinder correction is then placed before the patient's eye, with the axis parallel to the blurriest lines and perpendicular to the sharpest lines. As minus cylinder correction is increased, fogging is maintained by adding additional plus sphere, thus keeping both astigmatic focal points within the eye. The procedure is complete when all lines appear to be equally sharp (Plate 6–5,C). At this point the problem has been converted into a simple spherical refraction, and minus sphere is added until visual acuity is maximized, thus placing the focal point on the retina (Plate 6–5,D). At the conclusion of this procedure the astigmatic correction may be tested with the Jackson cross-cylinder.

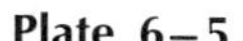

A   B   C   D

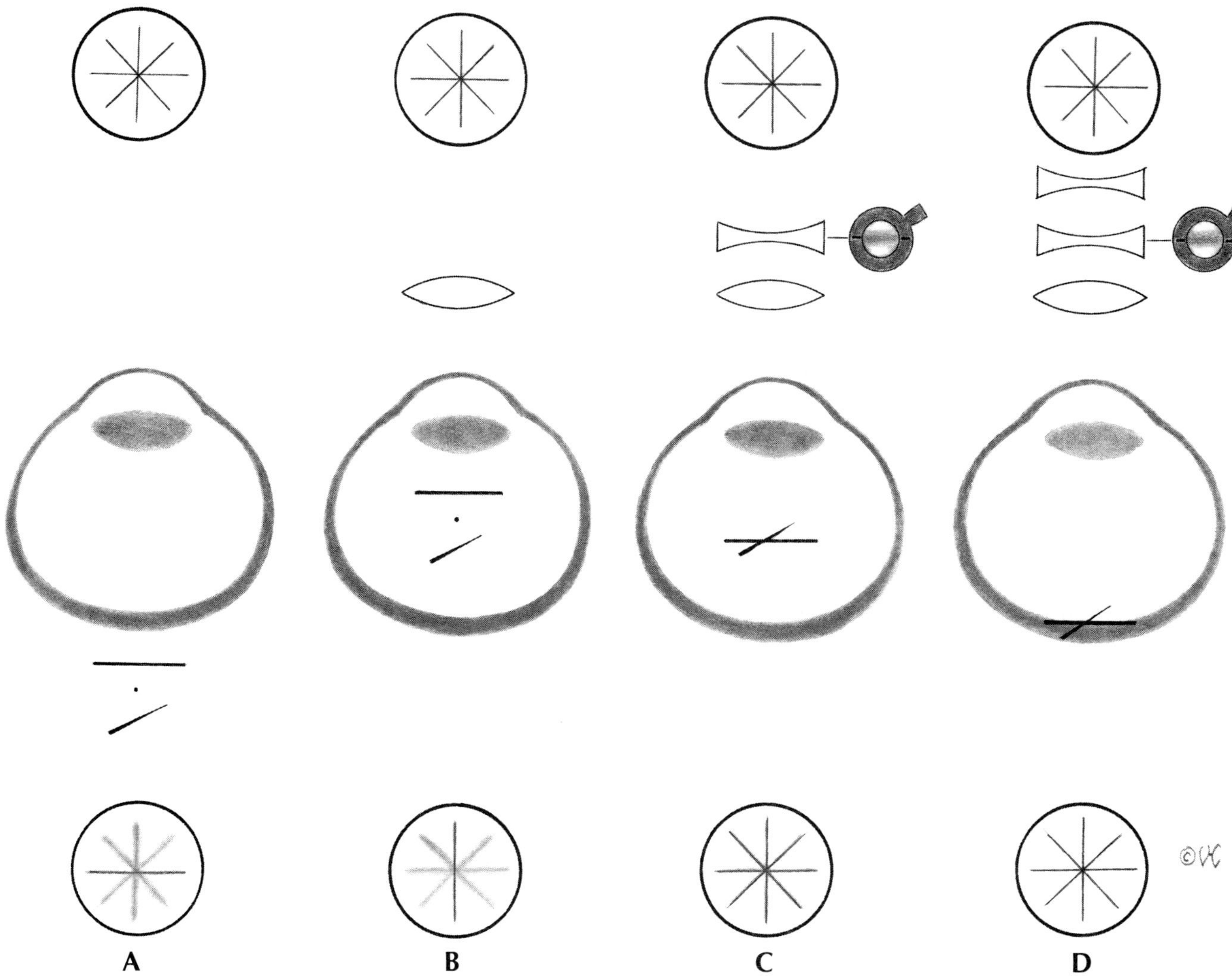

A, starting point of the fogging technique, with appearance of astigmatic clock. **B,** addition of plus sphere to move the astigmatic focal lines within the eye, and appearance of astigmatic clock. **C,** collapse of the interval of Sturm using minus cylinder lenses, and appearance of astigmatic clock showing symmetric blurring. **D,** addition of minus cylinder to move the focal point to the retina, showing symmetric sharpness of astigmatic clock.

KERATOMETRIC ASTIGMATISM REFRACTION

Although fogging can produce an acceptable refraction, it has several drawbacks that should be mentioned. First, it is time consuming and potentially confusing for the patient, and may result in an inaccurate representation of the astigmatic error if the patient begins to tire. In addition, it requires the use of minus cylinder lenses, which often are not available in an ophthalmology office or, if used, can cause significant confusion to technicians and others recording notations on the patient's chart. An alternative to these subjective methods of the Jackson cross-cylinder and subjective fogging technique is the use of keratometry readings as a starting point for the astigmatic refraction.

The advantages of using a keratometric reading as a starting point for the astigmatic refraction are simplicity, reduction of refraction time, and improved accuracy, because neither the refractionist nor the patient are tired by many recursive evaluations of clarity. Both the Jackson cross-cylinder method and the subjective fogging method can be used to quickly check the accuracy of the keratometric readings and further refine the astigmatic correction. In practice, however, we have found that the keratometric starting point invariably is close to the expected result and that the axis of astigmatism can be refined simply and accurately by placing the astigmatic correction in a trial lens set or the phoropter and allowing the patient to adjust the axis for optimal clarity. In most cases this will yield an axis close to the keratometric axis, and allows the patient to experience in a dynamic fashion the vector principles outlined above.

The keratometric readings in plus cylinder are placed in the trial lens set or phoropter. As a starting point, minus sphere is added equal to the amount of cylinder. For example, if the keratometry readings are 43.00 × 90/45.00 × 180, 2.00 D is placed in the phoropter at axis 180 in plus cylinder. In addition, minus sphere is added in the amount of −2.00 D. At this point, spherical refraction is performed to determine the spherical correction that will yield the best Snellen visual acuity. Although not required, the conversion of the starting point to a minus spherical equivalent is appropriate in most patients with myopic compound or simple astigmatism, and usually saves time.

The final refinement of the refraction proceeds as follows. The patient should be encouraged to rotate the trial lens slowly until blurring is encountered in each direction across the axis of correction, with gradually decreased amplitudes of oscillation around the clearest point until the appropriate axis is determined. This method is essentially the same as that used with the Jackson cross-cylinder, but obtains larger changes to the size of the correcting cylinder change (0.5–1.00 D for the Jackson cross-cylinder vs. full cylindrical correction (Plate 6–6). This technique involves the patient without requiring responses, rather than providing only one or

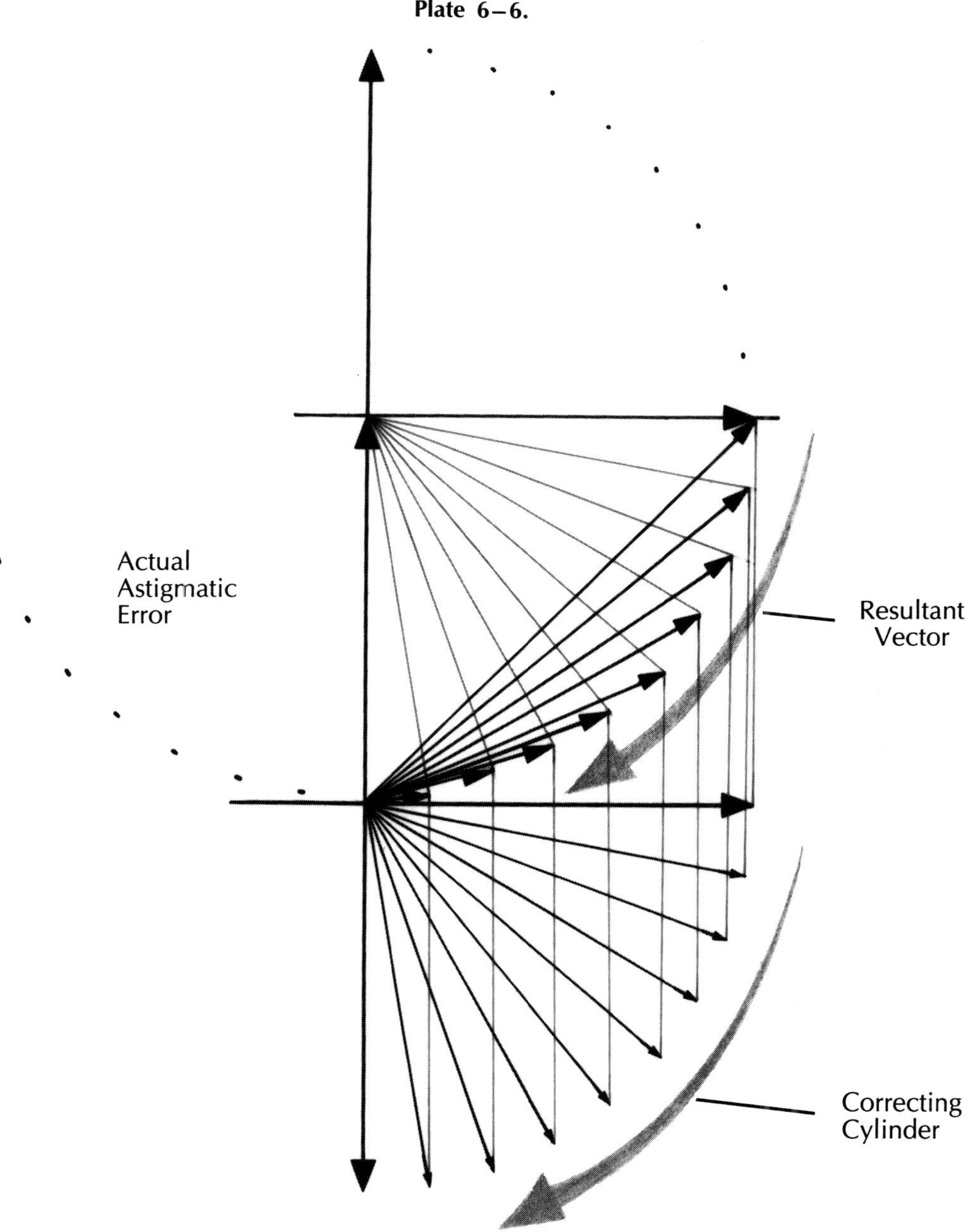

Vector effect of rotation of astigmatic correction, showing progressive reduction of the resultant vector as null point is approached.

two choices in a recursive manner, each of which requires a verbal response. In this manner the final refinement of cylinder axis can be accomplished rapidly without tiring the patient. The amount of astigmatism may then be adjusted using the principle of maintaining the spherical equivalent by adding minus sphere when plus cylinder is added. When the final astigmatic value is determined, the spherical component may be rechecked, as in a traditional spherical refraction, using fogging or the duochrome test.

REFRACTION OF IRREGULAR ASTIGMATISM

Two basic techniques exist for correction of irregular astigmatism; both involve the use of contact lenses. Regular-irregular astigmatism, such as keratoconus, has multiple focal planes that limit visual acuity (Plate 6–7,A). The goal is to regularize the surface and create a single focal point. These patients usually have myopia due to corneal steepening, and appropriate contact lens fitting will depress the cone, fitting the contact lens slightly flat, to absorb at least a portion of the myopia by physical flattening of the cone (Plate 6–7,B). This close contact between the cornea and contact lens can be seen, with the aid of fluorescein stain, in the form of the classic *bull's eye pattern* (Plate 6–7,C). Although the fitting of contact lenses in keratoconus is beyond the scope of this discussion, the principle of the use of rigid contact lenses to regularize the cornea in regular-irregular astigmatism is a key decision. Spectacle lenses, which cannot accommodate the multiple focal planes of irregular corneas, may provide adequate vision in darkened rooms under controlled conditions, but are not sufficient to meet the demands of ordinary life.

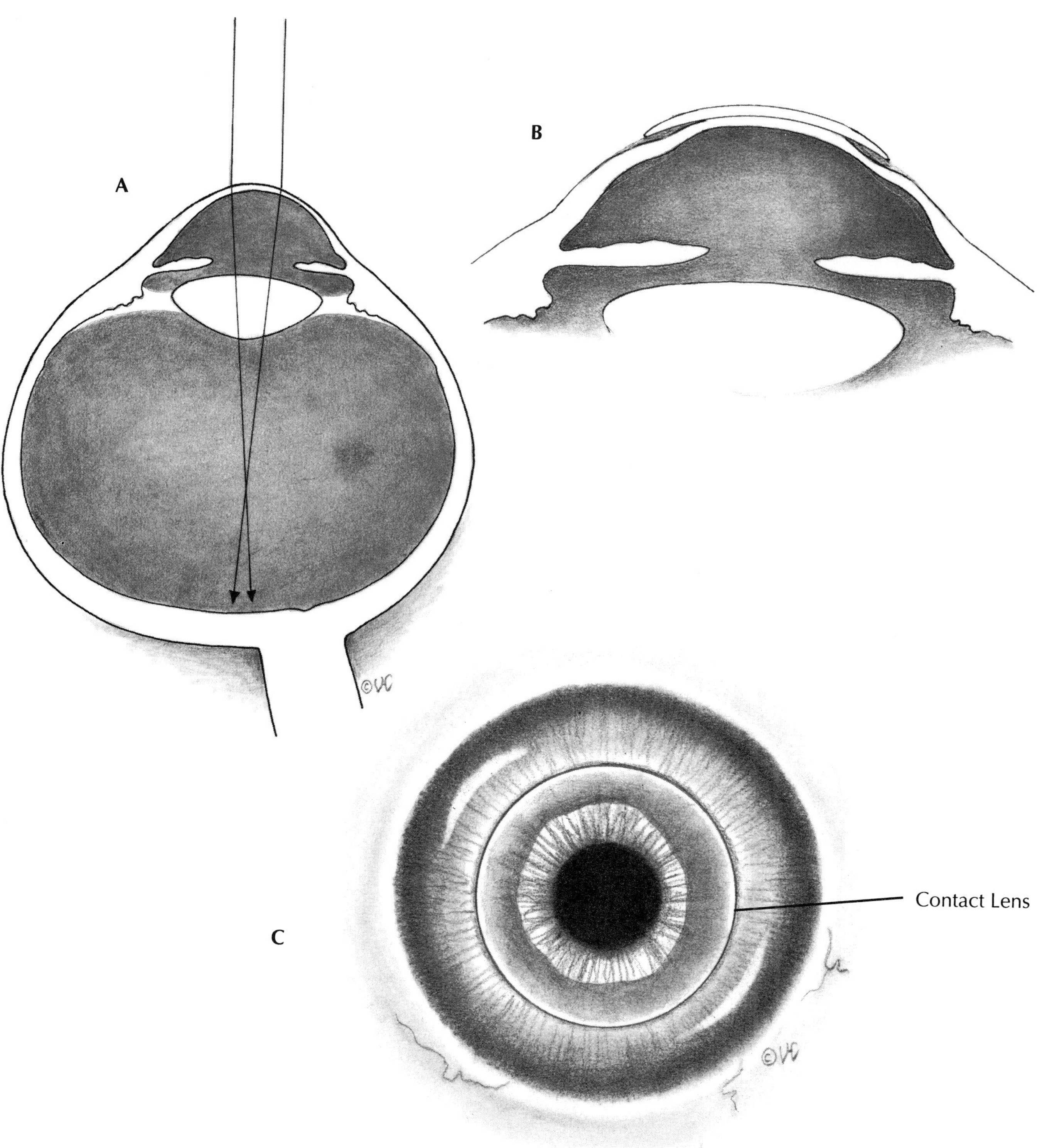

A, keratoconus with myopic irregular astigmatism due to steepened cornea. **B,** rigid contact lens fitting shows flattening and regularization of the cone. **C,** rigid contact lens fitting in keratoconus shows bull's-eye pattern of fluorescein stain.

The problem of irregular-irregular astigmatism is usually one of surface roughness leading to unacceptable glare (Plate 6–8,A). In this situation, the most common error is failure to recognize the problem. Mild to moderate surface roughness may not be immediately obvious, and the addition of a soft contact lens may produce a startling improvement in vision by producing a smooth anterior surface while filling the irregularities beneath the contact lens with refractively neutral tear film (Plate 6–8,B). The contact lens used in this circumstance may both improve vision and provide therapeutic healing of the surface. For more extreme roughness, a rigid contact lens may be used, fit slightly flat, to flatten the more extreme projections. Fluorescein stain may be used to observe the filling of irregular depressions and to assess proper fitting (Plate 6–8,C).

Contact lenses are particularly important in the diagnostic evaluation of corneal disease, because irregular astigmatism often distorts potential testing of visual acuity. The use of rigid or soft contact lenses in conjunction with the Guyton potential acuity meter test instrument or by interferometry may significantly improve predictability, particularly in corneal disease resulting in rough surfaces.

SUMMARY

The introduction of cylindrical correction into spectacles in the latter part of the 19th century represents a second approximation to the practical business of refining the human refractive error. Initially, spherical errors were the only correction possible, primarily because of the mechanics of actually producing spectacle lenses. As more sophisticated techniques were used, it became possible to produce a second generation of more sophisticated lenses that corrected astigmatism. Although this approach has, in general, been exceedingly productive and successful, assumptions are included in this model of the human optical system. One such assumption is that the plus and minus axes of astigmatism are perpendicular. In fact, astigmatic readings in cornea transplant patients, taken with a keratometer or the more sophisticated corneal topology units now available, clearly show that this assumption is not always true. In most corneas this assumption is valid enough to provide acceptable vision with the methods outlined.

A second controversy that remains hidden in our discussion of competing methods to determine astigmatic error lies in the location of this astigmatism within the human optical system. Gullstrand and others involved in physiologic optics found the cornea to be responsible for twice the overall effective power relative to the human lens. Moreover, because of the cornea's relatively exposed position in the eye and its dual role in mechanical support and refraction, it was surmised that the cornea accounted for the majority of asphericity or astigmatism in the human op-

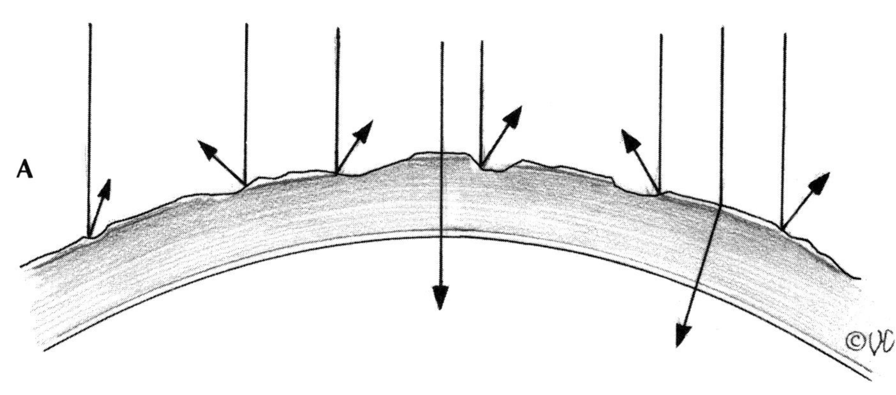

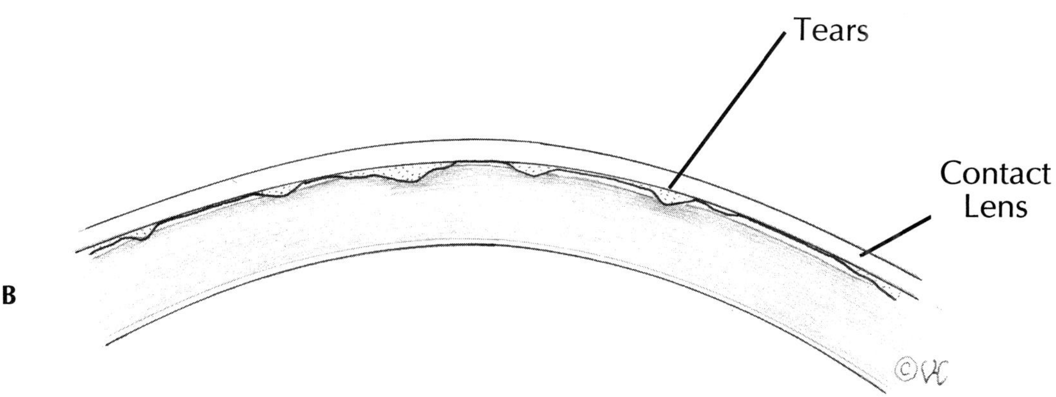

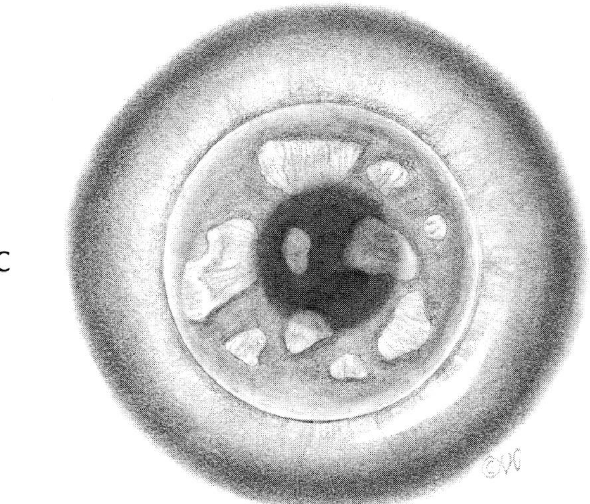

A, irregular surface with scattering of light, causing glare. **B,** contact lens over irregular surface, creating regular anterior surface. **C,** contact lens fitting over irregular surface shows pooling of fluorescein stain within surface depressions.

tical system. However, the development of the keratometer and comparisons between so-called corneal astigmatism and astigmatic error determined by subjective responses as to the clarity of a Snellen chart during manifest refraction often differed significantly. An immediate conclusion by clinicians observing this discrepancy was that significant astigmatic error might lie in the other major component of the human optical system, the lens. This controversy between those who believed astigmatism resides only in the cornea and those who believed astigmatism resides in both the cornea and the lens was not clearly resolved until the widespread use of the intraocular lens showed conclusively that the astigmatic error in a given patient did not change significantly when the natural lens was removed. Both Moore and Binkhorst originally found more astigmatism in patients with an intraocular lens than in those without. The topic was reviewed by Maltzman, whose conclusion was that astigmatism was primarily corneal in origin. In a study exploring the maximum amount of induced astigmatism by an intraocular lens tilted or displaced forward, Lakshminarayanan found a maximum induced astigmatism of 0.50 D, with an average of considerably less. Tschering found almost no tilt in the normal human lens, corresponding to <0.25 D.

These and other studies have shown that nearly all of human astigmatic error lies in the cornea, and the accessibility of the cornea to the keratometer makes its inclusion in the refraction process natural. By establishing a starting point that is essentially correct by means of a single objective measurement, the astigmatic refraction can be reduced to a much simpler spherical refraction.

The subsequent simplicity and saving of time translate into a more accurate and pleasant experience for both the refractionist and the patient.

Chapter 7

Microscope, Patient Preparation, and Instrumentation for Refractive Keratoplasty

Nowhere in ophthalmic surgery are microscopic magnification, microsurgical instruments, microsurgical needles, and suture materials more important to performance and results than in corneal refractive surgery. Ophthalmic microsurgical instrumentation is discussed in detail in *Microsurgery of the Anterior Segment of the Eye*, volumes 1 and 2. In this chapter, the highlights of the subject as originally presented are reviewed and specific details given of instruments and microscopes as they are used currently for prevention of corneal astigmatism as well as in corrective refractive surgical techniques. A number of new instruments have been introduced in recent years; others have been refined or modified. Because the number of manufacturers of microsurgical instruments has multiplied since publication of the two previous volumes, we have attempted to pick the best instruments generically rather than as produced by a specific manufacturer. It behooves the corneal refractive surgeon to examine carefully and compare specific instruments from several manufacturers. Not all manufacturers or instruments are created equal, although they may bear a strong superficial resemblance. Although the working end of an instrument should be similar with regard to its intended function, different manufacturers have a tendency to design a distinctive handle to distinguish themselves in the market place. The names of surgeon "developers" usually indicate only a difference in the handle; the function of the tip is essentially the same among broad groups. All other things being equal as far as intended function is concerned, the surgeon should choose the most ergonomically comfortable handle design.

MICROSCOPES

It is probable that most surgeons reading this volume will have at their disposal one or more modern surgical microscopes. For refractive surgery, the microscope used should incorporate zoom optics, have a working distance of not more than 175 mm, and have an inclined or folded binocular that limits eye-to-field distance to no greater than 350 mm. It should be fitted with a beam splitter to incorporate television, cine, or still photography equipment (Plate 7–1).

Although the microscope should have a tilt mechanism, the optics should be vertical to the cornea during refractive surgery, because the surgical keratometer or a centering device is not accurate in a tilted position. The microscope body should be suspended from a self-centering X-Y system, manipulated by a motorized foot control. The foot control also should actuate fine focus zoom and tilt and be fitted with on-off switches for oblique slitlamp or coaxial illumination.

For economy, most modern microscopes are configured primarily for extracapsular cataract surgery and have only coaxial illumination, which is difficult to use for corneal surgery. The high reflectivity of the corneal surface to direct illumination not only distracts the surgeon but also can be dangerous to the patient's eye as a result of prolonged direct exposure of the macula, because any protective device obscures the working field. Not only is oblique illumination safer and less tiring, it gives better shadow detail and stereopsis during performance of the precise cutting maneuvers and suturing necessary for accurate corneal and refractive surgery. A second focal-oblique illuminator convertible to a slitlamp is useful, especially in lamellar techniques.

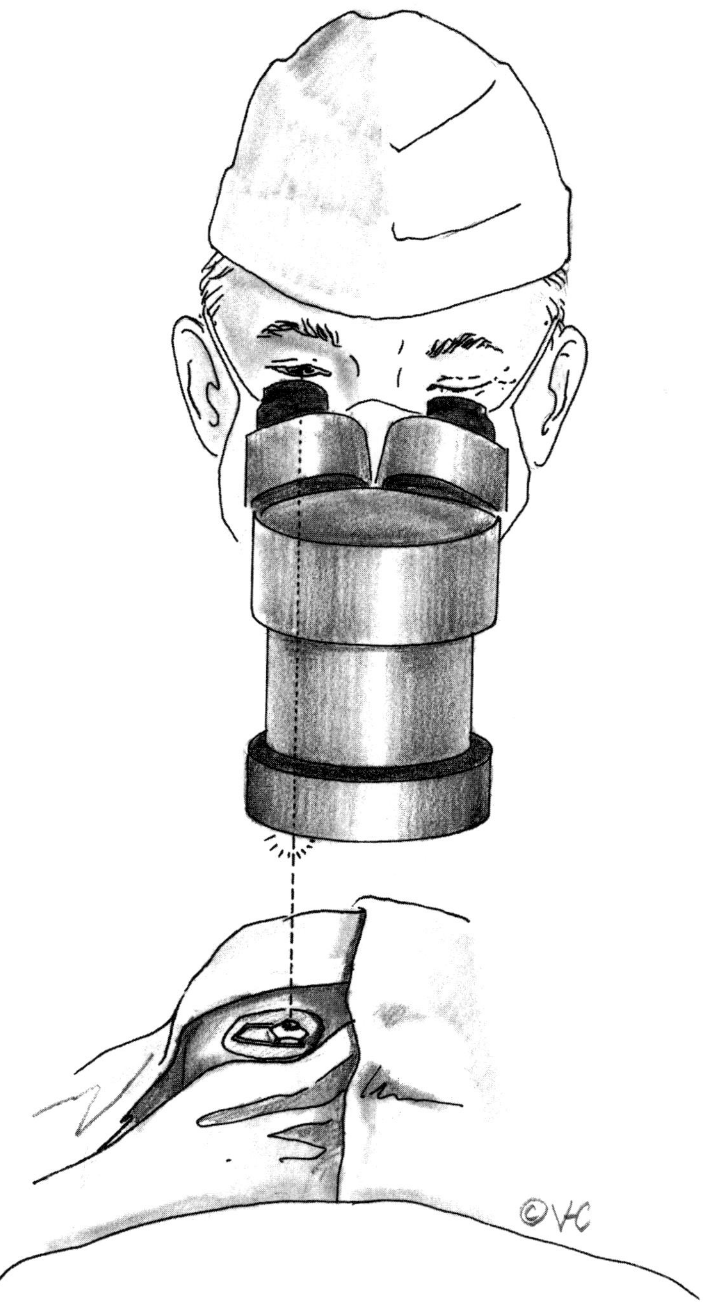

Surgical microscope. Surgeon centering fixation device for refractive surgery, microscope vertical to cornea.

A surgical keratometer attachment is an essential addition to the microscope for any corneal surgery, including cataract, particularly in surgery for astigmatism, to verify preoperative keratometry and to monitor intraoperatively the effect of incisions, excisions, and suturing (Plate 7–2). Qualitative keratometers are less expensive and almost as useful intraoperatively as quantitative keratometers, which are in the main used as qualitative instruments, because quantitatively they do not extrapolate better to postoperative results. The surgical keratometer is useful primarily to locate an astigmatic meridian, to identify areas for incision or excision, and to monitor effects of suturing, astigmatism compensation and compression sutures.

The zoom microscope system should have a range of magnification of approximately $4\times$ to $18\times$. The lower magnifications, up to $6\times$, are used primarily for identification purposes. Most surgery is done between $6\times$ and $12\times$. Magnification over $12\times$ is useful to enhance the accuracy of the surgical keratometer and to inspect for incision-suture irregularities or microdehiscences.

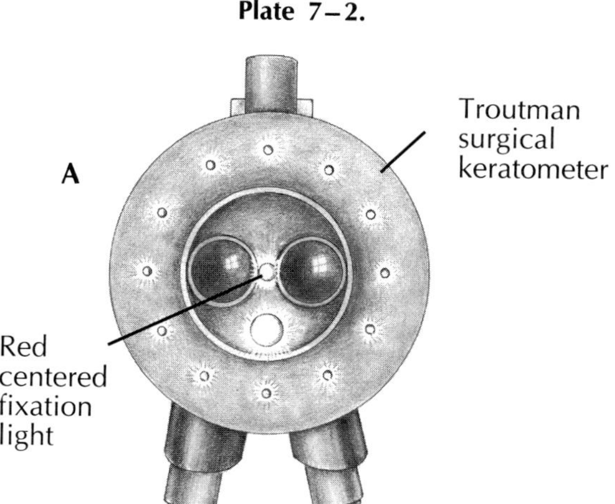

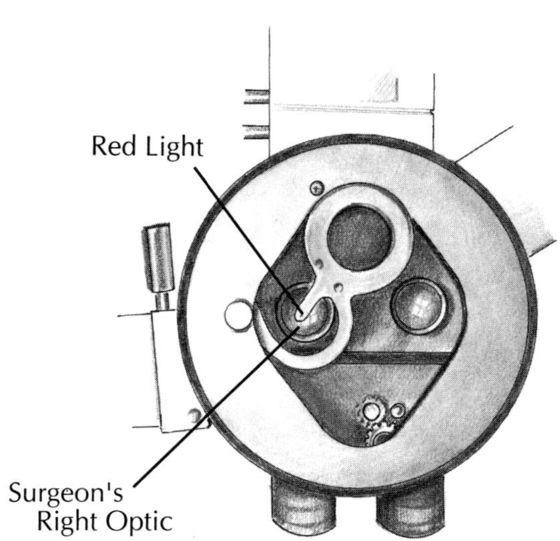

A, Troutman surgical keratometer. Centered fixation light, patient view. (Weck microscope). **B,** Troutman surgical keratometer. Centered fixation light (Topcon microscope).

SURGEON SEATING

As important as the microscope for magnification is the comfort of the surgeon during its use. The surgeon should select an ergonomically designed chair that provides forward-tilted seating without thigh pressure. It should be fitted with an adjustable back that provides support in the forward-leaning position assumed by the microsurgeon over the microscope binocular. Height adjustment should be under surgeon control, and the chair should be adjustable to accommodate surgeons of all heights and girths. A tilting, height-adjustable, platform for the foot-control stool should be provided for the shorter surgeon.

The operating table should have sufficient room to allow the surgeon's knees and foot controls to be directly under the patient's headrest. The footrest platform should be large enough to accommodate secondary controls for other instruments as required. The operating table should be height adjustable, within the range of the chair.

The patient's head should be comfortably immobilized, and draping should provide sufficient airway for patient comfort, especially under local anesthesia. Forearm support is essential to the required instrument control, and can be provided from the chair arms or by a ring support around the patient's head, at the surgeon's preference.

ANESTHESIA

Almost all refractive surgery, with the exception of that combined with extensive intraocular surgery, can be done comfortably with local or topical anesthesia. Refractive surgery and penetrating keratoplasty, with a few exceptions based primarily on general medical problems, can be done as outpatient surgery. The anesthesia department at our institutions preface administration of injection local anesthesia with a short-acting narcotic, such as methohexital (Brevital), so that the patient has no recollection of the local anesthesia administration. For penetrating keratoplasty, retrobulbar anesthesia with lid block is preferred to peribulbar anesthesia. When specialized general anesthesia is available, it can be better used than local anesthesia. Partial penetrating refractive surgery often can be done using a more superficial anesthesia. Sutures are removed easily with local drop medication in an office; an operating room setting is rarely necessary.

Devices such as the Honan balloon should not be used before corneal and refractive surgery, because the eye should be normotensive so that incision pressure will cause minimal corneal distortion.

In patients in whom extensive intraocular surgery must be done after the corneal recipient area has been excised, and medical condition permits, general anesthesia is preferable to local anesthesia, because of the more prolonged surgical procedure and because of the possibility of immediate or delayed retrobulbar extravasation that might promote intraoperative problems with vitreous or from subchoroidal bleeding.

Each patient must be carefully evaluated preoperatively for any drug sensitivities or other nonophthalmologic problems that might complicate anesthesia, the intraoperative period, and the postoperative course. This is particularly true of older patients, who have, on average, six unrelated medical problems.

DRAPING AND EXPOSURE

Draping with specialized ophthalmic paper drapes should leave adequate exposure around the orbit so that the drapes do not interfere with the instruments. Isolation of the lash line with plastic sheeting may be used unless it interferes with instrument insertion or use. Although ordinarily a wire speculum of the light Barraquer type is adequate, lid sutures or lid clips may be useful in an eye with small lid aperture or pathologic lid deformation. Lateral canthotomy occasionally may be indicated to relieve pressure on the globe.

INSTRUMENTS*

The development of specialized microscopes for ophthalmic microsurgery stimulated the refinement of the then-current instrumentation and the development of new instruments that could take advantage of the increased magnification. In recent years a number of new instruments have been developed, not only for microsurgical techniques for keratoplasty, cataract, glaucoma, and trauma, but also because of the increasing interest in corneal refractive surgery.

Because specialized microsurgical instruments are now made by a number of manufacturers, instruments from several different manufacturers are incorporated in a surgical set. These instruments are discussed in groups according to function, and new additions specifically used for preventive or corrective astigmatic surgery are illustrated and described in more detail. The axiom that surgeons are no better than their tools is true in particular in corneal refractive surgery.

*Principles and use of many of the instruments discussed herein are described in greater detail and are illustrated in Troutman RC: *Microsurgery of the Anterior Segment of the Eye*, vols 1 and 2. St Louis, Mosby–Year Book, 1974 and 1977, respectively.
Instruments in Plates 7–3 through 7–22 are shown actual size.

General Principles

To best use instruments, it is important to be aware of the principles of the design that facilitate or improve their intended function. Most of the new instruments, on careful examination, will be found to conform to these basic design principles. It behooves the surgeon who wishes more detailed understanding of these instruments to review these basic principles.

Metallurgy

Although high-grade stainless steel still is used by most manufacturers of microsurgical instruments, improved metallurgy has made it possible to substitute titanium for stainless steel in many cases. Titanium not only is strong, light, and noncorroding, but when well cared for can be more durable and longer lasting than stainless steel. However, the preferred material for scissors, because of better edge quality, is still stainless steel. There has been a proliferation of packaged sterilized disposable instruments made of various plastics and lower quality metals as well as ceramics and crystals. These materials are used for instruments such as trephines and razor blade knives and for ancillary items such as sponges, corneal cutting blocks on which corneal buttons are punched, drapes, and so forth.

Diamond Instruments

Since the days of the early diamond knife these predictably sharp, durable blades have undergone technical refinement. They are now much thinner, permitting a variety of cutting-edge shapes for more precise, specialized incisions. For example, a double-blade diamond knife has been developed for corneal wedge (block) resection. Especially with the introduction and popularization of radial keratotomy, a number of diamond blade knives have been developed that are incorporated in micrometric depth-setting handles for the more accurate performance of this technique as well as various astigmatism corrective procedures and corneal relaxing incisions. In both types, titanium is used extensively for the handles.

Instruments for Exposure and Fixation

Lid Speculum

The open light-wire Barraquer lid speculum still is the instrument of choice for most lid-retraction applications. In difficult situations and where the lid apertures are narrow and the exposure difficult, single or multiple lid sutures or clips may be used. When a rectus suture is used, it is inserted in the episclera anterior to the insertion of the superior rectus to minimize the possibility of hematoma, resulting in ptosis.

Superior Rectus and Scleral Expansion

The modified *Barraquer Llovera forceps* is used to grasp the superior rectus with minimum trauma to permit the episcleral needle passage just anterior to the rectus muscle insertion. The *Pierse scleral strap* fixation ring, affixed with a continuous suture, is preferred to a Flieringa ring fixed with interrupted sutures for perilimbal support. When a perilimbal suction trephine system is used, such as the Krumeich or the Hanna trephine, the ring may have to be omitted because it can interfere with the perilimbal suction. In certain instances, such as aphakic keratoplasty, when extensive vitrectomy is anticipated or when placing fixation sutures for a secondary intraocular lens into the scleral sulcus, the ring may be used with manual trephination or placed secondarily.

Instruments for Grasping and Suturing

Tissue Fixation and Needle Holders

Instruments for tissue grasping are available in two distinctly different tip designs: the Bonn 0.12 mm dog-toothed tip and the Pierse semicircular cupped tip. Pierse tips cause less tissue trauma and provide superior grasping than the Bonn. These forceps are available with curved or straight tips (Plate 7–3,A and B). Titanium is best for the *Pierse forceps,* whereas *Bonn forceps* are better made with stainless steel. Our preference is for short-handled titanium instruments.

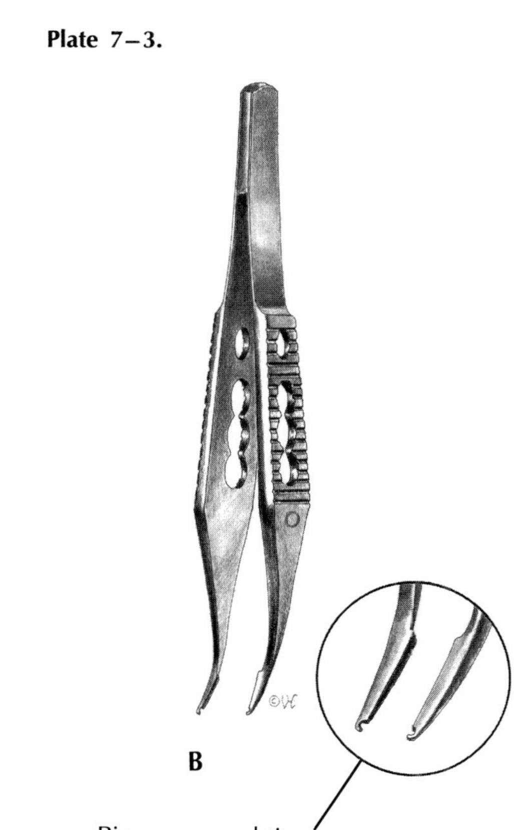

A, Pierse corneal forceps, straight tips. **B,** Pierse corneal forceps, curved tips. *Inset,* detail of cupped teeth.

The preferred needle holder has a short or medium length handle. The short handle type is exemplified by the *Pierse needle holders*, (Plate 7–4,A). These needle holders are available with fine tips, for use when firmer tissue is being penetrated, and ultra-fine tips. The short handle of this needle holder makes it possible to finger manipulate the straight, thin 0.75 mm tips through needle passage more readily than with a longer handled instrument. The *Troutman needle holder* (Plate 7–4,B), with intermediate handle length, is manufactured by Moria. This needle holder also has a very fine tip, 0.75 mm, that does not narrow as abruptly from the hinge to the grasping tips as the Pierse instrument, and allows somewhat better visualization during needle passage.

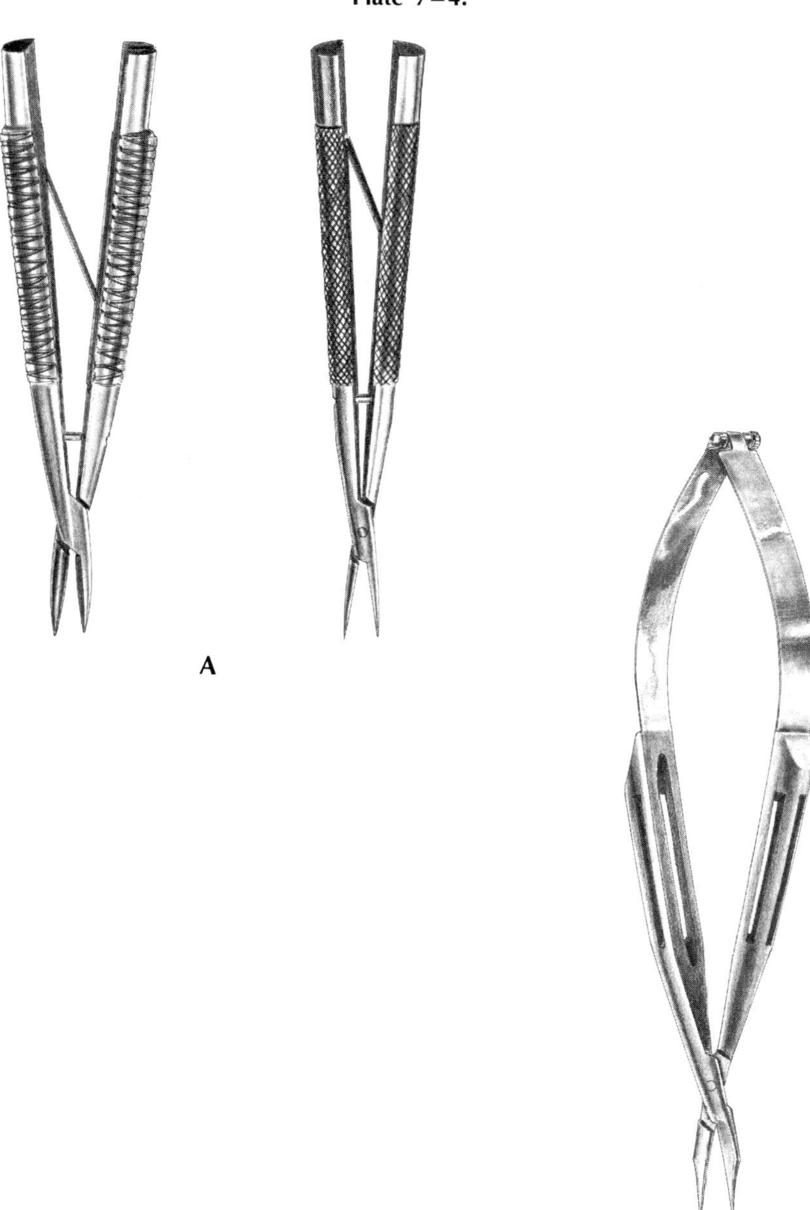

A, Pierse needle holder. *Left,* fine tips; *right,* ultra-fine tips. B, Troutman needle holder (Moria).

Tying Instruments

Fine monofilament sutures should be tied with special tying forceps rather than with a needle holder and necessarily heavier tipped platform tissue forceps. Such special tying instruments are less likely to damage the thread, and they hold better for tensioning and tying knots. The platform tips of the tying forceps have not been changed substantially, except for handle design, since they were first described by Harms. The *Harms forceps* held in the dominant hand should have curved tips to facilitate the slipknot tie (Plate 7–5,A). The forceps held in the nondominant hand should have straight tips (Plate 7–5,B). When selecting a set of tying forceps, it is important to ascertain that they will hold 10-0 or 11-0 suture without slipping. They should grasp the thread well enough to be able to break it by pulling it between the two forceps.

A   B

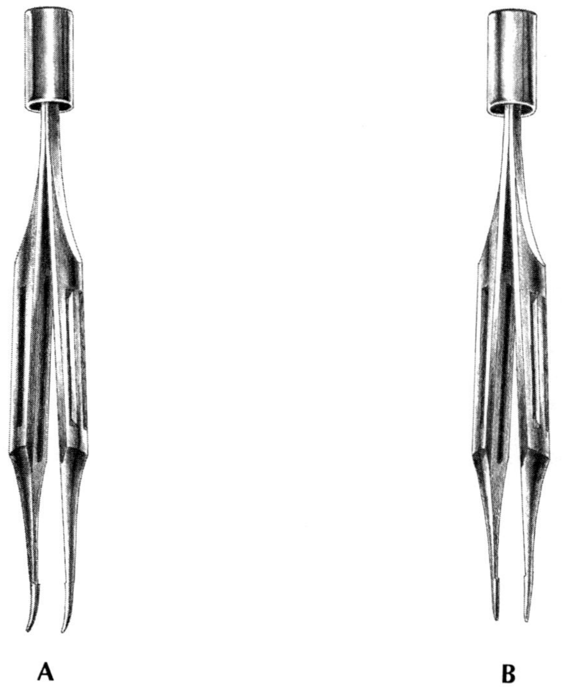

A, Harms suture forceps (Moria), curved tips. **B,** Harms suture forceps (Moria), straight tips.

Scissors and Knives

Corneal Scissors

Scissors for cutting the cornea should have delicate, exquisitely sharp blades supported by a strong hinge. Corneal scissors are rarely required to cut the full thickness of the cornea because after trephination, only minimal thickness of posterior cornea may remain. The scissors can have tips of equal length or a longer blunted lower blade. These are exemplified by the *Troutman corneal scissors* (Plate 7–6,A and B). These are advanced along the incision groove, tailor fashion, with the tips remaining slightly separated as the blades are advanced, to prevent displacement. When selecting scissors, it is important to ascertain that the lower blade is not pointed, hooked, or irregular, which may catch the iris. With smooth rounded tips, iris incarceration can be avoided by lifting vertically with the lower blade against the posterior lamella as it is cut. The hinge of the keratoplasty scissors is made so that the lower blade supporting the tissue is inside the curve of the upper blade as it descends to cut; this minimizes the shelving of the posterior incision commonly seen when the hinge and blades are reversed. The scissors blades are held vertical or slightly inverse to the corneal plane during cutting.

Conjunctival Scissors

Although conjunctival scissors are rarely used in cornea and refractive surgery, when they are required, angled, blunt-pointed, inverse-curved spring-handled scissors are used.

Intraocular Scissors

A fine, short-handled *Vannas scissors* is used for iris incisions and excisions and when excising small blocks of corneal tissue, for example, in corneal wedge or block resection (Plate 7–6,C). These scissors are used also for preliminary cutting of 10.0 sutures prior to razor cutting at the knot. The small, blunt-pointed *Galand scissors* is appropriately angled to cut under the corneal shelf, beneath the iris, and within the pupil (Plate 7–6,D). The angle of the blades permits better visualization of the slightly rounded tips during cutting.

Razor Knives

We use the hockey stick–shaped razor knife. Although it is easier to vary the angle and blade length for different applications than with a disposable razor knife, cracked blades are not as uniformly sharp as the disposable type. A unique use of the nonsharpened cracked edge of the blade is as a blunt lamellar dissector. When using the disposable razor knife, we prefer the type with a breakoff upper third of the plastic handle. The shortened handle facilitates blade manipulation and reduces risk of contamination.

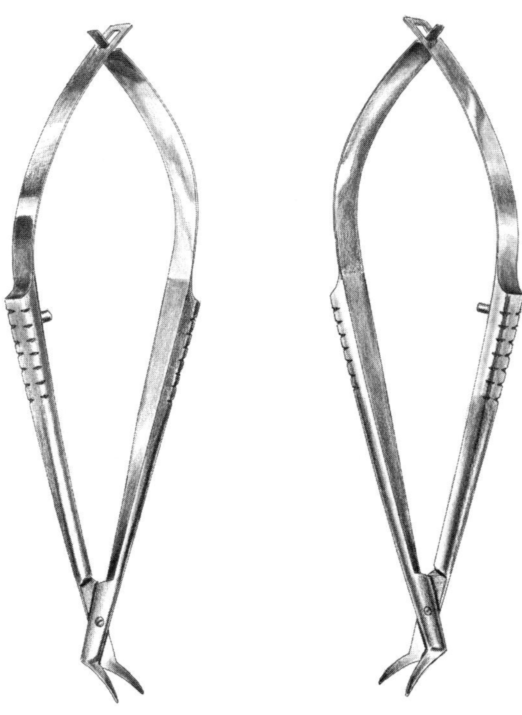

A. Right cutting   **B.** Left cutting

Note: lower blade cuts inside
of upper blade

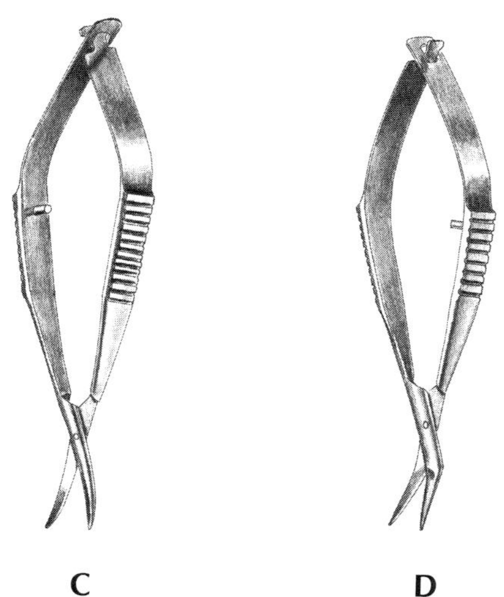

C   D

A, Troutman corneal scissors (Moria), right cutting. **B,** Troutman corneal scissors (Moria), left cutting. **C,** Vannas scissors. **D,** Galand scissors.

Microscope, Patient Preparation, and Instrumentation for Refractive Keratoplasty   **153**

Several instruments are particularly valuable for manipulating a lens into and within the eye. The *Duck-bill intraocular lens forceps* facilitates placement of the intraocular lens (Plate 7–7,A). The curved tips hold the lens in position for easier insertion across the edge of the recipient cornea to introduce the haptic into the distal sulcus. Once in place, the tip can be turned to readily grasp the proximal haptic for in-the-bag insertion. With the lens in place, one of three instruments, the *Osher Y shaped manipulator hook* (Plate 7–8,A), the *Sinsky hook* (Plate 7–8,B), and the *Kuglin hook* (Plate 7–8,C), is used to rotate, center, and position the lens. The Kuglin hook also is useful to retract the iris for better visualization of the peripheral sulcus. Finally, the *McPherson-Kelman forceps* is used to manipulate the lens haptics directly to avoid iris or transcleral sulcus sutures and to reposition the lens haptics in the sulcus or capsular bag (Plate 7–7,B).

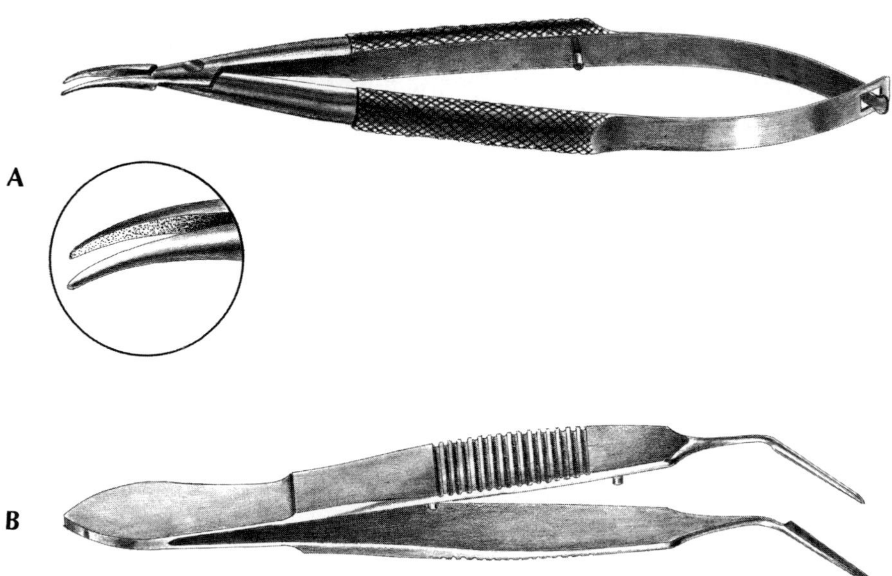

A, duckbill intraocular lens forceps. **B,** McPherson-Kelman forceps.

Plate 7-8.

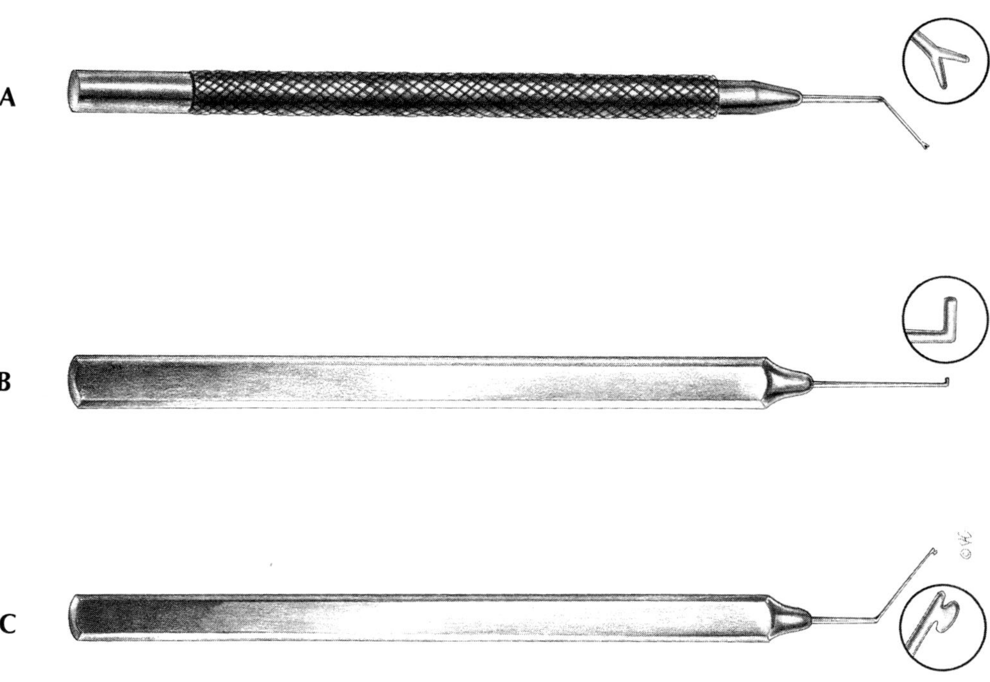

A, Osher Y-shaped manipulator. **B,** Sinsky hook. **C,** Kuglin hook.

Microscope, Patient Preparation, and Instrumentation for Refractive Keratoplasty **155**

Three types of handle support for diamond blades are used for refractive surgery and in surgery for the prevention or correction of astigmatism. An *unguarded diamond blade* is always preferable to a razor knife for both linear and curvilinear incisions (Plate 7–9,A and B). For this purpose, the thin single-edged blade has a 45-degree cutting angle. The knife blade should be retractable into its handle to protect it when it is not in use.

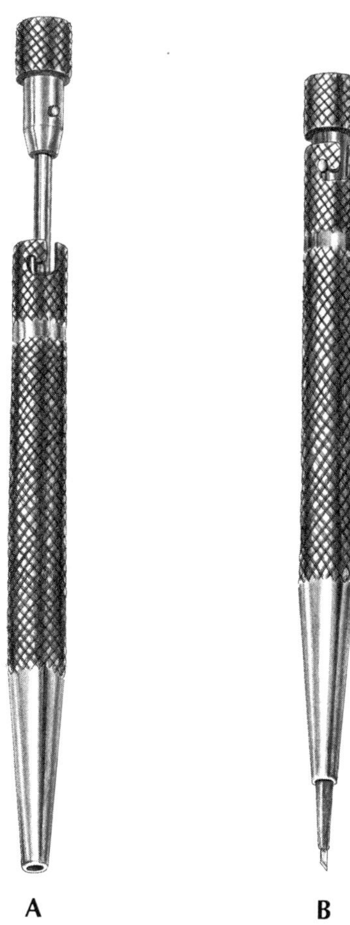

A   B

A, diamond knife (Metico), retracted. B, diamond knife (Metico), unguarded.

In partial penetrating incisions in which an accurate depth of cut is required, a *micrometer adjusting diamond knife* is used. This blade, which can have several angles and cutting edges, is fitted to a retracting handle with a micrometric adjustment for advancing the blade up to 1 mm (Plate 7–10,A and B). As the blade is extended beyond its guiding footplate, it has a 45-degree cutting edge on one side and a 90-degree vertical cutting edge opposite, to permit front or back cutting with the same instrument. An angled micrometric adjustable diamond knife designed by Osher permits better visualization of the cut as it is being made than straight-handled instruments do.

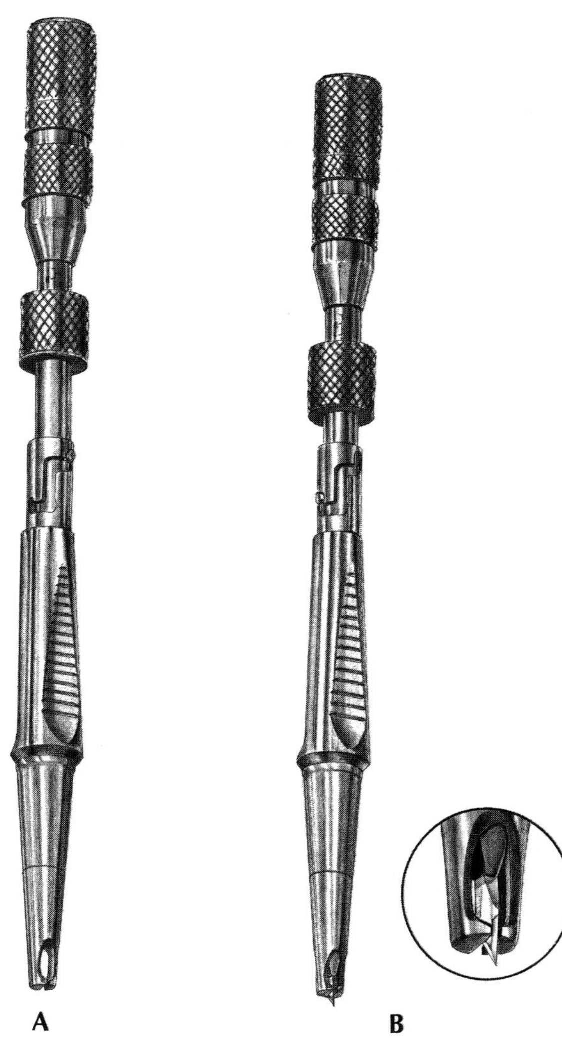

A   B

A, micrometer adjusting diamond knife (Metico), retracted. **B,** micrometer adjusting diamond knife (Metico), advanced for parallel cutting.

The *Troutman unguarded double-blade diamond knife* has an adjustable width, to make parallel incisions of the cornea for more accurate performance of block resections. As with other instruments, the 45-degree angle blades retract into the specially designed handle for protection when not in use (Plate 7–11,A and B).

Although handle designs may differ, knives from various manufacturers are made for the same functions and should be individually selected and examined carefully. The blade quality must be checked microscopically and depth calibration verified before each refractive surgical procedure. The footplate that guides the knife blade and limits the depth of cut should be free of any rough areas, dried tissue, or fluids. Although it is useful to place a small amount of hyaluronic acid (Healon) on the clean foot plates to facilitate smooth, uninterrupted passage of the blade across the incisional area, this must not be allowed to dry and roughen so as to impede later use.

Several additional specialized diamond knives are described in detail in Chapter 8.

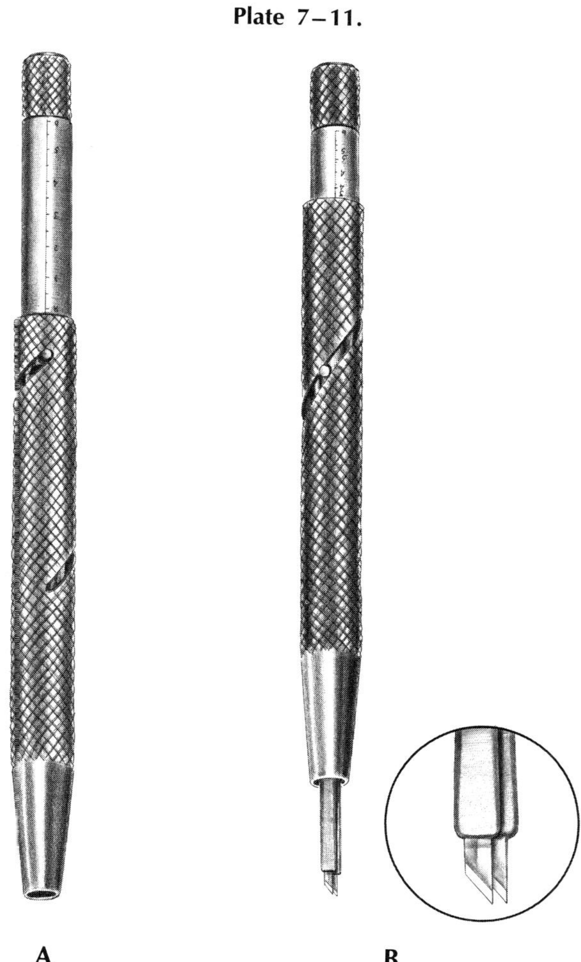

A, Troutman unguarded double-blade diamond knife (Metico) retracted. **B,** Troutman unguarded double-blade diamond knife (Metico), advanced for parallel cutting.

Suction Corneal Trephines for Penetrating Keratoplasty

Several suction corneal trephine sets have been designed to better cut the donor button or the recipient opening or both. These instruments include the Krumeich trephine set, the Hanna trephine set, and the Barron (formerly Hessberg-Barron) trephine. Use of these instruments and some of their design features are described in detail in Chapter 14.

Krumeich Trephine Set

The Krumeich trephine set consists of three basic units, the *artificial anterior chamber,* the *rotating micrometric adjusting trephine,* and the *suction recipient dovetail.*

The *artificial anterior chamber* consists of its base, the cornea retaining ring, and the screw compression ring (Plate 7–12,A). Assembled, with the scleral edge of the corneal graft compressed sealing the chamber, the pressure within the chamber is controlled through a three-way stopcock fitted to an intravenous set (Plate 7–12,B).

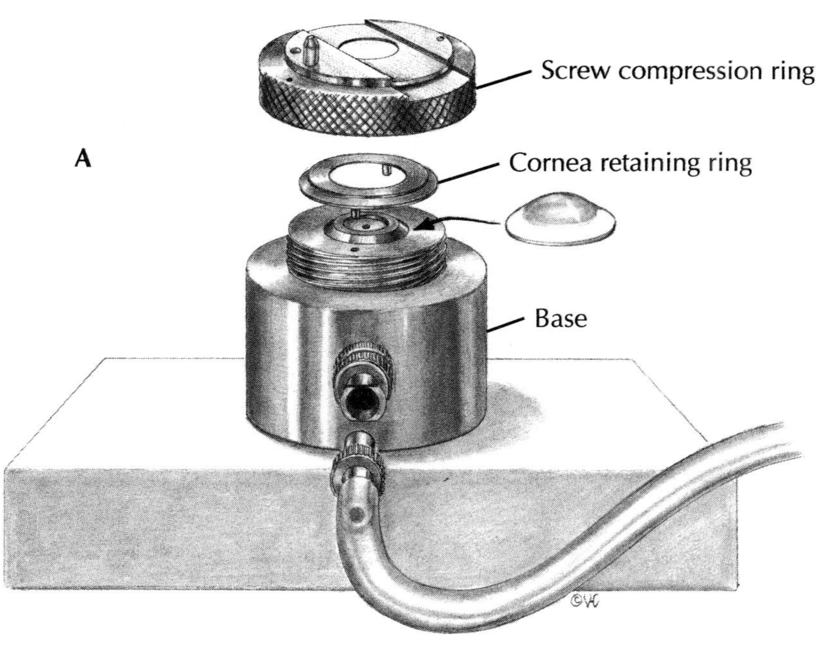

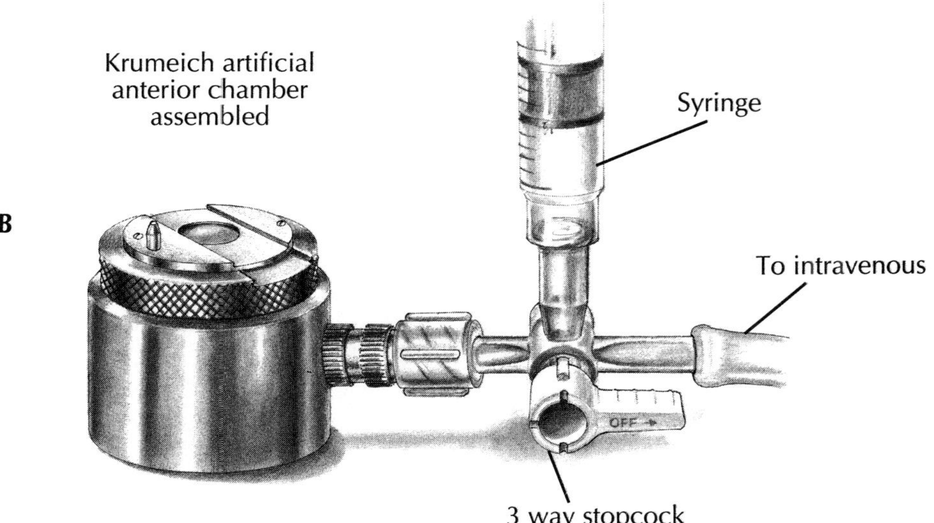

A, Krumeich artificial anterior chamber, exploded view. **B,** Krumeich artificial anterior chamber assembled with three-way stopcock.

The *micrometric adjusting trephine* consists of a base, the trephine (this unit uses a standard 8.00 mm trephine blade available from several manufacturers), the glass obturator, and the rotating micrometric adjusting trephine bezel (Plate 7–13,A). Assembled, the unit can be fitted either to the artificial anterior chamber or to the suction recipient dovetail (Plate 7–13,B). The micrometric adjusting screw is calibrated in 0.05 mm steps. Before the unit is fully assembled, the blade is set to zero in preparation for the trephination (see Chapter 14).

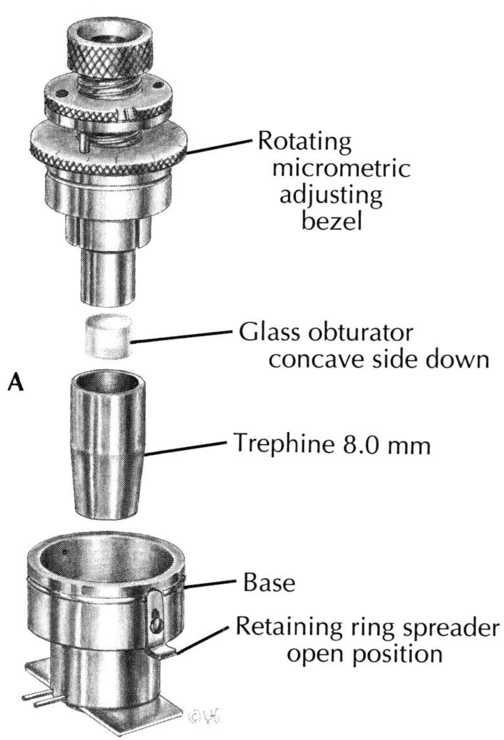

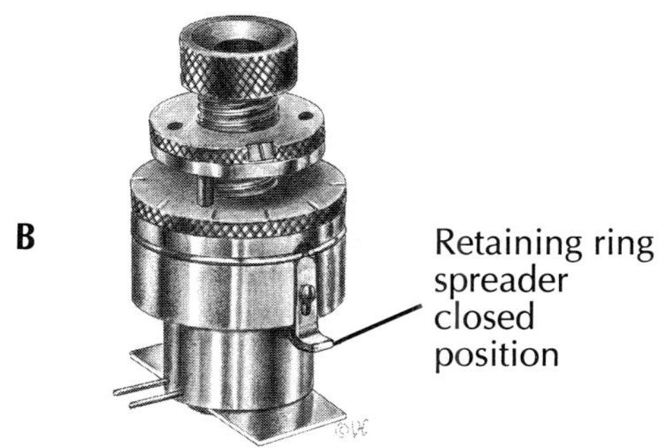

A, Krumeich micrometric adjusting trephine, exploded view. **B,** Krumeich micrometric adjusting trephine assembled for use with artificial anterior chamber or suction recipient dovetail.

The *suction recipient dovetail* consists of a knurled handle and the suction base (Plate 7–14,A). These are assembled and attached to a suction machine from which a suction of 800 millibars (600 mm Hg) is applied, fixating the unit to the anterior segment (Plate 7–14,B).

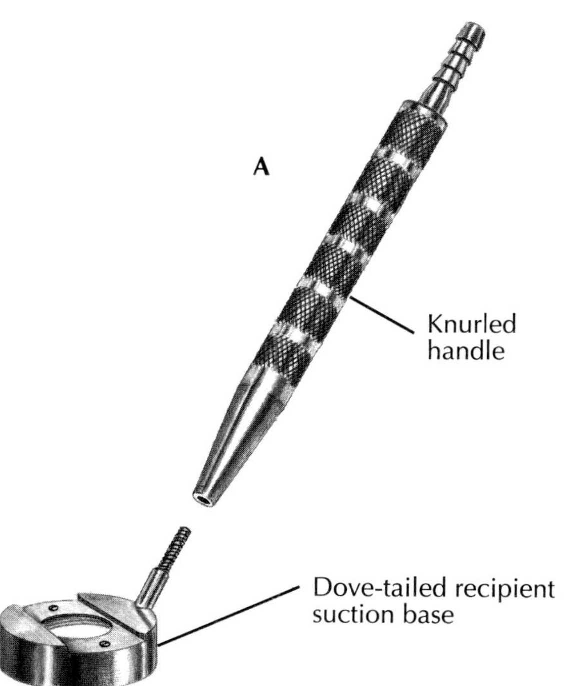

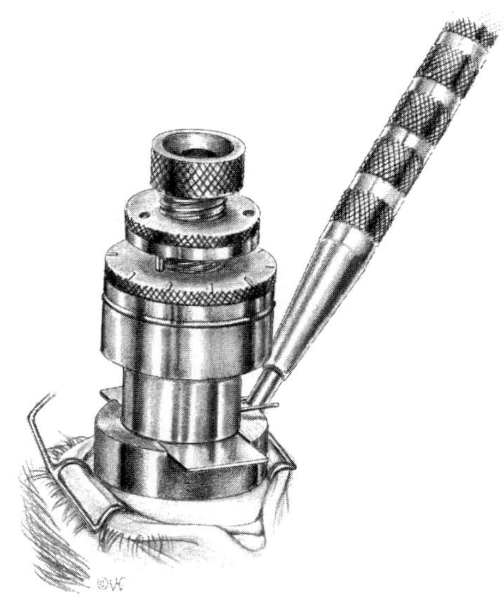

A, Suction recipient dovetail, exploded view. **B,** Suction recipient dovetail, and micrometric adjusting trephine assembled on recipient eye.

The Krumeich set also includes a *15 mm graft cutter* (Plate 7–15). This specialized trephine is fitted to a handle so that a donor cornea with a too wide scleral rim can be trimmed to fit the artificial anterior chamber. Rarely, the scleral rim of the donor cornea will be irregularly cut, necessitating the repositioning of the donor to the artificial anterior chamber.

It is important to keep this instrument scrupulously clean, especially the suction dovetail unit. This responsibility should not be delegated but should be the specific responsibility of the surgeon.

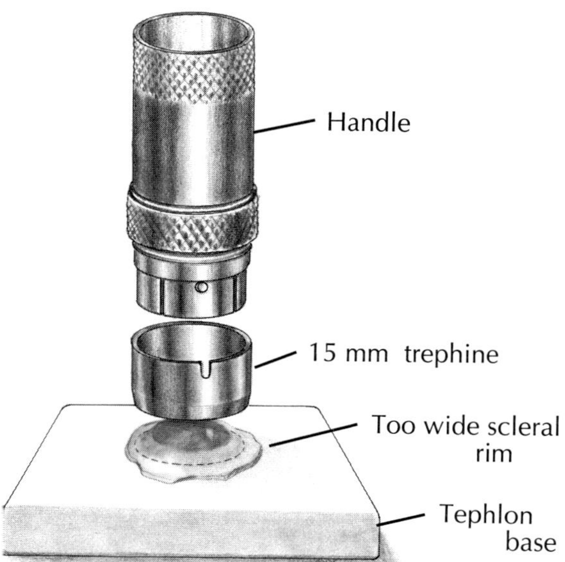

Fifteen-millimeter graft cutter (Krumeich).

The Hanna trephine set consists of the *recipient cornea suction trephine* and the *donor piston cutting frame*. The recipient cornea suction trephine is described in detail in Chapter 15. Assembled, the precision-manufactured trephine blade rotates to a preset position and stops (Plate 7–16). This permits cutting the recipient through its thickness with minimal possibility of iris damage.

Hanna Artificial Anterior Chamber

The Donor Piston Cutting Frame (Plate 7–17) recently has been modified as an artificial anterior chamber (not illustrated). This permits cutting of the donor from the epithelial surface with the Hanna suction trephine, using the same size trephine blade as used for the recipient cornea. Because of the ready availability of different diameter trephine blades, the Hanna set now can be used with increased versatility over the Krumeich set, in addition to the improved accuracy afforded by cutting the donor and recipient from the same aspect.

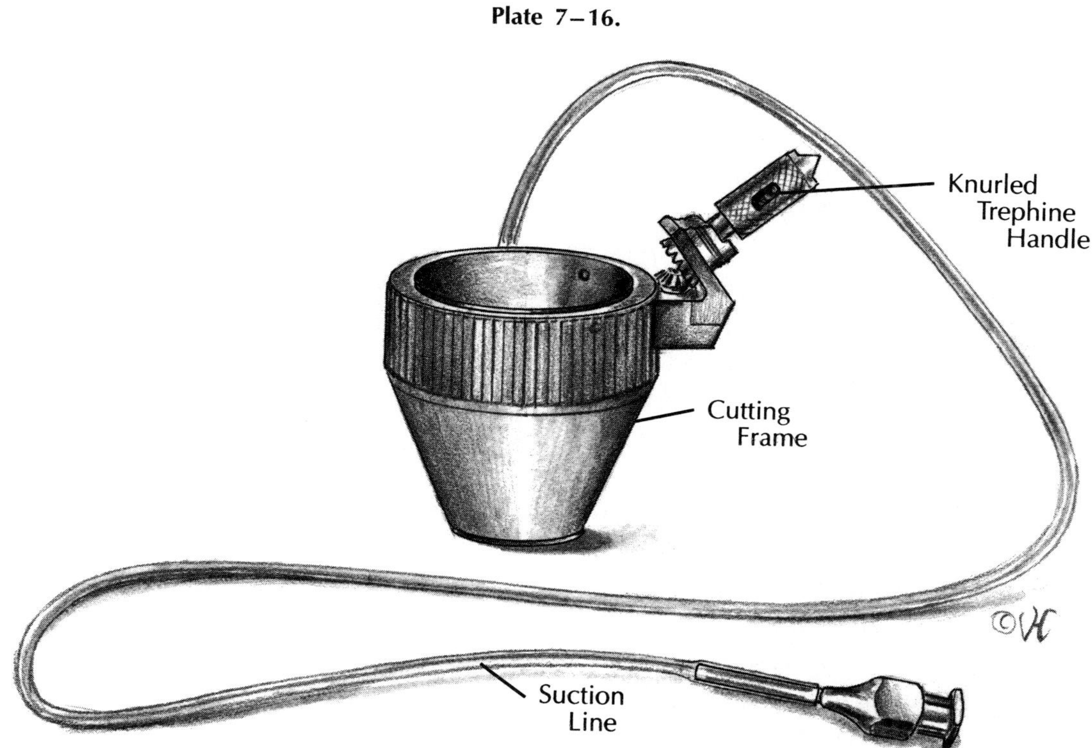

Hanna recipient cornea suction trephine.

The *donor piston cutting frame* uses the same precision blade (Plate 7–17). It consists of a screw base that includes a multiply-fenestrated cutting block that holds the donor cornea firmly against the concave Teflon base by suction applied with a foot pedal–controlled suction pump capable of creating 600 mm Hg or 800 millibars of suction pressure. The outer barrel of the piston is then screwed to the base, and the piston with the blade attached is passed to rest on the donor endothelium. With gentle pressure, the blade then is passed through the cornea onto the block.

This instrument is much more complex mechanically than the Krumeich instrument and requires even more careful maintenance. It has the advantage of having multiple diameter blades, 6.0 to 10.0 mm, with better visualization during trephination, than the Krumeich instrument. This makes it more useful for the preparation of variable donor and recipient diameters than the Krumeich instrument, which has only one diameter, 8.0 mm.

Barron Trephine Set

This instrument is described and illustrated in Chapter 14. It has the advantage of being disposable, and in its new configuration marks equidistant points on the recipient for more accurate suture placement. It has the disadvantage of significantly undercutting the recipient, making sizing and accurate edge-to-edge apposition difficult.

Instruments for Refractive Surgery

Specialized instruments for refractive modification of the cornea fall into three basic categories: crystalline knives and associated measuring or standardizing devices (see Chapter 8), instruments to fixate the eye, and instruments to mark the appropriate location for incisions. The instruments are best constructed of titanium for strength and durability. Any instrument that is used as a measure or marking device should be treated delicately, cleaned often, and checked for accuracy periodically with a device such as the *Baribeau micronscope* (see Chapter 8).

Fixation Devices

Because many refractive procedures are performed with only topical anesthesia, good fixation of the globe becomes even more important. Besides the level of fixation achieved with the instrument, the surgeon also must consider the degree of discomfort induced by fixation, because topical anesthesia will not completely anesthetize the tissues surrounding the eye. Initially, a simple Bonn forceps was used for this purpose. However, if used for radial keratotomy, the single-point fixation allowed a significant degree of lateral mobility, and erratic incisions often were obtained.

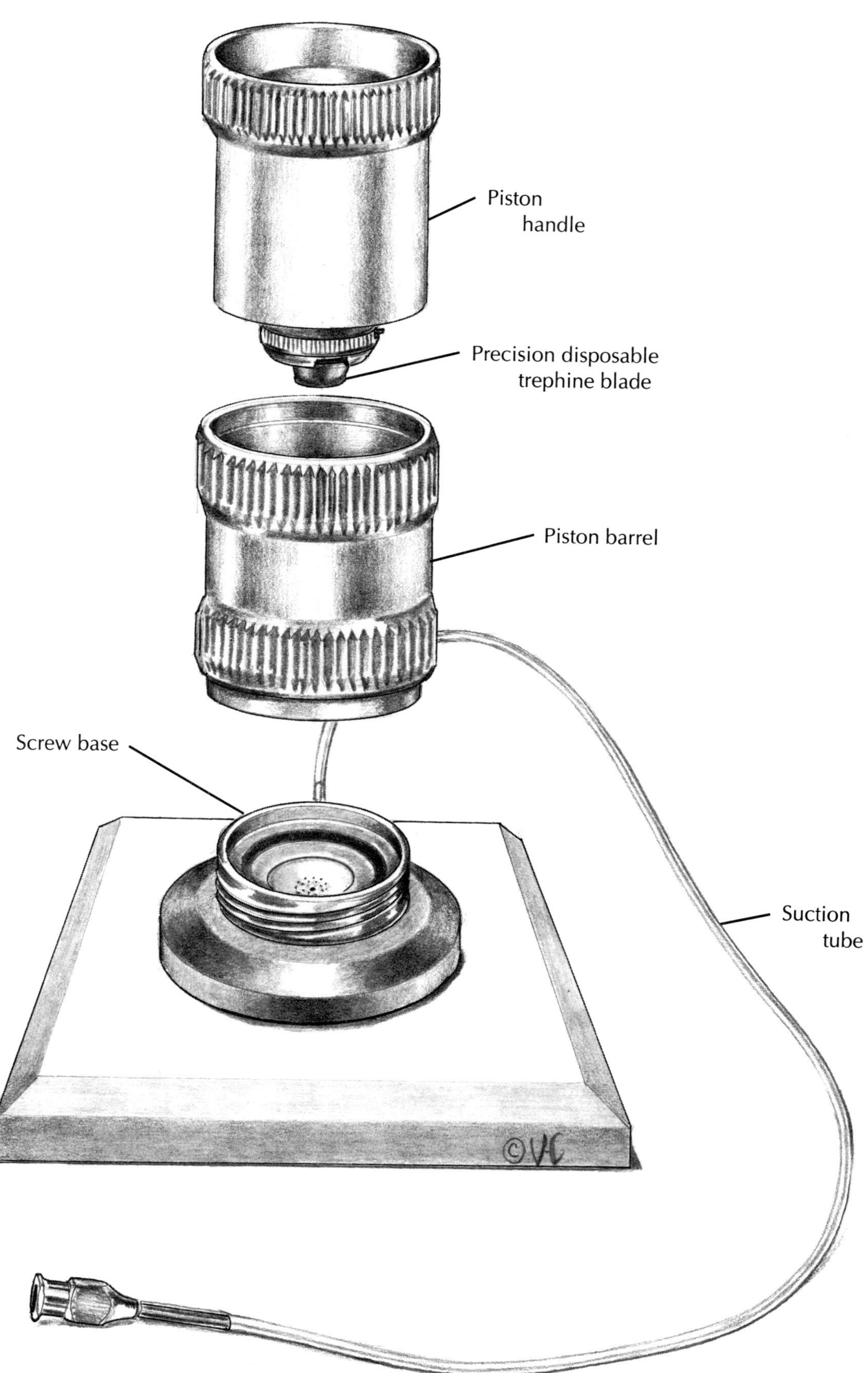

Hanna donor piston cutting frame, exploded view.

The two-point fixation forceps, as seen in the Bores forceps (Plate 7–18,A), provides more lateral stability but requires refixation before each radial incision. In addition, the pinching of the conjunctiva and episcleral tissue induces significant patient discomfort, making the procedure more difficult. The Kremer forceps fixates at two points, one on each side of the globe, and allows better lateral stability, with the added benefit that two incisions can be performed with each fixation. These are available in an angled version (Plate 7–18,B) to allow better hand position and in both locked (Plate 7–18,C) and unlocked configurations. The best choice to optimize hand position and ease of use is the locking, angled Kremer forceps.

Patient discomfort is a serious problem, even with the Kremer forceps, and the introduction of many astigmatic procedures requiring tangential and arcuate incisions revealed a serious problem with angular stabilization of the globe. Ring fixation devices, such as the Hofmann ring (Plate 7–18,D), provide excellent angular stabilization of the globe and significantly more comfort for the patient. These rings often have teeth on one side, which are not necessary and should be turned upward to avoid patient discomfort. In addition, a ring with a pivot on each side allows the surgeon better hand position during the procedure. This instrument also provides excellent stabilization for radial incisions, although a one-handed technique must be used in place of an opposed two-handed movement used to create radial incisions with the Bores forceps. An additional benefit is the induction of increased intraocular pressure, which aids the surgeon in creating more uniform incisions. It is our belief that the ring-type fixation device should be the first choice in astigmatic procedures and probably represents the best fixation device for all refractive procedures.

Marking Devices

Refractive procedures require a high degree of accuracy with respect to placement of incisions and sutures. To facilitate this process, a large number of marking instruments have been developed. These instruments are dipped in methylene blue and pressed on the cornea. The impression that remains after washing away excess dye provides a template for the surgical procedure. Although a multitude of such devices are available, certain characteristics are shared by a basic group of instruments, which can be enlarged with more specialized instruments as the need arises. These basic instruments can be most easily classified into optical zone markers, radial incision markers, angular degree markers, and transverse keratotomy markers.

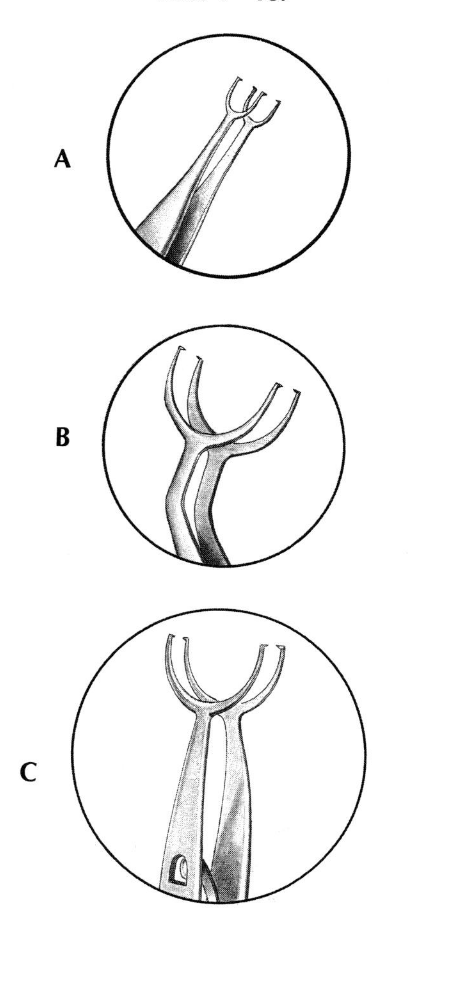

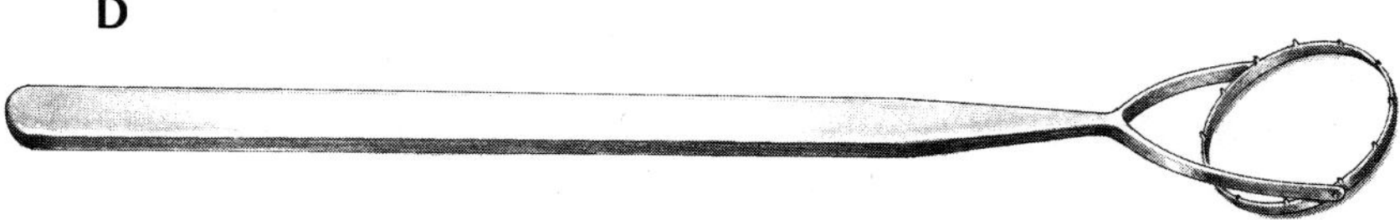

A, Bores-style two-point fixation forceps. **B,** angled Kremer two-point fixation forceps. **C,** straight locking Kremer two-point fixation forceps. **D,** Hofmann-Thornton ring fixation device.

Virtually every refractive procedure requires the use of an optical zone marker (Plate 7–19,A). The acquisition, familiarization, and care of a good set of optical zone markers is essential to every refractive surgeon. The application of zone markers requires a clear understanding of the benefits of various designs and the particular characteristics of the markers involved. After purchasing zone markers, the surgeon should measure each marker to determine accuracy of the device and whether the zone diameter is marked on the inside or outside of the individual marker. Because the mark can be 0.25 to 0.5 mm wide, considerable inaccuracy can arise if the mark is designed as an inside diameter and the surgeon uses the outside diameter. The edge of the marker should be sharp enough to give a well-delineated mark, but not so sharp as to cause an incision. The inexpensive plastic markers probably should be avoided because of the wide corneal impression obtained and their fragility. Markers should be examined for evidence of roundness and other localized deformations that could affect the surgery. Stainless steel markers are strong enough to resist damage by routine cleaning, but often corrode, leaving less than desirable impressions. These can be gold plated to reduce corrosion and improve function.

The indication of the optical axis is an important component of the optical zone marker. Several configurations are available that include cross hairs (Plate 7–19,B), needle tip (Plate 7–19,C), or no device at all (Plate 7–19,D) to center on the optical axis. The optical zone marker without a centering device can be reasonably precise, but this depends heavily on the surgeon's expertise. The cross hairs provide an excellent visualization of the zone, but are delicate and should be cleaned with great care to avoid disturbing the proper configuration. The needle tip is more durable, but can be bent or damaged. Any such device should be periodically examined to verify proper orientation, and the choice is a matter of personal preference. The authors prefer cross hairs, because this configuration seems to give a more symmetric geometric indication of the center of the zone.

For radial keratotomy, zone markers should be obtained with a range of 3.0 to 5.0 mm in increments of 0.25 mm. Most astigmatic procedures are performed at zones of 5.0 mm or more, indicating that a useful set of markers would be 5.0 mm to 7.0 mm in 0.5 mm increments. Zone markers can be used to delineate the length of tangential and arcuate incisions, indicating a use for markers from 2.0 mm to 3.0 mm in 0.25 mm increments (Plate 7–19,E). These general guidelines for useful increments and ranges may be modified by individual surgical technique.

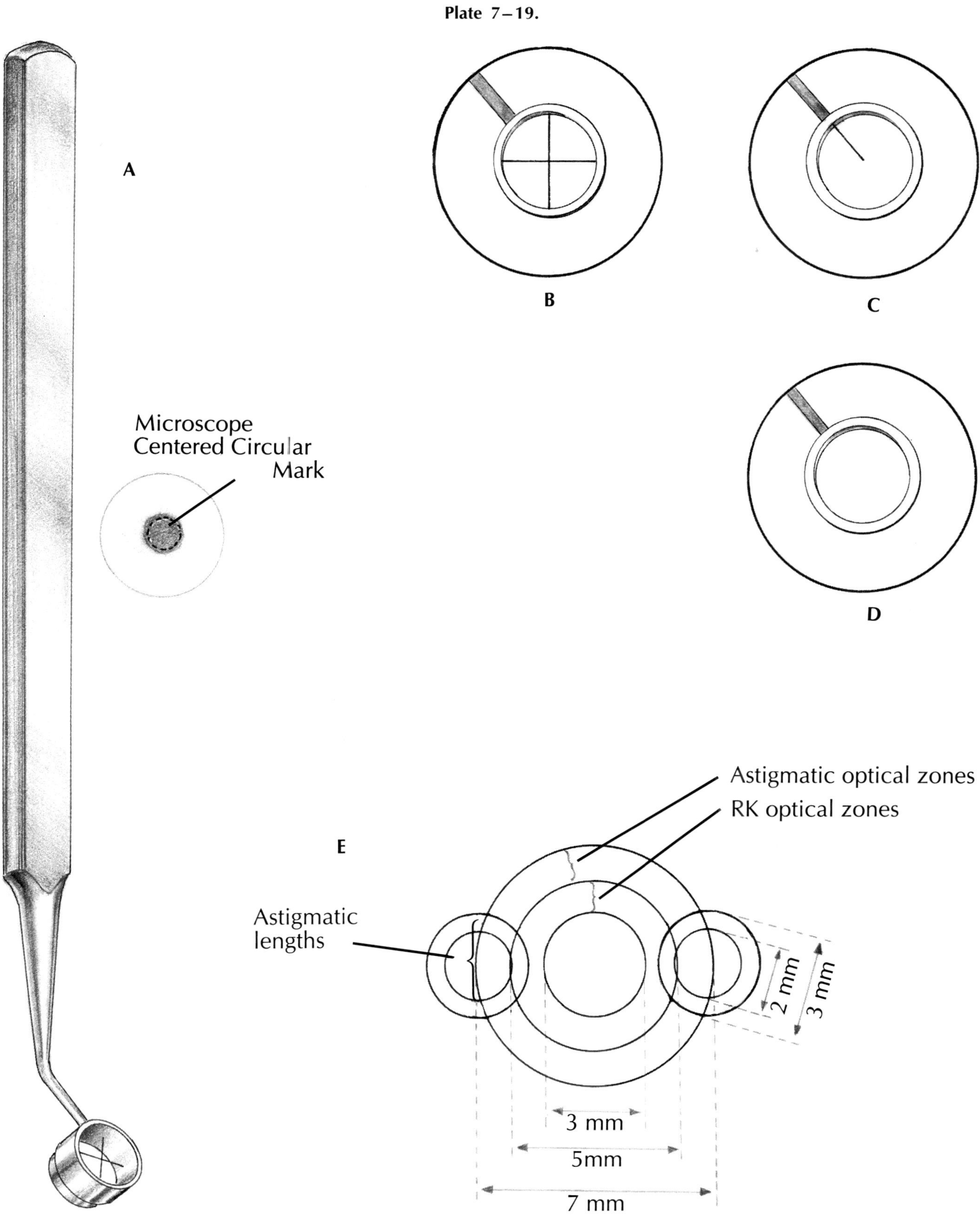

A, Hoffer stainless steel optical zone marker. **B,** Hoffer cross-hair centering device. **C,** Thornton needle tip centering device. **D,** Bores marker, no centering device. **E,** zones of the central cornea markers used in radial keratotomy and astigmatic keratotomy to indicate appropriate selection of optical zones and arcuate or transverse incision lengths.

Radial incision markers are an important part of precise radial keratotomy surgery. In the past, radial markers were not often used, and incisions were created without a template, relying on the surgeon's judgment. This approach was encouraged by the technique of creating radial incisions that emphasized the movement of opposed fixation forceps and the knife. With this technique, it was difficult to follow preset lines precisely. As patient demand for more precise refractive results grew and the understanding of the procedure improved, it became clear that accurate positioning of the radial incisions was not only desirable but necessary to prevent unwanted astigmatism. Moreover, to properly prepare the eye for astigmatic surgery and to avoid previous radial incisions, if additional incisions were contemplated, it was clear that equal spacing was a necessity.

Virtually all astigmatic procedures rely for effect on transverse or arcuate incisions. If a radial incision lies along the axis of astigmatism, the incision must be "jumped" to avoid wound dehiscence. The ability to rotate the pattern of radial incisions so that an open area appears along the steep axis is a desirable feature of the radial marker (Plate 7–20,A). Without a marker with this feature the ability to rotate the radial pattern is extremely difficult.

The radial marker rarely has a central device to locate the optical axis, and earlier ribbed designs made it difficult to properly align the marker with the optical zone. A smaller opening simplifies centration relative to the optical zone.

Radial incision markers may be used for a variety of purposes. They mark the location of radial incisions in radial keratotomy, and also play a role in marking the length of arcuate incisions. A six-cut radial incision marker divides the eye into six 60-degree segments (Plate 7–20,B). In the Troutman relaxing incision, this can be used to advantage to mark the extent of the incisions across the steep axis and the location of compression sutures along the flat axis. The eight-zone marker can be used for both four-incision and eight-incision radial keratotomy. Angular displacement in units of 45 degrees can be used for arcuate incisions, and provides an excellent marker to locate the position of sutures in the antitorque suture pattern. For the basic refractive set, only these two markers are required; most surgeons agree that a 12-incision radial keratotomy should not be performed, because of problems of corneal instability.

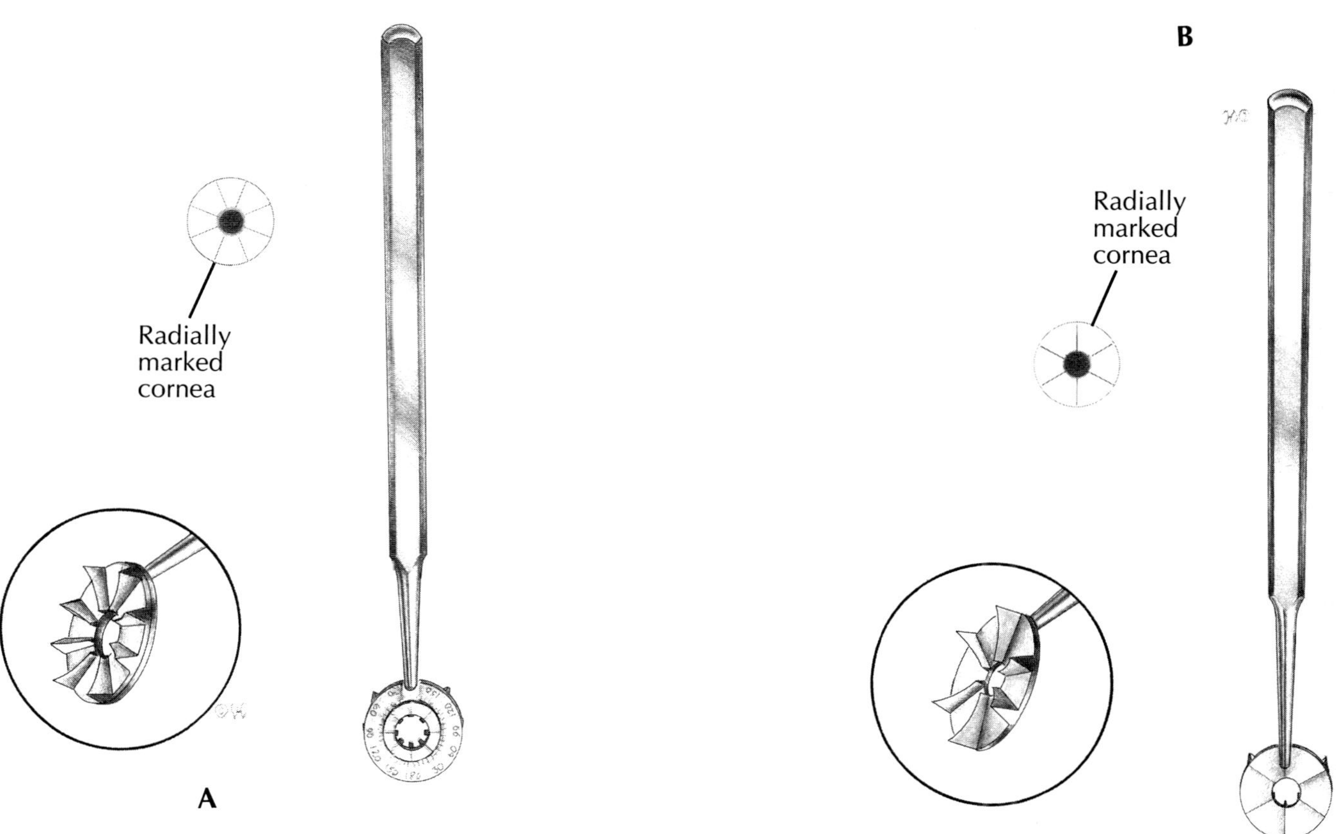

A, Grandon eight-incision radial keratotomy marker (Katena) with rotating head to align incision pattern to avoid astigmatic axis. **B,** Anis six-incision radial keratotomy incision marker (Katena) useful for Troutman relaxing incisions.

An important step in astigmatic keratotomy is location of the astigmatic meridians. This can be accomplished by means of a reticule in the operating microscope; however, orientation of the microscope relative to the patient is often less than perfect, resulting in errors of the axis of the astigmatic procedure. A better approach is to use a ring imprinted with an angular scale that orients the surgeon relative to the astigmatic meridian, such as the Mendez gauge (Plate 7–21,A). Before the operation the surgeon should mark the cornea at a known location, usually at the 6-o'clock position, to orient the scale relative to the eye. Failure to perform this simple maneuver may result in significant error in determination of the astigmatic meridian, due to the cyclotorsion often experienced by patients under stress.

After the position of the astigmatic meridian has been identified, the use of a marker to identify this meridian is prudent (Plate 7–21,B). This facilitates locating the marking for the actual incisions and prevents inadvertent incisions either in the wrong location or in locations not 180 degrees apart.

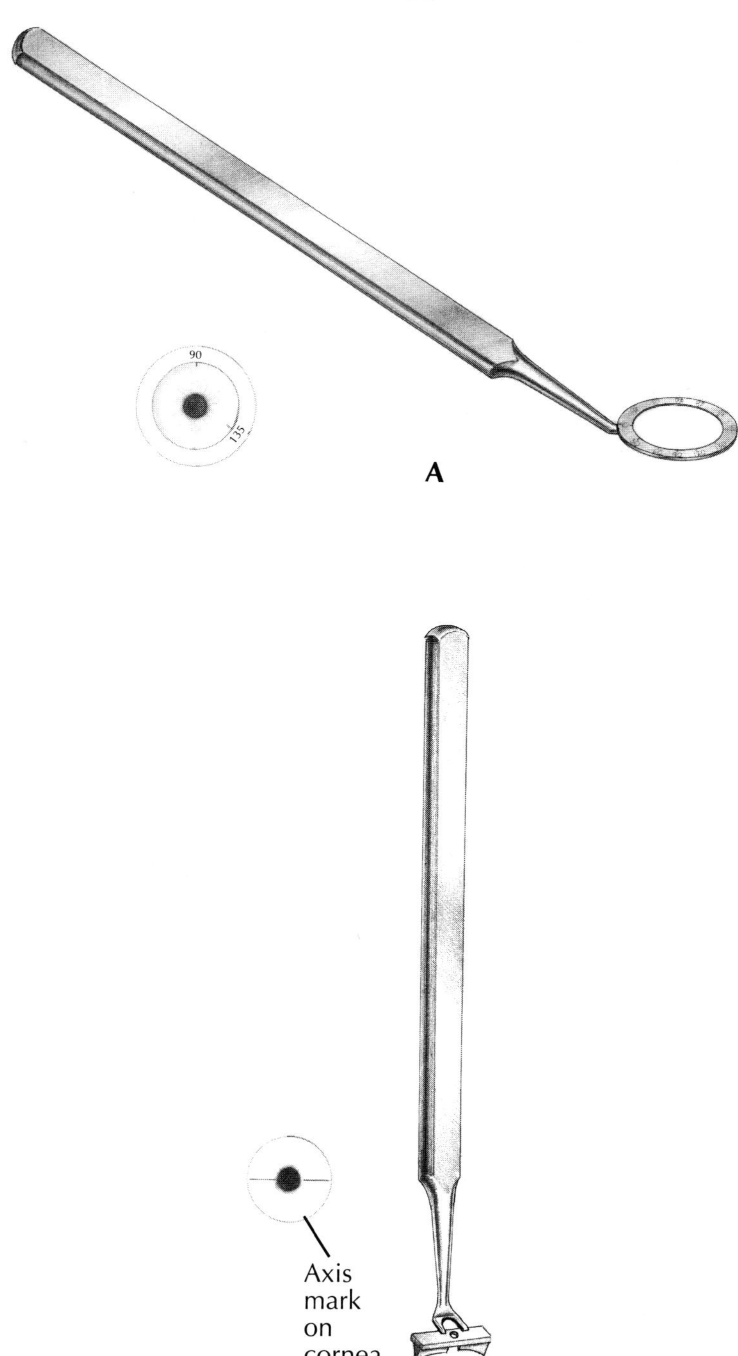

A, Mendez graduated ring (Katena) for determination of astigmatic meridian. **B,** Bores astigmatic meridian marker (Katena).

After marking the appropriate meridian of the incision, the length of the transverse incision must be marked. The simplest device for this purpose is a spatula of predetermined width, which is applied once on each side of the optical zone (Plate 7–22,A). This is a basic instrument, and every astigmatic surgeon should own several, with a range from 2 to 4 mm in increments of 0.5 mm. With the combination of this instrument and the radial incision markers, virtually all astigmatic patterns can be created, including the Ruiz procedure and its variants. An alternative to this instrument is to use an optical zone marker of the appropriate diameter (e.g., 2.5 mm) to make a straight incision within the marks created by the zone marker (see Plate 7–19,E). Most transverse incisions are greater than 2 mm, and straight transverse incisions longer than 4 mm begin to show wound healing abnormalities, thus the rationale for the range of markers.

A large number of specialized markers exist for transverse and arcuate incisions. For example, one marker obviates the necessity to mark an optical zone and places two transverse marks at a set distance apart with a needle-tip device to indicate the optical axis (Plate 7–22,B). This device also can be obtained with a gap to accommodate radial incisions that might be used in conjunction with radial keratotomy. Fewer marks on the cornea may lead to less confusion, but the decision to use it is purely personal. Another such marker creates three transverse marks 1 mm apart and was originally designed for the Ruiz procedure (Plate 7–22,C). The same result can be obtained with a combination of optical zone markers and spatula-type markers, but certainly this single device is more convenient. As the surgeon becomes more comfortable with the operations, the selection of specialized markers will become clear. One caveat concerns the device used to indicate the optical center. If the surgeon is comfortable with cross hairs and the new marker has a different device for indicating optical axis, errors may occur that can effect the procedure. New instruments should be considered carefully, and if possible should be tried on eye bank eyes before actual use in patients.

Instrument Care and Cleaning

Instrument care and cleaning should begin and end with inspection by the surgeon under high microscope magnification immediately before and after each use. Cleaning of instruments should be entrusted only to an experienced assistant. In some instances the instrument should be not only inspected but also cleaned and placed in its protective case only by the surgeon. This is particularly true for specialized instruments such as the Krumeich and Hanna trephines and for diamond knives. Every corneal trephine used, even though sterilized in a factory package, should be

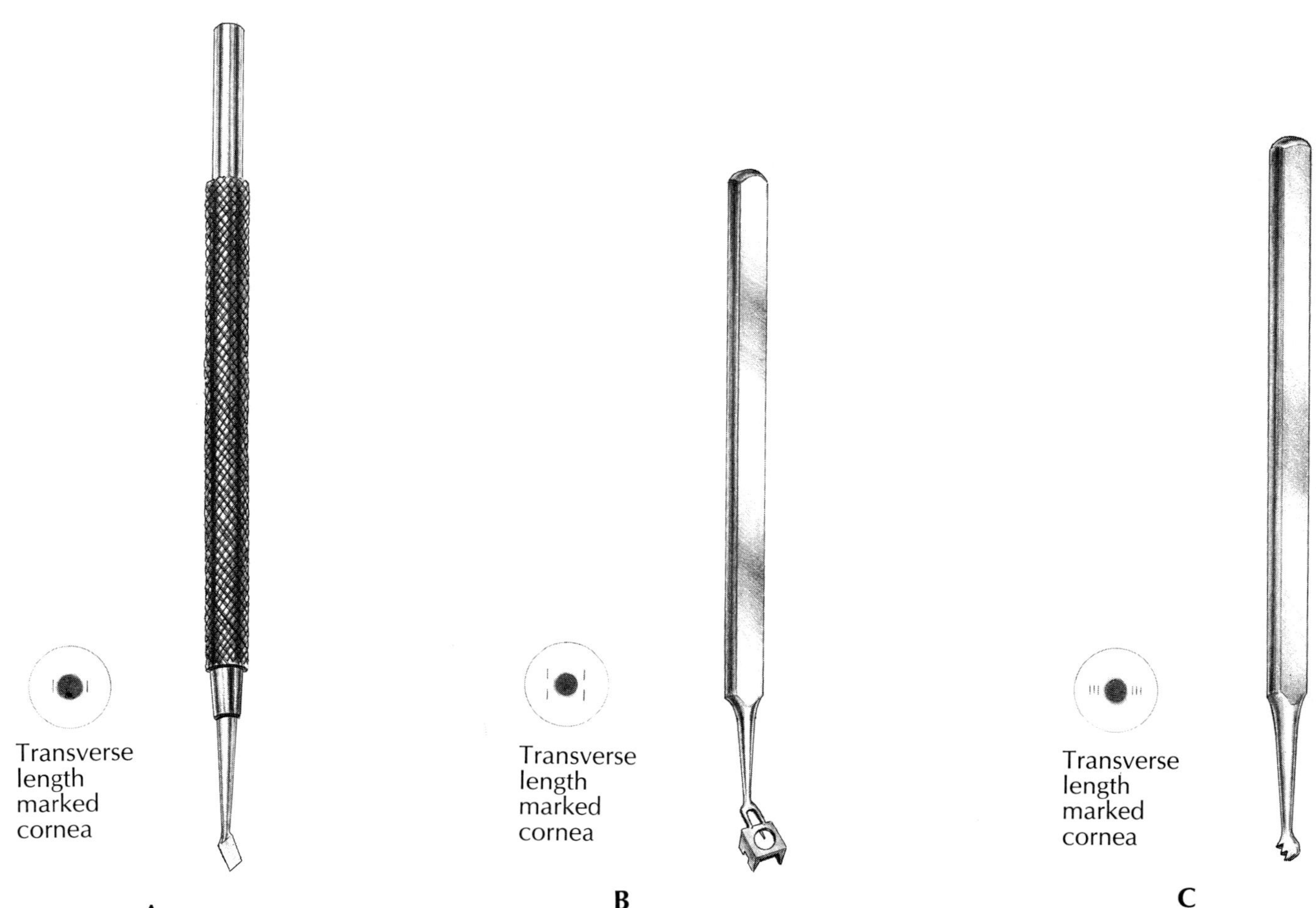

A, spatula marker with predetermined length for marking length of transverse incisions. **B,** Hoffman T-cut marker with needle tip device for determination of optical axis and gap to accommodate radial incisions. **C,** Bores stepped transverse marker with predetermined width and three transverse marks with 1 mm separation.

carefully inspected before use. A defective edge can damage or destroy a donor button or cause a defective recipient cut, or both.

The surgeon is responsible for the function of the instruments used during operative procedures. Only when careful attention is paid to their maintenance will the maximum result from the planned surgical procedure be obtained. *Understanding the instruments and their function in every detail is as essential as understanding the steps of the surgical procedure being performed.*

Incisional Techniques for Corneal Surgery

In its most elemental form, the process of corneal surgery can be divided into two parts: cutting (making incisions) and suturing (closing incisions). Each is equally important, because a poorly placed or inaccurate incision leads to a poor result no matter how carefully the incision is closed. The cornea cannot be discarded or replaced except under conditions that subject the patient and the eye to significant trauma and danger. The selection of proper instruments and their application therefore deserves great forethought and planning. Although instrumentation is discussed at great length elsewhere in this book, general principles of the instruments as they pertain to the specifics of incisions are discussed here.

KNIVES

The earliest knives used by humans were created from stones by the technique of *chipping* to create a sharp edge. In the stones that were used as knives, the natural structure of the rock (obsidian and quartz, among others) formed a relatively sharp edge. Irregular serrations along the sharpened edge, however, produced irregular cuts.

The next great advance in knife technology began with the ability to mold metal, leading to the ability to create a much smoother edge on the knife. However, a new property soon became apparent with respect to maintaining a sharp edge. Significant pressure was developed on the tiny area along the edge of the blade, and this led to the dulling of this surface even when it was applied to relatively soft materials. The introduction of hardened steel, which was folded and hammered many times, with immersion of the hot steel in water, thus increasing its rigidity or hardness, led to more durable knives that are used even today. Thus we see that although a knife may be created with a very fine edge, an equally important factor remains: the longevity of the knife in question. In ophthalmic use, the surgeon is well aware of the gradual loss of sharpness of metal needles and blades even when they are used to cut nothing denser than eye tissue.

Because refractive corneal operations often depend on maintaining the sharpness of the knife throughout the operation, so as to give equal and opposite effects in the cornea, metal knives soon were found to be inadequate because they caused ragged incisions. Crystalline knives, that is, knives created from precious crystals such as diamonds or sapphires, can be shaped to an extremely fine point by virtue of their intrinsic structure. If they are properly cut, the knife edge, theoretically, extends down to the molecular level. When such a knife encounters a substance, tremendous forces can be generated on the tiny area of its edge. Even a very hard substance, such as a diamond, can be damaged easily if it encounters even a fairly soft substance, such as nylon suture. Although sapphire can be cut to the required sharpness, it has been found that in clinical use application to even relatively soft corneal tissue will damage the knife after only a few uses. For sharpness and durability, the diamond crystalline knife remains the most appropriate for making refractive corneal incisions.

CUTTING WITH KNIVES

In the most general sense, a knife can be defined as an instrument for concentrating a force from a large area to a very small area. In engineering terms, pressure is defined as the force applied over a given unit area. In mathematical terms, this is force/area. We can see that if the force remains constant and the area decreases, the pressure will increase dramatically. If a large enough force is applied to a substance over a limited area, the ability of the substance to resist movement eventually will be lost, and the substance in question will be broken at the point at which the force is applied. This is then an operational definition of sharpness. Sharpness is a relative term, because at a given level of magnification all incisions involve a rough breaking of the substance to be incised. Certain other properties of incisions become immediately apparent. If a knife is applied point first (Plate 8–1,A), the area of the point of the knife will be exceedingly small, leading to a very high pressure at the point of the knife. Alternatively, if the knife is applied along a blunted edge (Plate 8–1,B), the forces will be distributed along the area defining that entire edge, markedly decreasing the pressure at any given point. Hence the entrance will be more difficult than if the knife is applied along an edge as opposed to point first, even if the edge is very sharp.

After entering the cornea, a knife as it creates an incision, must displace the incised tissue to move forward or backward. The movement of a knife through tissue is much like the movement of a rudder through water. The thinner the knife and the shorter the submerged portion, the smaller the resistance to forward or backward movement (Plate 8–1,C). As the knife becomes shorter the movement becomes more erratic, because the stabilizing effect of the knife, performing like a rudder on a boat, is lost. Thus, if the intention is to create a very straight incision, a wider, thicker knife or a knife with a shallow bevel is preferred, because this knife will receive extra stabilization during its passage through the tissue.

Conversely, to create a curved incision, the surgeon selects a sharply pointed, thin knife, which will have less tendency to proceed along a straight line in the tissue (Plate 8–1,D). In making decisions about the rudderlike considerations of the knife, we must accept certain compromises in terms of the cutting ability of the knife and the depth of the incision. If a thick, wide knife is used, the tissue will resist penetration, and the incision created may be shallower than the incision created by a thin, pointed knife. As we discuss later in the chapter, this compromise may be offset to some extent by the use of a second knife to deepen the same incision.

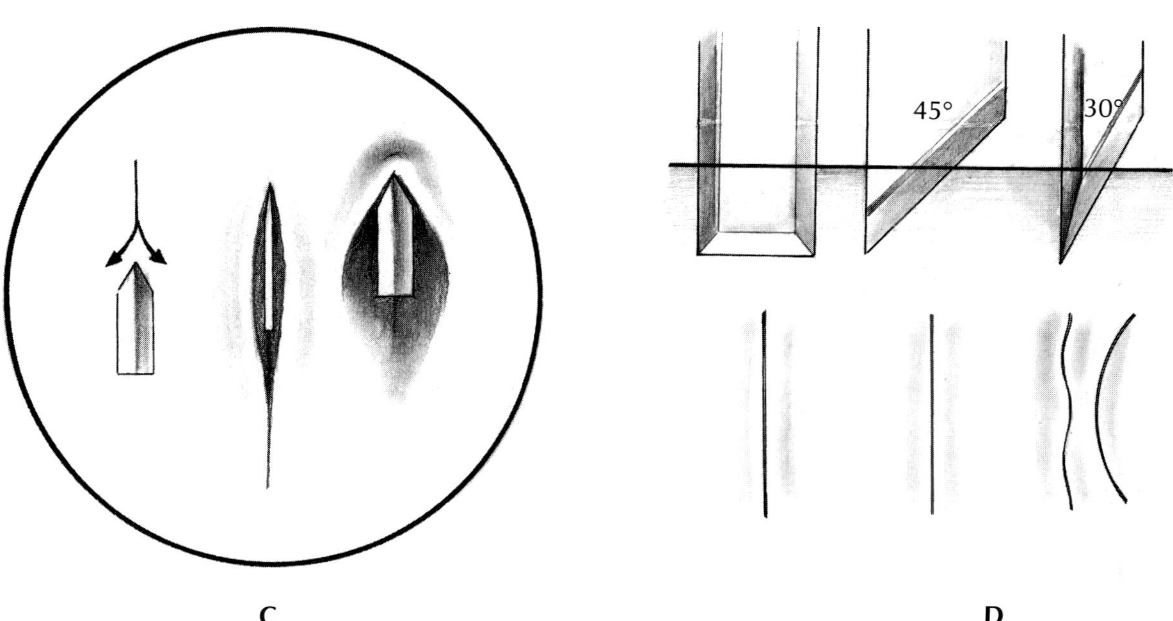

A, developing high forces at pointed tip of knife with minimal tissue distortion. **B,** increased tissue distortion caused by cutting with a blunt-edged knife. **C,** rudderlike action of knife in tissue showing less displacement with a thin knife and greater displacement with a thick knife. **D,** Cutting action of wide knife making straight linear incision, thin knife making irregular incisions, and thin knife making arcuate incision.

In general, crystalline knives used for refractive surgery are created with both a vertical edge and a diagonal edge. Either one or both edges can be sharpened, and the direction of cutting, that is, whether one chooses to use the vertical or diagonal edge, has a significant impact on the stability of the knife and the depth of the incision. If the vertical edge of the knife is used to cut, the tissue will bunch into the knife, creating a deeper incision (Plate 8–2,A). The trailing edge of the knife will then be stabilized by the sides of a deep incision, and this mode of cutting will inherently cause more irregular incisions because the knife will have a tendency to drift.

If a knife is used with the diagonal edge as the cutting edge, the tissue will tend to push away from the knife, creating a shallower incision (Plate 8–2,B). The larger the angle between vertical and diagonal edges the more prominent this effect will be. However, these incisions will tend to be more linear, because the sides of the knife are held more firmly by the incision edges. In addition, the beginning of the incision will be a shallow curve as the knife gradually reaches full depth. An exception to this is firm corneal tissue, such as that encountered in a scar, in which the tissue cannot push away and the knife achieves full depth quickly. Alternatively, a narrow-angled double-edged knife will achieve full depth more quickly, with a less rounded entry, even when cutting with the diagonal edge, because of the sharpness of the knife (Plate 8–2,C).

In short incisions, the rounded ends of the incisions created with the diagonal edge can seriously impair the effectiveness of the incision. Even with long radial incisions, it is desirable to have square ends, particularly adjacent to the optical zone. If an incision is created using the diagonal edge of the knife, for reasons of familiarity or because the knife used in this fashion creates straighter incisions, the issue of reproducible depth and rounded ends can present a problem. A solution is to return to the incision, cutting with the vertical face of the knife, to increase the depth of the incision reproducibly, and at the completion of the incision to create a square end (*tickle procedure;* Plate 8–2,D). This technique can be performed either at the time of surgery or later, and uses the best properties of both vertical- and diagonal-cutting knives to create straight, deep incisions with square ends. The tickle procedure described here can be performed at the time of the original surgery or in the postoperative period at the slitlamp to adjust the refractive effect of keratotomy incisions.

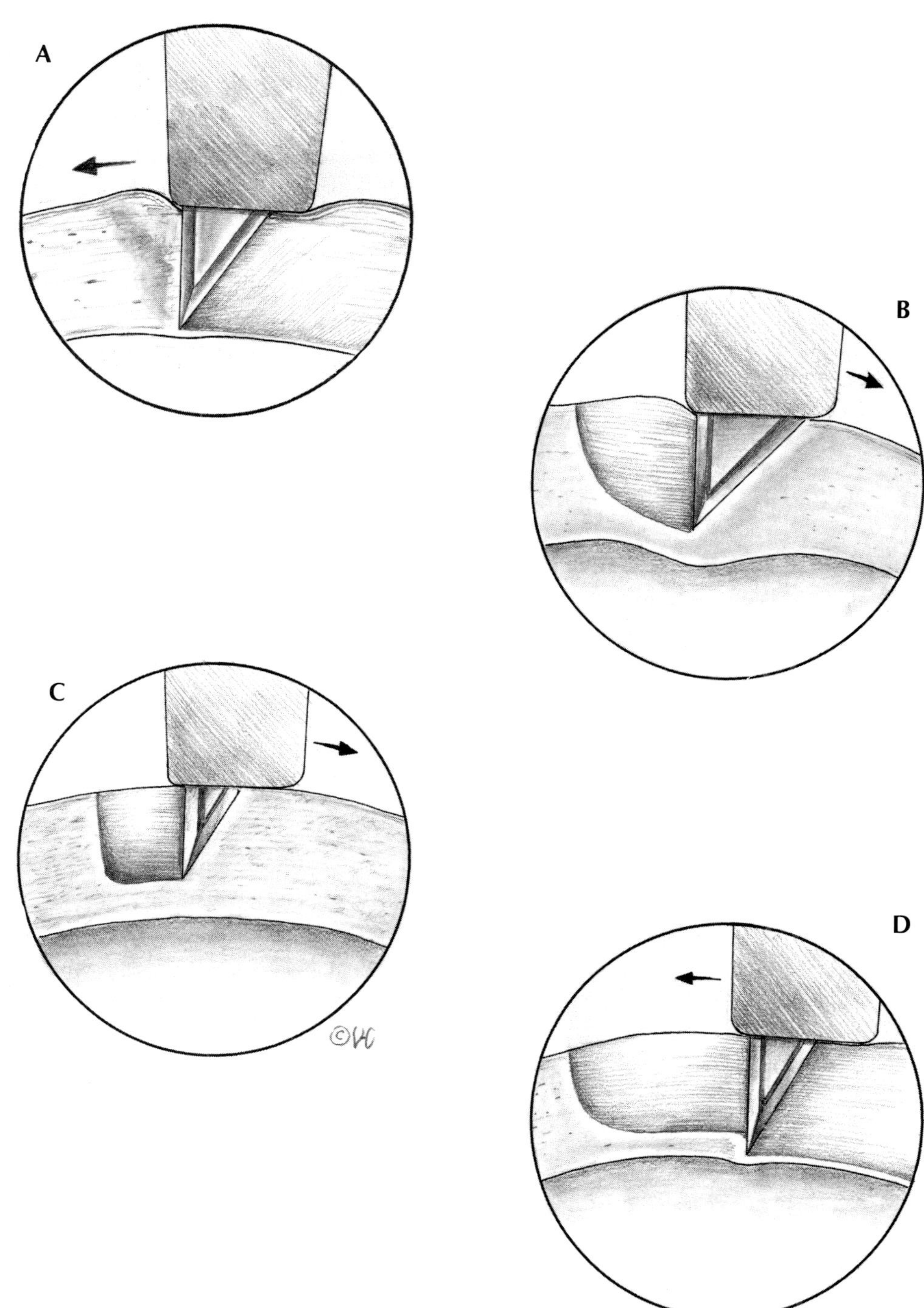

A, guarded 45-degree diamond knife used to create incision with vertical edge, showing bunching of tissue and tendency to create deep incisions. **B,** guarded 45-degree diamond knife with diagonal edge used to create incision, showing tendency to push tissue away from knife and rounded end of incision. **C,** guarded 30-degree diamond knife with decreased angle between vertical and diagonal edge, showing more rapid penetration of tissue and less rounding of end of incision. **D,** Tickle technique, in which a shallow incision with a rounded end is deepened and squared at the end of the incision, using a guarded 30-degree diamond knife cutting with the vertical edge.

Incisional Techniques for Corneal Surgery   **189**

CORNEAL STRUCTURE

From the standpoint of incisions, the cornea can be considered to be a *structural sandwich.* Descemet's membrane and Bowman's layer form a tough, strong envelope for the relatively soft stroma between them. It is clear that this arrangement allows a significant increase in strength of the entire cornea and limits the thickness required to resist the forces placed on it. If we examine a structural element that is fixed on each end and apply a force in the center, we can immediately see that the major forces are applied on the top and bottom surfaces. A stretching force exists on the top surface, whereas a compressive force is in place on the bottom surface. The area between the two surfaces experiences little force and therefore can be much less strong.

In the cornea, as in stiff structure, an incision is made in two steps: entrance through the tough Bowman's layer and extension through the relatively soft stroma. One complication is the compressible nature of the stroma, which is significantly stiffened by an intact Bowman's layer. Because incisions through Bowman's layer significantly weaken the corneal structure and subsequent incisions near the previous incision require the same force to penetrate Bowman's layer, careful planning is required to accurately create incisions in close proximity. Examples of situations in which this problem arises are the wedge resection and transverse incisions during radial keratotomy. If a transverse incision is attempted immediately after radial keratotomy, the block of tissue defined by the radial incisions will move, making the transverse incision shallow and distorted (Fig 8–3,A).

A useful technique for creating a secondary incision close to an existing incision involves use of the tip of the knife. Because we know that maximum forces are generated when the tip of the knife is used to incise the cornea, whereas lateral displacement is kept to a minimum, we may create the second incision by means of multiple punctures along its proposed path *(Multiple Puncture Technique,* Fig 8–3,B). In this way, an accurate incision can be created through Bowman's layer without concern for the distortion that would occur if the knife were continuously displaced laterally through the tissue. The stab incisions can then be connected in a reasonably accurate manner without significant distortion, as the stromal tissue will cut much more easily. In many cases, it is preferable to connect the stab incisions by means of gradually deeper, successive lateral movements, thus limiting the amount of stroma to be incised in any given path (Fig 8–3,C).

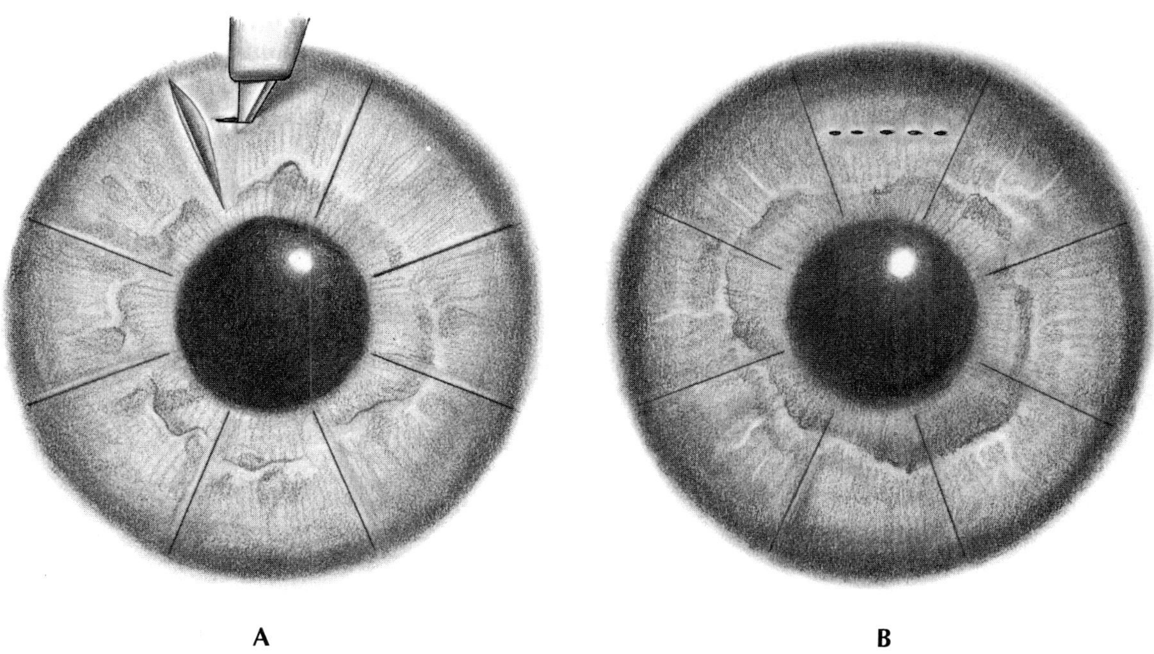

A   B

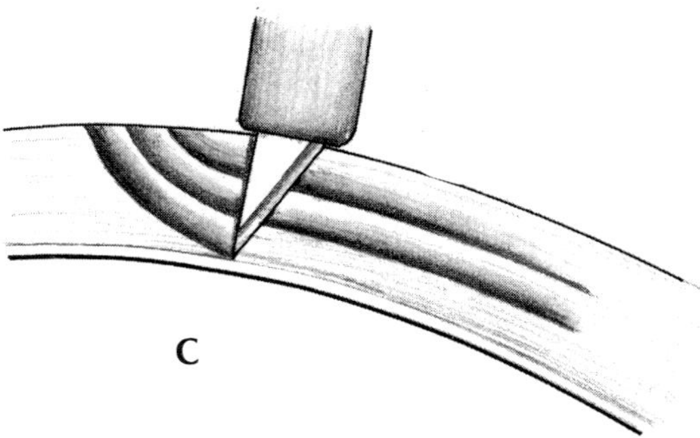

C

A, block movement of corneal tissue when attempt is made to create transverse incision immediately after radial keratotomy. **B,** *Multiple Puncture Technique* to avoid tissue distortion and block movement of corneal tissue, allowing corneal incisions to be created in close proximity. **C,** technique of successively deeper incisions used to connect multiple punctures or alone to minimize corneal distortion when creating keratotomy incisions.

In most refractive surgical procedures, the goal is to make deep but not penetrating corneal incisions. This is usually accomplished by the use of guarded diamond knives. The proper selection of handle, footplates, and diamond knife is an important component of the successful completion of incisional procedures. In addition, the micrometric adjustment of the knives relative to the cornea can mean the difference between success and failure in refractive surgery.

Guarded Diamond Knives

The essential components of a guarded diamond knife used for refractive surgery are the micrometer, the handle, the footplates, and the diamond (Plate 8–4). These components, working in harmony, allow the repetitive creation of incisions of predictable depth with a minimum of effort. Consideration of these elements in detail will illuminate the use of the guarded diamond knife.

The micrometer supplied with most diamond knives is made to allow small and predictable movements of the diamond relative to the footplates. Although these micrometers are calibrated, the harsh conditions to which they are subjected, including high humidity and high temperature during sterilization, virtually assure miscalibration over time. For this reason they should not be relied on; instead, the knife should be calibrated with a device such as the Baribeau Micronscope, discussed later.

The handle of the diamond knife should have sufficient length to allow proper grasping, with some degree of knurling or roughness to avoid slipping. Recently knives have been made with shorter barrels, which we believe allows a more complete degree of freedom with respect to hand position. An example of a short barrel knife is the Excaliber, from Magnum Diamond. In particular, when producing short incisions for astigmatism, the straight-barrel diamond knife requires hand position that obscures the entrance of the diamond into the tissue. The Osher handle from Metico (see Plate 8–4) has a unique design that places the handle at an angle relative to the diamond knife. This allows excellent visualization of the entry of the diamond knife without interference from the fingers surrounding the handle and makes it possible to use this knife at the slitlamp because it does not bump into the optics.

The design of footplates has a significant impact on the depth of the incision because the footplates protect the knife from unrestricted penetration of the cornea. Footplates that are too wide will interfere with other incisions and will cause unacceptable drag on the cornea. Footplates that are too narrow will not accurately determine the anterior surface of the cornea, but will sink into corneal tissue, possibly causing corneal abra-

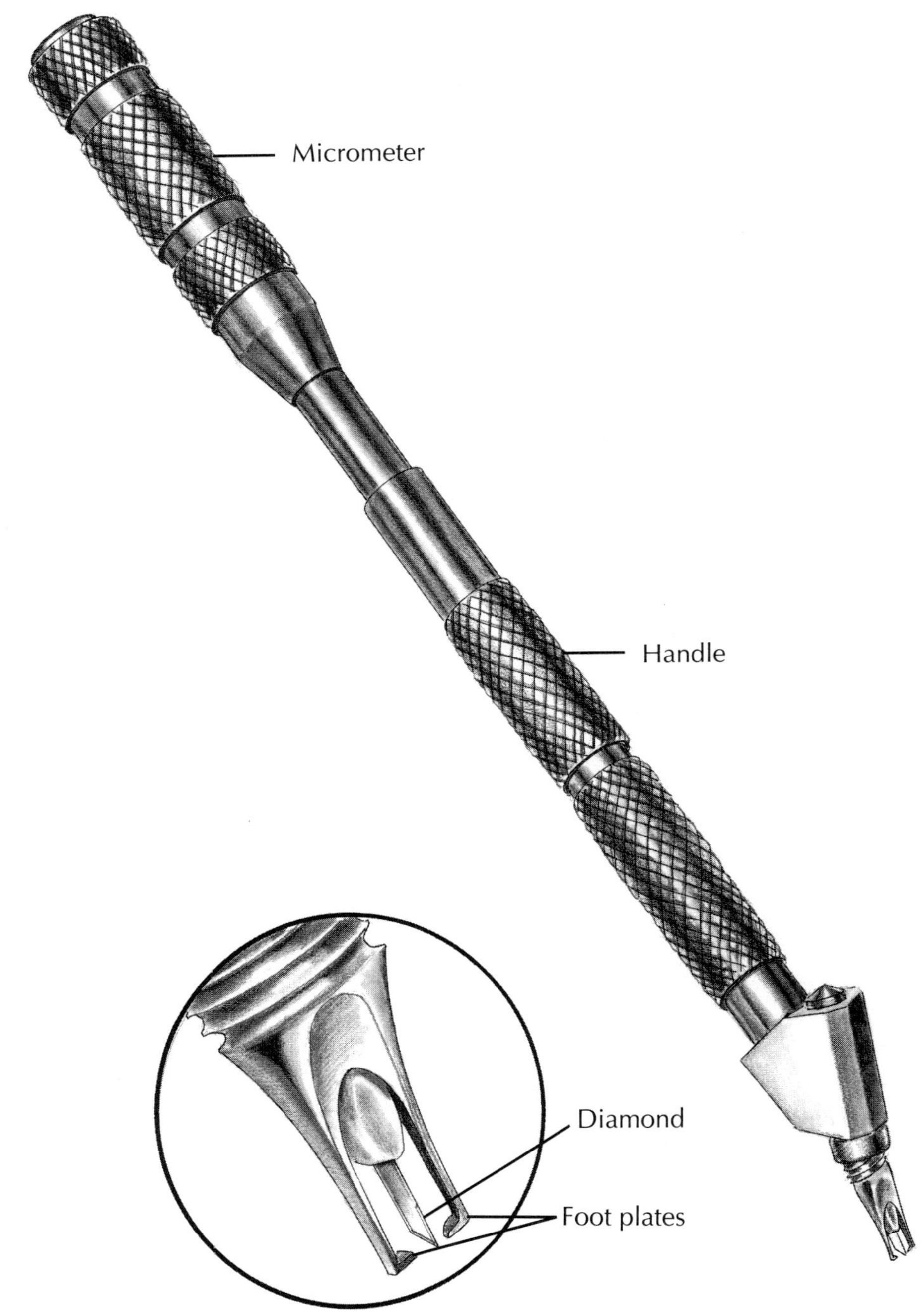

Osher angled guarded diamond knife illustrates four basic components: micrometer, handle, foot-plates, and diamond knife.

sions. A design that is convexly curved on the surface against which the cornea rests will allow rocking of the knife when cutting, causing an unacceptable variation of incision depth. Also, measurement of blade extension is more difficult with convexly curved footplates because a flat surface does not exist on which to center the cross hairs of the Baribeau Micronscope.

The mounting and design of the diamond represents the area of greatest choice to the surgeon and the greatest differentiation between competing knives. If the diamond is mounted so that it extends with the movement of the micrometer, it will be slightly less firm in resisting lateral forces than a design that mounts the diamond directly to the handle and moves the footplate instead. The Metico, Excalibur, and Pilling diamond knives have diamonds mounted directly on the micrometer, and the Katena knife has extensible footplates.

Diamond design represents the final choice in selection of an appropriate knife. Although we have mentioned other crystals, such as sapphire, gem-quality diamond is the only appropriate material for refractive surgery. In the past, the diamonds were relatively thick; the Osher knife is a good example of this older design. A thick diamond will tend to resist entry into the cornea and will necessitate a slightly wider angle between the faces of the knife (because the knife is thicker), thus creating a slightly duller instrument. In some circumstances this can be an advantage, as in incisional deepening, when the desire is to remain within the incision and to cut only at the tip of the blade. Advances in diamond cutting have given us ultra-thin diamonds that are sharper and penetrate the tissue better, but are more fragile.

The number of cutting edges also affects corneal penetration. Single-edged knives have sharpened edges along only the diagonal or vertical edge (Plate 8–5,A) and are slightly less sharp to vertical penetration than diamonds with edges along both the vertical and diagonal edges. Thus the entry of a single-edged diamond knife will give a rounded appearance to the end of the incision as the knife gradually sinks to full depth (Plate 8–2,B). A double-edged knife (Plate 8–5,B) will come to full depth almost immediately, entering more vertically and giving a squarer appearance to the end of the incision (Plate 8–2,C). Triple-facet knives, such as the Hofmann square blade (Plate 8–5,C), distribute forces along a fairly long, flat edge and thus require rocking of the knife to achieve corneal penetration. An advantage of the triple-facet knife is excellent, repeatable corneal depth on movement of the blade and vertical edges at the extremes of the incision, and it is particularly useful for deepening a shallow incision.

Finally, the angle between the vertical and diagonal edges has a significant impact on the vertical penetration of the blade, because a larger angle induces more displacement of corneal tissue than a narrow angle. The 45-degree diamond configuration (Plate 8–5,D) submerges a greater

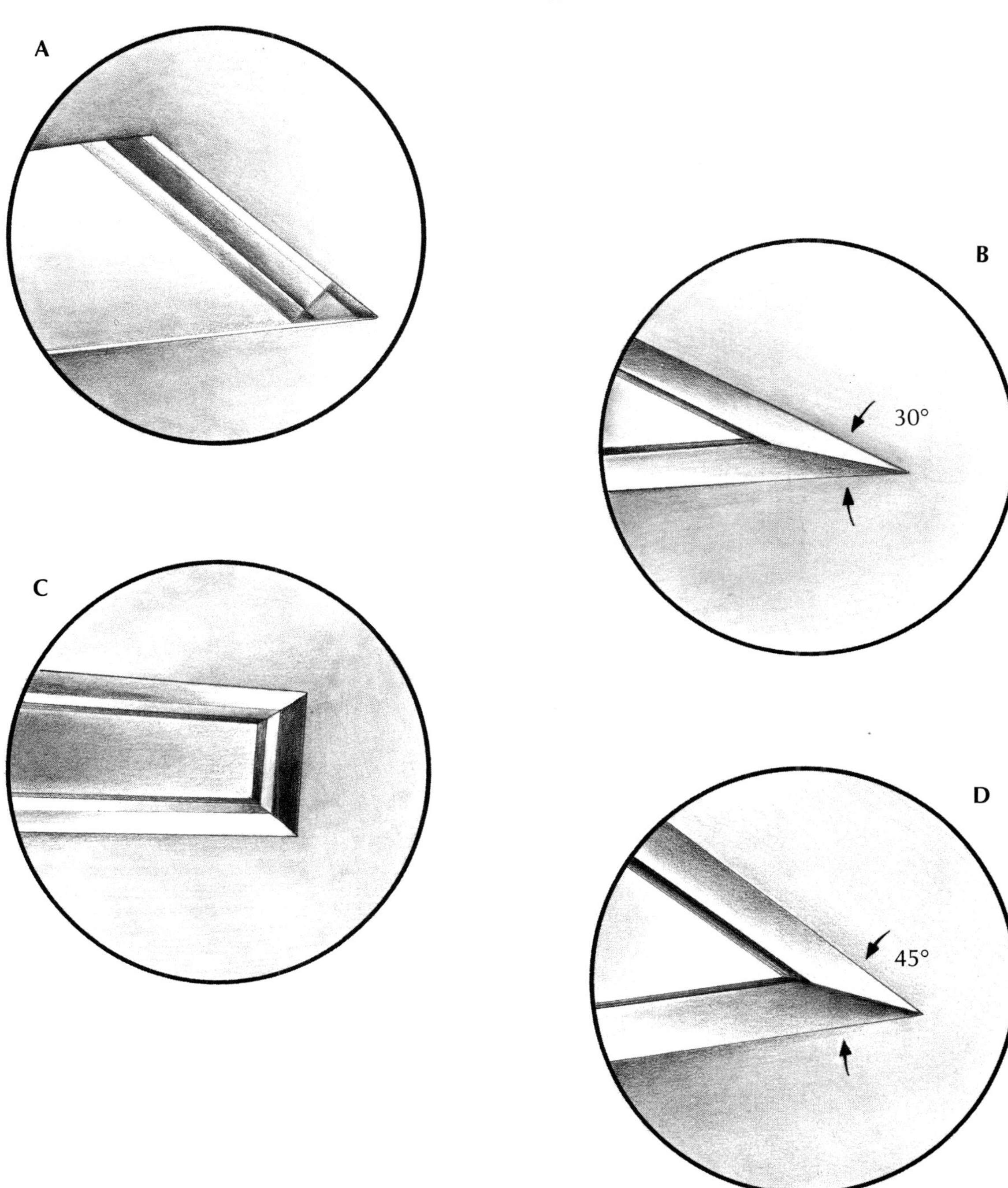

A, Single-cutting 45-degree diamond blade with cutting diagonal edge, which tends to make straight incisions with rounded ends and more shallow incisions, compared with double-cutting blades. **B,** double-cutting 30-degree diamond blade with cutting vertical and diagonal edges, which creates more square ends of incisions and deeper incisions but is more unstable in tissue and better for curved incisions or tickle procedure. **C,** Hofmann triple-facet square diamond blade with three cutting edges, which tends to penetrate cornea only if rocked but capable of creating short deep incisions with square ends. **D,** double-cutting 45-degree diamond blade with cutting vertical and diagonal edges with slightly poorer penetration of tissue but slightly more stable.

Incisional Techniques for Corneal Surgery   **195**

portion of the knife into the corneal tissue and thus creates more of a rudder effect, tending to direct the knife in a linear fashion. The 30-degree diamond configuration (Plate 8–5,B) submerges less diamond in the cornea and is more amenable to changes in direction.

Clinical Considerations

The combination of these four components can dictate the proper choice of guarded diamond knife for a particular refractive surgical procedure. No one diamond knife fulfills all needs in all situations.

The Osher diamond knife with the double-cutting 45-degree blade is a good choice for short transverse astigmatic procedures. Particularly in the presence of radial keratotomy incisions, its superb visualization of the entry point of the diamond enables excellent control of these incisions in a restricted area. With a straight handle, the fingers holding the knife interfere with proper visualization (Plate 8–6,A). With the angled design of the Osher diamond knife, the fingers are well out of view (Plate 8–6,B).

The thick diamond is slightly less sharp, which prevents unintended excursions. This knife is also a good choice for the tickle procedure or incisional deepening at the slitlamp because the slightly dull diamond splits the incisions open without tending to cut virgin tissue. In addition, the handle provides good visualization without bumping into the optics of the slitlamp. A modification of this knife with a triple-facet Hofmann square blade allows the production of short transverse incisions with square ends without the need for reversal of orientation of the knife.

This knife is not well suited to creating radial incisions, because it has a tendency to create beveled incisions if the knife is turned slightly in the hand (Plate 8–6,C). In addition, it is less intuitive and more cumbersome to tilt the knife through the normal excursion to create a radial incision. This knife, with either the double-cutting diamond provided or an ultrathin 30-degree double-cutting blade, is a good choice for most astigmatic procedures.

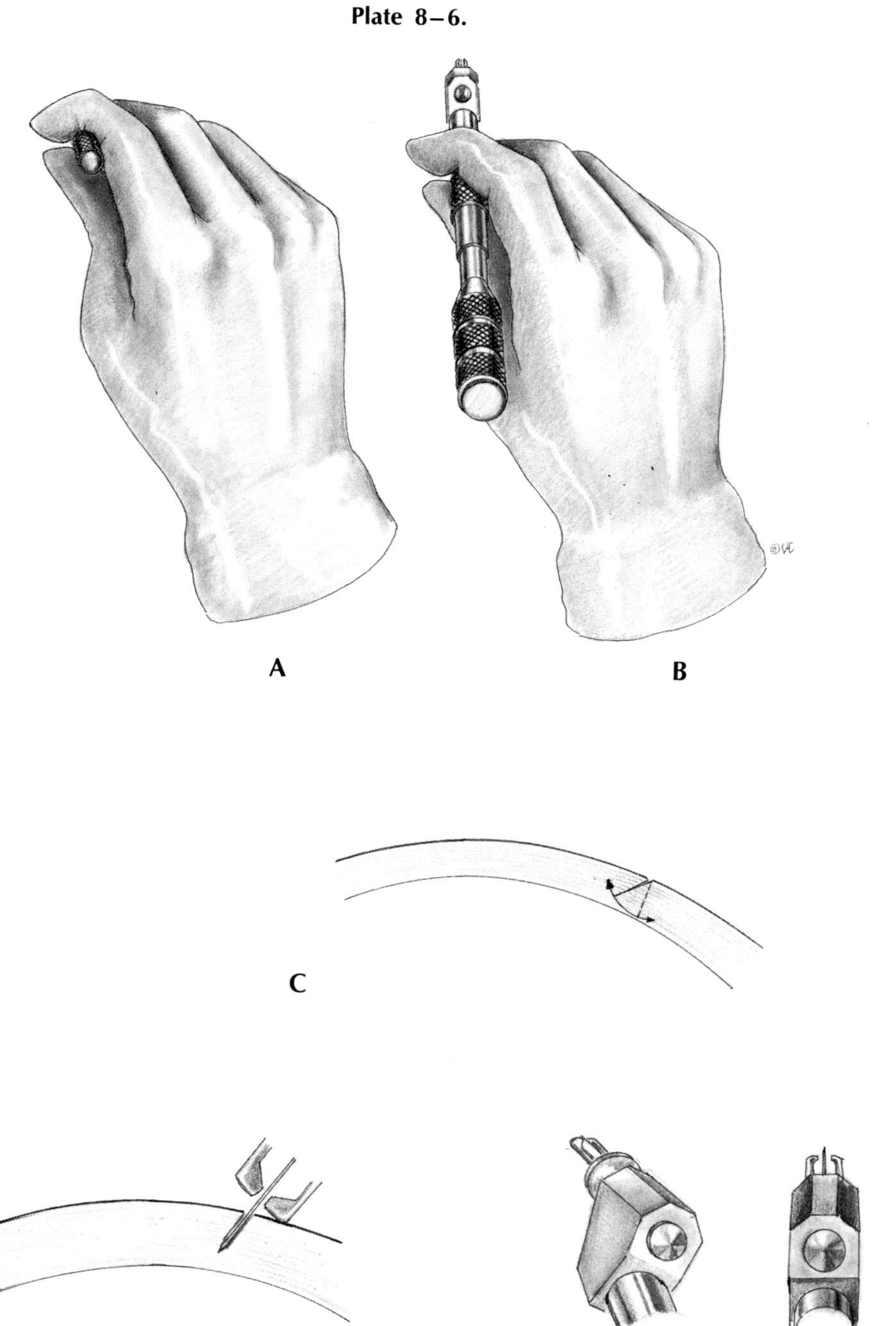

A, surgeon's perspective of straight-barrel diamond knife, showing obstruction of diamond cutting point by fingers wrapped around knife. **B,** surgeon's perspective of Osher diamond knife, showing advantage of tilted barrel and clear view of diamond penetration of cornea. **C,** disadvantage of tilted barrel on Osher diamond knife, showing tendency to create beveled incisions with slight rotation of barrel.

The Metico diamond knife has the advantage of titanium construction and a well-guarded diamond, which still allows good visualization (Plate 8–7,A). We prefer the KOI diamond knife for visualization relative to the footplates as a similar design, although the knife is constructed with stainless steel. These knives have the usual problem of having the diamond attached to the micrometer and, thus, it has a tendency to wobble with the incision. However, it is still a good choice in combination with a single-cutting diamond for creation of radial incisions from the optical zone to the limbus. For this purpose, a 45-degree diamond should be requested, as this will create straighter incisions.

A double-cutting diamond attached to these knives will have a tendency to create crooked radial incisions when used from the limbus to the optical zone, because of a slight instability of the diamond attached to the micrometer. When used from the optical zone to the limbus, the knife design is adequately stable, and can be used with a double-cutting diamond for this purpose. It would be wise to have a 45-degree angle on the double-cutting diamond to stabilize the knife.

A Katena (Plate 8–7,B) diamond knife has a more stable attachment of the diamond to the handle and is a good choice for a double-cutting 30-degree knife. The diamond is slightly more exposed and more subject to damage, but visualization is excellent. Even with this design, a radial incision created from the optical zone to limbus will be more difficult to keep truly straight because this diamond design has so little of its area in the cornea and, hence, is slightly unstable. In the operating room this knife or the Excalibur (with a stabilized blade) is preferred for secondary deepening of incisions with a 30-degree ultra-thin diamond to an Osher knife, because of the improved visualization of vertical orientation of the knife, enabling the avoidance of beveled incisions. These knives also are used to create long arcuate incisions, again because of improved appreciation of vertical orientation and the ability of these diamond and handle combinations to accurately follow curved incisions.

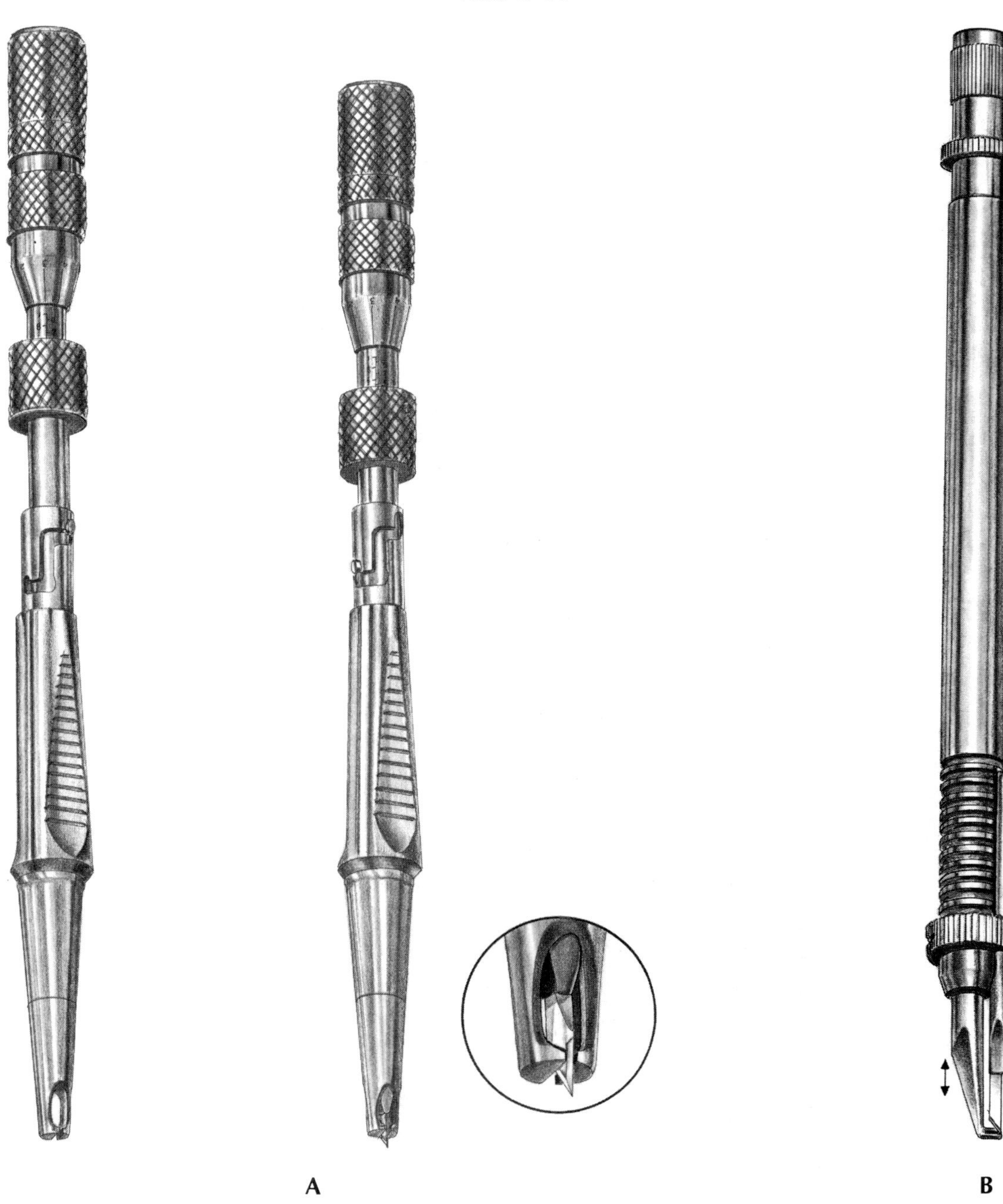

A

B

A, Metico titanium diamond knife, showing design with extensible diamond attached to micrometer. B, Katena diamond knife, showing design with diamond attached to barrel and extensible footplates.

Calibration of Blade Extension

One of the challenges of refractive surgery involves the degree of accuracy in terms of instrumentation that must be maintained to produce predictable refractive changes. The average thickness of the central cornea is only 0.55 mm, and to create the customary 90% to 95% corneal thickness incisions, the blade extension must be measured in microns to be reproducible. In the past, surgeons relied on blade extension that was measured by the built-in micrometer on most diamond knives made for refractive surgery. These knives undergo significant changes as they are repeatedly sterilized and subjected to the stress of continuous use. Thus the measurements indicated on the knife cannot be relied on for an indication of repeatable extension of the knife.

The blade gauge was developed as a secondary check of the measurement of blade extension and was produced in both bar form and as a coin gauge. The gauge consisted of an elevated metal edge of progressively varying thickness accompanied by calibrations indicating the thickness at each point. The diamond knife was placed above this calibrated metal edge, and by examining the knife over the gauge under the operating microscope, the blade extension could be verified. Many problems occurred with this instrument. For instance, the diamond knife is quite delicate, and any inadvertent contact between the diamond knife and the gauge would ruin the knife. Therefore, the knife was generally maintained some distance above the metal gauge to avoid damage to the knife. This technique was safer for the diamond knife but induced parallax in the measurement of blade extension, making the measurement virtually worthless. This approach was incapable of measuring blade extension more accurately than about 10%, or about 50 μm.

A significant development for the measurement and examination of the microsurgical instrumentation required for refractive surgery is the microscope with an attached micrometric stage, developed by Douglas Mastel. This Baribeau micronscope consists of a microscope with a reticule for definition of measurement points attached to a stage with 2 degrees of freedom controlled by high-precision micrometers capable of measurement on a scale of 1 μm (Plate 8–8). For measurement of guarded diamond blade extension, the knife is clamped on the stage with a special fixture, and the reticule is aligned with the footplates of the diamond knife. The micrometer is then moved to the desired blade extension, and the knife is extended until the tip is coincident with the reticule, which is now placed at the proper blade extension with an accuracy of 1 μm.

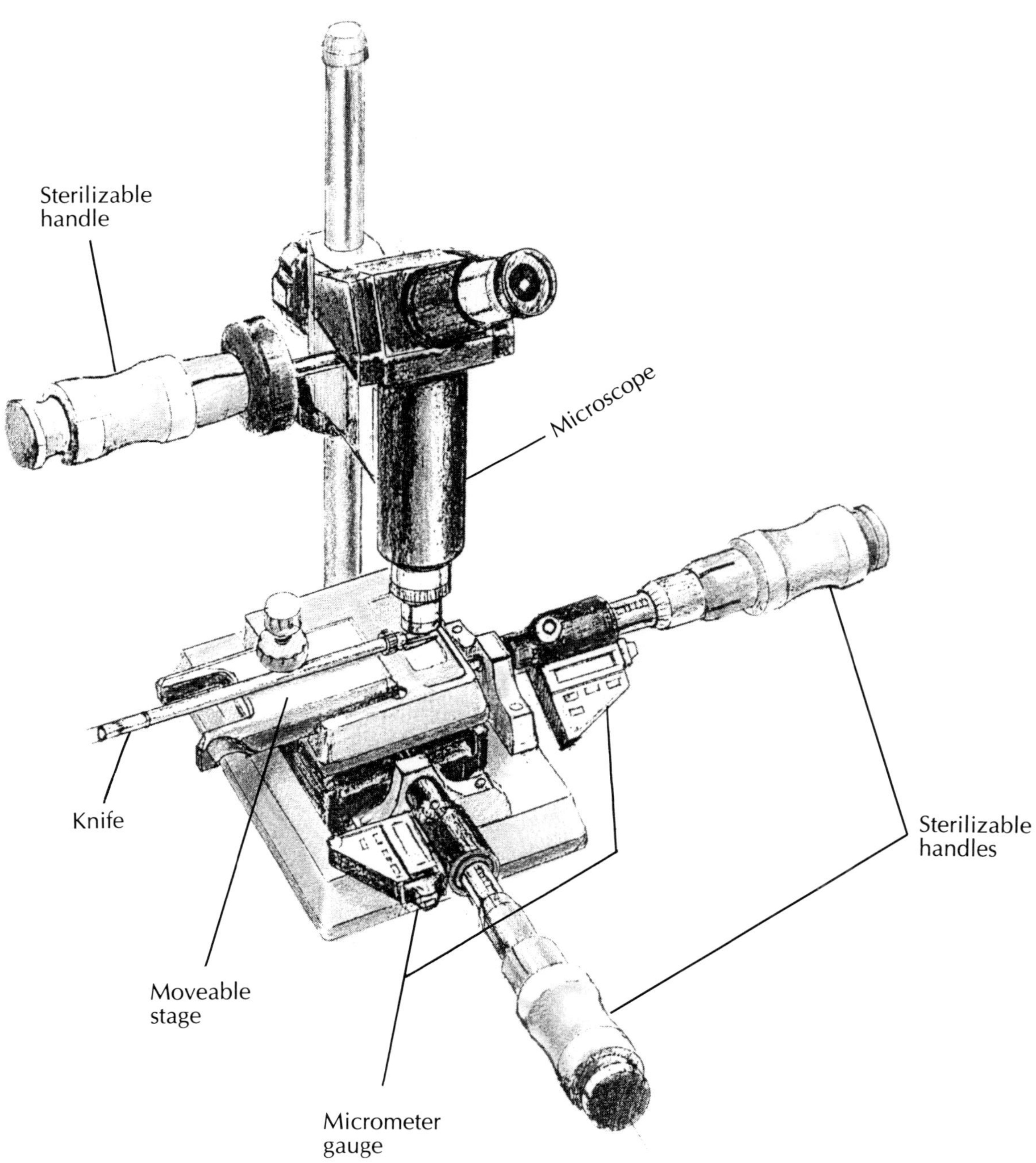

Baribeau Micronscope used for calibration of diamond knives and examination and calibration of microsurgical instruments, showing micrometer stage with 2 degrees of freedom and bracket holding the diamond knife.

Although this procedure is vastly more accurate than the coin gauges and blocks that preceded it, some problems remain. First, the proper alignment of the reticule with the footplates of the knife can be complicated if the footplates are curved. In addition, the proper point of focus on the footplates can be difficult to achieve, and in many cases, a blur pervades the edge of the footplate, making proper alignment with the reticule difficult. A different instrument, which in effect is a calibrated shadowgraph available from DGH, solves this problem by projecting a shadow of the knife, but this instrument does not allow direct visualization of the footplates, blade, and other instruments. As we discuss later, preventive maintenance of refractive surgical instruments by examination and measurement is extremely important and is facilitated by the Baribeau Micronscope, whereas similar measurements with the DGH instrument are possible but not so convenient. Several devices have become available (e. g., the Reti-cal microscope from Mastel) that although not so complete as the instrument described, function adequately, at significantly lower cost.

With the availability of these instruments, it is the belief of most active refractive surgeons that ongoing evaluation and calibration of refractive surgical instrumentation requires one of these instruments, and predictable refractive surgery cannot be performed without them.

Examination of Diamond Knives

The first observation should be an evaluation of the stability of the diamond blade as it is being extended. On diamond knives in which extension is accomplished by movement of the diamond, one often sees significant wobbling of the mounting during extension. This instability can manifest as S-shaped radial corneal incisions when used for radial keratotomy. Few guarded diamond knives with extensible diamonds have truly stable mountings, although most are adequate. However, they should be evaluated carefully before purchase and before each use.

Examination of the placement of the diamond relative to the footplates can give additional important information on the inner workings of the knife. Micrometers translate a twisting motion on the handle during linear extension of the blade. Within the knife is a stabilizing groove that keeps the diamond from twisting as the diamond is extended. This is a delicate assembly and often can be damaged, allowing the knife to twist relative to the footplates. If this condition is allowed to continue uncorrected, the knife will have a tendency to cut at a slight angle to normal, resulting in irregularly curved or jagged incisions.

Checking the footplates of the guarded knife is another important step for the knife being examined. Although they appear sturdy, they can be easily bent, resulting in a tendency to create beveled incisions. In addition, the footplates can come from the manufacturer with one footplate shorter than the other, which again, will cause beveled incisions (Plate 8–9,A). Finally, the footplates can become roughened or scratched with constant use or they can become coated with proteinaceous debris (Plate 8–9,B). Rough footplates can lead to shallow incisions and can tear the epithelium leading to postoperative wound-healing problems. A good protective measure against these problems is gold coating on stainless steel knives or the use of extremely hard materials such as titanium with highly polished footplates. Even with these measures, the footplates should be examined and cleaned after each use, preferably with an ultrasonic cleaner.

Examination of the diamond knife blade and tip are extremely important aspects in evaluation of the knife. Unless detected with a microscope, the tip of the diamond knife may have been broken without the knowledge of the surgeon (Plate 8–9,C). The only indication of this problem might be a sudden appearance of undercorrections and a tendency of the knife to *feel* dull. With abuse, the cutting edges of the knife can become damaged, and the change in feel can seem so insignificant that without the microscope, the surgeon may be unaware of the problem (Plate 8–9,D). Finally, dried blood and proteinaceous debris can accumulate on the diamond, reducing cutting efficiency and leading to trauma along the sides of the incision resulting in shallow incisions.

Thus, we see that the care and examination of a properly functioning, guarded diamond knife is a time-consuming and delicate procedure that must be undertaken to create repeatable results in refractive surgery. If any of these problems become present, the ability to create incisions of acceptable depth and configuration will diminish. The acceptable variation of depth in incisional refractive procedures is small. Shallow incisions produce progressive undercorrection, whereas excessively deep incisions can cause corneal perforation. To develop predictability, the refractive surgeon must be able to hold the variable of incision depth constant, to the level objectively determined by corneal pachymetry. This can be accomplished only with properly functioning and calibrated diamond instruments.

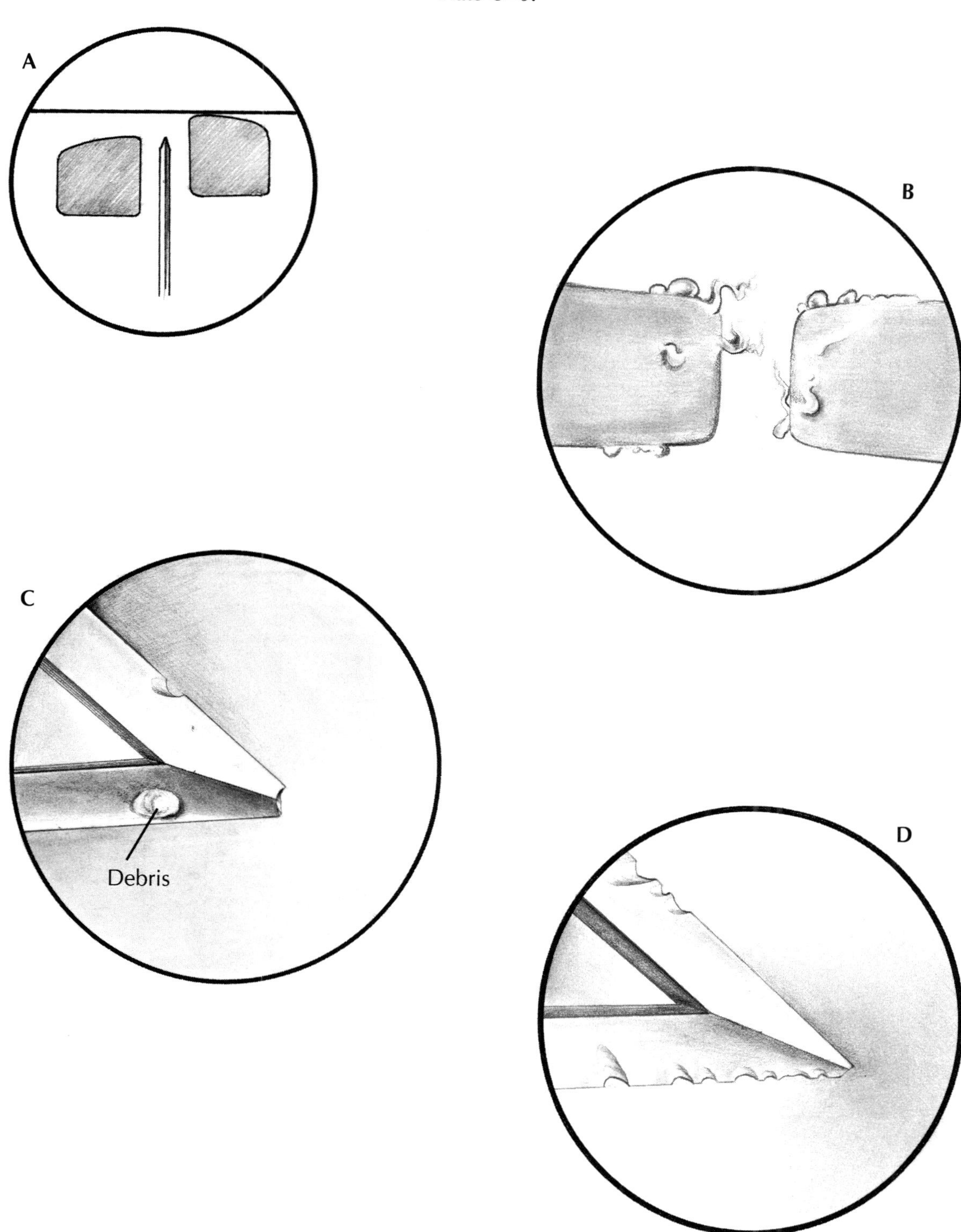

A, rounded and uneven footplates make calibration difficult and create a tendency for beveled incisions. **B,** accumulation of dried blood and proteinaceous debris on footplates of guarded diamond knife. **C,** broken diamond blade tip with view of proteinaceous debris on knife edge. **D,** abused and damaged diamond blade with multiple-edge serrations from trauma to cutting edges.

The goal of corneal trephination is to create a circumferential opening in the host cornea that matches the circumference of the donor cornea, with matching vertical incision edges. When considering variance from these goals, we should remember that very small incisional errors can result in significant changes in terms of astigmatism and spherical equivalent.

A third consideration is the location of the opening relative to the visual axis. As surgical techniques have improved, the perception of corneal transplantation as a refractive surgical operation has steadily gained prominence. Because the visual axis often is not located in the center of the cornea, this leads to a situation in which trephination occurs through areas of different firmness, such as in areas of arcus in the peripheral cornea. This can alter the performance of the incisional device or trephine along the perimeter of the incision, resulting in a sloping incision.

Examination of the corneal trephine reveals that the force applied to the trephine will be distributed along a very long edge. Thus even if significant force is applied downward on the trephine, we can expect little direct cutting. In fact, because the host cornea is flexible, excess pressure on the trephine will cause the cornea to well up within the trephine, causing a beveled incision. There are circumstances in which sufficient direct pressure can be applied to allow cutting of the cornea. If the cornea is supported against a firm surface, such as a Teflon concave cutting block, in cutting with the donor trephine, sufficient pressure can be developed to penetrate the cornea.

Cutting of the recipient is ordinarily accomplished primarily through rotation of the blade. This can lead to a significant problem during cutting, as rotating the blade creates a tendency toward drifting, both when trying to penetrate the firm Bowman's layer and later in the relatively soft corneal stroma. A punch incision creates characteristic incisions that are unlike incisions created by rotation of a corneal trephine, and this problem has been addressed in different ways as will be described.

Only the finest and sharpest trephines should be used for penetrating corneal transplantation. Modern manufacturing techniques have made extremely sharp trephines available on a regular basis. Before each surgery, the authors routinely examine each trephine that will be used in that operation. Only new, never before used, trephines are acceptable for surgery. If a defect in the trephine occurs at a given location along the edge, the incision will be impeded in that area, allowing the trephine to tilt and cause a beveled incision. Moreover, the defect will eventually rotate 360 degrees and cause excessive trauma to the cornea in the area of incision, leading to a poor-quality incision with subsequent poor wound healing. Although it has been common practice in the past to reuse corneal trephines, it is the opinion of the authors that the relative economy of trephines available today and the overriding importance of a regular and clean incision make the reuse of corneal trephines a false economy.

Finally, concerning the manufacture of circular trephines, it is quite difficult to sharpen a truly circular trephine evenly. When a flat portion of steel is sharpened and bent into a circular shape, sometimes two rough ends can be left that will cause trauma during trephination. Such trephines should not be used. Only truly circular trephines, which either begin as a tube or have no rough ends where joined, should be used for corneal transplantation.

One final concern regards the sharpened edge of the trephine. If the trephine is sharpened on the outer surface only, it will have a tendency to bevel slightly inward. It is preferable to have both the inner and the outer surfaces honed to balance cutting forces and promote vertical incisions.

Handheld Corneal Trephine

If the cornea is approached with a handheld corneal trephine, the problem of vertical orientation of the trephine to the cornea can be seen immediately (Plate 8–10,A). If the trephine is held slightly inclined, relative to the cornea, the pressure along a sector of the blade will be higher and that section of the blade will incise the cornea faster and at an angle. The cornea will be penetrated first at that level, and examination of the incision will show a bevel at the point of penetration with undercutting of the cornea 180 degrees away. This problem often can be appreciated at the time of trephination by careful attention to the level at which the trephine enters the cornea. If the cornea begins to wrinkle and move against the blade, an area of undercutting 180 degrees opposite is indicated (Plate 8–10,B). The surgeon should gently tilt the trephine away from this area while pulling back slightly. This problem is compounded when the consistency of the corneal tissue is not equal along the perimeter of the proposed incision, as in a corneal arcus. In such circumstances, the trephine must be watched very carefully to avoid both undercutting of the firmer cornea and beveling of the softer cornea.

The primary problem with the free corneal trephine, and in a sense its redeeming feature, is the degree of mobility of the trephine. The trephine is free to move laterally and to tilt relative to the surface. Modifications to alleviate these problems center on the addition of a supporting framework for the trephine that limits the mobility during the trephination.

Thus far we have concentrated primarily on the ability of the trephine to create steep, square incision edges. When excess pressure is applied to a trephine, the cornea may slide into the barrel of the trephine, thus, enlarging the proposed incision (Plate 8–10,C). If the corneal thickness and elasticity is equal along the perimeter of the trephine, this may occur in a uniform manner so that the final opening will be circular. More often, because of centration on visual axis or in corneal disorders in which the corneal thickness is not uniform, such as keratoconus, the tissue may slip more easily along one section of the trephine than another. This will result in an oval incision rather than a circular incision. This problem is exacerbated by the firm nature of Descemet's membrane, which makes the initial entrance into the corneal tissue difficult to achieve. A partial solution to this problem is to begin the incision with a free trephine with almost no pressure and to rotate 360 degrees in one direction before reversing. After a groove is established in the corneal stroma, slightly more pressure may be applied to facilitate completion of the incision.

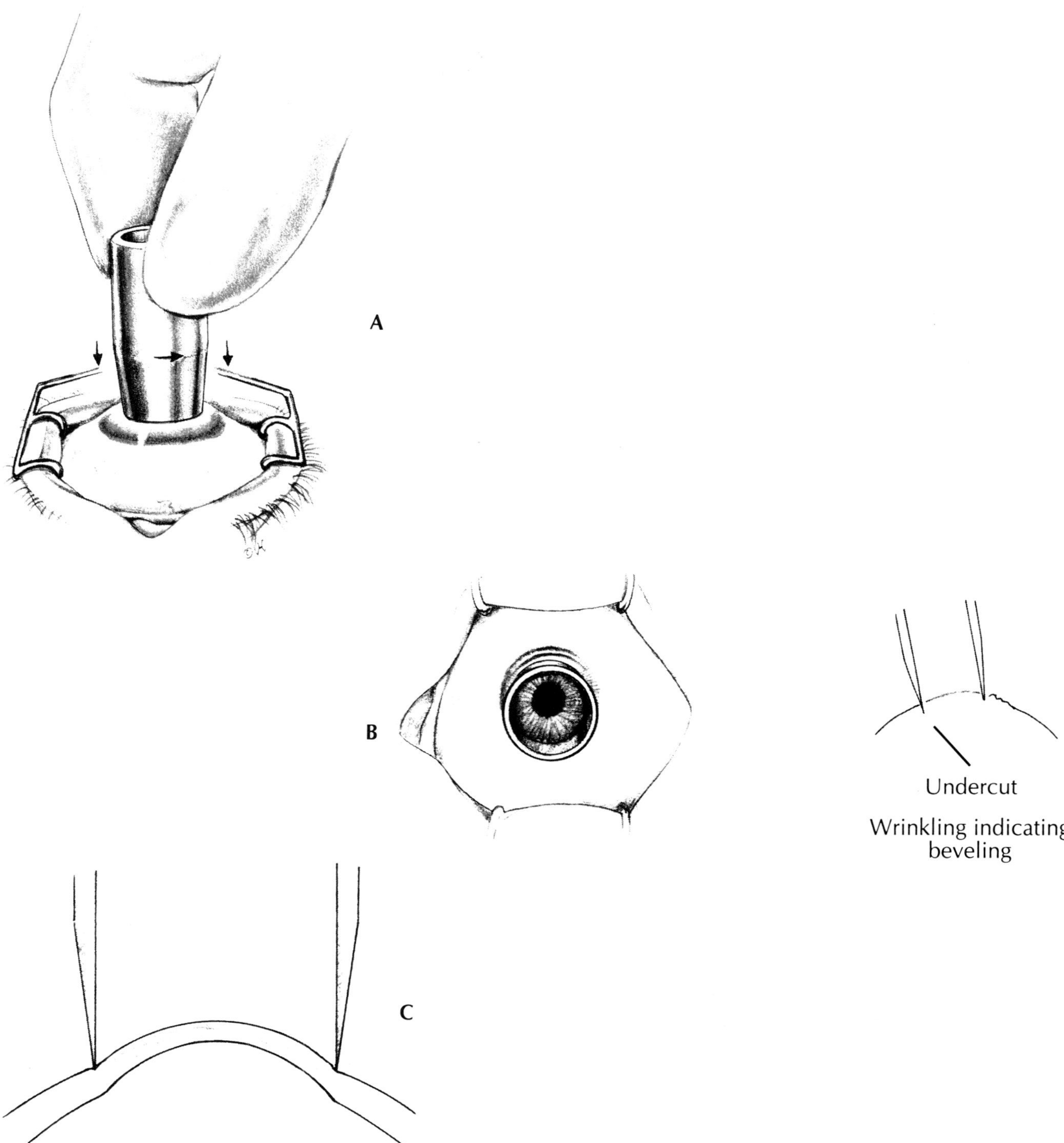

A, handheld corneal trephine showing degree of freedom and tendency to tilt during trephination. **B,** appearance of beveled incision during trephination, showing wrinkling of corneal tissue, indicating the need for corrective action by the surgeon. **C,** bulging of corneal tissue into barrel of trephine with excess pressure during trephination.

Incisional Techniques for Corneal Surgery   **209**

Suction Trephines

In an effort to control these problems, several devices have been introduced to fixate the trephine on the cornea and allow better trephination. These are discussed at greater length elsewhere, but some basic principles can be discussed here. The Barron *(Hessberg) trephine* creates an area of suction adjacent to the area being incised by means of a syringe mounted with a spring. This unmeasured suction variably fixes the trephine to the cornea, thus minimizing tilting relative to the corneal surface. As the cornea is cut, the suction tends to draw the central cornea into the trephine, causing a beveled incision. In addition, to prevent loss of suction and because the area of entrance is obscured, the surgeon will often apply excess vertical pressure to maintain suction during trephination. This results in additional lifting of the central portion of the cornea and undercutting of the incision.

The *Hanna trephine* solves this problem by means of a central obturator, which prevents corneal tissue from rising into the barrel of the trephine. The mechanism is more sophisticated, and the trephine can be preset to a predetermined depth where it can be rotated in place. The *Krumeich trephine* uses both a scleral suction ring and a central obturator to stabilize the trephine. By using fixation on the sclera, there is less corneal distortion, with the potential for a better incision and even the maintenance of the anterior chamber with perforation by the trephine, although both instruments perform excellent trephinations. An advantage of the Hanna trephine is the ability to use variable trephine sizes, whereas the Krumeich trephine is limited to a single trephine size.

A secondary issue revolves around the circularity of the incision. Because tissue is sliding within the barrel of the trephine, the same problems of oval incisions may occur with the Barron *(Hessberg) trephine* in corneas with thickness variation or corneal scarring. This can result in significant astigmatism following the procedure. The Hanna trephine will not allow sliding of tissue, but with an irregular cornea, suction can break during the procedure, leading to beveled incisions. The Krumeich trephine does not have difficulty with irregular corneas, but its application precludes the use of a stabilization ring sewn to the eye, which in itself can lead to astigmatic problems during suturing of the graft.

INCISIONS OF DONOR CORNEA

When the cornea is sufficiently supported to accept significant downward pressure, as in the Troutman punch, it is possible to incise the cornea without rotating the trephine. This method of incision creates a characteristic pattern that reflects the internal structure of the cornea (Plate 8–11). Because Descemet's membrane is more difficult to penetrate and

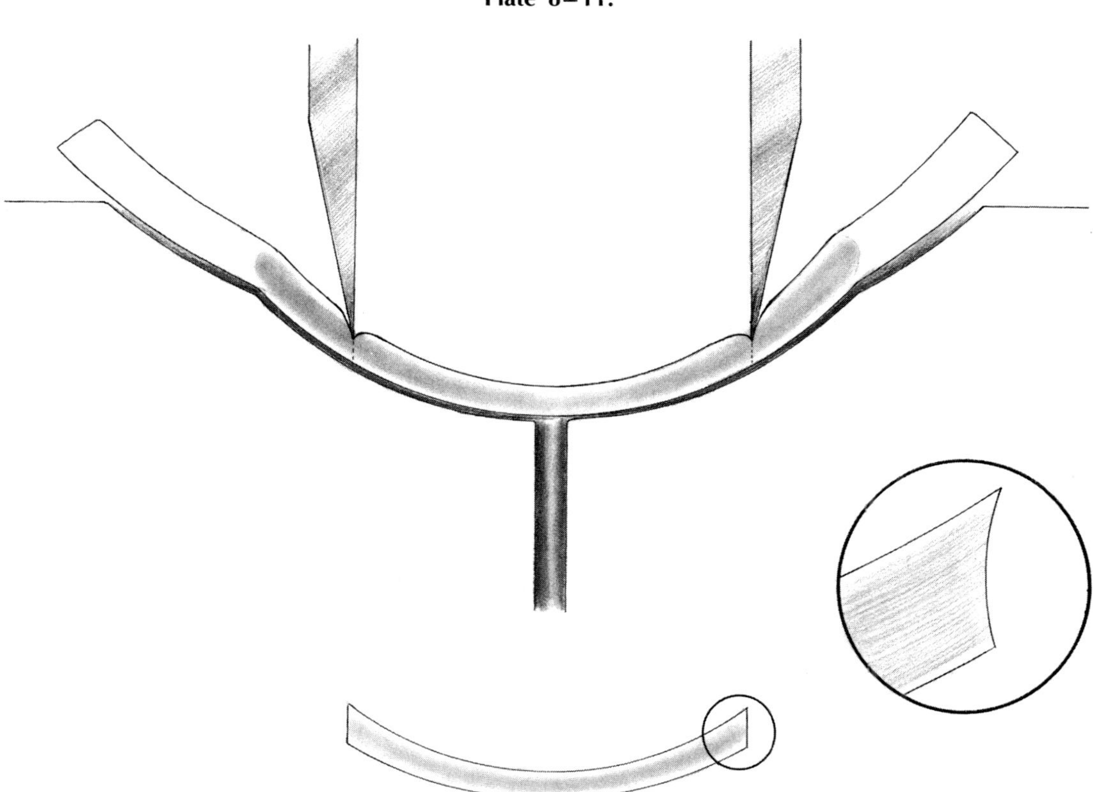

Preparation of donor button with handheld trephine, showing effect of tissue compression on incision.

the stroma is compressible, initial pressure on the cornea causes a flattening or compression of the cornea. At this point, the incision has not begun because the force exerted on the trephine is distributed along the entire perimeter of the trephine blade. Once penetration of Descemet's membrane occurs, the incision proceeds rapidly, and the cornea expands to its original thickness. A cornea incised in this manner under optimal conditions will always have a slight bowing inward from this cycle of compression and decompression. The effective diameter of the donor incision will therefore be slightly less than the diameter of the trephine blade.

This led Troutman in 1975 to the practice of oversizing the donor tissue with respect to the host incision, because of the flatter donor corneas he obtained with the same sized donor and recipient openings. Because the amount of bowing is approximately 0.1 mm along the perimeter of the incision, the usual practice is to increase the size of the trephine used for preparation of the donor cornea 0.2 mm relative to the trephine used to incise the recipient cornea. Because the recipient corneal incision is created using rotation of the blade, the diameter of the incision is approximately the same as the diameter of the trephine used to make that incision. In 1975 Troutman proposed using oversized donor tissue of 0.5–1.0 mm relative to the trephine used to make the host corneal incision to compensate aphakic ametropia. Since in phakic or pseudophakic eyes this leads to bulging of the donor cornea, with resultant steepening and unpredictable overcorrection the practice should be abandoned.

At least part of the rationale for using such oversized tissue was the lack of sharp corneal trephines available for regular use. If a dull trephine is used to create the recipient incision, excessive pressure may be necessary to facilitate the incision, allowing bulging of the cornea within the bore of the trephine and leading to a larger opening than the diameter of the trephine used to create that incision. Thus, early surgeons often compensated for this problem by using an oversized trephine for the preparation of the donor cornea. This should not be necessary with modern, sharp trephines.

In the early days of corneal transplantation, trephination of the donor cornea was accomplished using only a Teflon dish (multiple times) and a handheld trephine. Because the cornea was not well fixated, and a pool of fluid could collect beneath the cornea, the cornea would often slide laterally if the punch were slightly tilted. This would cause beveled incisions, resulting in an oval donor cornea (Plate 8–12). A major improvement in this situation was the development of the Troutman corneal punch. This used a disposable Teflon dish, which could be discarded after each use, with both a hole in the center to allow excess fluid to drain out and two separate curves to account for peripheral corneal flattening and for a tighter fit for the cornea. Finally, a frame set over the dish provided a stable, vertical orientation for the punch trephine (Troutman, 1977).

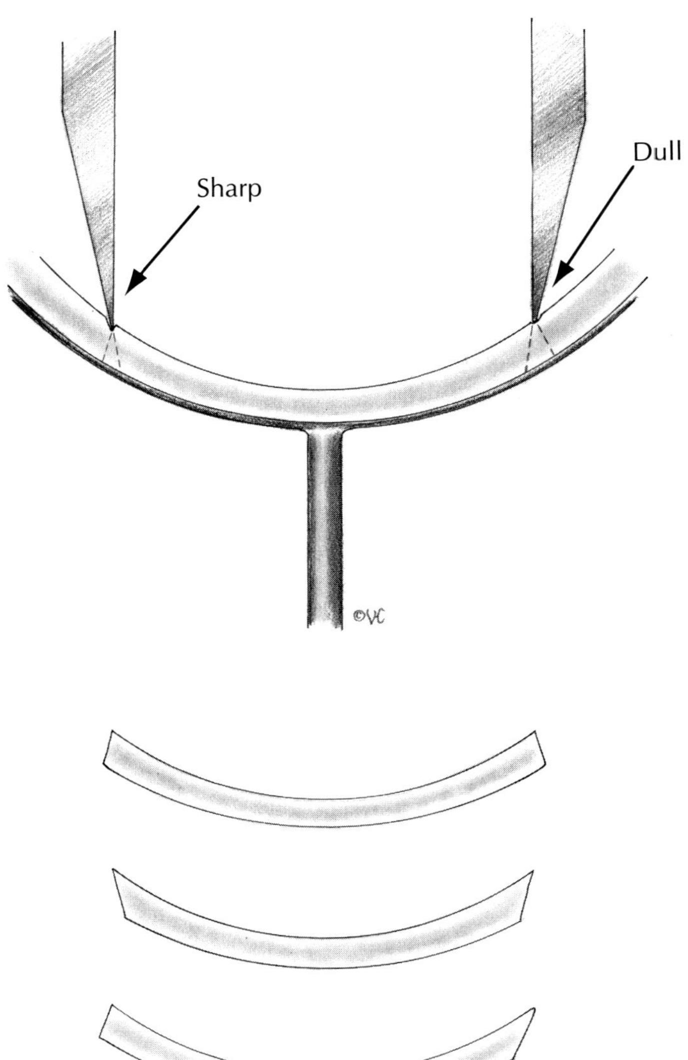

Problems encountered when trephine is tilted or donor cornea moves during preparation of donor button, showing beveled incisions.

Several variations on this design have been created over the years. One such design is the Liebermann guillotine corneal punch. This design uses the weight of a falling block to propel the trephine through the cornea. A serious drawback of this design is that if the uniform force resulting from the falling block is not sufficient to complete the cut at the first impact the trephine may bounce three or four times, causing multiple incisions in the donor cornea. Recently, Parel has suggested using suction beneath the cornea to hold it in place, and a heavier block, and this has shown improvement in the quality of incision.

A new approach to preparation of the donor cornea has been the introduction of the artificial anterior chamber. This device allows the donor cornea to be prepared under the same conditions as the incision for the recipient cornea; that is, from the anterior surface, using a turning, rather than punching, cutting action. Because the cornea is not punched, the size of the donor cornea is the same as the trephine and does not need to be oversized. Both the Krumeich and the Hanna trephine come with an artificial anterior chamber that works on this design. One disadvantage is the need for a significant scleral rim to permit operation of this artificial chamber, and this must be requested beforehand from the eye bank.

SCISSORS

Cutting the donor cornea with scissors is in many ways similar to cutting with trephines (without rotation). In both instances, the tissue is squeezed as the cutting progresses. In the case of cutting the donor cornea, the opposing forces are provided by the teflon dish, whereas in the case of scissors, the opposing force is provided by the opposing blades of the scissors. The actual cutting angle is somewhat different because it is caused by the shear action of the two blades.

Whenever tissue is compressed as it is being cut, a distortion can occur, resulting in beveled or S-shaped incisions. This is certainly the case with scissors blades in which the tendency for beveling increases as the thickness of the material increases. This is because there is a natural tendency for the material being cut with scissors to twist because the forces created by the scissors are, by necessity, not directly opposite each other. It is, therefore, a general principal that to create vertical incisions in the cornea, one should create as much of the incision as one can with a knife or rotating trephine, leaving the area to be cut with scissors as thin as possible to avoid beveling. Often countertraction can be applied to provide tension on the lamella being cut and thus avoid beveling (see discussion in Troutman, 1977). Certainly the scissors should be maintained in a vertical or inverse orientation, because tilting can easily create large bevels.

If the scissors are allowed to close completely, the ends of the scissors blades will cause a small irregularity in the incision. It is therefore a general principal in the use of corneal scissors to avoid closing the blades completely. As a corollary, it is useful to have fairly long blades to permit a reasonable length of cornea to be cut on each stroke of the blades. In the case of corneal scissors used after trephination of the cornea, there is a tendency for iris tissue to become impaled on the lower scissors blade, causing unintended iris trauma. The presence of a blunted longer bottom blade to lift the cornea slightly as cutting progresses can be helpful in the prevention of this problem.

Scissors can be self-sharpening if properly designed; however, the material of which they are made is an important consideration. Despite the strength and cleanliness of titanium used in many other instruments, titanium corneal scissors are difficult if not impossible to sharpen, and at the present time, stainless steel remains the material of choice for corneal scissors.

Incisions of the cornea often define the success of refractive corneal surgery. Although suturing techniques can be modified if they are unsatisfactory, a poor incision is usually irreversible, with the result that the remainder of the operation in question becomes more difficult or less satisfactory as a direct result. Although many factors are beyond the control of the surgeon, simple considerations can often make the difference in successful corneal surgery. The proper knife or application of the knife can make a difficult situation more amenable, and can make the difference between success and failure.

In this chapter we have outlined some of the basic principles of the design of cutting instruments and how the surgeon might choose a particular knife trephine or scissors for a procedure. In many cases, conflicting requirements make the choice difficult but illuminate requirements that may be met by some future instrument. Ultimately, our goal should not be to choose among available options but to be able to express our needs clearly enough so that instruments can be created that truly satisfy our needs.

Chapter 9

Sutures, Needles, and Suturing Techniques for Astigmatism Surgery

We have come a long way from the early days of corneal surgery when the only needles available were of such large diameter and so dull as to be incapable of penetrating the thickness of the incised cornea to allow edge-to-edge closure. The subsequent reduction in needle size and increased needle sharpness has been accompanied by a gradual reduction in the diameter of suture material and a new understanding of the dynamics of suture closure. One of the most significant developments in wound closure has been the change from readily biodegradable inextensible materials to more permanent monofilament elastic materials. These elastic materials were intially used because they were finer and relatively stronger than silk or gut. It was not realized until later that their elasticity was as desirable as the improved apposition and the reduced tissue trauma. Combined with their ability to hold the tissues firmly through a long period of healing, this elasticity allows a molding of the wound to its preoperative dimensions, affording for the first time a means to control optical as well as anatomical wound healing.

SUTURES

When suturing is required for the prevention or correction of corneal astigmatism, only an elastic, monofilament suture possesses the properties necessary to maintain the tissues in apposition with minimal reaction for a sufficient period of time to effect firm and accurate healing. At the present time, elastic monofilament suture is available in three materials: nylon, polypropylene (Prolene), and dacron (Merselene). Theoretically, if a suture material could retain corneal tissue apposition at optimal tension permanently, the desired anatomic as well as optical effects would be assured. The early promise of polypropylene as such a permanently nonabsorbable suture material has failed to materialize; eventually it loses its tensile strength and fractures or loosens, allowing the cornea to assume its unsupported curvature. Not only is the material too stiff, it is difficult to knot securely and over the long term, it loses its elasticity, becomes brittle, fragments, and is eventually absorbed. It has, however, seen extensive use for intraocular lens haptics, for iris, transscleral, and episcleral sutures.

More recently, another synthetic suture material, dacron was introduced in 10-0 and 11-0 sizes. It has the desirable elastic properties of nylon and is truly nonabsorbable. In practice, however, the 10-0–diameter dacron is stiffer and less predictably elastic than either nylon or polypropylene. Although less stiff in 11-0 diameter, it is more elastic than 10-0 nylon. Nevertheless, even when firmly tied, it tends to loosen and extrude. In addition, even with knots deeply buried, surface reaction along the external thread loops and sterile suture abscesses often necessitate its early removal.

Nylon in 10-0 diameter remains the suture of choice to maintain firm, nonreactive tissue apposition over the long term. We continue to use nylon in the 10-0 size both for astigmatism prevention and for closure of astigmatism-correcting incisions or excisions as well as for compensating or effect-enhancing compression sutures. Even if a truly nonabsorbable suture material existed that could maintain its tensile strength permanently, it would probably be undesirable over the long term.

To evaluate any technique used to prevent and correct corneal astigmatism, all appositional as well as all compression sutures must be removed after firm healing has taken place. Only by evaluating the suture uncompensated results by corneal topology can the permanent and final effect of any surgical intervention be accurately quantified. We have all seen penetrating keratoplasty patients with 20/20 uncorrected visual acuity and minimal or no astigmatism, with all or some sutures still in place, who acquire a debilitating astigmatism when a suture or sutures are removed. This can occur even when sutures are removed at 6 months, 1 year, or even longer after the primary surgery.

For this chapter and succeeding chapters in which suturing is discussed, monofilament nylon will be the suture recommended and used, unless another suture material is mentioned specifically as a substitute or alternative.

SUTURE NEEDLES

A needle featuring a compound curve and bent tip, as originally modified by Troutman (1974) from a full curved GS-9 needle, is recommended for placing the short deep suture bites suggested for full-thickness wound closure. Recently, Ethicon has introduced a commercial version based on this prototype. It is available in two wire sizes (0.006 in and 0.004 in) and is swaged to several thread diameters and materials. The larger needle tract of the 6-wire size facilitates burying the knot of the 10-0 suture material. The most recent versions are identified as TGW6C+ and CSC Ultima. The length of the needles is 5.5 mm to the swedge that holds the 10-0 or 11-0 thread. Its unique feature is a short (1 mm), straight tip obliquely angled to a shaft of gradually decreasing curvature. This straight tip and the following compound curve of the needle facilitate short, deep through-and-through needle placement and nondistorting needle withdrawal to place the thread for firm, full thickness apposition of a corneal wound.

Short, deep suture placement is difficult to achieve consistently with a conventional full-curve needle, especially when multiple bites are required in a long incision, such as with penetrating keratoplasty. In this case, the elastic monofilament suture loops will be placed too far anteriorly in the corneal stroma. In the usual longer bites, when tied for firm apposition, internal gaping of the cornea is induced creating a *lambda-shaped incision profile*. From anteriorly, the cornea is in apposition and appears to be closed. However, when the sutures loosen or are removed, the unapposed posterior wound tends to open. The resulting thin, superficial elastic scar induces flattening of the incisional meridian. With full-thickness through-and-through wound closure, these eventualities are prevented or minimized, not only promoting regular, firm wound healing but also resulting in an earlier, more stable optical result. For example, in keratoconus, with such deep sutures, the double, opposing, continuous sutures can be removed as early as 6 months postoperatively. Within 2 weeks of their removal, the corneal optics stabilize. Should any significant residual astigmatism occur, its correction is more predictable because of the full-thickness uniform scar. The quality, thickness, and vascularization of the recipient corneal bed is determined not by the surgeon but by the presenting pathology. In keratoplasty, at the very least a full-thickness vertical closure of the usually disparate wound edges should be maintained by through-and-through sutures during healing. Fortunately, the cataract surgeon is rarely faced with disparate wound edges. Nevertheless, accurate vertical wound closure is essential, or a lambda wound profile will result in *against the rule* flattening of the incisional meridian and sometimes a debilitating astigmatism.

There is the fear that epithelial downgrowth can result from through-and-through suturing, although it is probably more frequently the result of defective wound closure resulting from uneven, shallow suturing. Epithelial tissue enters the eye through wound dehiscences or tracts. When using nylon or any other suture material at any level, it is necessary to remove any loosened suture loop or exposed knot promptly. A loosened thread will promote softening and vascularization of the tissue adjacent to the loop and can become an avenue for both infection or for epithelium to enter the eye. A few days after placement of a through-and-through suture, the posterior loop of the tensioned monofilament elastic thread works into the softer posterior stroma. The anterior loop is prevented from cutting down into anterior stroma by the elastic condensed Bowman's layer. At this juncture, the posterior loop is effectively more distant from the internal eye than the posterior aspect of a shallowly placed suture loop, which may remain exposed in the lambda-shaped cleft behind it.

HANDLING COMPOUND CURVE NEEDLES

Correct handling of the compound curve needle with one of the needle holders, described in Chapter 7, is essential to its effective use. Because the needle is only 5.5 mm long and must be passed from entrance to exit through approximately 3 mm of tissue, a locking needle holder should never be used. With a straight tipped, nonlocking needle holder with fine 0.75 mm jaws, the needle may be grasped selectively during passage, and both bending and damage to the tip can be better avoided. To avoid regrasping during passage, the shaft should be grasped initially by its distal portion at three quarters of the distance from the tip to the swedge (Plate 9–1,A,B,C). If placed too far distally across the swedge, the needle will tend to twist in the jaws of the needle holder as it is passed. If placed too far proximally, the tip will be prevented from exiting without regrasping, and it can be more difficult to retrieve the needle without damage to the point or cutting edge. The 0.75 mm grasping tips of the needle holders, described in Chapter 7, enable the surgeon to avoid grasping the cutting tip and cutting edges.

The Pierse-style tissue forceps, with opposing laser-cut C-shaped grasping tips, requires less deforming force to grasp corneal tissue (Plate 9–2,A). When 0.1 mm Bonn-style dog-toothed tips are used, they tend to penetrate and lacerate the corneal tissue as pressure is applied.

Observation of compound or full curve needle passage under microscope magnification can be obscured by needle holder or forceps tips. Troutman has designed with Ethicon an **offset needle,** the shaft of which has been twisted to give 20 degrees offset of the point from the grasping area of the needle shaft, to allow unimpeded visualization of the wound area being sutured.

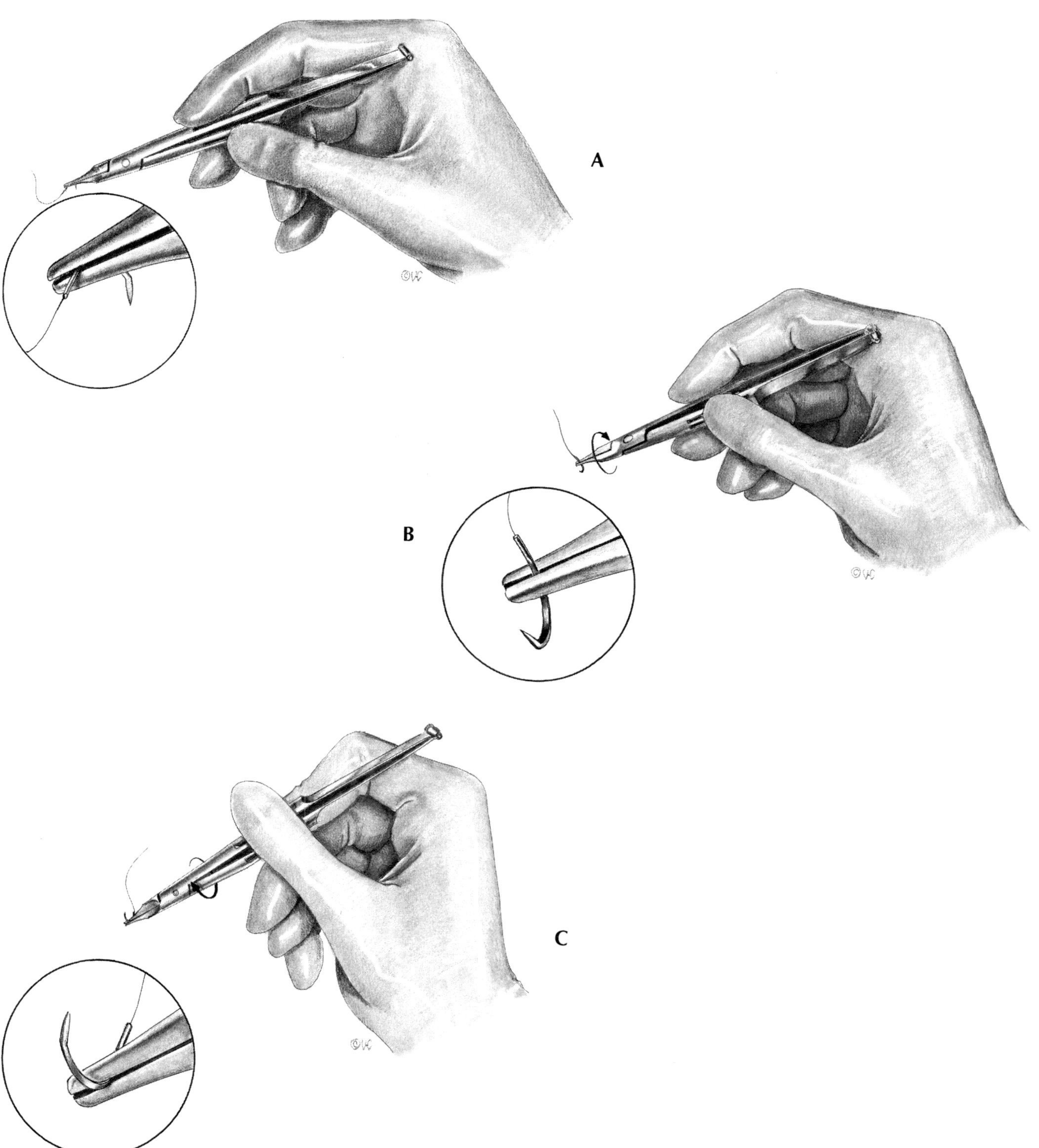

A, needle holder, straight, 0.75-mm tips, nonlocking. Needle grasped at three quarters of distance from tip for initial vertical penetration. Avoid grasping more distal, across the swedge. **B,** needle rotated to posterior penetration position. **C,** needle rotated to exiting position.

Sutures, Needles, and Suturing Techniques for Astigmatism Surgery **221**

In corneal and refractive surgery, both penetrating and partial penetrating incisions are almost always made in a single plane vertical to the corneal or to the iris plane. A single plane incision facilitates the placement of equal length, short, deep, or through-and-through suture bites. In a vertical wound, the compound curve needle can be passed accurately equidistant from both anterior and posterior apposing wound edges. To place a compound curve needle across a vertical corneal incision, the cornea or the donor button is grasped with the Pierse tissue forceps. With the needle holder securely grasping the needle shaft, the tip is directed vertically to engage the cornea at 0.5 mm, just behind the tip of the fixating forceps (Plate 9–2,A). *The needle point is driven directly, without rotation,* through the corneal thickness of the proximal wound lip to exit just distal to or at the posterior edge of the wound lip. Only then, as the needle exits, is it rotated beneath the wound to engage the posterior aspect of the distal wound lip (Plate 9–2,B). Then the straight point of the needle is driven straight up through the distal corneal lip, aided by counterpressure from the Pierse forceps, to exit 0.5 mm from the wound margin (Plate 9–2,C and D). This maneuver should be accomplished without regrasping the needle shaft. With the tip exited approximately 2 mm, the needle shaft is regrasped just behind the angle of the cutting tip (Plate 9–2,E). All parameters, entrance, passage, and exit with this maneuver are controlled to ensure the length and depth of the suture bite. As the needle is withdrawn, it will be seen that the wound edges remain in approximation due to the decreasing curve of the distal end of the compound curve needle, preventing wound gape and loss of the anterior chamber. The final position of the thread reflects the path of the needle equidistant from the incisional edges through-and-through the corneal thickness (Plate 9–2,F).

The needle is not turned when it is in the tissue; it is turned only when the tip exits behind the wound. Because of the proximity of the needle tip to the iris during its rotation under the cornea, the tip of the needle must be kept slightly turned up so as not to catch the iris. The ski-shaped tip of the compound curve needle facilitates this posterior passage, the angle distal to the needle tip tending to push the tip away from the iris. The underlying iris is more difficult to avoid with the tip of a full-curve needle.

With a shelved or multiple plane incision, such as that more commonly used for cataract surgery at the limbus and by some corneal surgeons, the length of the shelf and undercut make it necessary to place either the proximal or distal bite longer than the bite in the opposing edge. The disproportion created by the unequal length bites distorts the wound margin. This is compounded by the lambda wound profile induced when the bites are made at less than full thickness.

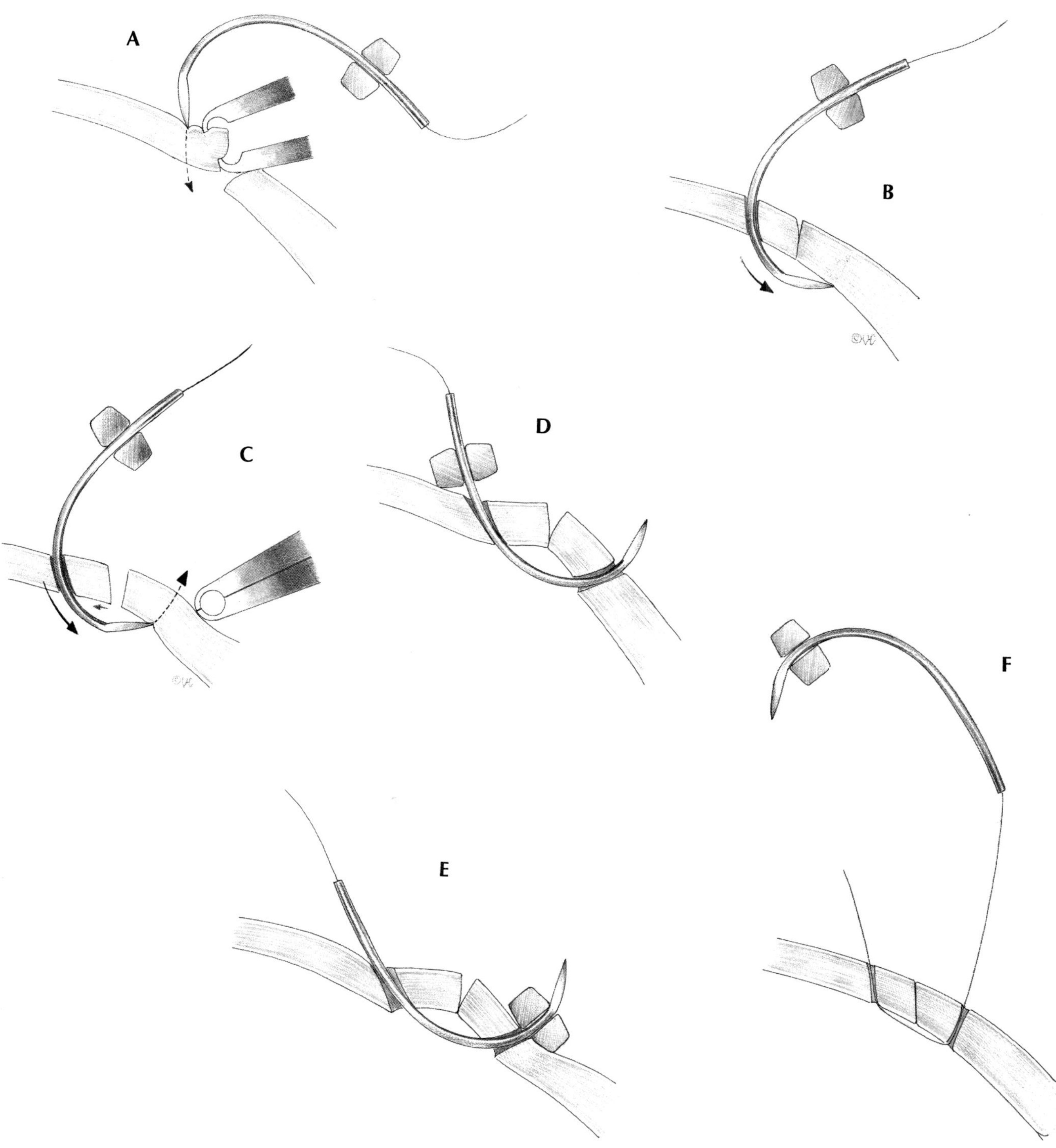

Suturing vertical wound edges. **A,** positioning compound curve needle proximal to Pierse forceps tips vertical to cornea. **B,** vertical needle entrance 0.5 mm from wound edge and rotation to opposing wound edge. **C,** engaging posterior wound edge for vertical needle passage. **D,** vertical passage to exit for needle retrieval, counter pressure with Pierse forceps. **E,** retrieval by grasping needle proximal to the cutting edge. **F,** thread position with needle exited.

Sutures, Needles, and Suturing Techniques for Astigmatism Surgery **223**

Through-and-through suture placement is essential to secure incisions of unequal vertical profile. Although a disproportion of the mating edges cannot be fully compensated, a full-thickness closure assures mating of the available opposing vertical wound dimensions, and a more secure healed wound results.

TYING THE SUTURE WITH SLIPKNOTS

When an interrupted suture loop has been placed or a continuous suture completed, the thread ends are secured with a slipknot so that the suture tension across the wound can be adjusted before completing the knot (see Plate 9–4,F and G). Elastic monofilament suture material is ideal to tension with a slipknot, as its smooth regular surface does not have the tendency to bind during adjustment as do braided or twisted materials. When wound tension cannot be maintained by a single slipknot, the knot may be doubled (see Plate 9–4,E). A completed slipknot is smaller than a surgeon's knot and is easier to bury in the suture tract.

There are several methods used to form a slipknot. Charleaux, who in 1970 described using the slipknot for wound closure, formed the knot by reversing and collapsing a square knot. This method often results in premature lock up of the square knot. Terry later popularized this concept using a more readily formed knot but still difficult to duplicate. This problem led us to design several methods to better assure routine formation of a single or double slipknot. By using one of these methods, depending on where the thread ends fall, slipknots can be quickly and easily formed singly and in series (Plate 9–3,A).

Single Slipknot

Step 1.—To begin any knot, the needle is passed through the tissue as has been described and the thread drawn until a short end, approximately 1 inch long, extends back from the distal wound edge. The short distal end of the suture, held with a straight tying forceps in the surgeon's nondominant hand, is brought back across the wound parallel to the needle-armed proximal end (Plate 9–3,B). (The artist has drawn the sequence for a right-handed surgeon.)

Step 2.—The curved forceps, held in the surgeon's dominant hand with the internal curve of its tip directed inferiorly, is passed under the proximal longer thread, turned, and hooked under the distal end to form a half loop, which is then brought back under the proximal thread (Plate 9–3,C).

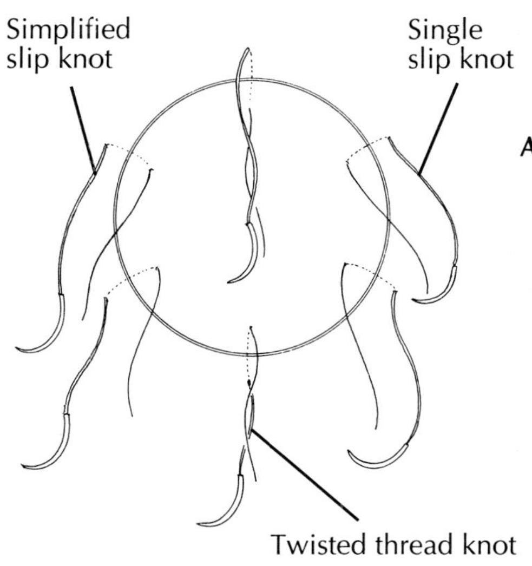

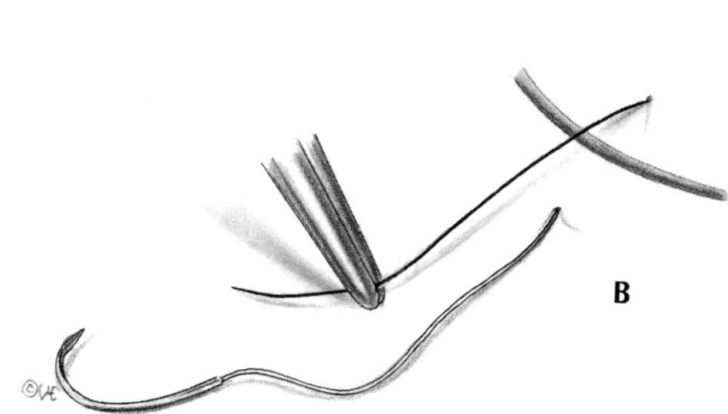

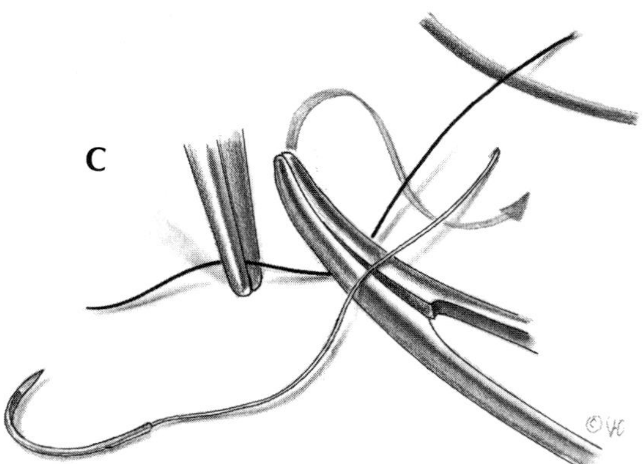

A, tying the suture, thread positions commonly seen prior to forming the slipknot tie. *Left,* simplified slipknot. *Center,* twisted threads. *Right,* single slipknot. **B,** tying from thread position, short end left (single slipknot). **C,** forming loop under longer thread.

Step 3.—The short suture end then is handed over with the straight forceps to be grasped by the slightly opened tips of the curved forceps (Plate 9–3,D).

Step 4.—The curved forceps grasps the short thread end as the straight forceps releases it (Plate 9–3,E).

Step 5.—The short thread end is pulled through the loop to create the slipknot (Plate 9–3,F).

Step 6.—The knot, thus created in the distal short end, slides easily along the proximal thread. Alternately pulling on the proximal thread to tighten the knot or on the distal end to release it adjusts the tension on the suture loop (Plate 9–3,F and G). Monofilament elastic thread, particularly nylon and dacron, and polypropylene only slightly less so, creates a readily adjustable secure knot due to the elasticity of the material. The thread diameter narrows within the knot as it is tensioned, like a knotted rubber band, locking the thread loop at the desired tension.

When the nonabsorbing characteristics of dacron or polypropylene are required, a slipknot can also be used to advantage. However, with 10-0 dacron or polypropylene the knot will be less secure because of the greater stiffness of the material. Care should be taken to jam the square knot down snugly, and an extra throw can be taken for security. Although 10-0 dacron is too stiff and difficult to manage, the 11-0 size has handling characteristics similar to that of 10-0 nylon. Although almost as strong as 10-0 nylon, it is less elastic, and its break point is reached more abruptly and unpredictably than with nylon, and greater care must be taken when adjusting suture loop tension.

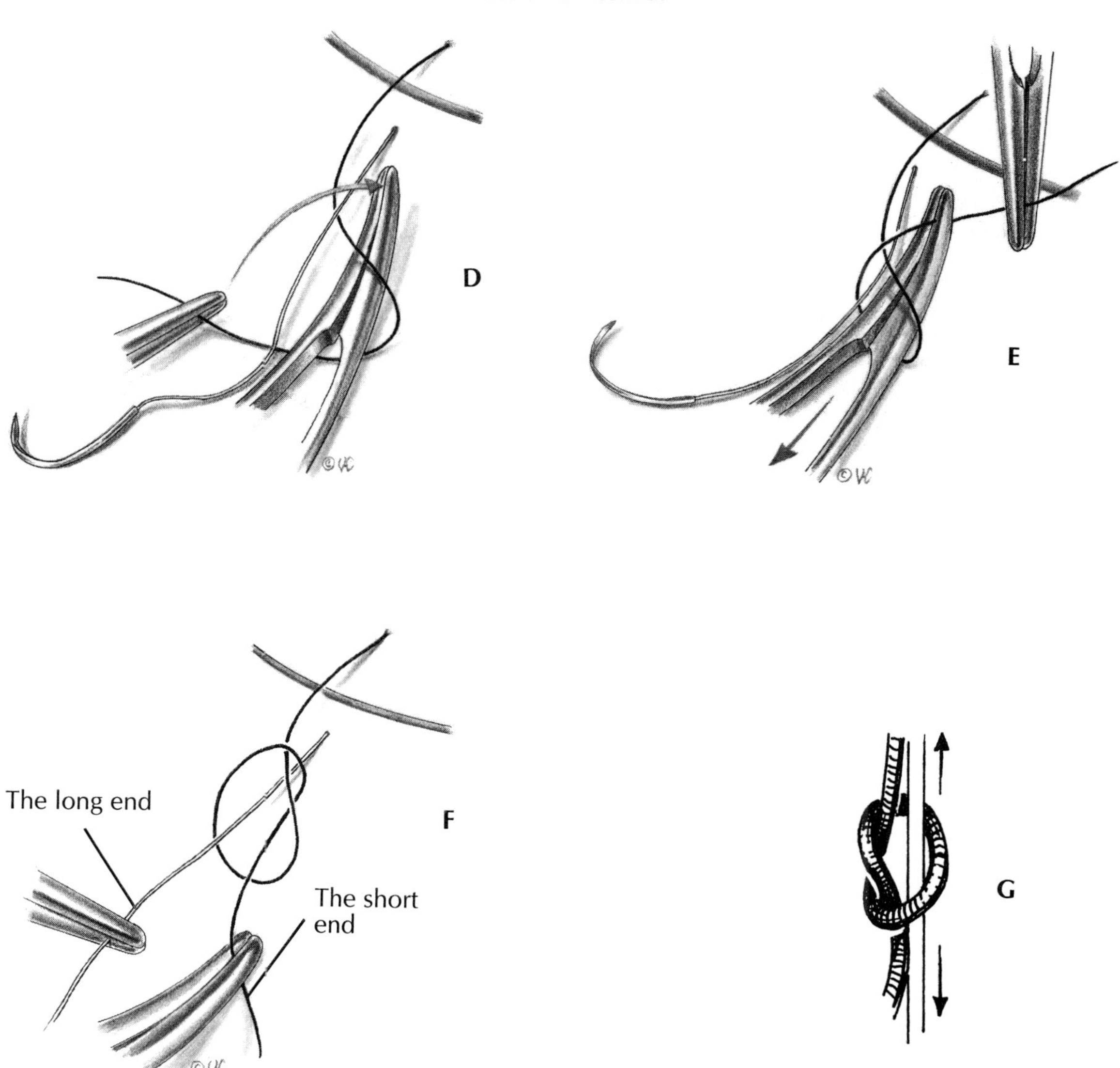

D, closing loop across longer thread. **E,** forming slipknot along longer thread. **F,** slipknot formed. **G,** adjustment of single slipknot. Pull on short end to loosen, longer end to tighten.

Simplified Slipknot

Step 1.— A simplified single slipknot can be formed by grasping the short thread end from under the longer thread end armed with a needle used with the straight forceps (Plate 9–4,A).

Step 2.— The curved forceps is then passed under the short thread end proximal to the longer thread to form a half loop (Plate 9–4,B).

Step 3.— The straight forceps brings the shorter thread proximal to the tip of the curved forceps (Plate 9–4,C).

Step 4.— The curved forceps grasps the shorter thread end while the straight forceps fixates the longer needle armed suture end. The curved forceps then pulls the shorter thread end through the loop to form the single slipknot (Plate 9–4,D).

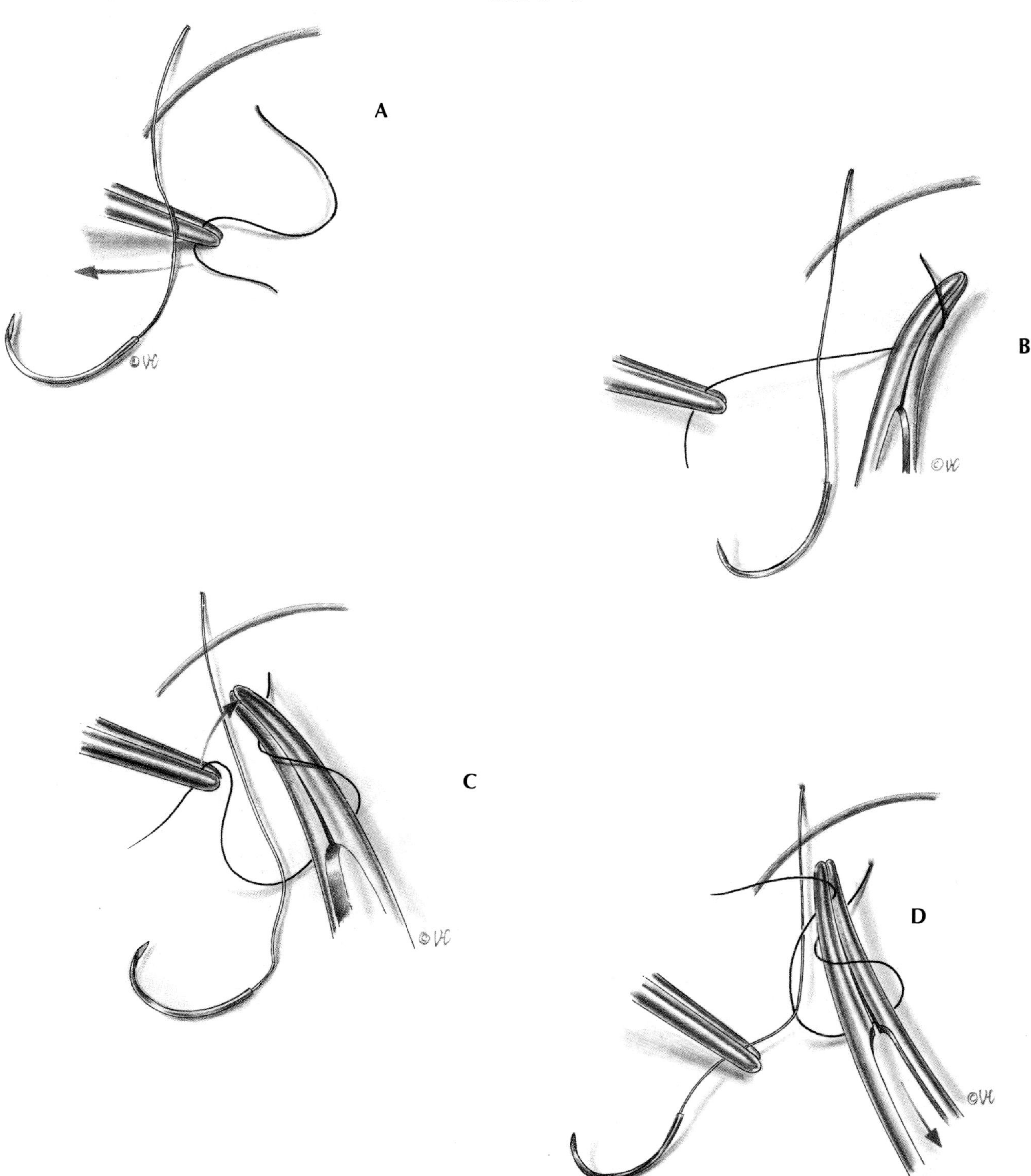

A, tying simplified slipknot, short end right. Short end retrieved under long thread end with straight forceps. (Simplified slipknot.) **B,** single loop formed in short end with curved forceps. **C,** short thread being passed to curved forceps tip to complete knot. **D,** slipknot formed around longer thread.

Special Slipknot Ties

A temporary lock may be put on a slipknot by forming a half bow. The slipknot is begun in a usual fashion, but leaving the short thread end long enough to be grasped by its middle rather than its end. As the knot is formed, the turned-over loop will be caught in the slipknot as it is formed. By pulling simultaneously on the longer thread end and the loop thus formed, the slipknot can be locked to form a half bow. The entire knot can be released by pulling on the free end, or the slipknot may be completed by pulling out the free end of the loop from the slipknot (Plate 9–5).

When the thread ends are twisted (see Plates 9–3,A [center] and 9–6,A), a secure slipknot may be formed by passing the curved forceps under the twisted threads to form a half loop (Plate 9–6,B). The curved forceps can then grasp the shorter thread end to form the knot (Plate 9–6,C–E).

Plate 9–5.

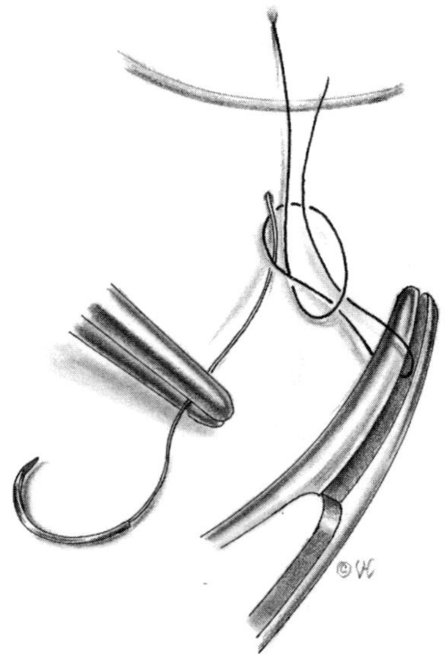

Shorter thread left, long loop of doubled thread held by slipknot to form a single bow knot; this knot can be left as a single bow knot for temporary closure, untied by pulling on the free end, or completed by pulling out the short thread end.

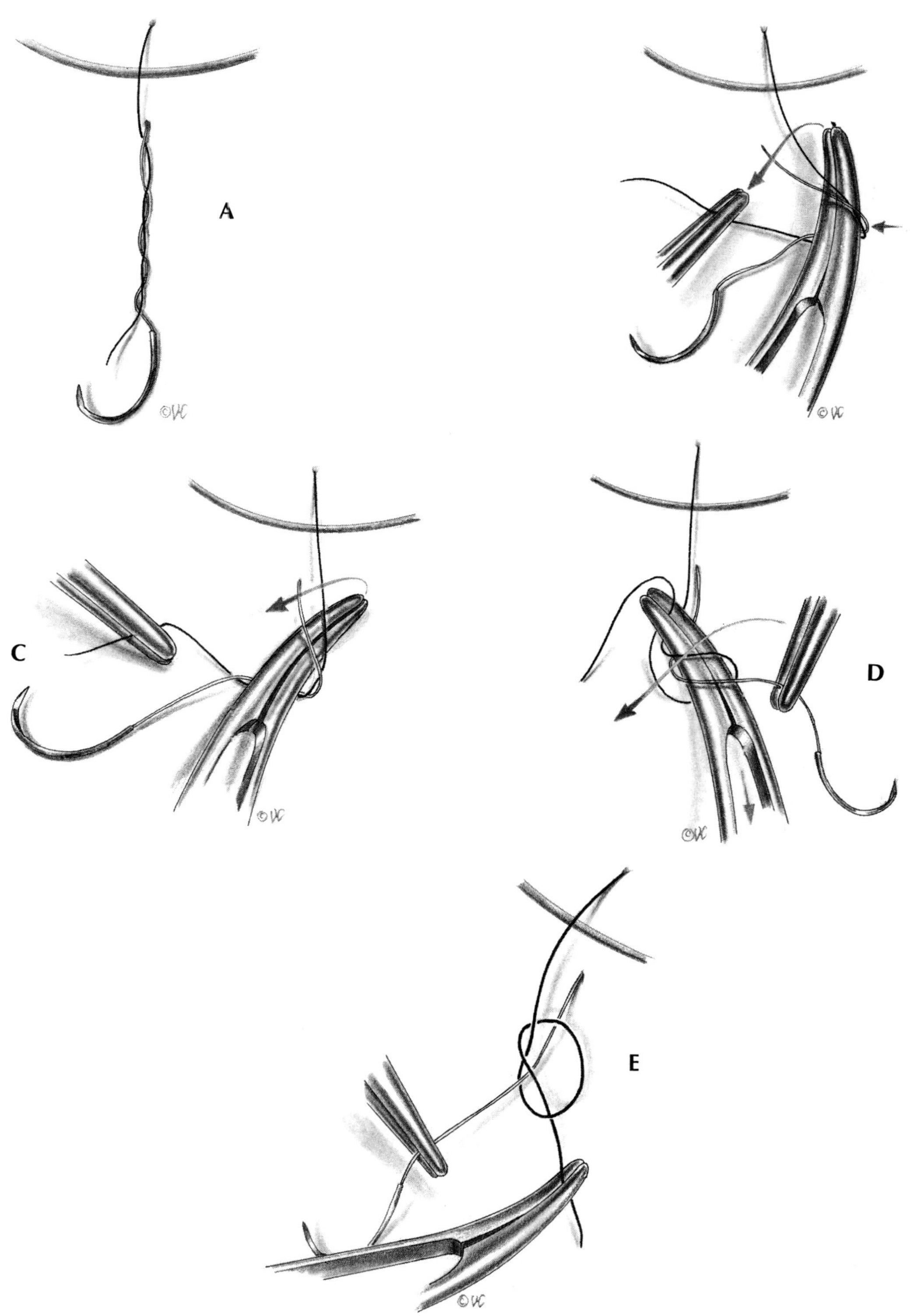

A, thread position prior to forming knot (twisted thread method). **B,** half loop formed by passing curved forceps under both threads. **C,** short end passed to curved tip. **D,** curved tip with short end grasped, curved tip in position to complete slip knot. **E,** completing the knot.

Sutures, Needles, and Suturing Techniques for Astigmatism Surgery   **231**

Double Slipknot

A double slipknot is used when the wound tension is too great to be adjusted and held securely by a single slipknot.

Step 1.—In this instance, a slightly longer length of the distal thread end is brought across the wound with the straight typing forceps. A single half loop of the short thread end is brought under the proximal thread as described before (Plate 9–7,A).

Step 2.—A second loop is created by again passing the end of the curved forceps, still bearing the first loop, back under both threads to form a second loop (Plate 9–7,B).

Step 3.—Then the straight forceps, holding the short end, hands the thread over to be grasped between the tips of the curved forceps (Plate 9–7,C).

Step 4.—As the straight forceps is released, the curved forceps draws the short end through the doubled loop to create the double slipknot (Plate 9–7,D).

Step 5.—As with the single slipknot, the thread can be tightened by pulling on the longer thread end or loosened by pulling on the shorter thread end (Plate 9–7,E).

Such knots are useful, for example, when closing a corneal wedge resection. They are placed in series and tensioned individually while observing the steepening effect with the qualitative surgical keratometer. They are then secured with square knots after the desired compression, along the extent of the wound, has been reached. The same technique is used when adjusting the tension of opposing compression or compensating compression sutures.

Completing the Knot

When optimal appositional tension with the slipknot closed suture loop is attained, the slipknot is locked down by placing a square knot carefully over it. The first loop of the square knot should not be tightly closed, because it may turn over to form a second slipknot on top of the first. When the first tie is firmly but not tightly in place, the square knot is completed and the second throw jammed snugly in place, in effect, squeezing the daylight out of the knot (Plate 9–6,E). For added security, a third throw may be placed. The resulting knot will be smaller and easier to bury than the less adjustable 3-1-1 surgeon's knot.

When the knot is complete, the thread ends are cut flush to the knot with a razor knife so that the short stiff thread ends do not protrude from the knot. The razor knife should be held so as to keep the knot in view as the thread is being cut. A razor knife is often sharper distal from its tip

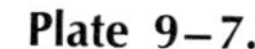

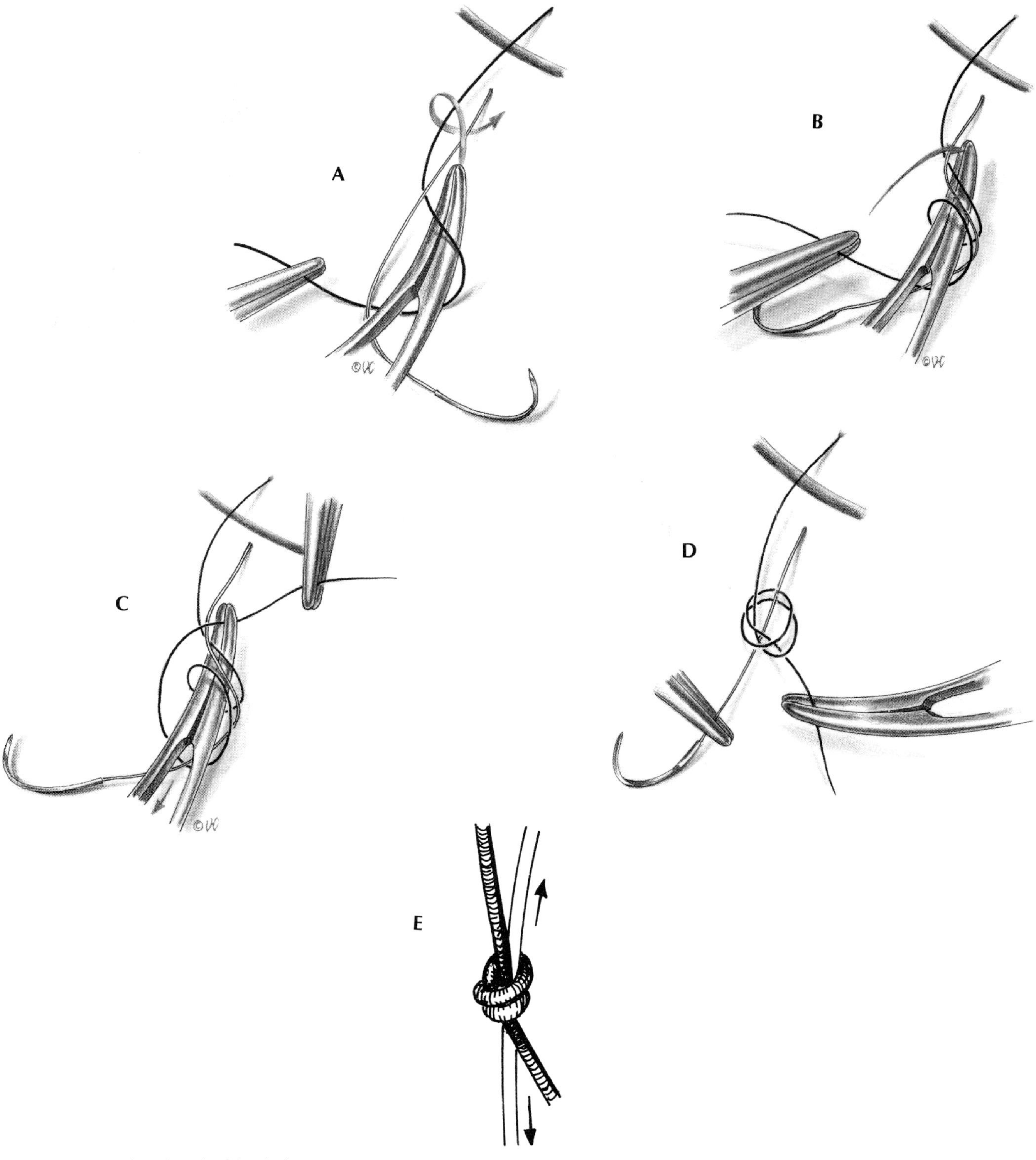

A, tying double slipknot; start with short end left. B, forming double loop, first loop formed with curved forceps. C, short end grasped by curved forceps. D, double slipknot formed around longer thread. E, adjusting double slipknot, pull on short end to loosen, long end to tighten.

Sutures, Needles, and Suturing Techniques for Astigmatism Surgery   **233**

than at its tip. If the blade is held flat against the knot and the thread end pulled up against the blade edge, the thread will be cut cleanly to the knot. The security of the knot is confirmed when it can be manipulated into the suture tract without ravelling.

BURYING THE KNOT

When a knot has been securely tied and trimmed, it is essential that it be buried in the corneal tissue as far from the limbus and blood vessels as possible. In keratoplasty, if the knot is buried too close to the limbus distal to the graft margin, neovascularization may be stimulated by irritation from the knot, and graft rejection may be initiated. Ideally, a knot should always be buried in the donor or proximal wound edge. If it is difficult to bury a knot on the proximal side, it will have to be buried in the suture tract on the distal side. For convenience in removing the knot of a suture loop closing a cataract incision, it should be buried to the proximal (corneal) side of the wound. In no event should a suture knot be left on the surface.

When burying the knot of a continuous suture closing a keratoplasty wound, sufficient slack should be provided in the thread proximal to the knot so that it can be entered from directly vertical to the tract. If a tight loop makes it necessary to pull the knot around the anterior edge of the suture tract, it is not only more difficult to bury, but the thread may be broken. If a knot cannot be buried readily, a dot of sodium hyaluronate (Healon) can be placed over the knot to lubricate it. The knot is then drawn into the hyaluronate and back into the tract. Gentle rubbing with a second instrument will facilitate entry and allow a resistant knot to be buried. Burying the knot between wound lips with the tie is not advisable in keratoplasty. Not only does it necessitate a less than full-thickness bite at the knot level, but it can prevent healing or fistulize.

REMOVING THE KNOT

A razor knife is used to remove an individual loop or successive loops of a continuous suture. The tip of the blade held on the flat depresses the epithelium just lateral to the suture loop and then is passed just under the suture and turned up to sever the thread from behind. Alternatively, the blade can be directed vertically down onto the thread, using the cornea as a block on which to cut the thread. Enough length of thread should be left on either side of the wound so that if the knot or thread cannot be dislodged proximally, it can be grasped and brought through the suture tract distally. It is important not to pull continuously to dislodge the knot but rather to use short jerking motions until the knot begins to move and only then to exit it. If the suture knot cannot be dislodged, the thread ends attached to the knot must be cut flush to retract under Bowman's layer and epithelium, or there can be an irritation, infection, or ulceration.

To remove a continuous suture, the thread should be cut first in the middle of the loop on either side of the knot, and then every second loop is cut. After the alternate loops are cut, the knot is removed by pulling on the thread end closest to it. Then with the back edge of a razor blade or a needle tip, the intermediate loops of the cut thread are successively lifted from beneath endothelium and removed with fine-pointed suture forceps. When removing double continuous sutures, the same technique is used. Here, after the knot loops are isolated, alternate loops of both threads can be cut simultaneously at their crossover on the donor.

SUMMARY

Elastic monofilament suture material and fine atraumatic needles, together with the increased magnification afforded by the surgical microscope, have been the major mechanical surgical factors contributing to the success of modern corneal surgery. We owe a great debt to Mackensen and Harms, who introduced this suture to ophthalmology, to Ethicon and especially to their ophthalmic products representative, Paul Haffey, who made it commercially available. Initially, the elastic properties of the monofilament thread were not as appreciated as they have come to be with wider use. Also, the nonreactive nature of the material was considered a problem; surgeons did not realize that it was the suture material, rather than their surgery, that kept eyes inflamed postoperatively. Also, in the beginning the firm closure of corneal wounds that the nylon thread afforded caused some surgeons to prematurely remove the suture before the cornea had healed. Because suture materials had always been placed in the anterior layers of the cornea because of their irritating properties, there still remains some resistance to the through-and-through placement of nylon and the excellent closure of the posterior wound that it affords. Accurate refractive surgery depends on full-thickness wound closure and healing, and this is emphasized throughout this volume.

Surgical needles have also improved greatly since the introduction of these finer materials. The needles one uses should be strong enough to be passed without bending and sharp enough to penetrate the tissues with minimal pressure. Several curvatures of needles have been designed for corneal surgery. A needle curvature should be selected that, in the hands of the surgeon, makes it possible for him or her to place the suture loops as close to the wound edges as possible and still penetrate the full corneal thickness. The monofilament suture threads lend themselves to being tied with slipknots, which provide better apposition and adjustment than the traditional suture ties. This has also made possible more regular adjustment of suture tension of wounds in refractive surgery.

Finally, the instruments used to place and tie sutures should be carefully selected and maintained so as not to damage the fine needles and suture material during placement or tying of sutures.

Chapter 10

Pathophysiology and Prevention of Astigmatism Secondary to Trauma

<table>
<tr><td>

Examination of trauma injury
Preoperative technique
Operative technique
Suture pattern
Compensating compression sutures
Penetrating iris trauma
Paralimbal wound

</td><td>

Mid-corneal wound
Central lacerations
Y-or stellate-shaped lacerations
Multiple corneal lacerations
Lost corneal tissue
Summary

</td></tr>
</table>

In many ways, corneal trauma represents both the most complex and simplest of the clinical situations the refractive surgeon may be required to face. In its simplest form, the process of closing a corneal wound without tissue loss is fairly straightforward. The wounds need to be cleaned and drawn together to avoid leakage of aqueous humor and to restore the intraocular pressure. As any surgeon who has encountered a severe trauma patient at odd hours of the evening or weekend can attest, even this fairly straightforward process can be quite difficult.

The process of corneal trauma can be viewed on a higher plane by the realization that virtually every form of corneal incision can be reproduced with trauma. Techniques that have been developed for corneal transplantation, overcorrected radial keratotomy, and astigmatic surgery can be applied to provide both immediate restoration of structural integrity and to maximize both the long- and short-term optical quality of the cornea. It is always difficult for the surgeon to expand concern for the short-term viability of the eye to include concern for the long-term refractive outcome, particularly when the circumstances are less than optimal and the pressure of family and associates creates a torrent of confusion surrounding the surgery. For these reasons, after the careful examination of the patient, it is always prudent to step away and on a sheet of paper outline the injuries and design a tentative surgical approach with the required instrumentation. In all cases, appropriate instruments and ancillary personnel should be present before the surgery begins. Within reason, every attempt should be made to create an optimal environment for the surgical procedure to the point that the patient could rest quietly in an emergency room or hospital bed for 1 or 2 hours prior to surgery rather than be rushed immediately to the operating room with inadequate preparation and support staff. On observing the eye initially in the operating theater, the first order of business will be to examine the eye closely and with great care, including appropriate cleansing of the ocular tissues and debridement to obtain the clearest possible picture of the injuries that are present.

In this chapter, we confine our attention to problems of the cornea and the surrounding relevant structures as they pertain to astigmatic complications in the postoperative period. Our approach is to draw parallels between common traumatic injuries and well-recognized surgical principles that can be found in other corneal and ocular surgery. Approached in this manner, ocular trauma can be a tremendous learning experience, and the interplay of knowledge applied from more common everyday surgery can enrich our expertise with trauma surgery and result in better surgical and functional outcomes.

EXAMINATION OF TRAUMA INJURY

At presentation, the patient usually has pain and the eye is extremely sensitive to light. Examination often will be quite limited, even at the slit-lamp, because of photophobia and swelling of periocular tissue. If evidence of a penetrating injury is present with softening of the globe and possible prolapse of uveal tissue, the examination should not be overly long because of the possibility for prolapse of ocular contents by pressure on the lids or by the patient's own squeezing of the lids. Additionally, a more thorough examination can be performed in the operating room. Precise details of the injury together with the object of the injury should be obtained if at all possible. Previous ocular surgeries, medications, and the patients most recent meal should also be documented. Often, the patient is seen directly by the ophthalmologist, and tetanus booster information is not obtained. Ocular injuries, as with other trauma induced by foreign objects, require a tetanus booster if one has not been recently given.

Significant questions that must be answered include:

1. What is the vision?
2. What is the ocular pressure?
3. Location and configuration of corneal incisions?
4. Conjunctival laceration with or without conjunctival chemosis and bleeding?
5. Is there an anterior chamber?
6. Does the penetration break the lens/iris diaphragm?

7. Is evidence of prolapsed uveal tissue present?
8. Is there missing corneal/scleral tissue?
9. Are foreign bodies present in the eye?

After the examination, reconstruction of the details of the accident in the form of drawings often leads to practical solutions for closing the wounds. Careful notations regarding orientation and depth of the wound can often make subsequent closure more appropriate. In addition to simply observing the trauma patient, it is often helpful to physically determine the depth of corneal wounds with the aid of sterile instruments. In some cases, the apparent nonpenetrating injury will be found to have fully penetrated the cornea and often the length of the penetration can be better determined at this time.

Consideration of possible ocular foreign bodies should always be kept in mind and if none are visualized, an orbital x-ray series, at the very least, should be obtained to rule out this possibility. Metal fragments will usually make a significant finding on plain films, and, prior to surgery, the surgeon should examine these x-rays to make certain no evidence of an ocular foreign body is present. If even a question of abnormality with respect to a foreign body is seen or if a foreign body is visualized on the examination, a computed tomography (CT) scan of the eye should be performed prior to surgery. In most modern hospitals, these tests are readily available, even at night and on weekends, and should not delay the surgery beyond a reasonable time period. If these tests are unavailable, the surgery should of course proceed; however, the practitioner should take extra care to locate and remove foreign bodies. Removal of these objects within the eye should not be attempted at the slitlamp despite the inviting nature of removing a large foreign body, such as a nail or a metallic fragment deep within the wound. If the patient is to be taken to the operating room in any case, such maneuvers should be postponed until appropriate steps can be taken to protect and repair the eye.

As the maxim states, "forewarned is forearmed." The initial examination of the patient with trauma should be designed to allow the surgeon to plan in fair detail the course of the proposed operation. Supplies, instruments, and personnel that will be required are all determined by this examination. For instance, the need for a magnet, vitrector, phacoemulsifier, intraocular lens, and even corneal tissue should all have been determined prior to taking the patient to the operating room. Of course, some aspects of trauma are not predictable, and some conditions that are present at the time of trauma can be relegated to a later time for repair. However, these decisions are better made prior to surgery, perhaps in consultation with various specialists, and in many cases, delay of the surgery, even for several hours, is preferable to entering into the operation without appropriate preparation.

PREOPERATIVE TECHNIQUE

The surgery should be performed under general anesthesia because the open eye may be compromised by the pressure induced by retrobulbar block. All operative room personnel should be informed as to the presence of an open eye, and appropriate precautions should be used in terms of moving the patient and avoiding undo pressure on the abdomen or the eye. The eye shield should remain in place at all times, and should be removed only by the surgeon. The preoperative preparation of the eye with respect to povidone-iodine (Betadine) or alcohol should be performed using a no-pressure technique in which the disinfectant is lightly brushed across the lid. Often the use of a dilute Betadine™ solution is helpful in terms of an actual wash of the conjunctiva and eye. This will effectively decrease the bacteria count in areas in which contamination may well have occurred. An additional precaution is the use of preoperative intravenous antibiotics.

OPERATIVE TECHNIQUE

Immediately on opening the lids, a careful examination should be performed to confirm or amplify the examination performed preoperatively. We will restrict our considerations at this point to corneal lacerations, although similar principles of wound closure also apply to sclera. The wound should be carefully cleaned of extraneous debris. Prolapsed intraocular material, such as uvea, should be reposited unless it appears that the degree of contamination of the uvea is unsuitable for repositing. Prolapsed lens and vitreous should be excised. In general, removal of iris material in excessive amounts, particularly if the pupillary ring is broken, will lead to peripheral anterior synechiae and abnormal wound healing. Every attempt should therefore be made to conserve and repair iris tissue. In addition, it generally is poor policy to attempt significant surgical manipulations through the wound, because this area may be unsterile and additional trauma may make closure more difficult.

At this point, the wound should be temporarily closed with interrupted sutures both to restore intraocular integrity and to allow reformation of the anterior chamber. This will allow more appropriate tissue closure without the intrusion of uveal prolapse, complicating the surgery. The surgeon should create a stab incision well away from the trauma wound to allow the uncontaminated introduction of fluid and viscoelastics. Additionally, this opening can serve as a convenient point to introduce a cyclodialysis spatula, which can sweep prolapsing uveal tissue away from the wound during suturing and at the conclusion of the surgery (Plate 10–1). Having reestablished intraocular pressure by a gross approximation of the wound the surgeon can now direct his or her energy toward the various problems of wound closure.

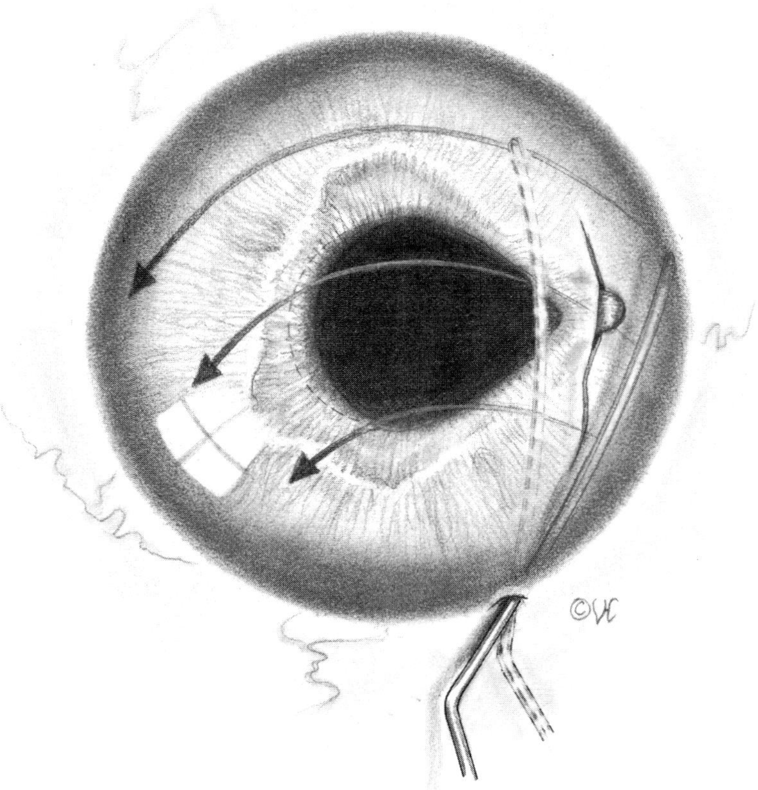

Stab incision peripheral tc trauma allowing introduction of cyclodialysis spatula to sweep incarcerated iris.

SUTURE PATTERN

In general, the first responsibility in closing corneal trauma is to reestablish intraocular integrity. Although astigmatic considerations should play an important role, the importance of proper closure should be the first consideration. Usually this will imply the conversion of corneal astigmatism from a condition with the flat meridian along the axis corresponding to the laceration (Plate 10–2,A) to a condition in which the steep meridian lies along the axis corresponding to the sutured laceration (Plate 10–2,B). If the principles of proper corneal closure are correctly followed and if the laceration is reasonably clean, this iatrogenically induced astigmatism (Plate 10–2,C) will resolve with the removal of the sutures (Plate 10–2,D). Buzard has presented a technique involving the use of compensating compression sutures, similar to those recommended by Troutman for corneal wedge resection, that can alleviate the problem of induced astigmatism during the interim *sutures in* period, which can accelerate visual rehabilitation in the trauma patient.

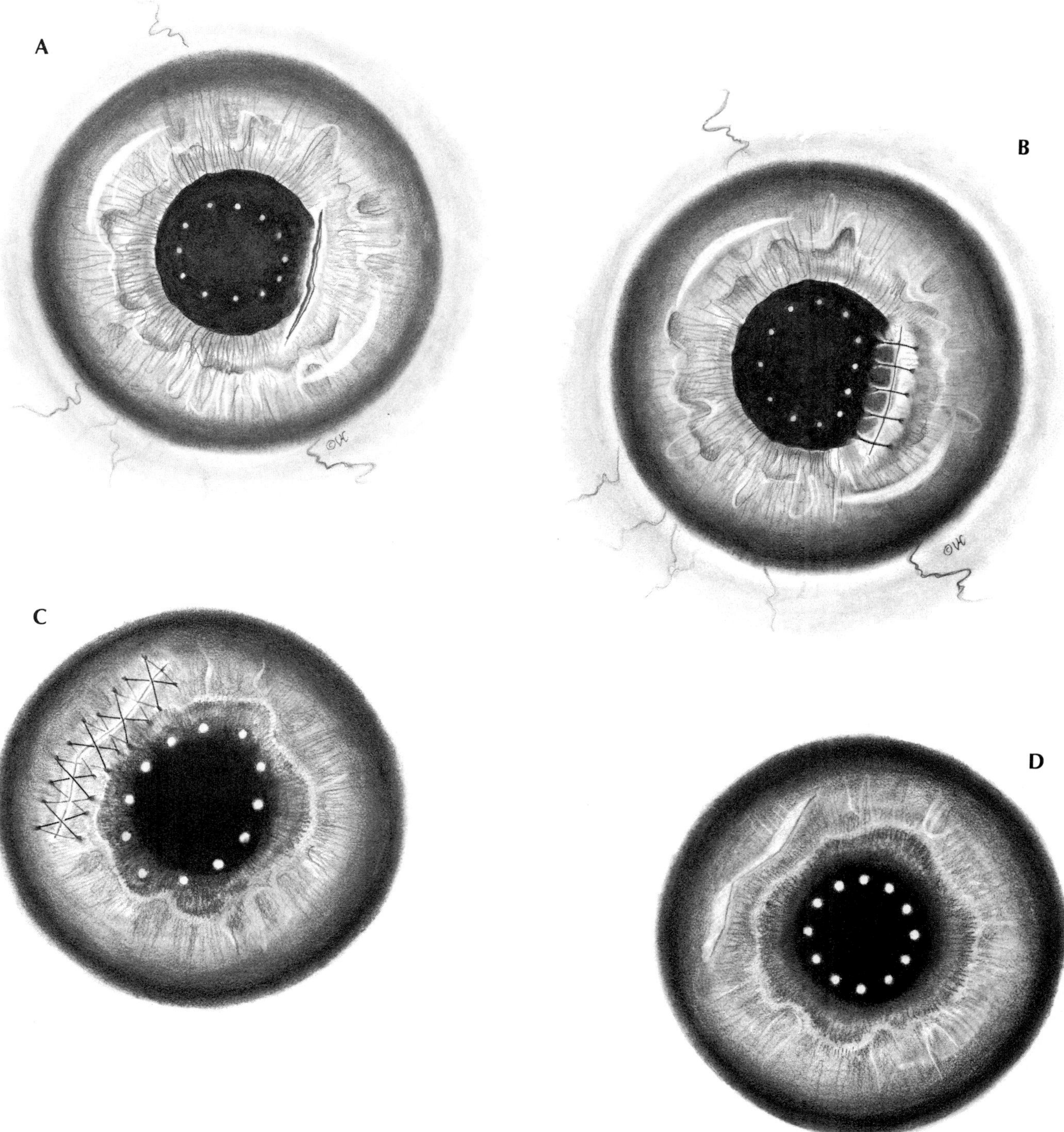

A, mid-corneal laceration showing dehiscence and central astigmatism with flat meridian in axis of laceration. **B,** properly sutured mid-corneal laceration showing steep meridian in axis of sutured laceration. **C,** mid-corneal laceration showing persistence of central corneal astigmatism with sutures in place. **D,** restoration of spherical cornea after removal of sutures from well-healed laceration.

Pathophysiology and Prevention of Astigmatism Secondary to Trauma **243**

The general principles of wound closure dictate a distinct advantage of running sutures over interrupted suture closure. Interrupted sutures have the disadvantage of many knots, which may be difficult to bury and may contribute to vascularization of the cornea by their presence. In addition, removal is often difficult, leading to broken sutures along the wound that can incite areas of differential wound healing long after the repair of the corneal lacerations has occurred. Interrupted sutures do not provide anterior support between the sutures and can lead to areas of anterior or posterior malposition with subsequent problems of edge lift and differential healing. Moreover, the interrupted sutures may have to be placed in many different directions to close the wound orthogonally, and because they do not actively interact with one another, irregular astigmatism may result (Plate 10–3,A). In contrast, a running-suture pattern has some ability to adjust itself to the requirements of the eye and can be adjusted by the surgeon at the conclusion of the surgery. The running suture can provide a predictable and regular band of force that can regularize or linearize an irregular incision, thus preventing an irregular astigmatism at the conclusion of the surgery (Plate 10–3,B).

The precise method of producing the running closure is also of concern. A simple running suture will tend to shift the sides of the wound laterally in opposite directions, which can cause wound apposition problems and even puckering of the wound both at the ends of the incision and in areas of irregularity. A shoelace-type closure, similar in a linear fashion to the opposing continuous suture, is better able to provide adequate perpendicular pressure across the wound and at the same time provide anterior corneal support.

The eye is circularly symmetrical around the visual axis maintained by its corneal optical ring. When closing corneal lacerations that are paracentral, an attempt should be made to increase the length of the bite peripherally and, if possible, to make the bites radial with respect to the optical axis of the eye. Of equal importance, is the need to close the incision with the bites placed as perpendicular to the wound margin as is practical. If the length of the bites are kept short in the central portion of the wound and lengthened as the bites extend toward the limbus, one can satisfy both criteria to some extent because there will tend to be a circular symmetry to the suture pattern even though the individual bites are perpendicular to the wound. In short incisions, these considerations are less important, particularly if the laceration is far in the periphery.

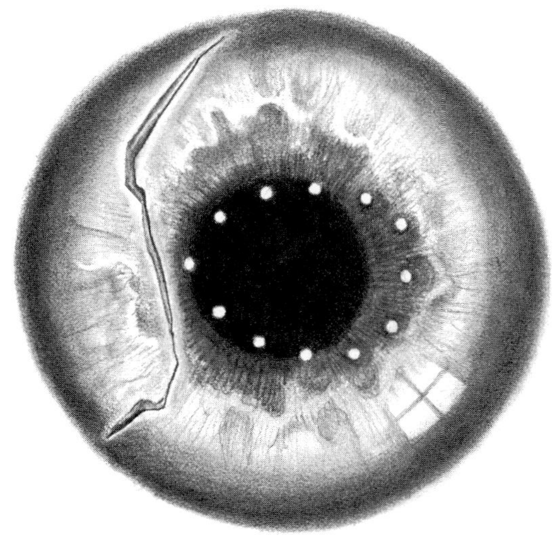

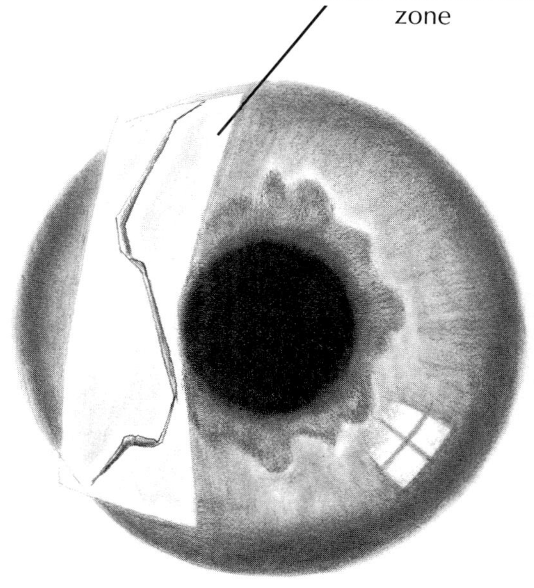

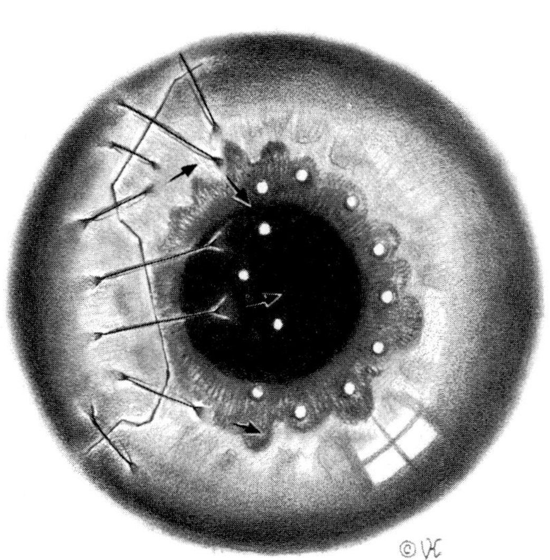

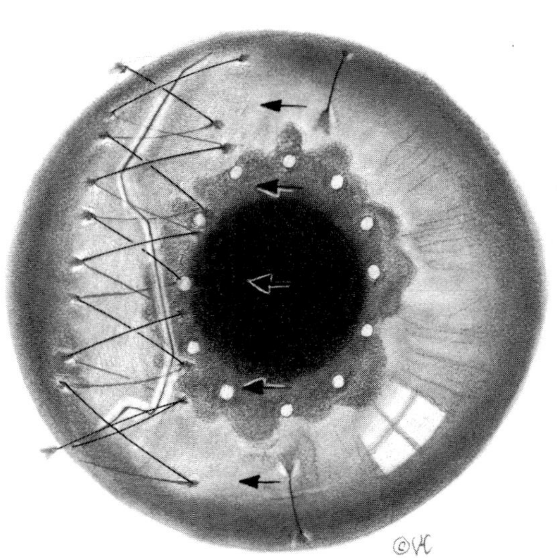

A, irregular mid-corneal laceration with interrupted suture closure and resulting irregular central astigmatism. **B,** irregular mid-corneal laceration with running suture closure showing creation of regular band of forces creating regular central astigmatism.

Pathophysiology and Prevention of Astigmatism Secondary to Trauma **245**

The closure of the penetrating laceration should adhere to the same principles used in penetrating keratoplasty. Perforating incisions should be closed with through-and-through monofilament nylon sutures to prevent posterior lambda effects discussed at length elsewhere in this book. Short partial penetrating incisions may be left unsutured if less than 50% depth because our experience in refractive surgery has shown us that without suturing these incisions heal well with little residual refractive effect. In deeper, nonpenetrating incisions a closure should be performed, particularly for the longer incisions because these will often have a significant refractive effect. The procedure for injuries that have both partial and fully penetrating injuries requires a slightly different approach. If the entire incision is not fully closed, there will be a tendency for the incision to leak. Therefore, in incisions of this type, the entire extent of the incision, regardless of its depth, should be closed and in the section of penetrating injury, the bites of the suture should be created through the entire corneal thickness to prevent the posterior lambda effect.

Beveled incisions represent an area of special consideration because a simple through-and-through closure will apply forces on the wound that tend to create either edge lifts or edge depressions (Plate 10–4,A). In these situations, the needle should be placed so that it exits through the tip of the extended bevel and is reinserted close to the posterior edge of the wound (Plate 10–4,B). This technique is more difficult but is well worth the effort to avoid relative sliding of the wound. If the suture is overly tightened, the tissue will bunch and slide creating poor wound apposition (Plate 10–4,C). If care is not taken to go through the tip of the bevel, the tissue will gape inferiorly causing a posterior lambda effect (Plate 10–4,D). For proper tightening, the tissue should appose on visual inspection and a slight elevation of the tissue will indicate appropriate tightness, preventing leakage of aqueous humor (Plate 10–4,E).

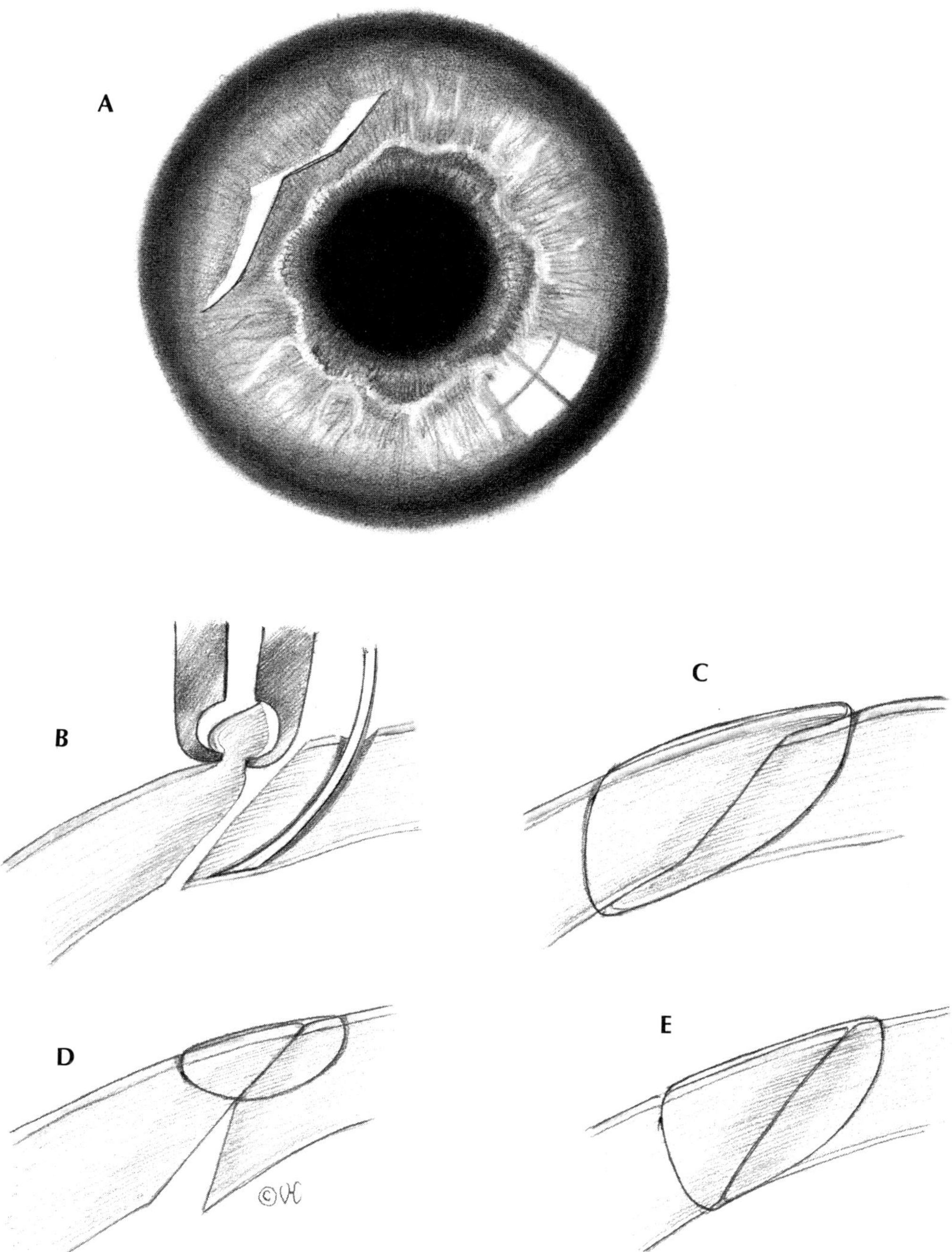

A, beveled mid-corneal laceration. **B,** needle placement through tip of beveled laceration aided by retraction of anterior corneal tissue. **C,** excessively tight closure of beveled laceration showing displacement of proper tissue apposition. **D,** shallow closure of beveled laceration showing posterior lambda effect. **E,** closure of beveled laceration with appropriate suture tension allowing proper apposition of corneal tissue.

COMPENSATING COMPRESSION SUTURES

After closure of the wound, one might be tempted to end the operation. However, the patient will invariably have a significant degree of regular astigmatic error due to the compression induced by closure of the corneal wound (Plate 10–5,A). This astigmatic error can be neutralized while the corneal sutures remain in position by the use of compression sutures placed at the time of the repair. The application of these compression sutures is relatively straightforward and will be described later.

At this point, the stab incision previously made in an area of uninvolved cornea should be used to normalize intraocular pressure during the application of the compression sutures. In addition, this entry can be used to verify the absence of vitreous or iris tissue incarcerated in the penetrating wound. Using a blunt instrument, such as a tying forceps, pressure is applied along the limbus while observing the reflex of the Troutman keratometer. If pressure is applied directly along the flat axis of the astigmatic pattern projected on the cornea, a correction will be seen to occur (Plate 10–5,B). If a suture loop is placed in this location and tied under keratometric control, the same effect can be maintained on a long-term basis (Plate 10–5,C). Using the same technique of pressure at the limbus, the flat axis 180 degrees away is now identified, and a suture is placed and tied in such a way that all remaining astigmatism is corrected, as verified by the Troutman keratometer. These sutures are left in place during the time that the primary sutures closing the laceration remain in place. Significant improvement in *sutures in* astigmatic error can be accomplished in this manner.

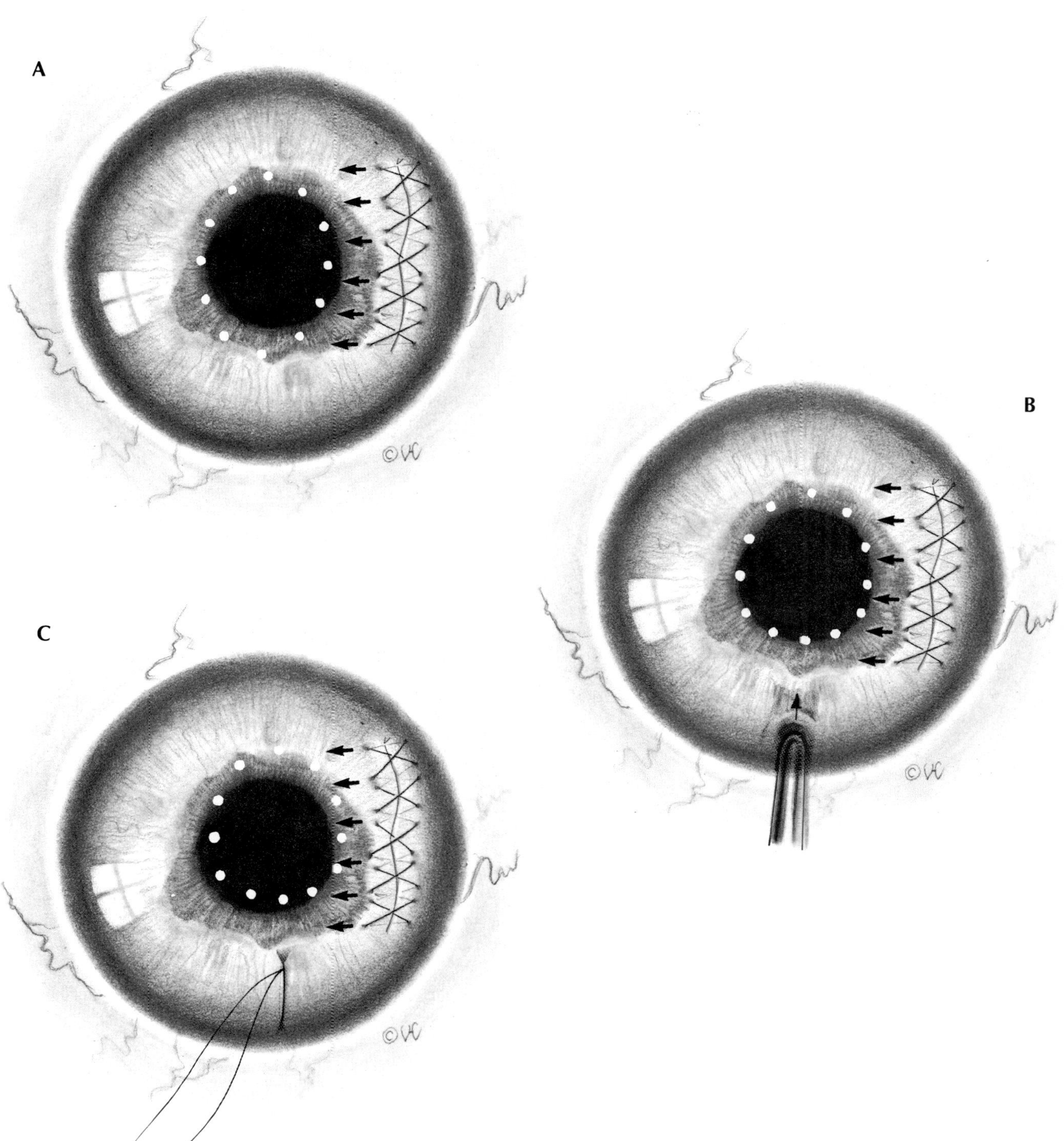

A, induced central corneal astigmatism by running suture closure of mid-corneal laceration. **B,** use of blunt tipped tying forceps at limbus to identify proper location for addition of compression suture showing reduction of central astigmatism as seen with Troutman keratometer. **C,** placement of interrupted compression suture left untied pending placement of remaining compression sutures for the purpose of simultaneous adjustment.

If pressure is placed away from the flat axis, the astigmatic pattern will be seen to worsen and will be displaced along the axis of the indentation (Plate 10–6,A). If when a suture is placed and tied in this location it only partially corrects the error, any residual astigmatism can be reduced further by additional suture. To find the appropriate point for the second suture, one must press at various points along the limbus until the reflex from the keratometer becomes round, which in many situations is a case of trial and error (Plate 10–6,B). A permanent suture is then placed at the second location. The vector forces from the two sutures taken along the original flat axis will then add up to the vector forces of the single suture placed directly along the original flat axis (see Plate 10–5,B). The appropriate location(s) for the compression suture(s) can be determined in this interactive manner, without the trauma of placing unnecessary compression sutures.

The compression suture should be placed so that it lies in its entirety in the cornea and is approximately 2 mm to 3 mm in length. Placement should be deep, but not penetrating the cornea. A slipknot should be placed, and the suture should be tightened so that approximately one half of the astigmatic error is corrected with the Troutman keratometer. The remaining error then is compensated by a compression suture 180 degrees opposite. When appropriate tension is applied, striae may be observed perpendicular to the area of the suture.

A slight overcorrection should be present at the conclusion of the procedure to allow for stretching of the compression sutures. Occasionally, more than two compression sutures may be required to produce a round reflex, and in this situation, additional sutures are placed in the manner described above. At this point, all of the compression sutures have been closed with slipknots to facilitate final adjustment to obtain a round reflex from the surgical keratometer. When this condition is achieved, each knot is locked sequentially with a square knot and buried. It should be noted that "overtightening" or premature locking of the compression sutures will often result in the need to place additional sutures. If more than four compression sutures are required it is likely that either the compression sutures are poorly placed or overly tight.

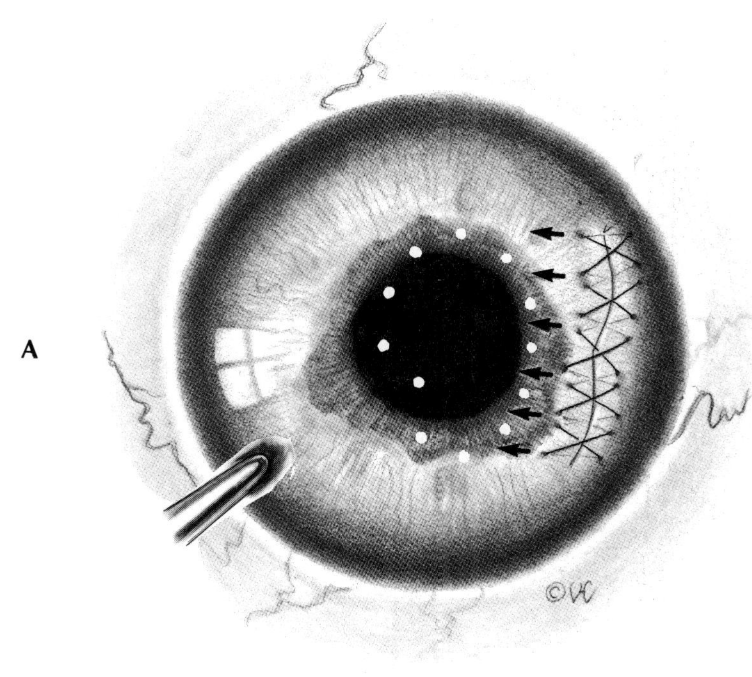

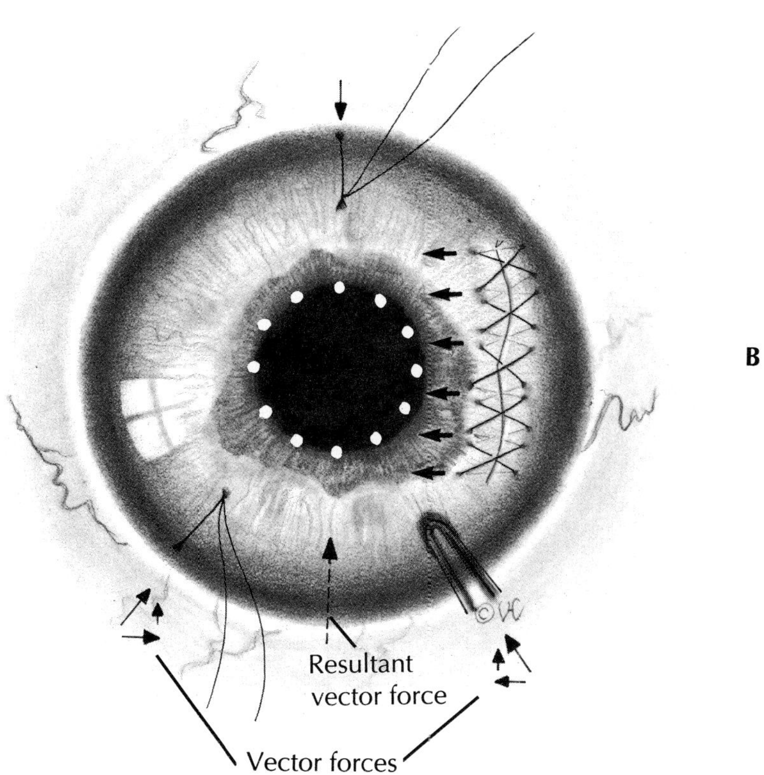

A, appearance of cornea with placement of limbal pressure in incorrect position showing indentation and movement of reflex from operative keratometer. **B,** appearance of cornea with limbal pressure at appropriate location to balance placement of compression suture in the incorrect location noted previously, showing vector addition of forces to equal forces that would have been created by proper suture placement.

In situations in which lacerations either involve the iris sphincter or extend close to it, the iris wounds should be closed to reestablish tension across the iris. If this is not performed, there will be a tendency to create synechia between the iris and the "sticky" corneal wound, which may affect wound healing. Moreover, a deformed pupil or an iris with a large laceration proximal to the pupil may cause diminished vision, glare, and even diplopia.

The closure of iris tissue is a delicate procedure that should be performed with the smallest needle available. Use of a large or cutting needle will cause unacceptably large tracts and even iris shredding. We have found the BV 100–4 by Ethicon placed on a 10–0 polypropylene suture to be an appropriate combination for the repair of iris trauma if adequate exposure for mobilization and tying exists through the wound. This can be tied with a simple square knot, which should be left above the iris if the patient is phakic and below the iris if the patient is aphakic or pseudophakic.

If the wound is too small, closure of an iris defect can be accomplished with a long, straight needle, such as the ST 6 Ethicon, used in the following manner. Stab incisions should be placed on each side of the cornea at the level of the iris laceration. The anterior chamber is filled with sodium hyaluronate. The needle is introduced into the anterior chamber from one of the incisions, and the iris edges are transfixed successively with the needle. A 25 g bent cannula is introduced from the second incision. The tip of the needle is placed within the cannula and drawn with it out of the cornea (Plate 10–7,A). A hook is used to draw the unarmed distal end of the suture through the second stab incision now occupied by the needle-armed proximal end (Plate 10–7,B). A slipknot is tied and tightened, using a Y-shaped Osher hook to push and close the knot and the iris coloboma (Plate 10–7,C). Next, two additional throws are placed and pushed sequentially into position with the Osher hook. Finally, the sutures are cut with a sharp cystotome, or better with a fine retinal scissors, introduced in the opposite stab incision (Plate 10–7,D). When long suture ends are left that impinge on the endothelium, an Argon laser can be used to shorten the suture ends.

This technique is awkward, and if the laceration is reasonably close to the periphery of the cornea, a third stab incision can be created in line with the laceration, and the suture threads can be bought through this laceration, tied down, and then cut directly with scissors. This technique is more convenient, but if used on lacerations at or near the iris sphincter or when closing a wide dehiscence, the knots may tear the iris during tying.

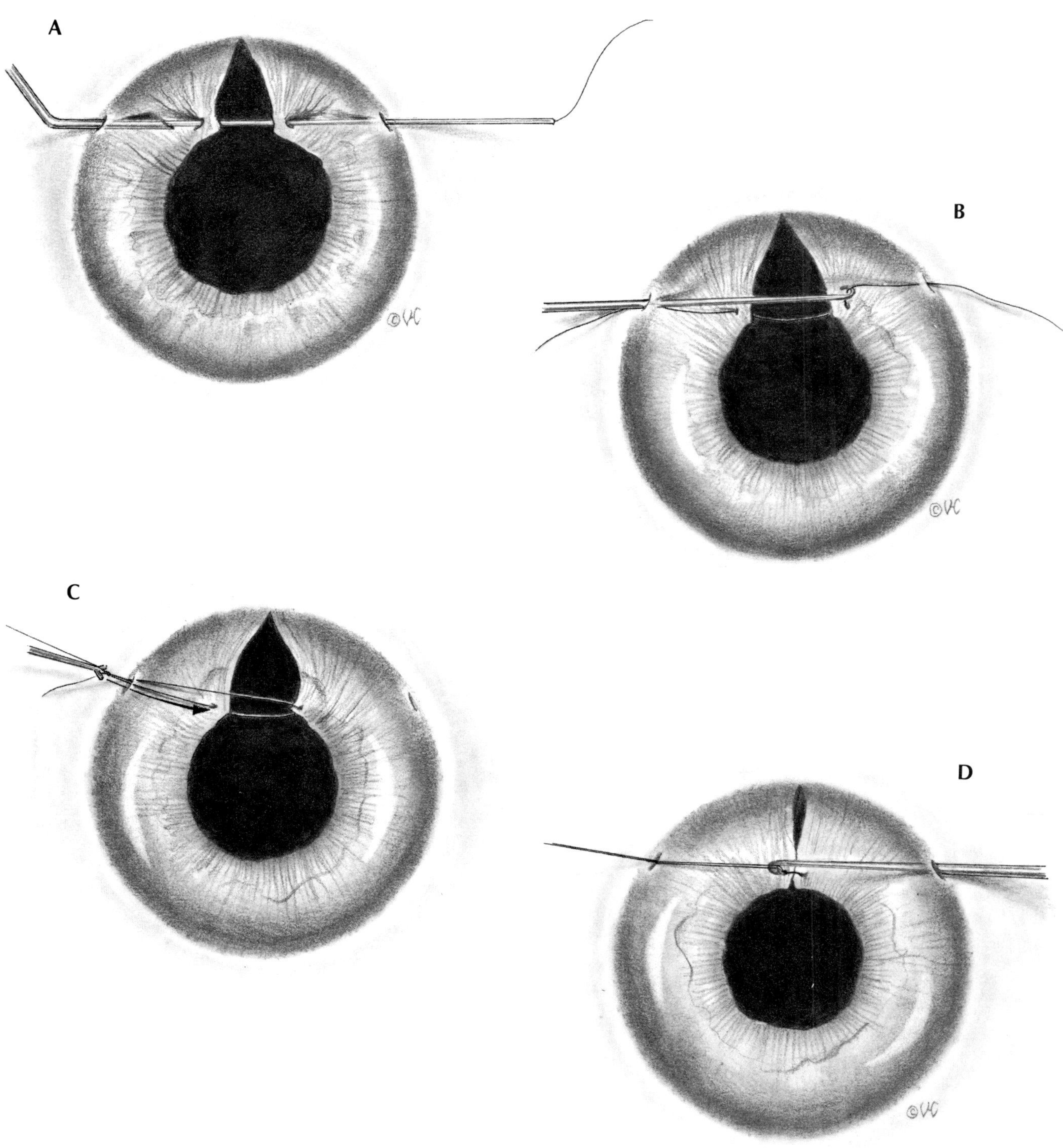

A, repair of iris tear by introduction of straight needle through a stab incision, passing through iris edges, and lodged within a canula for simplified extraction through a second stab incision. **B,** retraction of suture end through stab incision by means of a hook. **C,** tightening of slipknot with Osher hook drawing iris edges together. **D,** cutting of sutures with cystotome.

PARALIMBAL WOUND

This wound is quite common with blunt objects, such as nails or table corners, and occurs because of the change in curvature between the cornea and sclera at the corneal optical ring (Plate 10–8,A). Such trauma often causes significant damage to the iris, which in many cases is either prolapsed or severely contused (Plate 10–8,B). If a break in the iris is present, it is better to create an iridectomy at this location rather than to leave iris shreds in position that later may cause peripheral anterior synechiae (Plate 10–8,C). This approach must be balanced by the concern for glare or diplopia disturbing vision if the injury is in the inferior portion of the cornea.

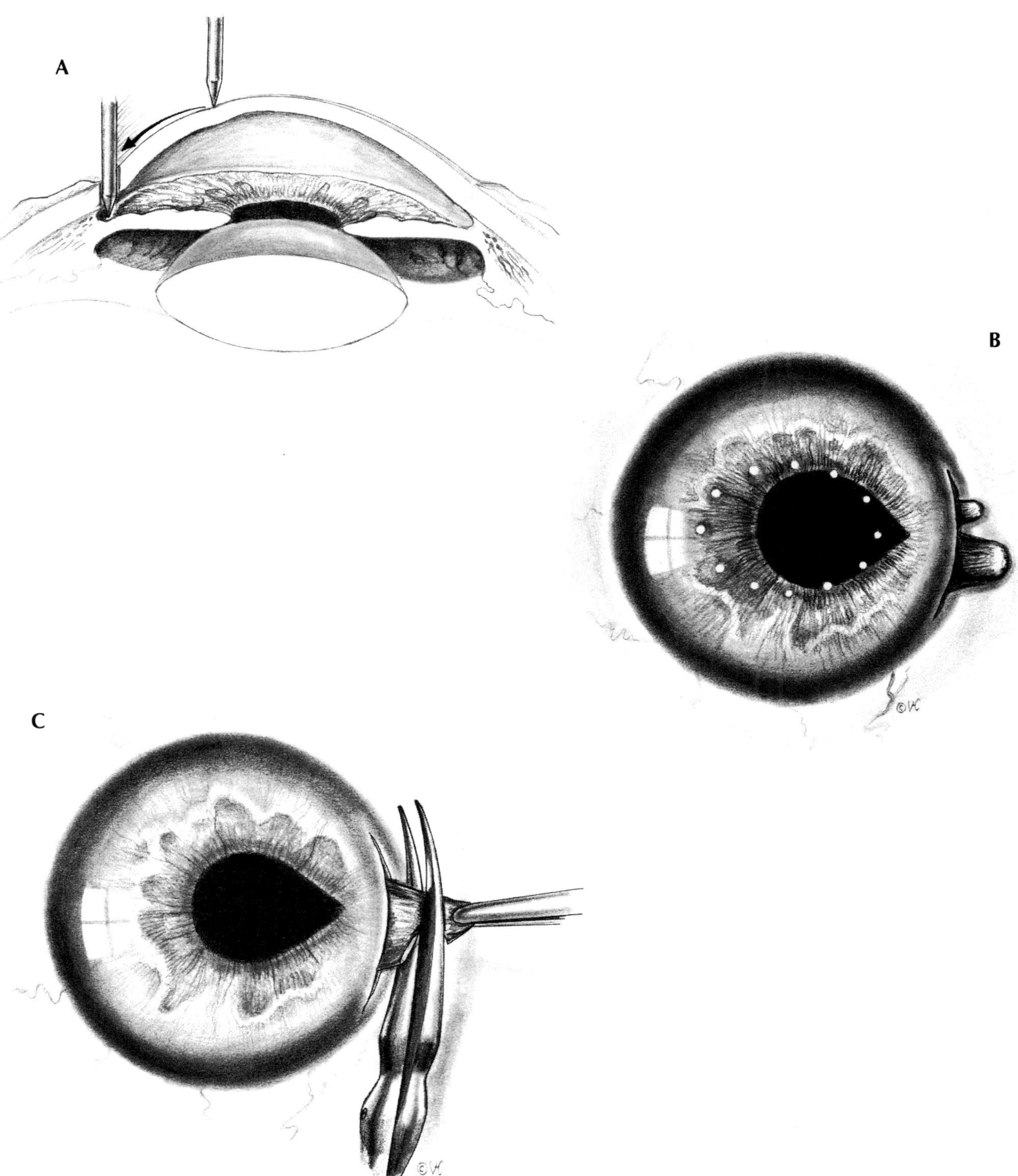

A, origin of peripheral corneal trauma due to sliding by blunt objects, such as nails, to limbus. **B,** uveal prolapse with macerated tissue. **C,** peripheral iridectomy to remove macerated uveal tissue and prevent peripheral anterior synechiae. *Continued.*

Pathophysiology and Prevention of Astigmatism Secondary to Trauma **255**

Often, the ciliary body may be damaged, and if excessive bleeding is encountered, a scleral extension can be performed posteriorly to expose this area and to resect the involved tissue with the help of cautery. It is best to avoid this approach when possible. The closure of such trauma is much like that used for the running closure of a corneal cataract wound, and these eyes often do quite well from the standpoint of permanently induced astigmatism as with a cataract incision in the same location (Plate 10–8,D). As an adjunct to more rapid visual rehabilitation, compensating compression sutures may be placed after closing the wound (Plate 10–8,E,F). Corneal sutures should remain in place for 3 to 6 months, depending on proximity to the limbus, and rapidity of wound healing.

D

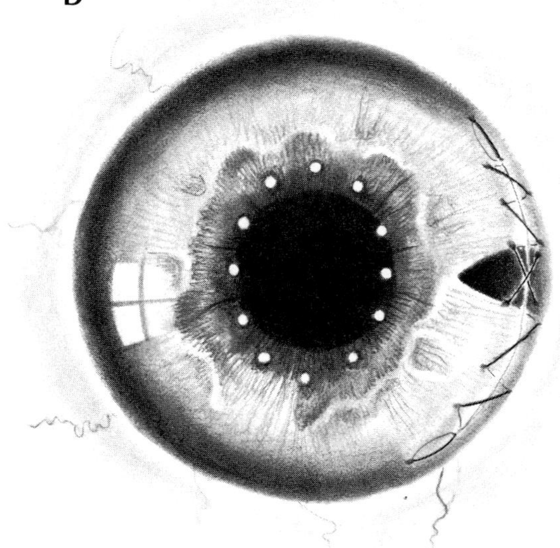

E

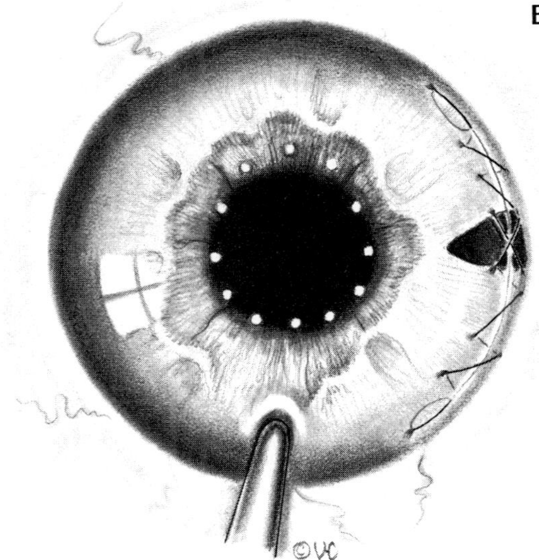

F

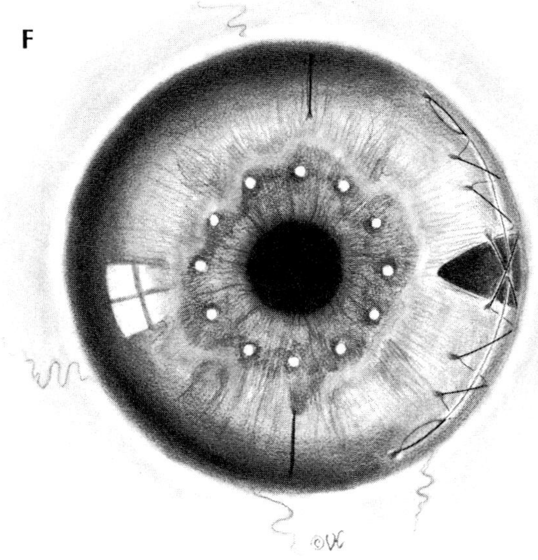

D, closure of peripheral corneal laceration with running closure used in corneal cataract incision. **E,** use of limbal pressure to identify proper axis of compression suture. **F,** final result with round reflex from operative keratometer following placement of compression sutures.

Pathophysiology and Prevention of Astigmatism Secondary to Trauma   **257**

MID-CORNEAL WOUND

Lacerations in the mid-cornea are often associated with sharp instruments that penetrate at the point of impact and cause the laceration. Beveled wounds and even loss of tissue are common in this location. These wounds are closer to the central cornea and induce more marked central corneal astigmatism in both the unsutured and the sutured wounds (Plate 10–9,A). Iris incarceration into the wound is often encountered, although iris laceration is not common because the pliability of the iris leads to contusion rather than rupture. In these wounds, the first consideration should be to reposition the incarcerated iris with a viscoelastic substance. Interrupted sutures should be placed to restore intraocular pressure. A stab incision placed at the paralimbal area will aid in the maintenance of intraocular pressure and will serve as a site for the introduction of a cyclodialysis spatula to replace the iris incarceration.

Suture technique should take into consideration the proximity to the optical axis. This dictates shorter suture bites centrally than peripherally, both to avoid direct trauma to the visual axis and to respect the circular symmetry of the eye (Plate 10–9,B). The closure of beveled incisions should be performed as discussed previously, and overtightening of the sutures should be avoided. The addition of compression sutures to enhance *sutures in* rehabilitation is highly effective in this group of patients (Plate 10–9,C). Sutures should be left in place longer for this group of patients than for more peripheral trauma because healing is slower in the mid-cornea. As with penetrating keratoplasty, more centrally placed sutures should be left in place for 6 to 9 months.

Trauma in the mid-corneal region often results in lens trauma, and even though the incision may seem large enough to express the lens or its fragments without creating another incision, the approach will be unfamiliar and the results are likely to be less than satisfactory. For this reason, it is better to completely close the trauma wound and to remove the lens fragments later in the procedure through a paralimbal incision in the manner to which the surgeon is accustomed. Occasionally fragments, or indeed entire objects, causing the laceration may still be in place at the time of surgery. When extensive manipulation is not required, such fragments can be cleaned from the wound and anterior chamber. Even when more extensive debridement including vitrectomy is required, it is still preferable to enter from a paralimbal or pars plana approach with positive control of intraocular pressure and with the assistance of a vitreoretinal surgeon.

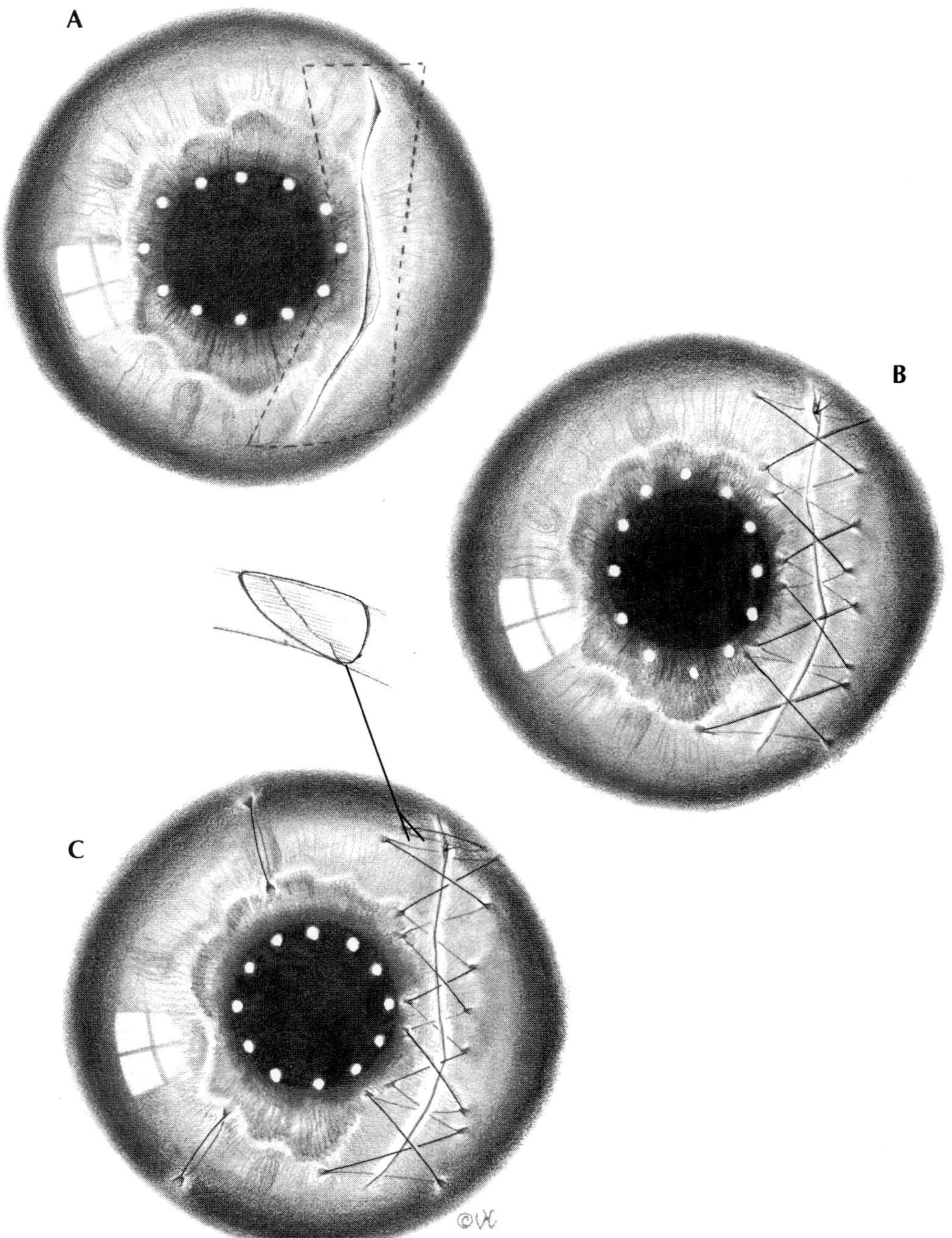

A, mid-corneal beveled laceration. **B,** running suture closure with shorter bites centrally to avoid optical axis and to create a curved incision pattern. **C,** final appearance after placement of compression sutures with round reflex from operative keratometer.

CENTRAL LACERATIONS

The repair of central lacerations passing through or very near the visual axis is a problem in which full visual rehabilitation may be difficult or impossible at the primary procedure. Often, such lacerations occur in children in whom at least partial visual rehabilitation during the healing of the wound would be desirable to avoid amblyopia. Shortening the length of the bites of the sutures centrally can often avoid contact with the optical axis as can slanting of the bites of the running suture to avoid directly impinging on the optical zone. Significant distortion can occur even if this is done. Another solution has been the use of two running sutures, leaving an open area without suturing in the central 3-mm zone (Plate 10–10). If the wound is sufficiently clean and atraumatic, this closure often is sufficient to prevent leakage, particularly if a soft contact lens is used in the immediate postoperative period. If necessary, a hard contact lens can sometimes provide surprisingly good vision after the incisions have healed for 1 to 2 weeks.

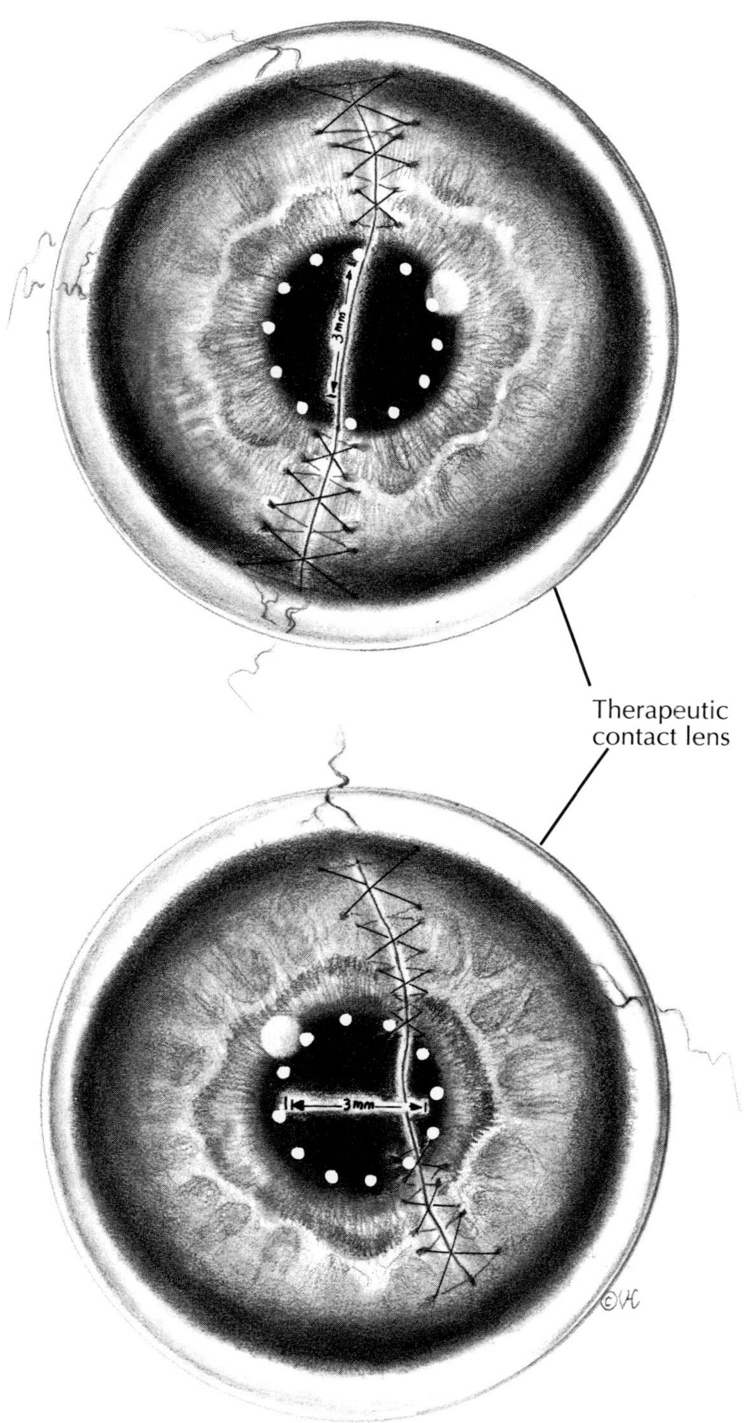

Central corneal laceration showing sparing of central 3-mm optical zone, with closure peripherally with running sutures to improve *sutures in* visual acuity with the use of soft contact lens.

Y- OR STELLATE-SHAPED LACERATIONS

Frequently a laceration will split into two or more directions, leaving a sharp corner, or two to three lacerations extend outward from a central point. The tendency is to place a suture in the very friable tissue at the "point" of the laceration (Plate 10–11,A), where the tissue is often avulsed, causing a loss of substance at a critical location. The principle used in closing such areas is to provide circumferential force, drawing the tissue toward the central point of laceration and avoiding sutures at the friable ends.

In a Y- or T-shaped laceration, a rectangular or trapezoidal suture pattern can perform a pursestring function, drawing the tissue together while being anchored in more durable tissue some distance away from the center of the laceration (Plate 10–11,B,C). If a stellate pattern is encountered, a similar principle is used, simply crossing each incision with a bite and drawing the area together with the pursestring (Plate 10–11,D). This situation is similar to the problem of crossed incisions in radial keratotomy in which the radial and transverse incisions cross each other, leading to a wound healing abnormality at the area of crossing. As this example illustrates, a partial penetrating incision crossing a second partial penetrating incision should be closed using this procedure because long-term instability may result even if the penetration is relatively minor.

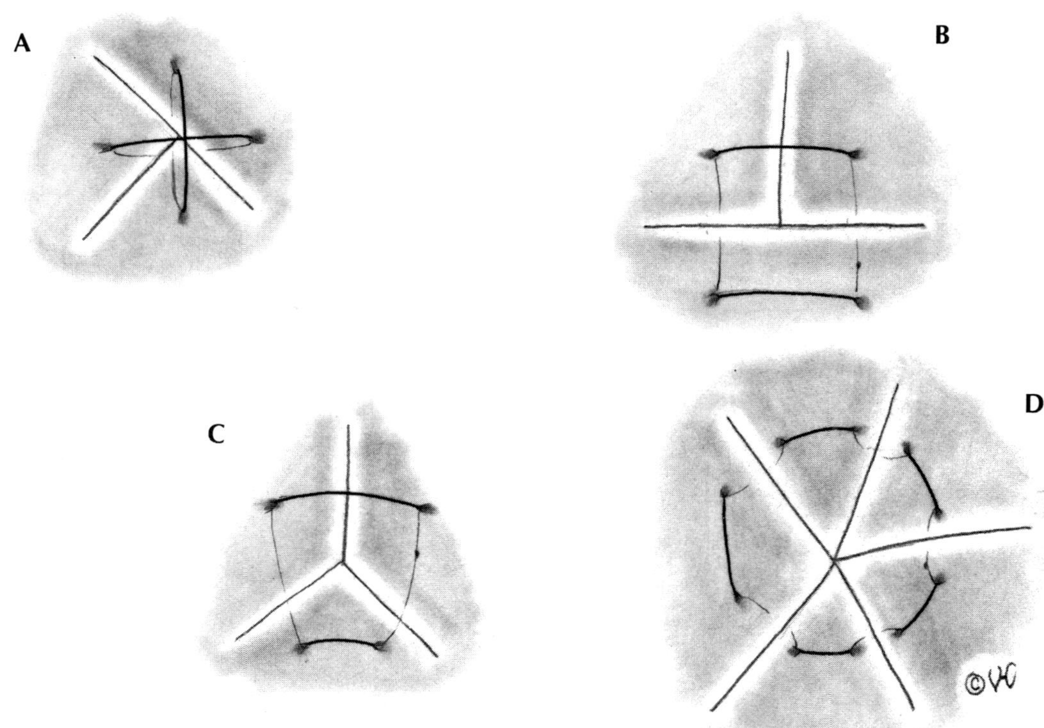

A, improper interrupted suture closure of stellate laceration. **B,** rectangular *pursestring* closure of crossed corneal incisions or lacerations showing central compression of tissue. **C,** trapezoidal *pursestring* closure of Y-shaped corneal laceration showing avoidance of fragile tip of flap. **D,** circular *pursestring* closure of stellate corneal laceration through firm peripheral tissue providing central compression and closure.

MULTIPLE CORNEAL LACERATIONS

Often the cornea will present with many lacerations in a restricted area, for example, from glass. These injuries are problematic from a number of standpoints. First, the glass is not well-visualized on x-ray unless it contains a large amount of lead; preoperative magnetic resonance imaging (MRI) scanning of the eye may illuminate glass fragments in the eye more clearly. Second, the multiple lacerations may be quite difficult to close, and even if the majority of the lacerations are partial penetrating incisions, corneal instability may result from the injury. Our experience with 16- and 32-incision radial keratotomy has taught us that the cornea can tolerate only so many incisions in a given area. When too many incisions are present, and particularly if a combination of radial and transverse incisions are used, the cornea becomes unstable, and severe healing abnormalities become apparent. Homoplastic lamellar keratoplasty using the microkeratome has been used to stabilize the cornea and promote healing in this circumstance (Plate 10–12,A).

With these facts in mind, the best treatment is a lamellar keratoplasty with interrupted sutures closing the lacerations in the lamellar bed to stabilize the remaining posterior cornea (Plate 10–12,B). Fresh corneal tissue prepared with a microkeratotome or by hand dissection is preferred, although the lyophilized keratopatch material from AMO has been a useful alternative. If neither of these options is available, all surgeons who encounter trauma in their practice should keep a vial of glycerin-preserved corneal tissue available.

The approach to lamellar keratoplasty should begin with a partial approximation of the tissue to restore intraocular pressure. The importance of a stab incision away from the area of laceration is reemphasized. If possible, the area involved should be encompassed by a trephine that is used to provide a smooth and atraumatic edge with which to begin the lamellar dissection. It is not absolutely essential to include all of the lacerations within the area of the lamellar transplant. A stray laceration extending beyond the lamellar bed can be sutured separately. The goal of this surgery is to provide sufficient mechanical stability to allow the cornea to heal. After partial trephination with a free trephine, the incision should be deepened with a diamond knife to at least 50% of the corneal thickness to provide a clear step in opposing the lamellar transplant. When the dissection involves the corneal periphery, as with a pterygium, a peritomy is performed. A semisharp rounded spatula, such as the Troutman or Paufique, is then used to dissect the lamellar bed. As sutures are cut in this process, they should be replaced to maintain intraocular pressure and corneal stability and to enhance the creation of a level lamellar bed. The dissection should be carried just beyond the limbus and cut with a diamond knife.

The donor tissue can be incised with a trephine 0.5-mm larger than

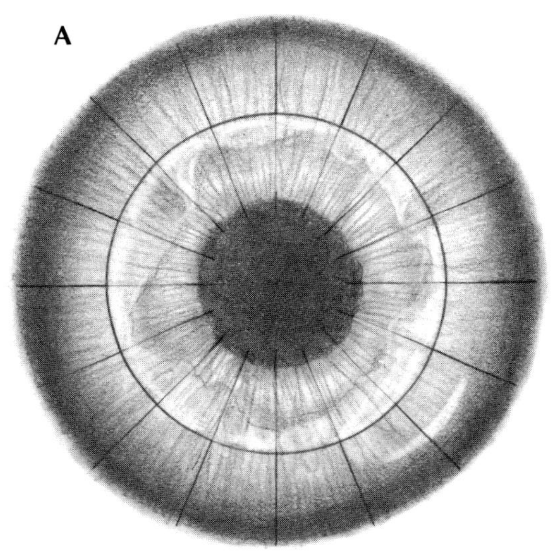

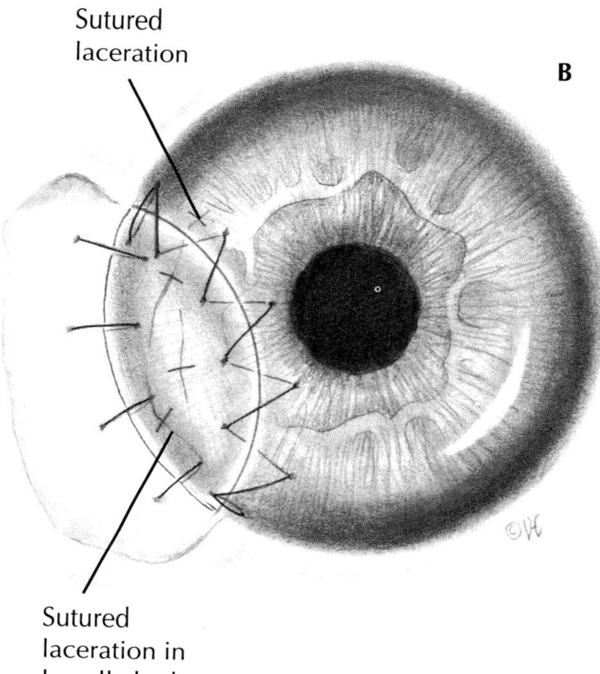

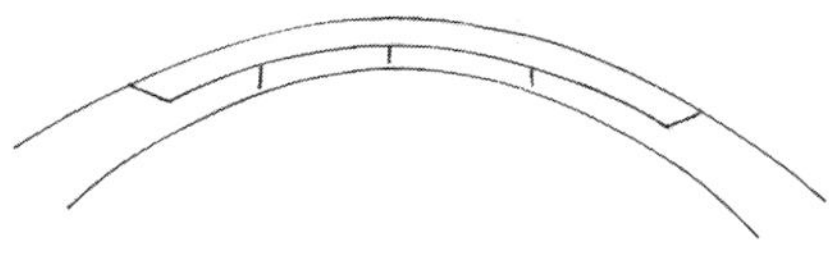

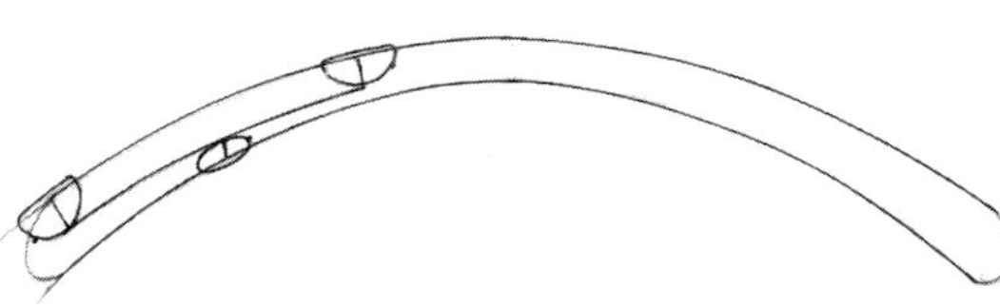

A, lamellar homograft used to treat overcorrected 16-incision radial keratotomy. **B,** lamellar transplant to stabilize cornea with multiple lacerations in limited corneal area. Note sutured lacerations extending beyond graft and also in bed of lamellar transplant.

the trephine used to create the lamellar bed and sutured into place with interrupted cardinal sutures. We prefer the larger graft because creating the bed in a soft or relatively soft eye often leads to a slightly larger bed than the trephine that is used for the primary dissection. A running suture is placed along the curved anterior corneal edge of the graft, and the graft should be trimmed with scissors to extend approximately 2 mm behind the limbus. Several interrupted 8:0 Vicryl absorbable sutures or 10-0 nylon can be used to close the limbal edge of the graft. The conjunctiva should be closed with horizontal sutures to complete the procedure. At the conclusion of this surgery, the operative keratometer should be used to examine corneal astigmatism, and compression sutures should be applied to round the corneal reflex and to speed postoperative visual rehabilitation. This technique is further discussed and illustrated in Chapter 11.

In the extreme example, corneal tissue may actually be avulsed, creating one of the more challenging situations for the trauma surgeon. In this situation, the temptation is to proceed to corneal grafting immediately without restoring intraocular pressure. This temptation should be avoided, because preparation of a circular and regular graft incision is extremely difficult in the soft eye. The first step in such cases is to ascertain the actual loss of corneal tissue. Surprisingly, traumatic incisions of the cornea often retract by the time the patient reaches the emergency room, and careful reapproximation of the tissue may reveal an intact cornea.

In circumstances in which corneal loss clearly is present, the preparation should be similar to an ordinary corneal transplantation. If tissue is not available, the use of glycerin-preserved corneal or scleral tissue can often reestablish ocular integrity until such tissue becomes available. A ring, such as the Pierce or Flieringa ring, should be sewn to the sclera to provide good control of the corneal surface. Often, this technique alone will reestablish a semblance of normal corneal contours that will aid in trephination.

If the area of tissue loss is small, cyanoacrylate glue (Histoacryl) can provide a temporary plug long enough to reestablish intraocular pressure and complete the trephination. Often, the addition of a soft contact lens or plastic drape material, in conjunction with the glue, will provide an adequate patch over slightly larger areas of corneal tissue loss. In terms of application, one should keep in mind that the area to be glued must be dry and clean and that excess glue within the anterior chamber can be toxic and can cause adhesions to the iris and lens.

One technique used to avoid these complications with a larger hole is the introduction of a small piece of plastic drape within the anterior chamber against the posterior cornea (Plate 10–13,A). This is held in place with viscoelastic or air introduced from a stab incision peripherally to push the plastic material up against the cornea to create a seal. Weck sponges dry the external area grossly, and Histoacryl glue is applied along the bottom edge of the opening, creating a temporary seal (Plate 10–13,B). The area is then additionally dried with Weck sponges, creating a small well, which is filled with histoacryl glue (Plate 10–13,C). We prefer to use a micropipette to apply the glue to avoid using an excess amount. Plastic drape material can then be applied to the surface creating a sandwich that provides a secure plug for moderate-size corneal openings. Trephination can then proceed in the usual manner (Plate 10–13,D).

In the large corneal tissue-loss situation, it may be necessary to sew a temporary patch graft into position, reestablish intraocular pressure, and proceed with the usual corneal trephination. Although extensive preparation is not required for this temporary patch graft to create a seal over the irregular dehiscence, one should keep in mind that significant distortions of the cornea will reflect equally significant distortions in the graft margin, which can create large amounts of astigmatism. In this technique, the tissue is sutured over the corneal surface with mattress or overlying sutures, *Greffe Bouchon*. In each of these techniques, the importance of a stab incision for introduction of viscoelastics to maintain the chamber and intraocular pressure until a seal is secured cannot be overemphasized.

SUMMARY

Trauma surgery can be one of the most rewarding and challenging areas of ophthalmic surgery. The key to success in this area centers on careful preoperative observation, evaluation, and planning. Nothing is more disturbing than being confronted in the operating room with a situation that requires a particular instrument or person, which is unavailable simply because it was not anticipated. We have given some basic strategies to aid the surgeon in this planning process. Ultimately, the most valuable source of information for trauma surgery is the surgeon's own experience and the association of trauma situations with more common surgical situations. This process can work equally well in the opposite direction. Some of the greatest advances of modern ophthalmology, including the intraocular lens and radial keratotomy, have come when the surgeons reflected on their experiences in trauma surgery and transformed this experience to create new procedures. Certainly, trauma surgery is the crucible of ophthalmic theories and practice.

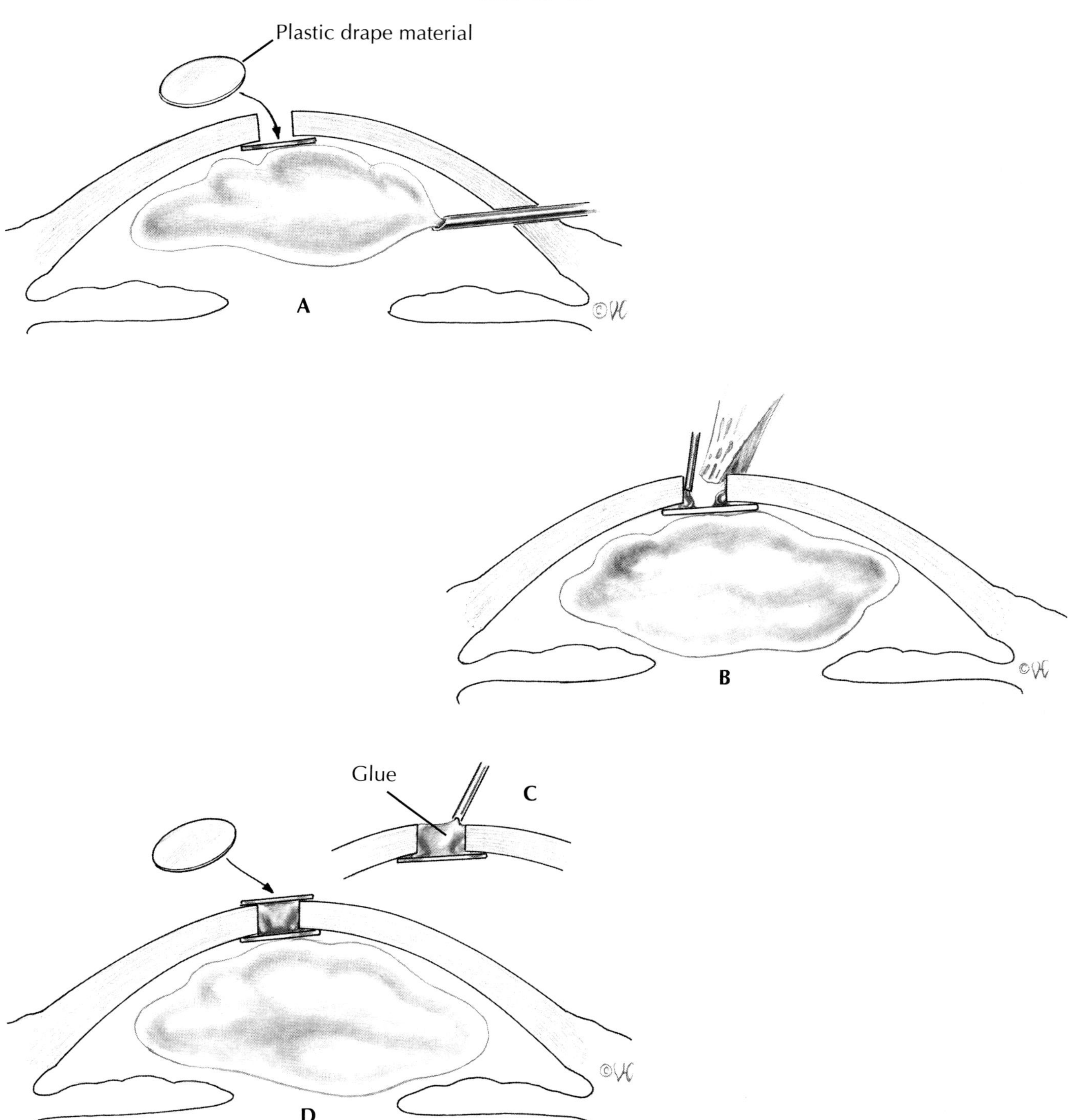

A, introduction of plastic disc to block large corneal opening made from drape material held in place by viscoelastic material or air in anterior chamber. **B,** application of tissue adhesive around posterior edge of opening to allow better drying of tissue with sponges. **C,** filling of well created by corneal opening with tissue adhesive. **D,** application of plastic disc from drape material on surface of cornea to complete corneal plug and normal intraocular pressure to facilitate trephination of the cornea.

Chapter 11

Pathophysiology, Prevention, and Surgical Management of Astigmatism in Lamellar Keratoplasty

Lamellar keratectomy and lamellar keratoplasty, first performed successfully by von Hippel in 1877, preceded penetrating keratoplasty as a surgical procedure. For many years, even after the first successful penetrating keratoplasty was performed by Zirm in 1905, it remained the procedure of choice, especially when the corneal opacity was present only in the anterior layers of the cornea. Surgery for pterygium was and remains probably the most commonly performed lamellar keratoplasty procedure. The French school, led by Paufique, Sourdille, and Offret, championed lamellar keratoplasty in the 1930s and 1940s as a means of avoiding the severe surgical and immunologic complications of penetrating keratoplasty as performed during that era. Cornea splitters were designed (e.g., Paufique knife) for improved manual dissection, particularly of the recipient bed. However, the relatively crude dissection of the recipient as well as the donor cornea often left the interface so scarred and irregular that the vision results were disappointing as compared with those obtained with the occasionally successful penetrating keratoplasty. Castroviejo, a champion of penetrating keratoplasty in full-thickness pathology, also performed lamellar procedures and, to lessen the interface scar, devised a motorized lamellar *keratotome* that could excise a more regular lamella from both donor and recipient. At about the same time, José Barraquer independently developed a *microkeratome* with which a precisely graded thickness of cornea could be removed from recipient or donor cornea for refractive modification as well as for lamellarization and replacement of corneal scars. The motorized keratotomes tended to follow any anterior irregularity, recreating it in the dissected bed. Nevertheless, lamellar keratoplasty had to be confined to those corneas that had relatively normal endothelial function and had opacified tissue extending no deeper than two thirds of the corneal thickness.

Astigmatism in an eye requiring lamellar keratoplasty though often irregular, is not excessively high in a given meridian unless the corneal optical ring is involved in the presenting pathology. When the corneal thickness within the optical zone can be restored, postoperative astigmatism is not a significant problem. This was yet another reason why many early corneal surgeons preferred the loss of several lines of vision from the lamellar interface scar to the then-insoluble postoperative problems of high astigmatism and anisometropia after penetrating keratoplasty.

Lamellar pathology peripheral to the central optical zone is often the cause of moderate-to-severe central astigmatic errors, for example, from pterygium and, in particular, from recurrent pterygium. Some dystrophies and degenerative diseases such as marginal dystrophy, keratoglobus, and Mooren's ulcer, which attack the cornea primarily in the periphery preserving the optical zone, are also productive not only of high and sometimes irregular astigmatism but also, as in the case of keratoglobus, corneal myopia as well. Scars from superficial central and peripheral trauma or from deep or penetrating peripheral trauma can also be productive of excessive central corneal astigmatism.

Some lamellar and incisional refractive keratoplasty procedures that are primarily designed to correct spherical myopia or hyperopia may produce excessive astigmatism. Among these are the procedures of Barraquer as well as epikeratoplasty and epikeratophakia that may induce astigmatism from unequal healing around the corneal cap periphery. When used to manage severe keratoconus, epikeratoplasty may induce astigmatism from the compression of irregular underlying keratoconic tissue.

PREVENTION OF ASTIGMATISM IN LAMELLAR KERATOPLASTY

As with any corneal surgical procedure, exclusive of uncontrollable tissue factors, accuracy in the preparation of the lamellar donor tissue and in the dissection of the recipient eye is essential to the prevention of astigmatism at the primary procedure. When combined with precise edge closure, these precautions will be a major deterrent to the development of residual astigmatism, ametropia, or both.

For purposes of this discussion, the primary surgeries for prevention of astigmatism in lamellar keratoplasty are divided into two categories: circumferential total and subtotal lamellar keratoplasty and partial or segmental lamellar keratoplasty. These divisions are based in part on the fact that the individual categories differ in their potential to induce or correct astigmatism.

TOTAL AND SUBTOTAL CIRCUMFERENTIAL LAMELLAR KERATOPLASTY

Circumferential lamellar keratoplasty, whether total or subtotal, is inherently less productive of meridional distortion than segmental or partial surgery. First, the dissection of donor and recipient can be facilitated by automated instrumentation such as the Barraquer microkeratome. Second, using current suture-closing techniques, a circumferential incision is easier to balance and adjust and to manipulate segmentally should sector apposition or healing be deficient.

PREPARATION OF RECIPIENT CORNEA

In contradistinction to penetrating keratoplasty, in lamellar keratoplasty it is usually advisable to prepare the recipient bed before preparing the donor replacement tissue because there is a greater possibility of or need for intraoperative variation of depth or diameter. Whether the recipient dissection is better done by the microkeratome or manually depends on two factors: the extent of the corneal scar to be resected and the regularity and thickness of the recipient cornea. The goal of the procedure is to excise the scar tissue and replace it with donor cornea in the optical and midperipheral zones. It is not always necessary to remove scar tissue external to the central 4 to 6 mm. The more accurately and regularly one can dissect the central optical zone, the better the final optical as well as the tectonic or the reconstructive result.

Superficial lamellar corneal dissection may eventually be better managed by the use of excimer laser photoablation. Using fill-in techniques to regularize the anterior surface, a smooth recipient bed can be prepared to the depth and diameter required to remove the scar. Unfortunately, with the present technology of excimer laser delivery systems, the beam of the laser flattens the corneal curvature as the tissue is ablated to the depth of the scar. This creates a flatter or hyperopic anterior corneal surface and has resulted in significant and debilitating hyperopia and anisometropia in early cases. This problem is in addition to the one caused by the glare induced by the removal of Bowman's layer. It is probable that even after a corneal scar is successfully removed by photoablation, the anterior corneal curvature may need to be restored by a lamellar graft.

Manual Dissection of Recipient Cornea

For most ophthalmic surgeons at the present time, the only method to prepare a lamellar graft bed is by manual dissection. If the Barraquer microkeratome or a modification (e.g., Barraquer-Krumeich-Swinger, Draeger, or Ruiz microkeratomes) is available, the lamellar cap may be precisely and regularly removed from the donor, and for accurate matching from the recipient as well. Removal of a cap from the recipient by one of these instruments is more complicated when the anterior surface is irregular because the instruments tend to follow the irregularity, recreating it in the bed. If this is anticipated, then the donor lamella is better cut by the manual method because all of the microkeratomes taper the edges of the lamellar resection, both in the donor and in the recipient, and those edges will not match the edge of a manually cut recipient. Because of this problem and because of the cost and relative unavailability of these automated instruments, we will not illustrate them or describe their use.

When performing a lamellar keratoplasty by the manual technique, the dissection begins with the recipient excision because the possibility of misdirection of the dissection or of perforation may require a change in the depth, size or shape of the donor lamella. To begin the manual dissection, one must first determine the depth and peripheral extent of the scar and then outline the incision circumference with a trephine blade of appropriate diameter. The Hanna trephine has the possibility to use blades of a range of diameters (6–10 mm) to create an accurate vertical incision to the depth necessary to allow complete lamellar removal of the scar tissue (Plate 11–1,A). The dissection depth required to reach clear cornea is not always immediately apparent at the preoperative examination. To determine the maximum depth of dissection, it is important to know the approximate corneal thickness so that dissection to whatever level will not risk accidental perforation. An ultrasonic pachymeter is used to make such a determination. If a Hanna trephine is not available, the cut is made with a manual trephine, preferably one fitted with an obturator to prevent perforation.

After the trephine mark is made to the desired depth, dissection should begin at that depth at the edge of the circumferential trephine cut. The manual dissection should begin with a sharp, angled corneal splitter to establish the plane of dissection (Plate 11–1,B). Once a plane is established, a semisharp dissector should be used to complete the dissection. As one dissects into the corneal scar tissue, the plane can be lost, and it is sometimes necessary to begin the dissection at another quadrant to complete the lamellarization. It is useful to create a tunnel across the cornea with a long, inverse-curve semisharp dissector and then to proceed laterally from the tunnel to complete the dissection. The dissector is advanced by short, lateral wobbling motions that lift the cornea as the lamellae are gently separated (Plate 11–1,C). A sharp dissector should be avoided because the curve of the cornea will cause the dissector to move out of the plane into the deeper or superficial layers of the cornea. When the bed is completed to the deepest level possible to include the scar but not to penetrate the posterior lamella, the dissection of the donor button can proceed.

Manual Dissection of Donor Cornea

The manual technique for the dissection of the donor proceeds in a similar fashion to that of the recipient cornea. Unless one has an artificial chamber such as that supplied with the Krumeich or the Hanna system, it is best done on a whole eye. Because the condition of the endothelium is not essential to the survival of the lamellarized donor cornea, viable donor tissue not suitable for penetrating keratoplasty may be used. The dissection of the donor will be found to be somewhat easier than that of the re-

Plate 11–1.

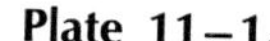

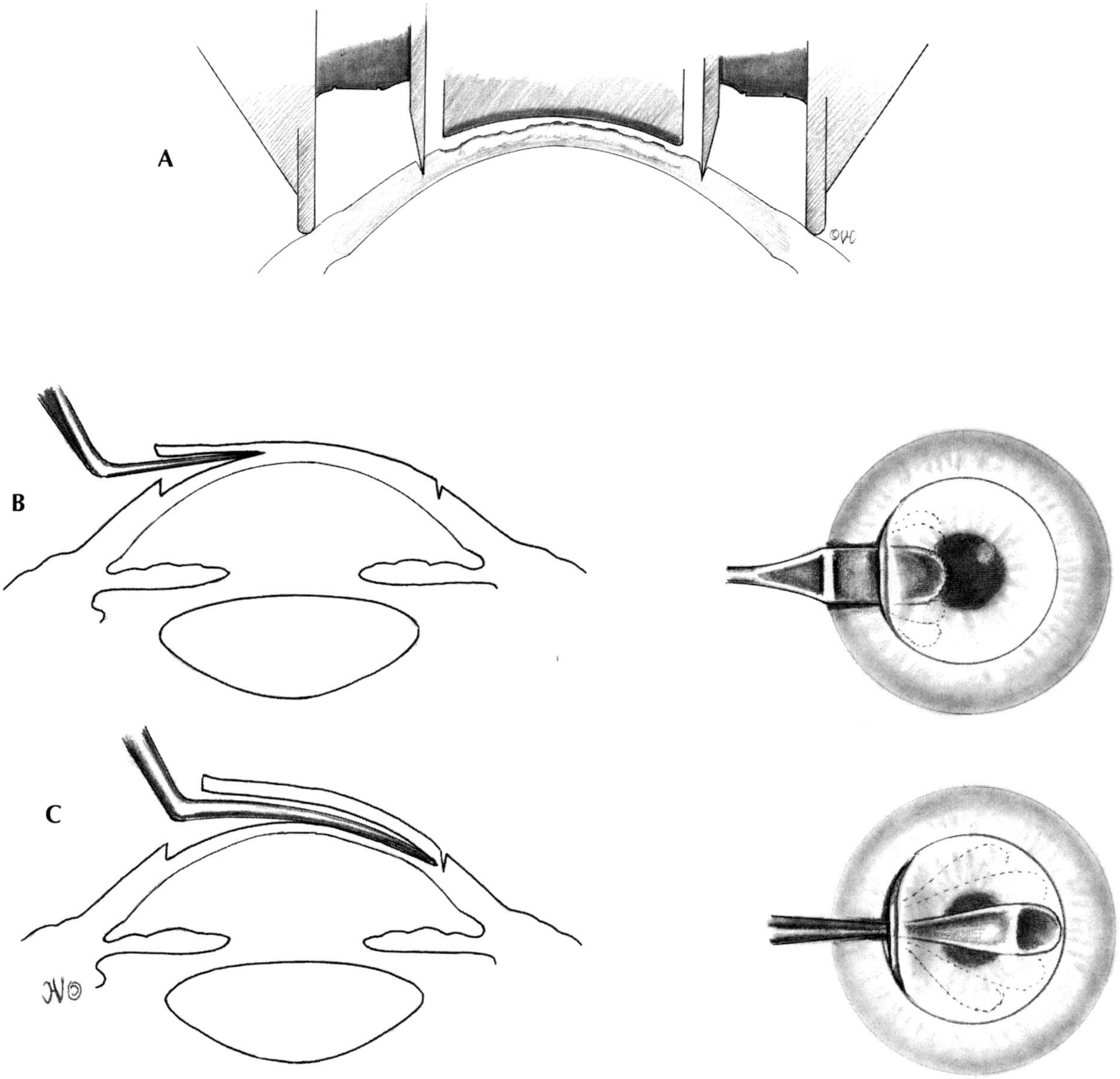

A, use of Hanna trephine to create accurate vertical incision depth in the recipient cornea. **B,** beginning the lamellar dissection. **C,** completing the lamellar dissection of the cornea prior to trephination.

cipient because of the more regular lamella in the absence of scar tissue. In larger lamellar dissections, the diameter of the trephine used to cut the donor graft should be larger (from 0.25 mm to as large as 1.0 mm) than the diameter of the trephine used to outline the recipient zone. Depending on the diameter of the lamellarized recipient, 0.25 mm usually is sufficiently large between 7 and 8 mm, 0.5 mm larger between 8 and 9 mm, and 1 mm when the diameter is in excess of 9 mm.

The preferred method for manual dissection of the donor begins by establishing the depth of the dissection, using a Hanna or Krumeich trephine and proceeding with lamellarization as outlined above. Alternatively, a short 5 mm dissection to the desired depth external to the circumference chosen is made with a single-blade guarded diamond knife. Then with a short, sharp corneal splitter, the plane is established (Plate 11–1,B). Then using the longer, inverse-curve corneal splitter, the dissection is carried across the cornea past the intended graft circumference (Plate 11–1,C). A trephine blade of the diameter chosen cuts from the donor lamella from anteriorly to the desired circumference.

The graft is sutured in place with a continuous antitorque suture. A useful technique for accurately placing an eight-bite antitorque suture is to use an eight-incision radial keratotomy marker as a template for the suture pattern (see Plate 7–25). The suture bites are then placed with equal lengths so that the overlying bite intersects the graft margin at each radial mark at an angle of 45 degrees (Plate 11–2,A). A second suture, placed in reverse, should be used in grafts larger than 8 mm in diameter (Plate 11–2,B). Alternatively, double opposing, radially placed, continuous sutures can be used, as in penetrating keratoplasty (see Plate 14–20). The suture loops can be adjusted under the surgical keratometer and, as necessary, adjusted postoperatively during the early weeks after surgery to reduce any suture-induced astigmatism. Because of the support of the posterior lamella, astigmatism is easier to control with suture adjustment following lamellar keratoplasty than it is after penetrating keratoplasty.

In scarred corneas in which the anterior surface is regular and the corneal thickness, determined by ultrasonic pachymetry, is uniform, a microkeratome, when available, produces the most uniform mechanical excision of both the recipient and the donor button. When a corneal cap is necessary to restore regular anterior corneal curvature or the lamellar dissection of the donor cap by one of the mechanical methods cannot be done, the manual technique should be used.

As with penetrating keratoplasty, corneal curvature will not stabilize and residual astigmatism will not become manifest until all sutures are removed. Following lamellar keratoplasty, sutures can usually be removed by 3 months postoperatively. They should be removed sooner if they loosen or if peripheral vascularization is present. Management of residual astigmatic errors after central lamellar keratoplasty is similar to penetrat-

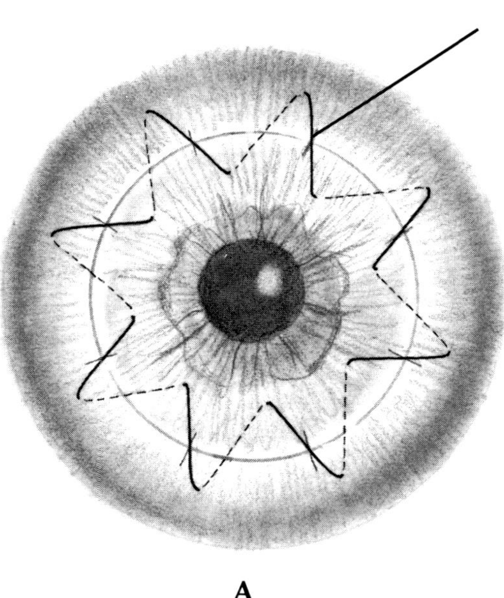

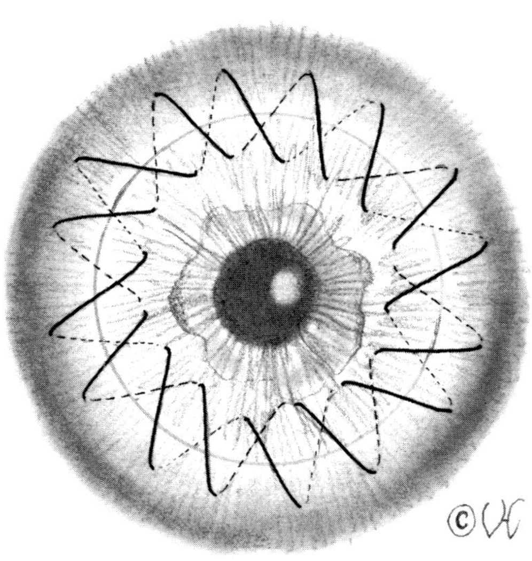

A, single clockwise antitorque suture, overlying suture loops crossing at 8 zone marker points. **B,** second clockwise antitorque suture, used for lamellar grafts larger than 8 mm.

ing keratoplasty (see Chapter 15). The Troutman relaxing incisions or wedge (block) resection can be used as appropriate to correct these errors.

PREVENTION OF ASTIGMATISM FROM PARTIAL OR SEGMENTAL LAMELLAR KERATOPLASTY

By far the largest category of partial or segmental lamellar keratectomy and keratoplasty is performed for pterygium. Other partial lamellar procedures are done for the peripheral dystrophies and for Mooren's ulcer. Lamellar procedures for peripheral penetrating and partial penetrating trauma inducing astigmatism are discussed in Chapter 10.

Pterygium

Exacting surgery of the primary pterygium is the best means to prevent astigmatism from this pathology because it is the recurrent pterygium that is most productive of meridional errors. In pterygium surgery, as in all ophthalmic surgery, the less trauma to the tissues during surgery the better the result and the lower the rate of recurrence. There is a tendency in pterygium surgery to remove the head by a deep dissection from the corneal side, followed by a wide resection of the conjunctiva and the episcleral tissue nasal to it. However, in areas of the United States and in other countries where pterygium is endemic because of local atmospheric and weather conditions, corneal surgeons tend to be minimalists in their pterygium surgery to prevent recurrence. The more radical approach usually achieves success only because the patients are not exposed again to the precipitating causes.

Pterygium is primarily a scleral conjunctival, not a corneal, disease. Initially, the head of the pterygium is only a secondary manifestation of the more peripheral problem. Only later does the cornea become involved. Often the cornea is damaged unnecessarily during attempted removal. As the pterygium progresses from its origins near the inner canthus onto the cornea, Bowman's layer and anterior stroma are minimally involved. As it crosses the limbus, the head of the pterygium loosens in the small area of the cornea at the limbus just distal to the head. This perilimbal cornea area and the normal episclera immediately adjacent to it must be preserved to prevent regrowth. The subconjunctival portion of the pterygium, inflamed tissues, and scar tissue must be excised and allowed to retract from this area. A barrier of normal conjunctiva may need to be interposed to prevent its regrowth while the cornea recovers, and accelerates healing by its protective function.

In later stages, when multiple procedures have failed and Bowman's layer is destroyed central to this zone, it must be replaced and corneal thickness restored by a lamellar graft to prevent regrowth. This will also prevent reestablishment of the strong fibrous band originating from the inner canthus, which often induces 3 to 5 D of *against the rule* astigmatism from flattening across the pterygium meridian.

Dissection of Head of Pterygium

Contrary to the usual practice, removal of a pterygium should begin at its base at the limbus, not at its head on the cornea. The dissection is begun by grasping the conjunctival portion of the pterygium as it crosses the limbus. Using blunt dissection with conjunctival scissors, a tunnel is made under the conjunctiva across the limbus. The head is cut free from the conjunctival portion of the pterygium at the limbus (Plate 11–3,A). The cornea under the proximal end of the head at the limbus will usually be found relatively smooth and free of scar tissue. The pterygium is grasped by its cut end at the corneal scleral limbus and lifted away toward the corneal apex to establish the dissection plane (Plate 11–3,B). In primary cases and most secondary cases, the head can be pulled away from the cornea without the necessity for instrument dissection, leaving Bowman's layer intact or with only a superficially roughened but regular surface where Bowman's layer has been compromised by the head. No attempt should be made to further excise the tissue exposed beneath the head, although it can be smoothed gently with the flat of a number 15 Bard Parker blade. A diamond burr should be used with caution or avoided because it can catch and tear adjacent normal tissue and make a roughened surface out of a relatively smooth one.

Free Conjunctival Flap

The operation proceeds to the superior fornix in which an injection of saline or buffered salt solution is made beneath the conjunctiva, and a small sector of conjunctiva, corresponding roughly to the retracted area of the conjunctival portion of the pterygium, is excised. A template of paper or a plastic drape will aid in accurate matching of the graft to the recipient area, as described by Shaw. To avoid inserting the graft with the epithelial side down, a small dot from a marking pen is made on the face of the graft before dissection. This tissue is placed over the bared sclera and sutured to the cut edge of the conjunctiva, using 10–0 monofilament nylon suture, in a running pattern to oppose the conjunctival edges. It is not sutured to the corneal margin. Absorbable *silk or dacron sutures should never be used because their very presence sometimes causes sufficient irritation to induce early recurrence of a pterygium.* The monofilament thread should be removed as soon as the graft has begun to heal and the sutures have become loosened, about 1 week postoperatively.

If the operation has been done as described, minimal or no astigmatism should be induced. If astigmatism has been induced primarily by the pterygium, it will regress immediately following the surgery. A faint corneal haze over the head area may persist for a few months but it eventu-

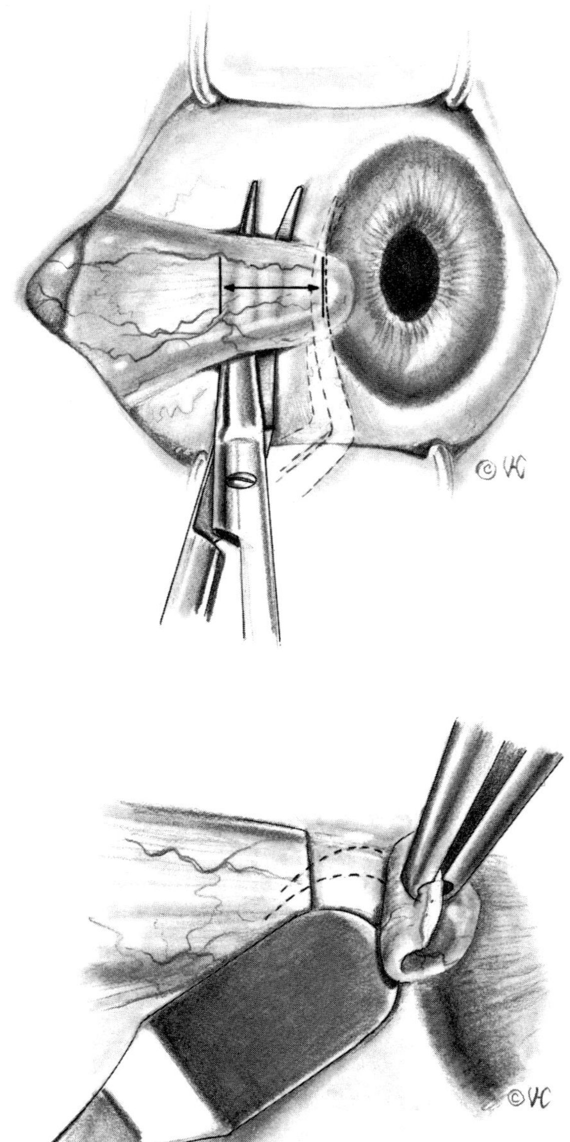

A, subconjunctival dissection and incision of pterygium at limbus. **B,** dissection of pterygium head from its base, avoiding Bowman's layer.

ally clears, and the cornea resumes its normal contour. Smoothing the superficial cornea with the excimer laser after mechanical removal has been performed has recently been advocated. Extreme care should be taken if this is done because Bowman's layer may be unnecessarily removed making recurrence more likely.

CORRECTION OF INDUCED ASTIGMATISM BY LAMELLAR KERATOPLASTY

Lamellar keratoplasty may be used to correct meridional distortions of the central cornea associated with previous lamellar or sector corneal surgery and for disease processes such as the peripheral dystrophies and degenerative diseases, for example, Mooren's ulcer. Because each of these entities is treated somewhat differently, they will be dealt with on an individual and consecutive basis.

ASTIGMATISM RESULTING FROM RECURRENT PTERYGIUM

Infrequently, in about 10% of cases, a pterygium will continue to recur, invading and expanding from the area of the original pathology. An additional attempt at minimal surgery combined with radiation therapy should be contemplated before proceeding with lamellar replacement unless it is certain that Bowman's layer has been destroyed and the corneal stroma has been excessively thinned at the primary procedure. The head of the pterygium should be removed with as little additional dissection as possible and the area carefully inspected. An 8-mm diameter trephine blade (or larger as required) is used to outline the scarred area of the cornea in which Bowman's layer and the stroma are obviously missing or involved. The blade is allowed to penetrate approximately 50% into the corneal thickness (Plate 11–4,A, cross section; Plate 11–4,B, front view). Beginning at the depth of the trephine cut, a lamellar dissection is made toward the limbus up to, but not including, the corneal optical ring (Plate 11–5,A). A vertical incision is made just inside the corneal ring to release the lamellarized scarred tissue (Plate 11–5,B).

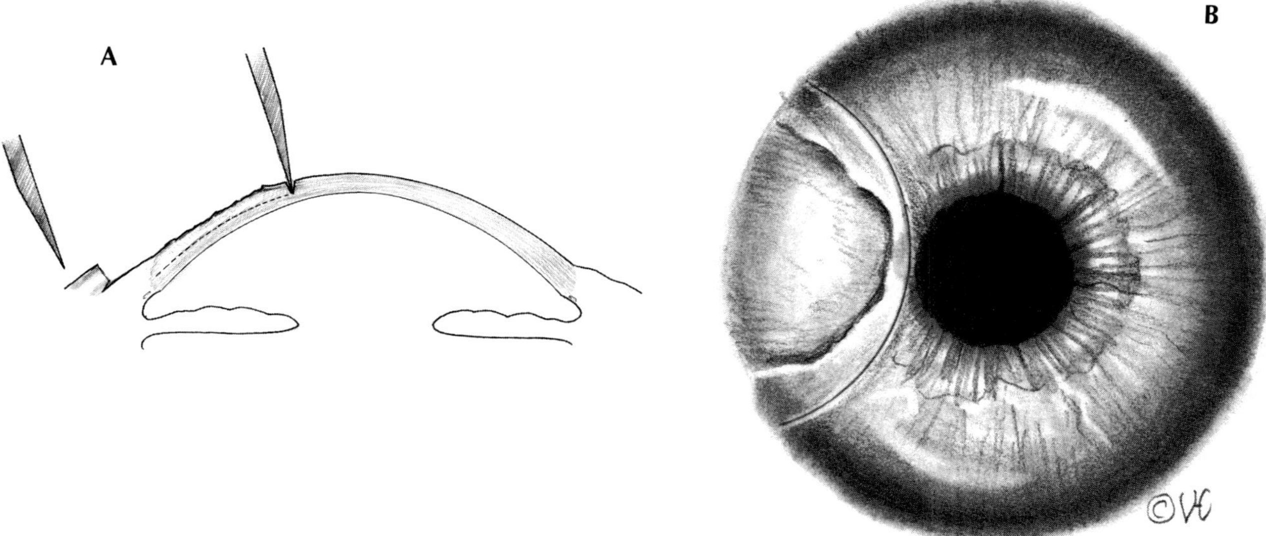

A, partial penetration of recipient cornea for dissection of recurrent pterygium scar, cross section. **B,** anterior view, avoiding pupillary zone.

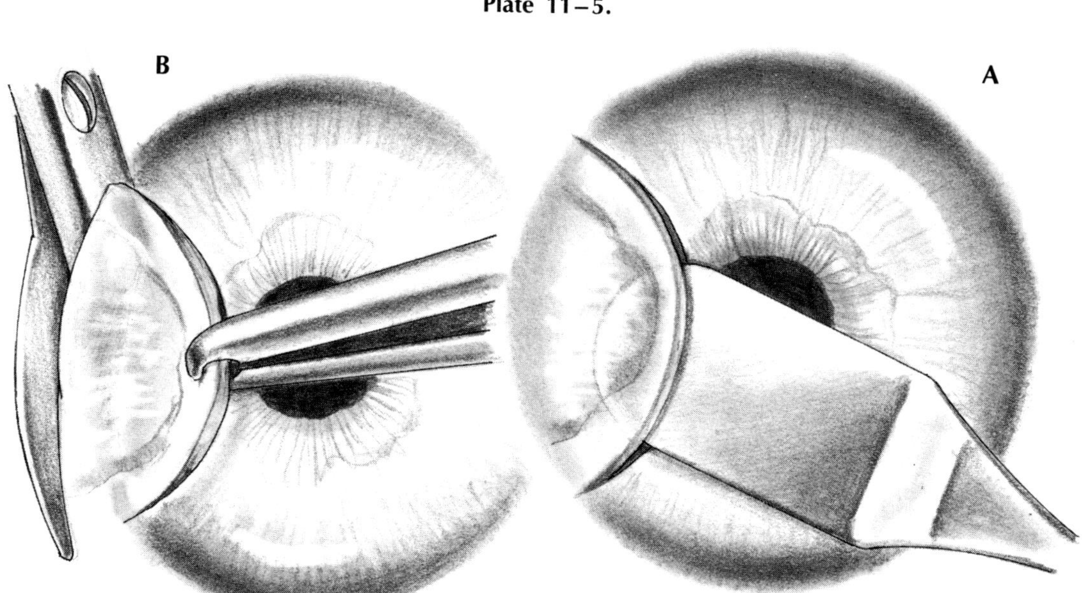

A, dissection of lamellar scar to optical corneal ring. **B,** resection of lamellarized scarred cornea.

Pathophysiology and Prevention of Astigmatism in Lamellar Keratoplasty   **283**

Using a whole eye or a cornea mounted on an artificial anterior chamber, a partial penetrating incision with a trephine is made of the diameter selected for the recipient. If available, a Krumeich or Hanna trephine with its artificial anterior chamber makes the most precise lamellar cut and allows the use of preserved donor cornea. An 8 mm lamellar donor button is dissected at the same depth as from the recipient cornea. An edge of the donor button is sutured to the edge of the recipient cornea lamella at its junction with the limbus, using two interrupted 10–0 monofilament sutures. With the graft thus fixated, corneal scissors are used to trim the excess to the limbal edge of the dissection. A hemicontinuous antitorque suture closes the corneal side of the incision (Plate 11–6,A). Additional interrupted sutures are placed along the limbus. The knots are always buried in the donor tissue. Suture loops should not be placed directly opposite to the visual axis (Plate 11–6,B). Suture loops should be short and at full lamellar thickness in both donor and recipient edges. A conjunctival free graft may be used, as described earlier, to fill in the bared sclera.

Preoperatively, these corneas will often have high astigmatic errors, 3 to 5 D, with flattening in the horizontal meridian. This will partially release immediately and will usually disappear over a period of several months following surgery.

The fixating suture loops should be removed immediately if loosened, and all of them should be removed by 3 months postoperatively. By restoring Bowman's layer and reconstituting the thickness of the cornea, vascularization and recurrence is also almost always prevented.

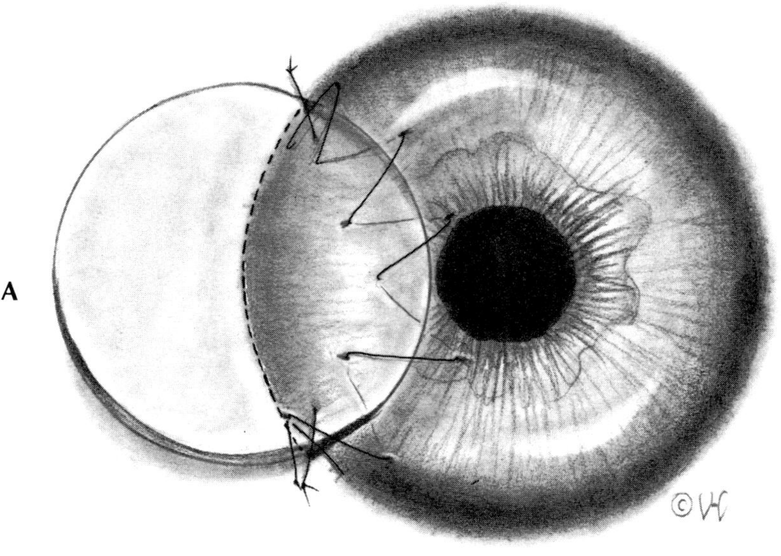

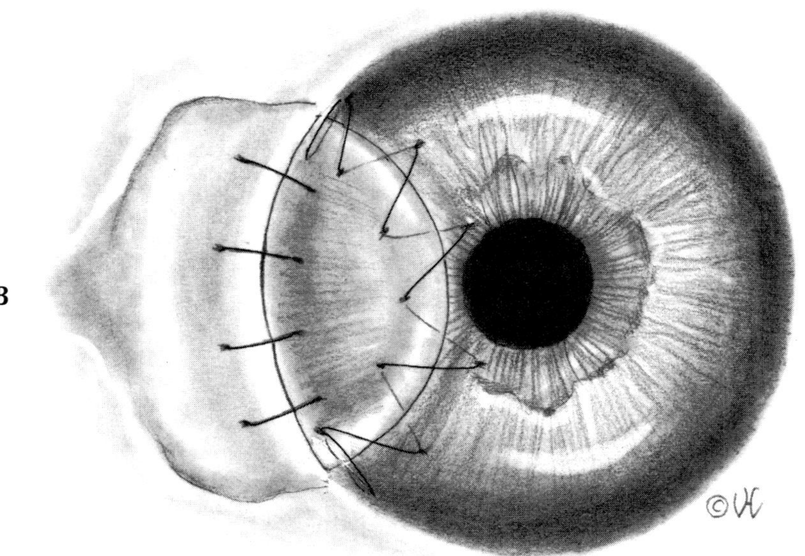

A, leading edge of donor lamella sutured to recipient cornea. Avoid placing suture loop across pupillary zone. **B,** donor cornea trimmed to fit scleral edge of recipient. Interrupted sutures fixating donor cornea to scleral edge of recipient inside optical corneal ring.

LAMELLAR KERATOPLASTY FOR PERIPHERAL CORNEAL DYSTROPHIES

Peripheral corneal dystrophies, especially when in a sector, often induce severe meridional defects and in addition may cause sufficient anterior movement or curvature change of the optical center of the cornea to cause an ametropia. The purpose of the lamellar graft is not primarily to restore central clarity, but rather it is reconstructive to reconstitute the thickness and integrity of the peripheral support zone and relieve the induced distortion of the central optical zone.

Dissection of Recipient Cornea

In this case, the corneal marks delimiting the area to be resected are made with disparate diameter trephines corresponding to the diameters of the inner and outer limits of the peripheral defect, for example, 6-mm central, 10 mm peripheral, leaving a 4 mm intermediate zone to be lamellarized and replaced (Plate 11–7,A). The deepening of the curved superficial incisions to an equal depth along the trephine marks is done with the double-blade diamond knife or with a guarded-blade micrometer diamond knife. With one technique, multiple punctures to the same depth are made with the guarded knife along the trephine marks *(multiple-puncture technique)*. These are then connected, using either the single- or the double-blade knife. In the lamellar dissection of a peripheral dystrophy, one may often encounter descemetoceles between thinned areas of cornea. To avoid perforations, the internal and external cuts should be made in relatively normal-thickness corneal or limbal tissue, dissecting from the edges of the peripheral incisions only as much of the intermediate tissue as possible to avoid perforation or too deep dissection at the level of the corneal optical ring. The conjunctiva should be released from its attachment at the limbus to facilitate dissection and suturing.

Preparation of Donor

When the recipient area has been lamellarized, a lamellarized donor doughnut of the same internal and external dimensions is cut from a whole eye. It is also useful here to make a pattern, using the same trephines to cut a piece of drape material to the same dimensions as the recipient area. The larger trephine is then used to outline the peripheral extent of the donor. A lamellar dissection is begun from the periphery toward the center of the cornea. The second trephine then cuts the internal diameter of the doughnut. The donor doughnut is sutured into the lamellarized zone with interrupted sutures. It is trimmed with a diamond knife to fit the ends of the incomplete annular lamellar dissection. Continuous sutures are used to approximate the longer borders of the incision.

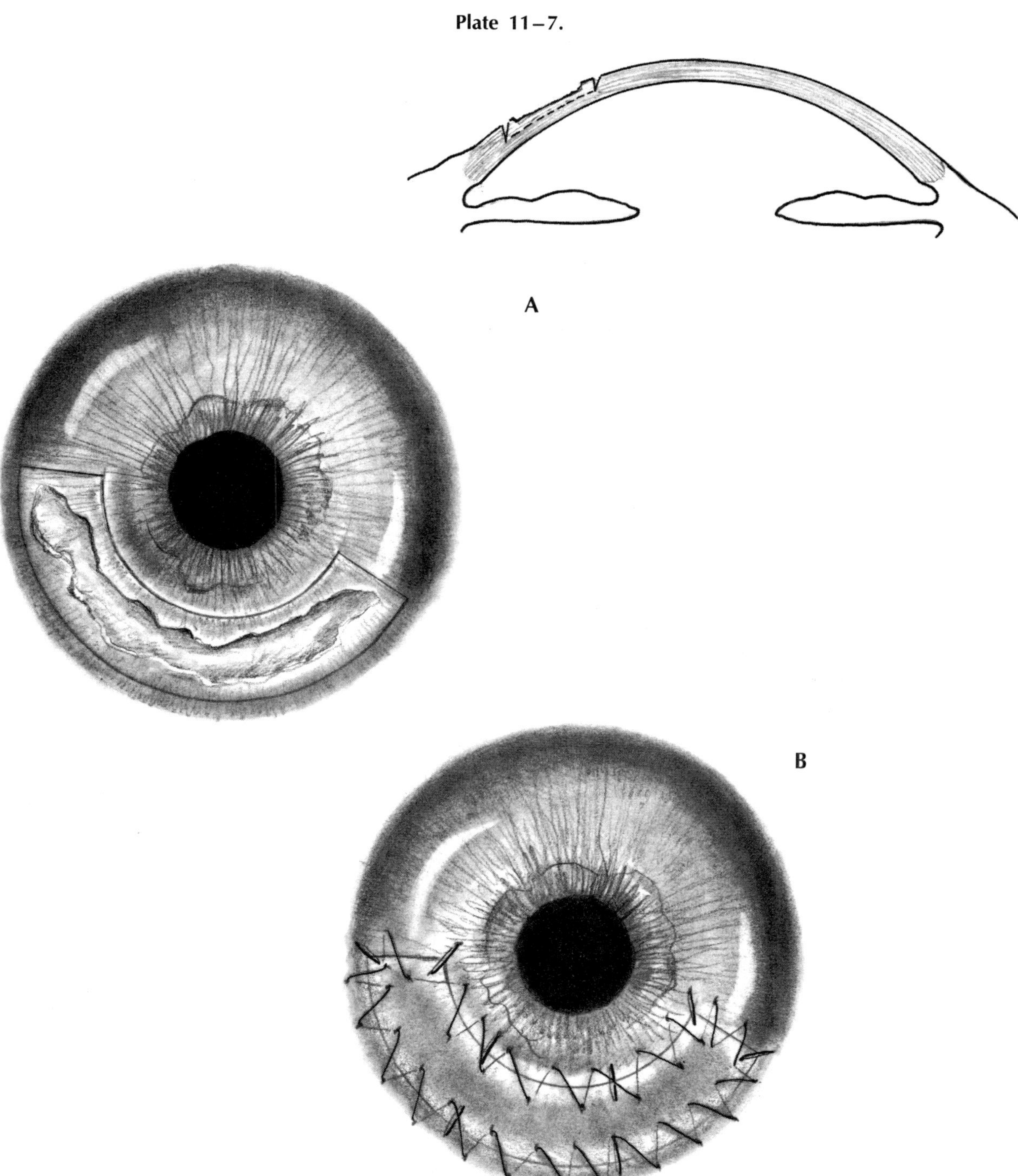

A, outline of dissection of peripheral dystrophy in preparation for lamellar dissection. **B,** donor lamella sutured in peripheral recipient lamellar bed.

Knots should be buried in the recipient rather than the donor lamella (Plate 11–7,B).

The retracted conjunctiva is freed and brought across the peripheral cornea to cover the graft. In severe peripheral degenerative disease, free limbal conjunctival transplants may be done in preparation for the graft to improve epithelialization of the peripheral cornea (Thoft).

The sutures may be removed relatively quickly from the scleral edge as the conjunctival flap retracts. These peripheral reconstructive grafts usually flatten the cornea and significantly reduce astigmatism as well as ametropia. It may be necessary, after the corneal thickness has been reconstituted and all sutures removed, to perform a sector corneal wedge resection in the relatively normal peripheral cornea to reduce a residual error. It is not advisable to use corneal relaxing incisions to correct astigmatism, because of possible poor wound healing from local pathology. In peripheral degenerative pathologies, considerable improvement may occur following conjunctivoplasty alone (Thoft), and lamellar keratoplasty may not be required if the disease is arrested.

MANAGEMENT OF ASTIGMATISM SUBSEQUENT TO LAMELLAR REFRACTIVE AND RECONSTRUCTIVE PROCEDURES

The management of astigmatism resulting from primary lamellar refractive surgery is typically less severe than that seen following penetrating keratoplasty. For the most part, it seems to occur primarily as a result of sector incisional or suture deficiencies and is best approached initially by resuture or suture addition.

In the case of epikeratoplasty, it has been advised to release a sector of the wound from its insertion into the anterior corneal stroma. The host edge of the peripheral corneal incision in the steeper corneal meridian is identified and opened with a Suarez spreader. Using a lateral motion, a sector of the wound is broken open with blunt dissection. A Pierse forceps is used to grasp the edge of the epikeratophakic lenticule, and with firm traction the cap will begin to release its attachment to the cornea. A cyclodialysis spatula can then be used to bluntly dissect a sector of the epikeratophakic lenticule from the host. It has been suggested that this opening be left without sutures for an effect similar to a relaxing incision. However, this may invite epithelial ingrowth, and the lamellar cap should be resutured with a circumferential antitorque suture adjusted under keratometric control.

In general, relaxing incisions are less advisable than resuture or resection procedures when the surgery involves a sector of lamellar tissue. However, to control a residual *with the rule* astigmatism following surgery for pterygium, relaxing incisions should be made in the steeper meridian of the cornea to avoid wound healing problems in the pterygium meridian.

MANAGEMENT OF OVERCORRECTED RADIAL KERATOTOMY

The overcorrected radial keratotomy often involves an excessive number of incisions that are either unhealed or poorly healed, leading to dehiscence and excessive corneal hyperopia. In addition, significant astigmatism often accompanies these conditions due to differential healing of the incisions. The patient is often visually incapacitated due to glare. Even with contact lenses, which are difficult to fit, visual acuity may be inadequate.

One approach to stabilization of the radial keratotomized cornea is lamellar resection of the anterior cornea with the microkeratotome and replacement with a donor cornea cap. It may be possible to include a spherical correction to compensate for the myopia by optical lathing of the replacement cap. However, it can be difficult to determine the power requirement, because the cornea is unstable and only the astigmatism may be compensated. This approach is identical to the management of multiple lacerations in a restricted area (see Chapter 10).

SUMMARY

Lamellar keratoplasty is a powerful but underutilized means to compensate for both meridional and axial corneal ametropias. Barraquer has revived interest in this technique through his development of lamellar refractive surgery for myopia and hyperopia. Indeed, these techniques have created their own problems with regard to astigmatism. Excimer laser photoablation promises renewed interest in lamellar keratoplasty. A combination of the Barraquer techniques for the resection of the corneal cap and precision photoablation may be used to optically modify either donor or recipient cornea, or both, to achieve optical correction. Even in severely scarred corneas, penetrating keratoplasty no longer may be necessary, and astigmatism may be minimized as well.

Some reconstructive lamellar techniques remain for which manual dissection and donor preparation are still preferable. These include most prominently pterygium and peripheral corneal dystrophies.

Pathophysiology and Prevention of Astigmatism Secondary to Cataract Surgery

The paralimbal incision used in cataract surgery is perhaps the most studied incision in all of ophthalmology, both because of its prevalence and because of its potential to cause both temporary and permanent central astigmatism. The limbus forms a natural anatomic landmark for this type of incision, and the effect of paralimbal incisions cannot be approached without consideration of the anatomy and biomechanical implications of the surgical limbus. Other considerations that must enter into any discussion of paralimbal incisions are the method of extraction of the natural lens and the artificial intraocular lens that replaces it. The incision must therefore be utilitarian in the sense that the size and configuration of the incision facilitate the operation and provide optimal characteristics for healing after the incison is closed. To achieve good wound closure, the surgeon must think not only of the incision after the cataract is removed and the intraocular lens is in place but also of the intraoperative implications leading to appropriate closure, including the initial preparation of the operative wound.

BIOMECHANICS OF THE LIMBUS

The limbus represents a two-dimensional stiffened structure resting on a three-dimensional spherical shell (Plate 12–1,A). Stiffening of this structure is accomplished by a variety of means. First, the material content of limbal tissue is significantly different than that of the cornea or the sclera. Water content is decreased, and internal collagen structure is correspondingly increased. On light microscopy, the artifactual lacunae seen in the

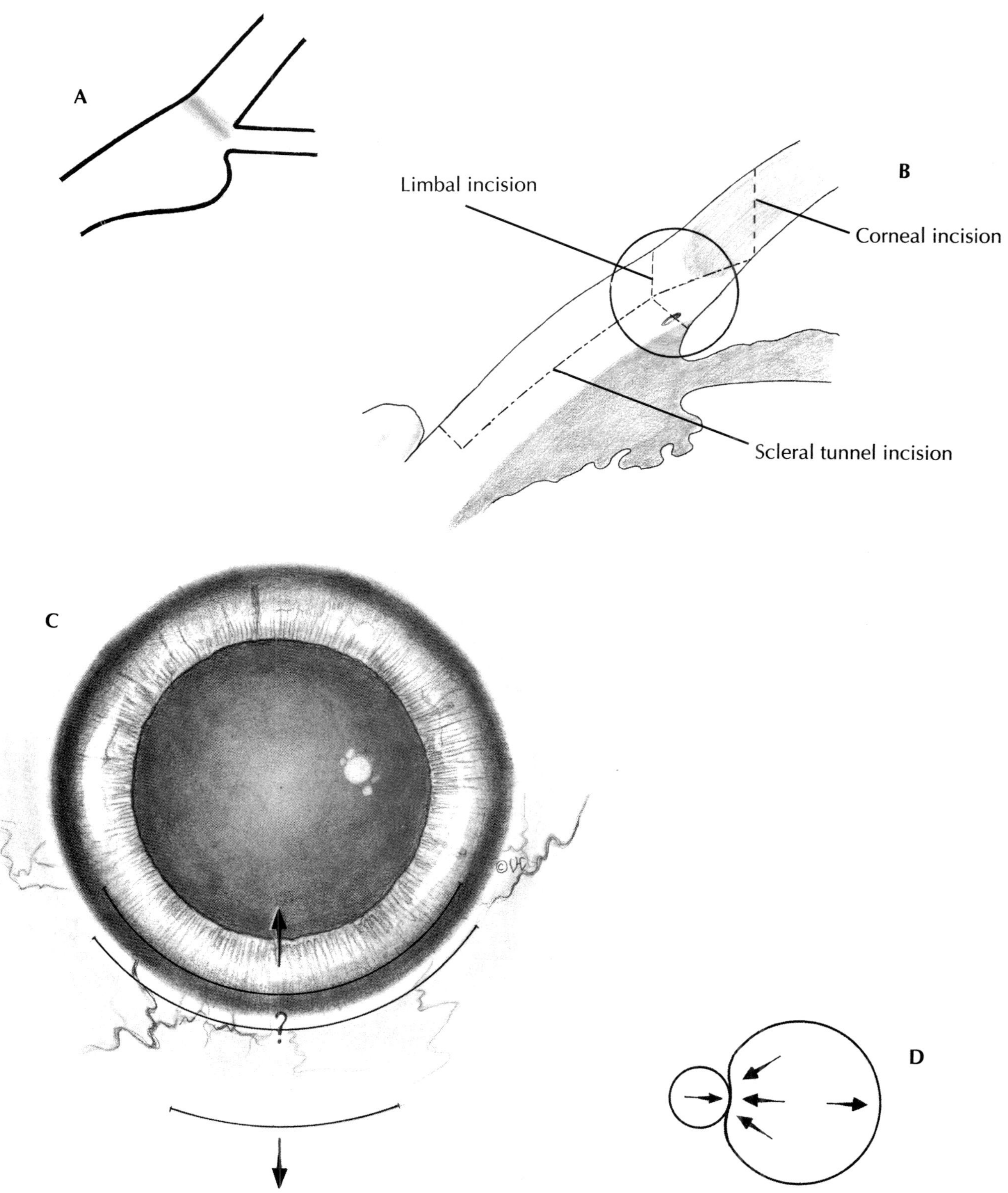

A, stiffened limbal structure. **B,** locations of scleral tunnel, limbal, and corneal incisions for cataract surgery. **C,** direction of effect of limbal incisions. **D,** sphere resisting indentation.

cornea when the tissue is processed, representing potential spaces filled with fluid, are absent in the limbal tissue due to the dense nature of this tissue. This compaction, coupled with the structured orientation of collagen fibrils, adds considerable strength to this ringlike structure. In addition, the scleral spur adds still more bulk and strength. Incisions directly into this structure can have a lasting detrimental effect to the stability of the surrounding tissue, because wound healing will weaken the structure and disrupt the orderly composition of collagen fibrils in this area. In addition, the scleral spur may actually be eliminated by the incision and the ensuing healing, resulting in thinning and weakening of the corneal optical ring (Plate 12–1,B). Additional stiffening is achieved by the uveal tissue adherent to the limbal and scleral support in this area. Although uveal tissue does not have great innate resistance to deformation, orientation of this tissue in the human eye produces a structure that is analogous to the I beam used in the construction of many buildings. The stiffening prevents mechanical weakening outside the corneal optical ring from affecting the cornea within the ring by virtue of the mechanical stiffening achieved by this combination with relatively weaker materials. Inversely, incisions anterior to the corneal optical ring affect the cornea and not the area outside the ring. As stated, incisions through the limbus destroy the structure of the limbus and result in unpredictable astigmatic effects (Plate 12–1,C).

One final principle that must be discussed is the concept of *least energy*. A law of thermodynamics states that nature seeks the lowest possible energy for a given situation, thus a ball at the top of a hill will naturally go down the hill to reduce the total energy of the ball and, similarly, mountains will eventually be reduced by erosion to the lowest possible level. Any deformation of a sphere produces a changed local radius of curvature, which then experiences a higher internal force to restore it to a sphere (Plate 12–1,D). Tight sutures can distort the spherical nature of the eye, flattening the area under the suture. Localized high forces will then come into play in the area of distortion to force the eye back into a spherical state. Similarly, localized distortions of the circular corneal optical ring by sutures will be resisted by the eye, and an attempt will be made to restore the corneal optical ring to a more even contour. If more inelastic sutures such as dacron are used, the result will be a tearing of the tissue with inappropriately tight sutures. Although a complete discussion of these matters is beyond the scope of this text, it is clear that sutures placed overly tight to the point that the normal anatomy of the limbus and globe are distorted will certainly be resisted by the thermodynamic law of least energy.

CAUTERY

Cautery has been used in different forms since the inception of cataract surgery. The most common modern device is a bipolar cautery that achieves the same effect as the original heated glass rod, which is to develop thermal energy in the area of bleeding and thus close capillaries, arterioles, and venules. Although the immediate effect aides the process of surgery, making visualization more convenient and the postoperative appearance more acceptable, the long-term effects of cautery can lead to unacceptable levels of postoperative astigmatism. If we examine the effects of cautery closely, we can identify unwanted side effects related to astigmatic problems. The first problem relates to the application of thermal energy on collagen. As we know, heat tends to contract and cross link collagen in the eye, leading to uneven shrinkage of the wound and difficulties with even closure if both sides of the wound do not shrink in an identical fashion. If this situation is taken to the extreme, we may even see leakage along an incision that has tight suturing. If the cautery is lightly applied, the shrinkage will be superficial and the effect on the bulk of the sclera will be minimal. If the cautery is excessive, the collagen shrinkage will extend into the depths of the sclera, resulting in unpredictable long-term shrinkage of the involved collagen. As we have seen in thermal alterations of the cornea, such shrinkage will probably reverse in time, but the possibility of gradual continuing changes in the astigmatic portion of the refraction over a period of several years is quite possible (Miyajima, unpublished data).

The second significant side effect of cautery has to do with its role in closing both capillaries and larger vessels. If excessive cautery is applied, the small capillaries, which are essential mediators in the wound healing process, will be damaged and, although they will eventually regenerate, the process of wound healing will be significantly slowed. In patients with vascular abnormalities, such as rheumatoid arthritis or diabetes, cautery may actually induce melting of the scleral tissue in the wound, resulting in a wound dehiscence. Even if such a drastic outcome is avoided, excessive cautery can delay wound healing and soften surrounding tissues to such an extent that the sutures are loosened and clinical wound dehiscence occurs.

The necessity for cautery has often been called into question because in many circumstances, appropriate dissection along tissue planes, coupled with pressure and patience, will often resolve minor bleeding problems. Precise application of cautery only to affected areas with instruments that are properly cleaned of dried blood and tissue remains can significantly lessen the amount of cautery necessary. When a scleral flap is prepared, light cautery over the surface may be necessary, but after the flap is opened, the surgeon should avoid cautery to the flap or to the interior wound because this will inevitably cause differential shrinkage, resulting in poor wound closure. The possibility of melting will increase if the flap is cauterized because the energy cannot be dissipated into the bulk of the stroma and the flap may melt in the postoperative period.

INCISION LOCATION

The location of a cataract incision can most easily be divided into three positions: corneal, limbal, and scleral. In terms of the utility of the incision, the corneal position has certain definite advantages. First, because it is removed from the iris root, iris prolapse tends to be less of a problem than with other incision locations. Second, bleeding is not a problem, and cautery can be entirely avoided. This can be a particular advantage if there is preexisting disease along the limbal border (e.g., severe scarring from herpes or other trauma, a preexisting filtering bleb that one might not wish to disturb, or cicatricial ocular pemphigoid that if disturbed might trigger an attack of the disease process). In patients with glaucoma, a triple procedure with a filter operation can be performed in which the mechanical constraints of the cataract of wound closure can be separated from the fistular aperture of a filtering procedure. Finally, extraction of the nucleus in extracapsular cataract surgery and subsequent aspiration of cortex remnants can be accomplished in a particularly convenient manner due to the relative angle of approach to the cataract. In particular, aspiration of superior cortex remnants can be approached from a reverse angle, thus facilitating this difficult maneuver.

Suturing of corneal incisions within the limbal *guy wire* of the corneal optical ring can induce significant astigmatism while the sutures are in place (Plate 12–2,A). This effect is reversed when the sutures are removed. Running sutures are removed in 3 months, and the two interrupted stay sutures are removed when healing is complete, as indicated by keratometry readings. Although the potential for astigmatism is high with this approach due to the location of the incision within the limbal guy wire, proper healing results in minimal astigmatism due to the precise through-and-through apposition of wound edges possible with corneal tissue (Plate 12–2,B). The temporary astigmatism during the *sutures in* phase of the corneal incision can be countered effectively with compensating compression sutures placed approximately at the 4- and 8-o'clock positions.

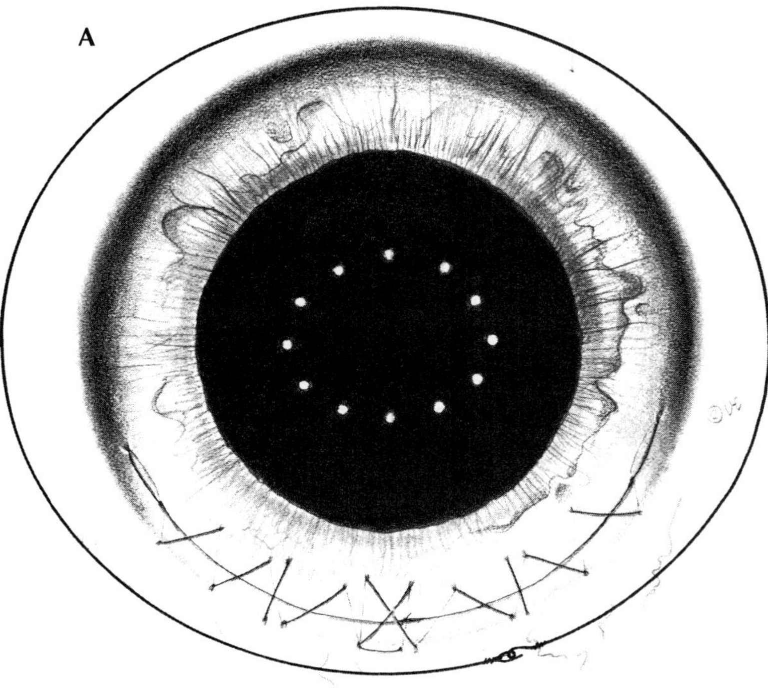

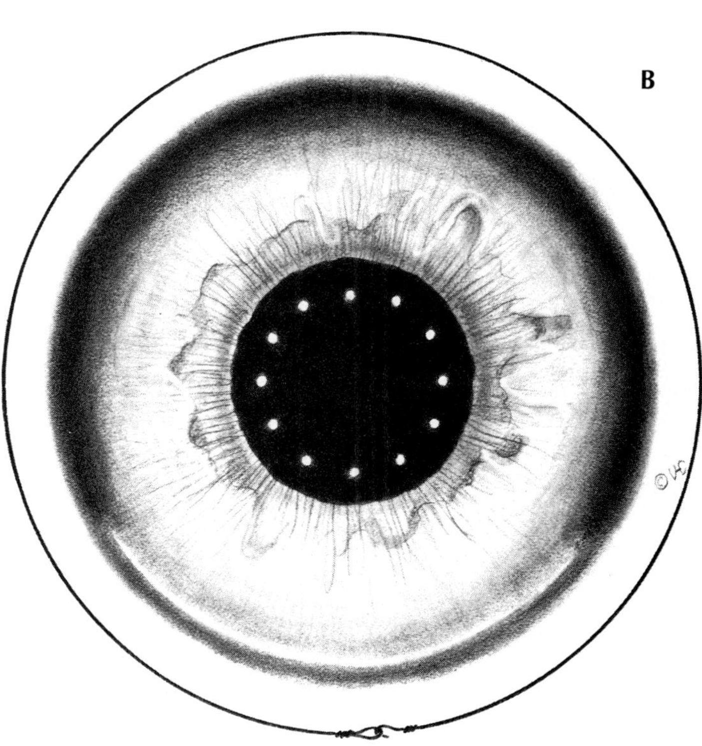

A, sutured corneal cataract incision with significant *with the rule* astigmatism; inside intact optical corneal ring. **B,** healed corneal cataract incision without astigmatism.

Pathophysiology and Prevention of Astigmatism Secondary to Cataract Surgery   **295**

A scleral incision, outside the limbal *guy wire,* must be associated with a scleral tunnel, because direct posterior dissection beneath a scleral incision will collide with the ciliary body (Plate 12–3,A). The internal exit of the scleral incision should be identical to the corneal incision because exit at the iris base will promote iris prolapse during cataract surgery. Thus the benefits of a corneal incision, from the standpoint of anterior entry with diminished iris prolapse, can be obtained while avoiding an external incision through Bowman's layer and the cornea. Avoidance of corneal incisions by this approach also reduces the potential for delayed astigmatic errors entering outside of the limbal *guy wire.* Surgical exposure is quite different, and although it is possible to perform extracapsular cataract surgery through a posterior scleral incision, it is somewhat simpler to perform phacoemulsification from this location, thus influencing the choice of technique for cataract removal.

Significant benefits are derived from entering the anterior chamber anterior to the iris root. Both the corneal and the scleral tunnel incisions share this desirable characteristic. The corneal incision lies internal to the limbal *guy wire* and will by its nature affect late corneal astigmatism less, whereas the scleral incision lies posterior to the limbal *guy wire* and by its nature will affect early corneal astigmatism less significantly (Plate 12–3,A) when healed operatively (Plate 12–3,B). The relative instability of the corneal incision can be offset by good surgical technique and, in some cases, may be used to advantage, when placed in the proper meridian, to achieve correction of preexisting corneal astigmatism. The final incision that we will discuss is the limbal incision used for cataract surgery, which we feel offers the most liabilities of any of the options mentioned here.

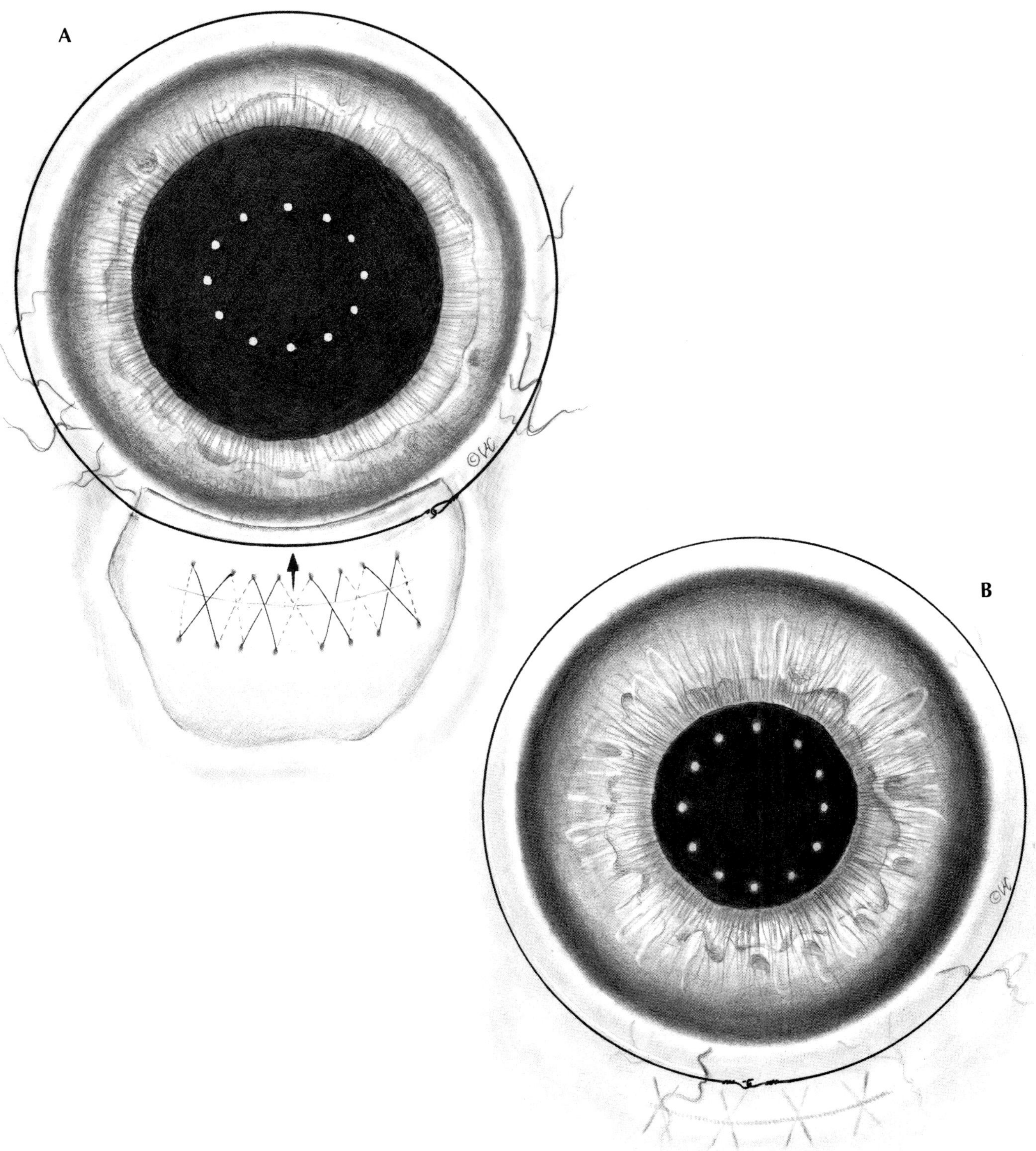

A, sutured scleral cataract incision with slight *with the rule* astigmatism; intact optical corneal ring.
B, healed scleral cataract incision with minimal *against the rule* astigmatism.

Pathophysiology and Prevention of Astigmatism Secondary to Cataract Surgery   **297**

As we have previously discussed, the limbus is a complex biomechanical structure that is responsible for maintaining dimensional stability of the cornea. Any damage to this limbal structure will affect the stability of the cornea and in turn central corneal astigmatism, often in an unpredictable and progressive manner. In addition, the change in curvature from the cornea to the sclera in the limbal area presents difficulties in terms of appropriate suture closure that we will discuss later. Historically, the limbal incision for cataract surgery was the most common method used to open the eye. Initially the incision was created with a Graefe knife, which created a beveled incision that tended to be somewhat corneal in its posterior penetration. As instruments improved, the tendency was to make the incision more vertical, entering just anterior to the iris root, which encouraged iris prolapse during the operation and often led to problems with wound stability in the postoperative period. To assure a more anterior corneal entrance internally, the *two-step* limbal corneal incision was introduced, which involved a partial penetrating vertical incision at the limbus, followed by the use of scissors to create a so-called *valved* incision, which was supposed to be self-sealing. Anatomical work by Straatsma and Foos demonstrated the fallibility of this theory in that internal closure of the limbal-based wound was often incomplete. The limbal-based cataract incision creates a wound that has theoretical deficiencies in terms of both damage to the corneal optical ring and problems with appropriate closure. Combined with clinically apparent problems at the time of surgery (Plate 12–4,A), this also affects long-term wound healing (Plate 12–4,B). This has been expressed in studies by a number of authors, including Stark, who observed astigmatic instability of the postoperative extracapsular cataract-extraction patient for more than a year after surgery. It is our belief that the limbal cataract incision should be rejected in favor of either corneal or scleral approaches for the reasons we have presented here.

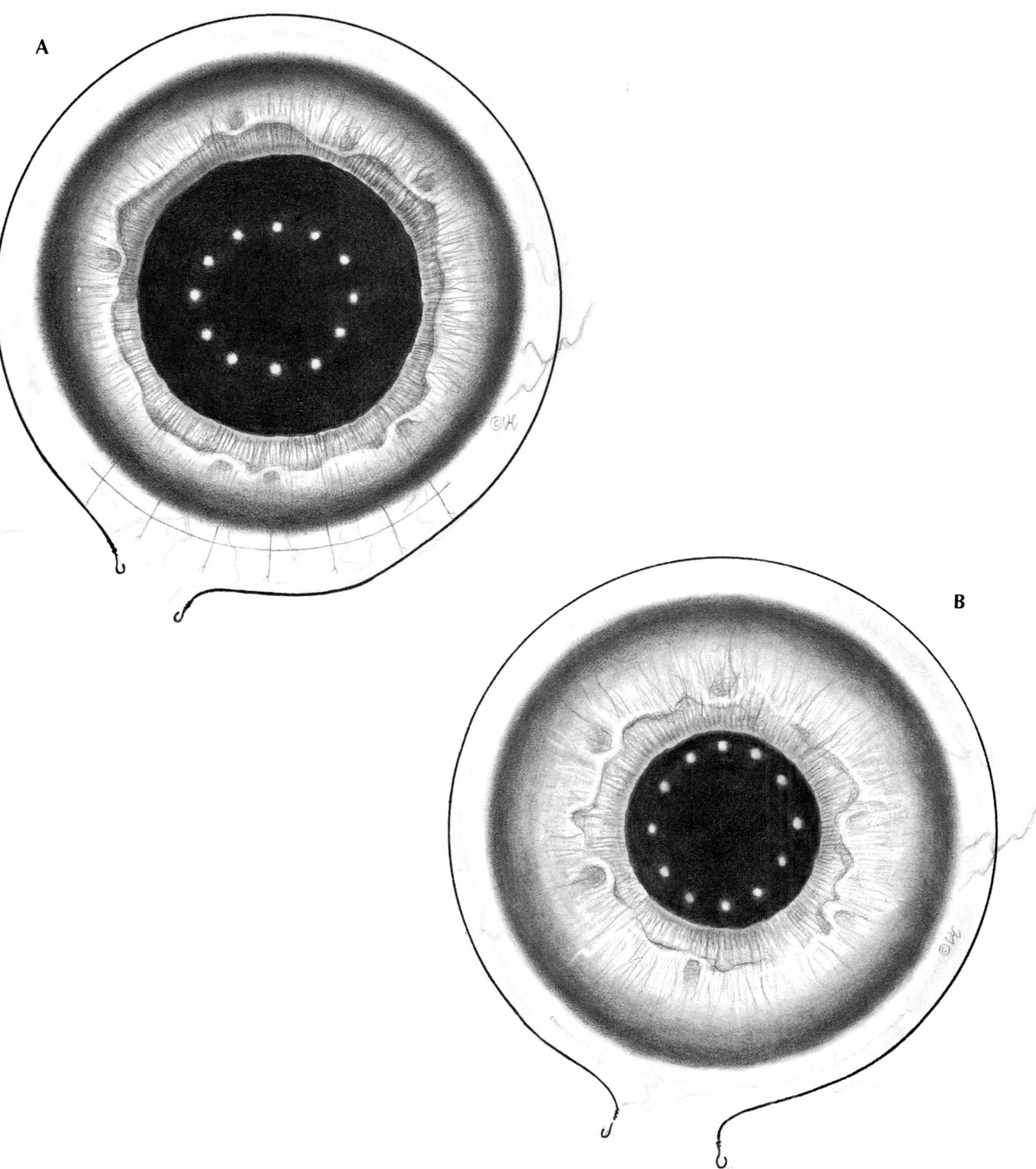

A, sutured limbal cataract incision with broken corneal optical ring. **B,** healed limbal cataract incision with continuing change in astigmatism.

Pathophysiology and Prevention of Astigmatism Secondary to Cataract Surgery   **299**

SCLERAL TUNNEL INCISION

The purpose of the scleral tunnel incision is to incise the exterior portion of the globe outside the corneal optical ring and the internal portion within the ring from within the cornea. The farther one begins the incision external to the limbus the less effect, theoretically, it will have on corneal astigmatism. Practically, however, it is more difficult to operate through a tunnel incision longer than 2 to 3 mm. Creation of the proper scleral tunnel incision depth is important. If the flap is too thin it may tear during surgery, requiring repair and possibly damaging to the integrity of the scleral portion of the globe. If the anterior flap is too thick, one may penetrate the vascular structures lying beneath this portion of the sclera.

The creation of a scleral tunnel incision begins with the peritomy. Light cautery is applied over the area of the proposed flap to prevent bleeding from deep vessels that may be encountered during splitting of the scleral bed. The second step involves marking the appropriate width of the incision with calipers, 10 mm for extracapsular cataract surgery and 6 mm or less for phacoemulsification. A rounded blade, such as a Beaver 69 or a Grieshaber, is used to create a shallow vertical scleral delimiting incision 2 mm behind the corneal optical ring for phacoemulsification and 1 mm behind the ring for extracapsular cataract surgery (Plate 12–5,A). A guarded diamond blade is better for this purpose. The scleral flap can be created without a delimiting incision; however, achieving appropriate depth often is difficult. The risk of penetration of the eye is higher because of difficulty in finding the appropriate surgical plane. When sewing the thin flap back in position, the margins may become friable and tissue may be lost.

The final step in creating the scleral flap involves dissection forward through the corneal optical ring into the cornea. This is accomplished by using blunt dissection rather than by using the knife in a cutting mode. Entering along the delimiting incision, the rounded blade is introduced at a 45-degree angle to start the dissection plane. The edge is then grasped with a toothed forceps and lifted slightly as downward pressure is exerted on the blade, now oriented parallel to the scleral plane (Plate 12–5,B). The combined upward and downward pressure tends to split the tissue along a plane, only gentle sweeping motions of the blade being required to advance the dissection. Dissection is continued until the rounded tip of the blade can be clearly seen in the cornea (Plate 12–5,C). At this point, a super-sharp blade can be used to enter the anterior chamber at the most anterior portion of the dissection into the cornea approximately 1 or 2 mm internal to the corneal optical ring. If phacoemulsification is planned, a calibrated 3 mm triangular knife may be used to enter the chamber to create an appropriate internal incision for phacoemulsion and for a water-

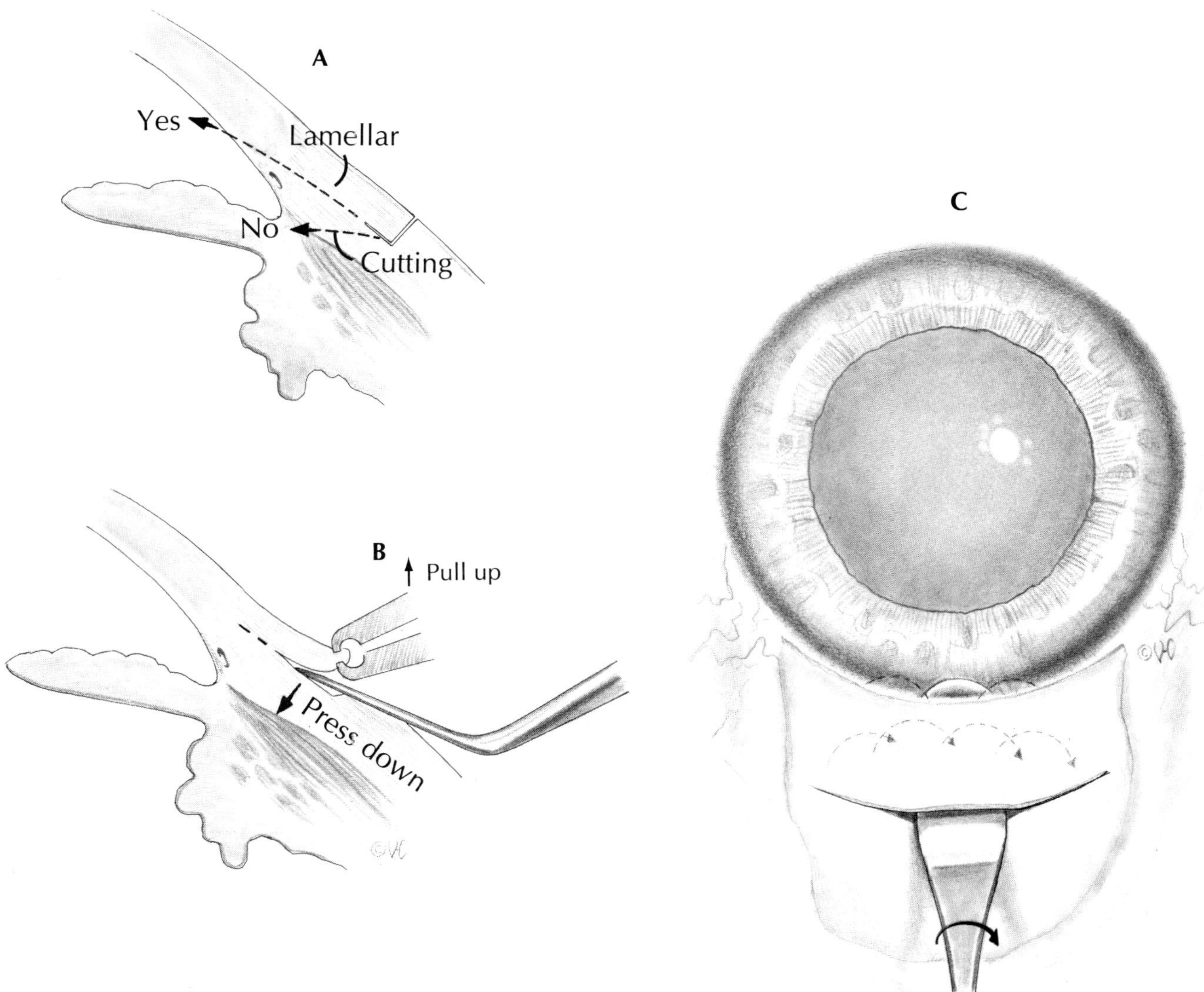

A, preparation for scleral tunnel with 50% incision in sclera. **B,** dissection technique using traction and blunt dissection. **C,** proper end point of scleral tunnel dissection showing tip of blade at limbus through cornea.

tight seal. The incision then can be opened with a super-sharp blade for insertion of the intraocular lens.

When extracapsular cataract surgery is planned, the scleral incision will be delimited at 10 mm. A variety of flap configurations may be used. One approach is to create a so-called miniflap, which is made approximately 1 mm behind the surgical limbus. This has the advantage of ease of manipulation of the nucleus during extracapsular cataract surgery but suffers, although to a lesser degree, from many of the problems of limbal incision due to its proximity to the corneal optical ring. Another approach is to create a 6-mm scleral tunnel approximately 2 to 3 mm behind the surgical limbus and then to create extensions to either side, for a full 10-mm incision with a peripheral flaps of approximately 1 mm. The 2 to 3 mm × 6 mm central flap gives good astigmatic control. Creation of the flap is simplified and exposure is improved by the short lateral extensions. A less desirable method of enlarging the incision involves making a standard 6-mm scleral flap and extending the sides with scissors or a super-sharp blade, thus creating a beveled edge on the lateral 2 mm of the wound on each side of the central 6-mm flap. This incision is often used when converting from phacoemulsification to extracapsular cataract surgery. Essentially, it has the same properties as the incision described previously, with the exception of the beveled margins along the lateral aspects of the wound. Care should be taken to place the sutures deeply, because it is easy to *cheese wire* through the narrow flap.

An unproved dictum of contemporary cataract surgery is that the wound should be as small as physically possible, primarily to prevent postoperative astigmatism and to speed wound healing. Stark has demonstrated that even well-sutured extracapsular cataract wounds demonstrate gradual changes in central corneal astigmatism over a period of 1 year. It follows that the potential for wound-healing abnormalities remains high for the 10-mm wound required for extracapsular cataract extraction performed at the limbus. The introduction of phacoemulsification makes it possible to significantly reduce incision size, limited only by the size of the phacoemulsification apparatus, which is approximately 3 mm (Plate 12–6). In fact, by separating the infusion and phacoemulsification tips, the size of the required incisions can be reduced to two 1-mm incisions, as shown by Shearing. After the decision to perform phacoemulsification has been made, the real limitation of smaller incisions is dependent on the choice of the intraocular lens, which will be discussed later.

Both Masket and Buzard and Shearing (1988) have shown, after approximately 6 weeks, stabilization of the standard 6 mm phacoemulsification wound closed with radial or semiradial running sutures. With proper suturing technique, induced astigmatism averages approximately 0.5 D and is not significantly different from preoperative astigmatism. The 3-mm scleral incision has been shown, both theoretically and clinically, to be stable without sutures, and this represents a practical minimum-incision length for which to aim. The 1-mm scleral tunnel incisions reported by Shearing were not sutured and encountered no significant postoperative astigmatism after approximately 1 week. Both Shepherd (1989) and Buzard and Shearing (unpublished data, 1988) have shown that 4-mm in-

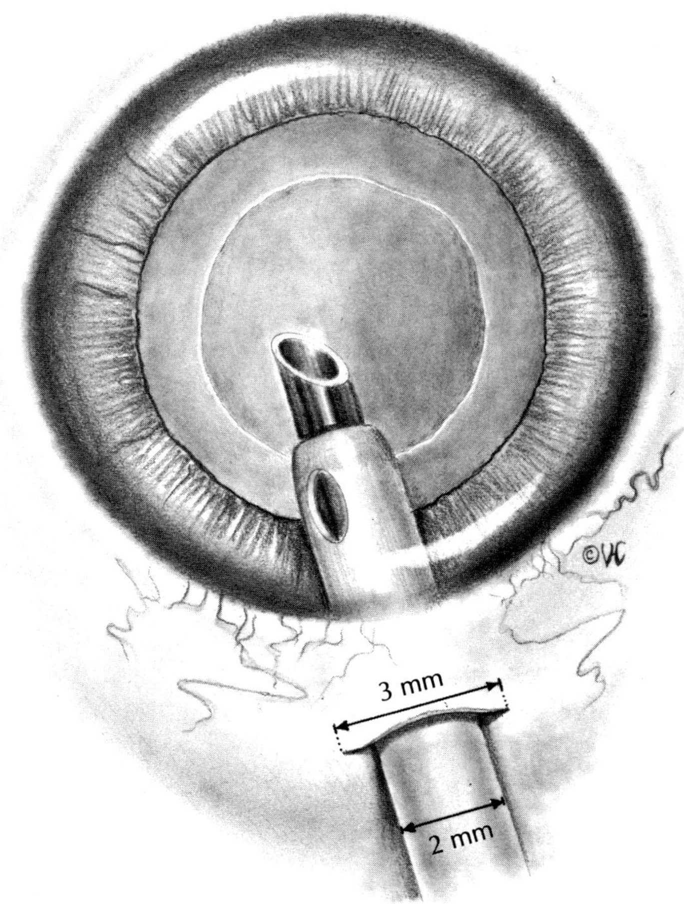

Three-millimeter incision produced by standard phacoemulsification cf cataract.

cisions closed with interrupted radial and/or cross sutures stabilize in terms of astigmatism in a period of approximately 3 to 4 weeks with little change from preoperative astigmatic values.

A significant development that parallels the continuing reduction in incision length has been the introduction by Shepherd of horizontal suturing techniques resulting in the single horizontal closure and the infinity closure, including several variants. With horizontal suturing, astigmatic stabilization, even in 6.5-mm wounds, has been reported (Buzard and Shearing) in as little as 1 week with no induced astigmatism. We discuss this development in more depth in a later section, but at this point, we make the significant observation that reduction of incision size below 6 mm may be less important than the contribution of suture technique.

The intraocular lens is the major determinant of the length of the cataract incision, because no available intraocular lens can be placed through an incision of less than 3 mm. At this time, the standard intraocular-lens optic diameter and incision size is 6 mm, although both larger and smaller optics are available (Plate 12–7,A). Considerable effort has been expended in reducing the size of the required incision needed to insert the intraocular lens, because the 3-mm incision of phacoemulsification is enlarged only to accommodate the intraocular lens. The Starr Surgical Silicone Intraocular Lens was the first widely available lens to be folded and inserted through a small incision. The original lens design did not incorporate the compressible loops introduced by Shearing, and the lens suffered from torsion and expulsion from the location in which it was placed ("Z" syndrome). This experience demonstrated the importance of proper lens design along the lines of the original Shearing-style lens, and subsequent foldable intraocular lenses have adhered to this principle. In addition, the lens really did not fit through a 3 mm incision. Both the AMO silicone lens and the improvements of the Starr Surgical lens have compressible haptics but still require a 3.5 mm incision (Plate 12–7,B). The development of acrylic lenses by Alcon has made the introduction through a nearly 3 mm incision possible, and acrylic compounds may well be the proper choice of material for this type of lens. Even these lenses have problems, including the sticky nature of the lens, which if touched to the endothelium can cause endothelial cell loss.

Ultimately, the surgeon should be aware that the use of foldable lenses may require accepting a slightly higher incidence of complications and possible loss of best-corrected visual acuity due to the very fact that the lens is flexible and may be subject to forces within the eye, even within a secure capsulorrhexis "in the bag placement," causing irregular astigmatic refraction in the lens itself.

Recently, the concept of oval optical zones for the intraocular lens has been explored with a series of 5 × 6 oval PMMA intraocular lenses with compressible loops. A lens such as this can be inserted through a 5-mm incision, and by using a simple technique of creating a radial incision in the central base of the phacoemulsification tunnel, the incision can be further reduced to 4.5 mm (Plate 12–7,C,D). The lens provides stable optics, and the manufacturing costs are comparable to a standard intraocular lens. This oval lens is essentially a 6 mm round optic intraocular lens trimmed to an oval shape. Thus the thickness of the lens is such that this becomes a factor in the introduction of the lens through a scleral tunnel incision. In addition, decentration may be a problem. A thinner 5-mm optic intraocular lens has also been developed, which solves this problem and gives comparable results. Because flexible intraocular lenses are fre-

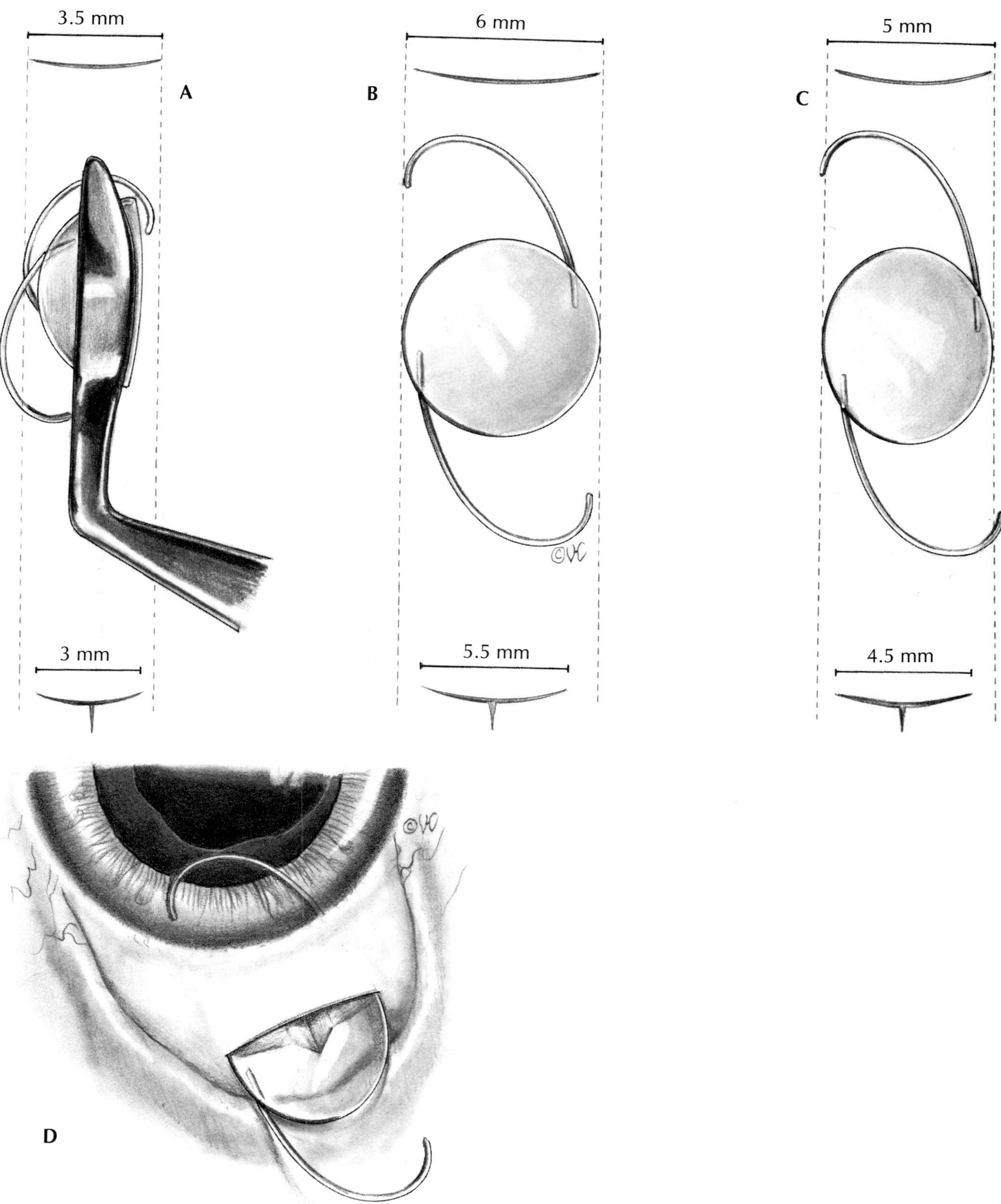

A, incision size required for foldable silicone lens with reduction in incision size using *T* incision. **B,** incision size required for oval 5 × 6 mm optic with reduction in incision size using *T* incision. **C,** incision size required for standard 6-mm round optic with reduction in incision size using *T* incision. **D,** insertion of oval 5 × 6 mm optic using 4.5-mm incision with *T* incision showing spreading of posterior incision.

quently inserted through a 3.5 to 4 mm incision, these lenses can give incision reduction comparable to that with a flexible intraocular lens without compromising lens stability or best-corrected visual acuity. In a small series, Buzard and Shearing demonstrated stabilization of central astigmatism in 1 to 2 weeks with incision lengths of 5, 6, and 6.5 mm. This indicates that the choice of PMMA optics may have identical results in terms of astigmatism as the insertion of a flexible intraocular lens, without the difficulties of insertion, the increased cost, and the concerns over long-term best-corrected visual acuity due to optic stability.

SUTURE TECHNIQUES

The most meticulous incision, when closed with inappropriate suture technique, can lead to an unsatisfactory result. Conversely, a poorly made incision may resist even the most elegant suture closure and result in wound instability. Suture patterns can be grossly divided into interrupted, continuous, radial, and horizontal. For any suture pattern, the course of the suture over and through the cornea/sclera must be appropriate to the forces exerted on the suture strand or tissue buckling will occur, with subsequent wound dehiscence in the adjacent area.

The third dimension of the cornea, which is often overlooked, is the depth of suture placement, perhaps one of the most important considerations in the placement of the suture. For corneal sutures, we believe that the suture should penetrate the cornea and exit from the anterior chamber, a so-called through-and-through suture closure (Plate 12–8,A). The concern of creating a track through which infections or aqueous humor may travel is unfounded because with appropriate tension, the elastic nylon monofilament suture easily buries itself in both the anterior and posterior cornea in a few days. Corneal suture placement should be equally balanced across the wound, and the tracks should be as vertical as possible with short bites. The sutures should be tied tightly to provide good healing, and this will inevitably cause steepening anterior to the suture placement because the suture lies within the limbal *guy wire*. The amount of steepening can be minimized somewhat by keeping the suture bite as short and deep as possible, thus preventing excessive *bunching* of the tissue beneath the suture and excessive steepening anterior to the suture.

Errors in centration of the bite relative to the wound can lead to differential compression of the wound, with the possibility of subsequent poor wound healing on the basis of override of tissue or *cheese wiring* of the suture through an inadequate bite through the tissue (Plate 12–8,B). Failure to make a full-thickness bite will result in a so-called posterior lambda effect (Plate 12–8,C). When this occurs, the posterior lamellae of the cornea fail to meet, and because wound healing has been demonstrated to be slower in the posterior cornea, this can result in a posterior wound dehis-

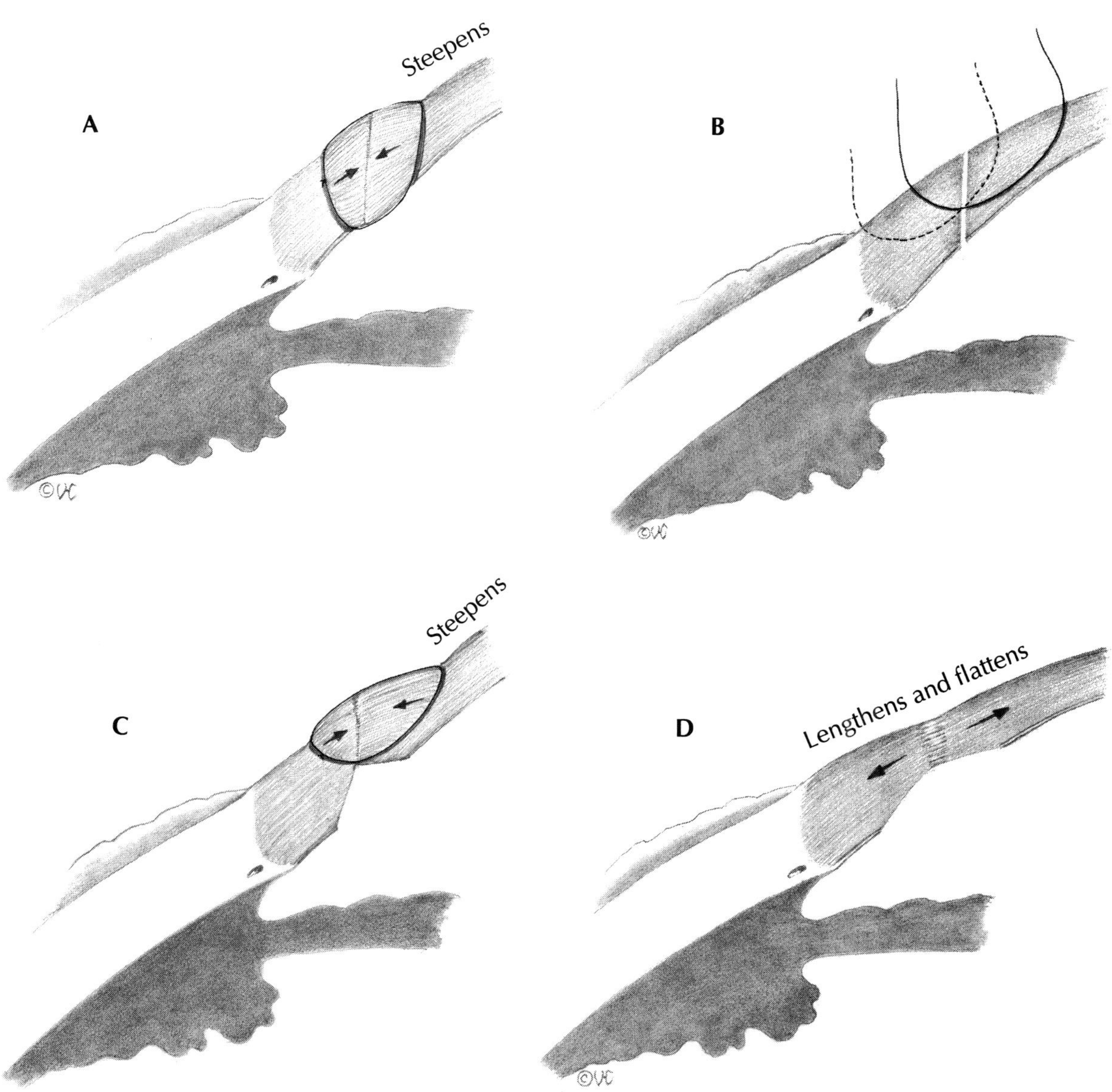

A, proper *through-and-through* closure of corneal cataract wound. **B,** improper centration of suture on corneal cataract wound. **C,** *lambda* effect caused by shallow suturing of corneal cataract wound. **D,** wound thinning caused by *lambda* effect in corneal cataract wound; progressive *against the rule* astigmatism.

cence, and removal of sutures ultimately causes flattening of the cornea in this meridian (Plate 12–8,D). This problem can be quite difficult to repair because excision of too much tissue with a wedge resection will cause steepening in this meridian, and excision of the abnormal tissue within the wound may cause additional dehiscence due to thinning and abnormal healing of the tissue.

The proper choice of suture in this situation is essential. Monofilament 10–0 nylon suture has enough elasticity, enabling it to give slightly during the initial swelling in the postoperative period, and can then retain sufficient tension across the wound to allow good wound healing; 11–0 nylon suture has insufficient strength to close such a wound and will result in wound dehiscence. Dacron suture, which is relatively inelastic, will loosen too quickly during the 3-month period in which the sutures remain intact and, in loosening, may allow wound dehiscence and/or infection. For corneal incisions, we believe that 10–0 nylon suture possesses the best balance of strength and elasticity currently available for closure of the corneal wound.

A single interrupted suture should always be placed in a radial position relative to the cornea and perpendicular to the wound involved. If the wound has been created appropriately, these two requirements will coincide in the same suture loop. If the incision has not been made to curve parallel to the limbus but has been made straight or otherwise deviating from the natural curvature of the eye, a decision must be made as to whether the suture should be made perpendicular to the wound or radial relative to the eye. Usually, it is better to compromise in this situation and place the suture midway between the two positions. Failure to respect the circumferential symmetry of the eye will result in forces that will tend to pull the wound in directions in which the suture no longer supports it. This will result in *fish mouthing* of the wound with subsequent wound dehiscence in the postoperative course. This situation is particularly critical with respect to the limbal cataract incision, which we will not discuss at great length. The potential instability in this region makes proper suture placement essential to minimize long-term wound instability.

The problem with interrupted sutures is the inability to support the anterior surface of the cornea or sclera. Particularly in the cornea with significant variability in thickness due to osmotic considerations, the anterior surface can develop wide incision gaps that can lead to inappropriate healing between suture bites. Running sutures cross anteriorly, providing anterior support and preventing gaping between the bites. For this reason, we feel the running closure of the corneal wound (Plate 12–2,A) and scleral tunnel wound (Plate 12–9) are superior closures to interrupted radial sutures. With the use of a Troutman operative keratometer, running suture patterns can be better adjusted by the surgeon at the close of the operation. Because the corneal sutures induce central corneal astigmatism, compensating compression sutures may be added to correct this induced astigmatism and to accelerate visual rehabilitation during the *sutures in* period of the postoperative course. In the corneal cataract wound, the running sutures are removed at 3 months, whereas the remaining interrupted sutures (two sutures in the operative wound and the two compensating compression sutures) are removed sequentially to con-

Plate 12–9.

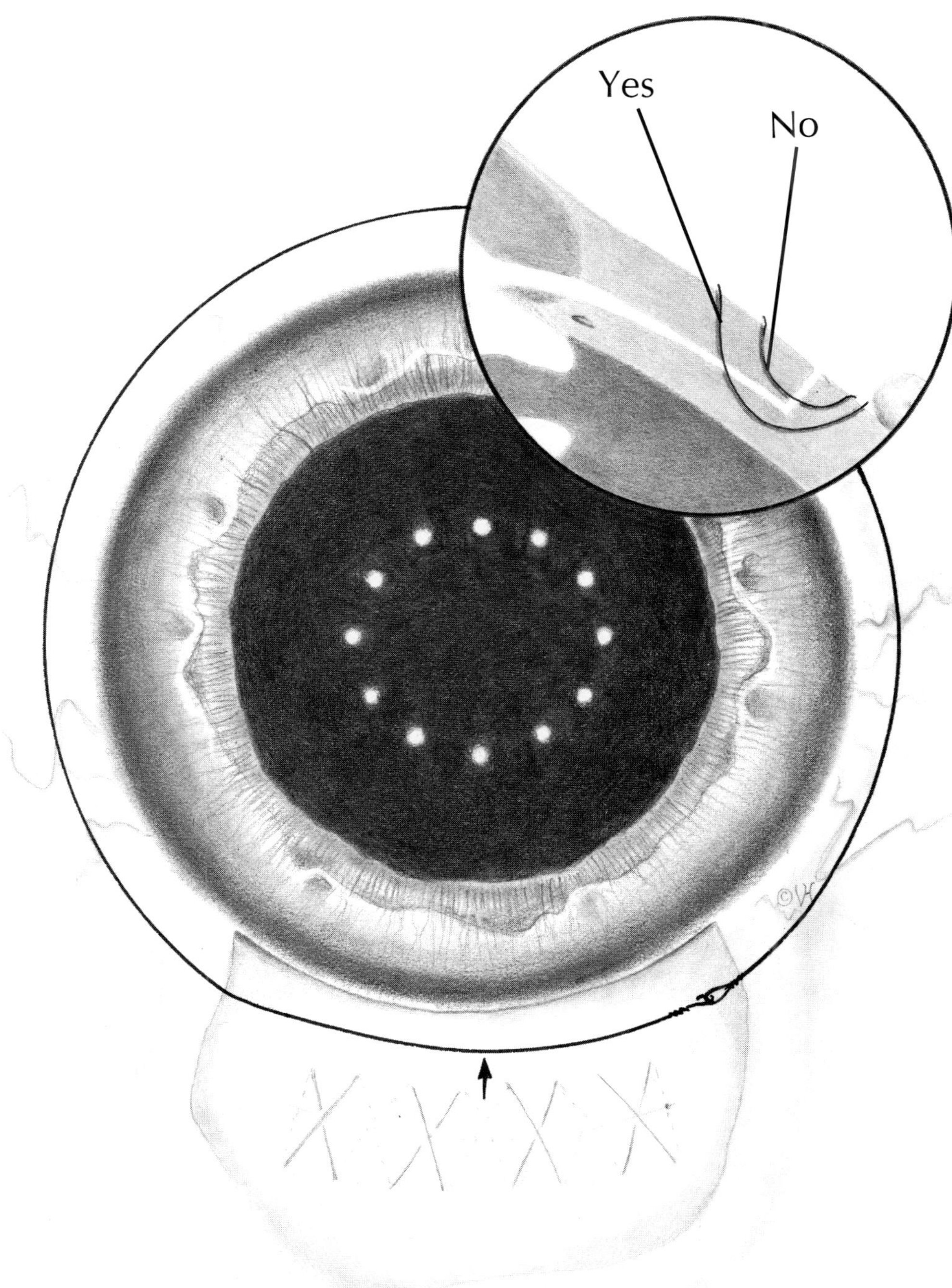

Running suture closure of scleral tunnel incision with proper placement of suture bites.

trol astigmatic error with the aid of a keratometer and/or photokeratoscope.

In the scleral tunnel wound, the bite cannot be placed through the full thickness of the sclera; however, the surgeon should resist the tendency to close only the tip of the tunnel (Plate 12–9). The scleral tunnel incision has two distinct openings, the exterior entrance into the sclera and the internal exit from the cornea into the anterior chamber. This incision is self-sealing if the internal extent is short enough to prevent gaping. This assumption is correct for the 6-mm and smaller phacoemulsification wounds, but has been shown by Foos and Straatsma to be a problem in the extracapsular cataract extraction wound. If a wide scleral tunnel is performed, the internal entry of the incision should be closed through the corneal optical ring to prevent gaping.

Closure of the scleral tunnel incision depends on compression of the tunnel to prevent leakage of fluid. The forces in this area should be quite small, because the corneal opening of the incision is self-sealing and the anterior scleral opening is outside the limbal *guy wire*. In the past, this closure has been accomplished with a running or interrupted suture that placed significant radial forces on the wound (Plate 12–10,A). Because the scleral tunnel has intact sides and is outside the limbal *guy wire*, the tendency of the eye is to resist astigmatic deformations along the meridian of the incision. Temporary astigmatic errors were created that tended to dissipate gradually as the distortion caused by the radial forces of suturing the scleral tunnel incision were counteracted by loosening of the suture material. This time period has been shown in several series to be approximately 6 weeks. Attempts to create a permanent astigmatic change by means of combining wedge resection with a scleral tunnel incision have generally met with failure, due to the strength of the limbal guy wire.

The development of horizontal suturing techniques was coupled with the continuing search for smaller incisions with the scleral tunnel technique. Rapid *astigmatic neutralization,* a term used to denote a return to the preoperative astigmatic error, was observed by Shepherd with the 3.5-mm incision that had been closed with horizontal suturing. Horizontal suturing provides vertical closure of the scleral tunnel without inducing radial forces external to the limbal guy wire (Plate 12–10,B). The astigmatic neutralization, at first attributed to the 3.5-mm incision, was soon felt to be at least partially due to the improved suturing technique. Larger incisions could be closed with the so-called *infinity closure* (Plate 12–10,C), although a single horizontal suture has equal benefit. In a small series, Buzard and Shearing have demonstrated rapid astigmatic neutralization in wounds as large as 7 mm closed with a single horizontal suture (Plate 12–10,D). Creeping against the rule astigmatism with this closure remains a possibility, and variants on the infinity closure to include a radial bite at the 12-o'clock position have been debated. Siepser has even

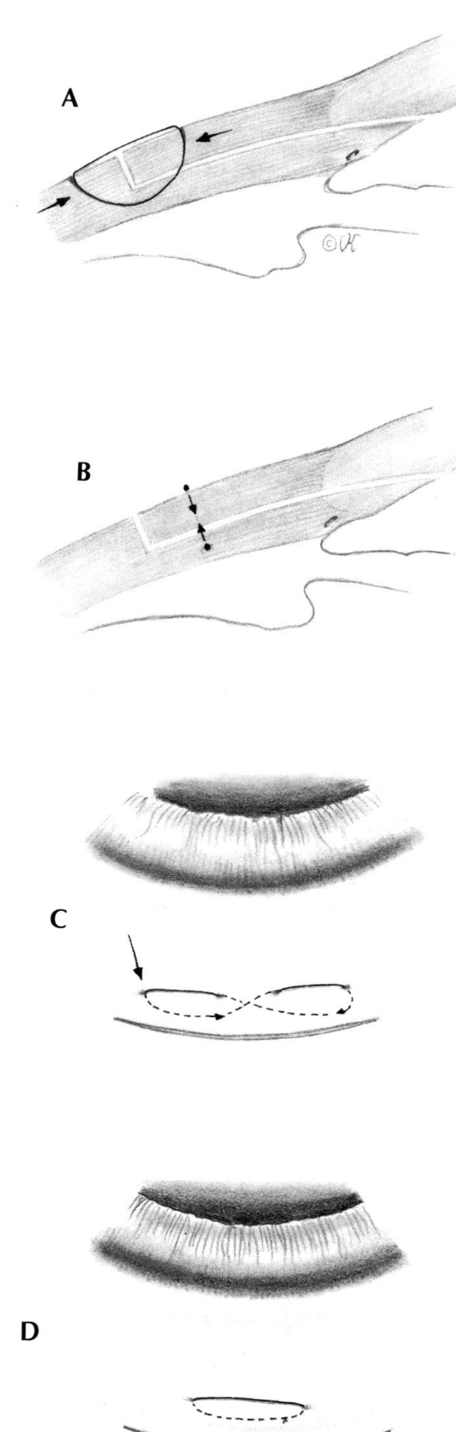

A, radial forces induced by radial interrupted or running suture closure. **B,** compression of scleral tunnel without radial forces created by horizontal suturing. **C,** *infinity closure* of the 6-mm scleral tunnel incision for cataract surgery. **D,** horizontal suture closure of the 6-mm scleral tunnel incision for cataract surgery showing closure of central third of incision.

Pathophysiology and Prevention of Astigmatism Secondary to Cataract Surgery   **311**

suggested a radial anterior scleral incision for the scleral tunnel incision, which simplifies horizontal closure and provides even more radial stabilization of the tissue. The horizontal suture should be short and central in the scleral tunnel incision to avoid distortion of the wound and subsequent wound leak.

As incision size has gradually become smaller and horizontal suturing techniques have demonstrated the problems of induced astigmatism with the suturing of the cataract wound, some surgeons have begun to question whether the self-sealing scleral tunnel incision needs to be sutured at all. Anecdotal reports of 3- and 3.5-mm unsutured cataract wounds reported no leakage and no induced astigmatism without short-term development of against the rule astigmatism. Shearing and others have investigated the use of the round 5 and 6 mm optic intraocular lens inserted through a scleral tunnel incision left unsutured at the conclusion of the case. In a large series of patients, no wound leaks were observed. In these patients, the scleral tunnel was carried well into the cornea, and at the conclusion, in many cases, corneal edema was observed surrounding the internal entrance of the wound. The combination of a self-sealing corneal entrance and mild corneal edema effectively closes the interior portion of the wound. Central corneal astigmatism was noted to be essentially the same as that observed preoperatively, and over a short follow-up, against the rule astigmatism has not been observed. The probability that a properly formed scleral tunnel incision can be left unsutured as a solution to the problem of induced astigmatism during cataract surgery must be considered pending long-term studies.

Horizontal suturing techniques, avoiding radial forces external to the limbal guy wire, have thus been demonstrated to be a factor as significant as incision size in the search for rapid astigmatic neutralization. Combined with the T incision for the scleral tunnel incision, which is closed nicely by horizontal suturing, the surgeon can implant a 5 × 6 mm oval intraocular lens or a 5 × 5 mm round intraocular lens through a 4.5-mm incision and, using horizontal closure, obtain astigmatic neutralization in as little time as 1 week. The benefits of *small incision* cataract surgery are made available without sacrificing the dimensional stability and long track record of PMMA optics of the intraocular lens. Certainly innovations in cataract surgery will continue, but the importance of basic principles of incision location, orientation, size, and closure can be applied to any new technique to aid the surgeon in evaluating the contribution.

After the surgery is completed, variations in wound closure will manifest as both immediate and long-term alterations in central and peripheral astigmatism. If the variation is more major, an actual short-term wound instability can result with subsequent wound leakage and the necessity for further surgical intervention. Corneal topology has been helpful in identifying both individual tight and loose sutures that point the way to further surgical intervention. Wound dehiscence should be repaired early, because identification on peripheral corneal topology can indicate pathology that will not regress spontaneously (Plate 12–11,A). The findings on photokeratometry are most easily observed if the patient is asked to look downward so that the area of the wound is more evenly covered by the photokeratometer. If this is not done, the peripheral wound dehiscence of cataract surgery may often be missed. The typical finding of a *V*-shaped abnormality pointing toward the area of greatest weakness has been termed the *microdehiscence* by Buzard. As in the finding of this abnormality in other situations, the solution requires an in-depth evaluation of wound healing, including the possibility of scleral melting associated with collagen vascular diseases. In many cases, inappropriate suture tension or placement is responsible for the abnormality and simply opening the incision and resuturing will correct both the peripheral microdehiscence and the central astigmatism.

Conversely, removal of tight sutures should be approached with caution, even more so if the incision is longer than 6 mm. Tight cataract sutures can be visualized on photokeratometry with the same technique used previously, namely, to have the patient look downward to bring the area of the wound more in line with the photokeratometric mires. Tight sutures will manifest themselves after photokeratometry by the flattening of the usual round contour of the mires (Plate 12–11,B). Inappropriate removal of sequential sutures before the wound has reached effective stability, at approximately 6 to 10 weeks, may result in wound dehiscence and central astigmatism. With running sutures, this problem can be managed if the running suture is adjusted to release excessive tension of tighter suture loops. Even this approach should not be considered before 1 month for running patterns with radial components to the suture pattern. Horizontal sutures do not have a radial component and thus theoretically can be left in place indefinitely. Through-and-through corneal continuous sutures should not be removed before 3 months because of the avascular supply of the cornea. Compression sutures and additional interrupted sutures in the wound should be left in place and removed sequentially.

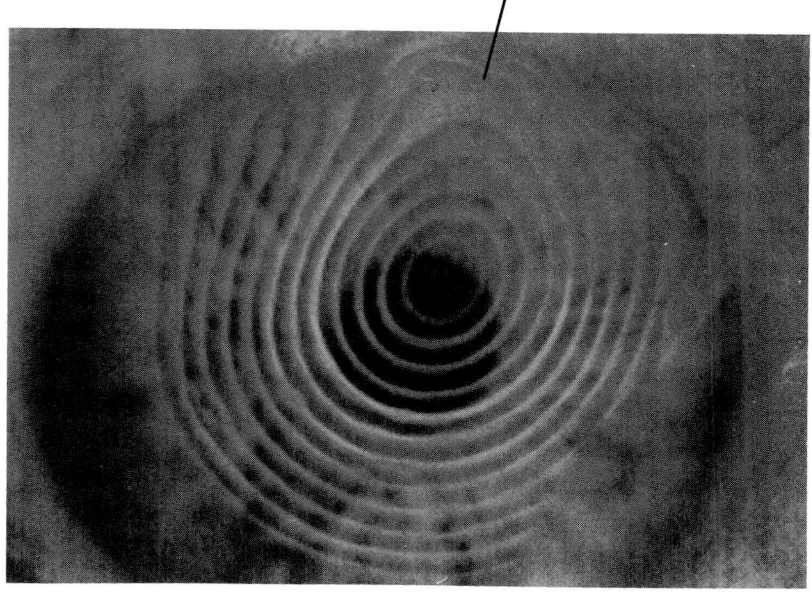

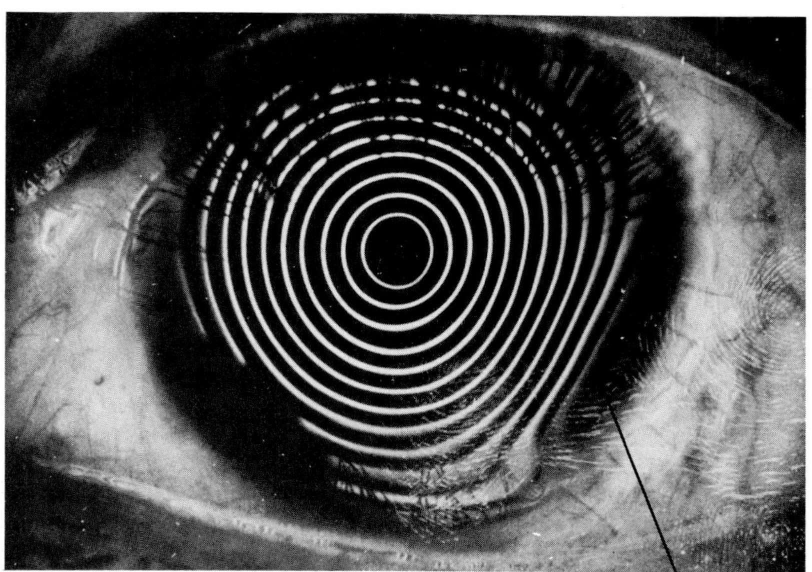

A, Photokeratometric appearance of the *microdehiscence* of a cataract wound showing a *V*-shaped abnormality at the area of wound weakening. **B,** Photokeratometric appearance of tight sutures in a cataract wound showing flattening of the round contour of the photokeratometric mires.

SUMMARY

Because of its proximity to the corneal optical ring and limbal guy wire, the cataract wound is a potential source of an unstable astigmatic error. The authors believe that limbal incisions through the corneal optical ring destabilize this area and contribute to progressive astigmatism, which carries with it a significant incidence of visually debilitating iatrogenic astigmatism.

Over the long term, both corneal and scleral tunnel incisions provide a more stable wound and facilitate the intraocular surgery by inhibiting internal incarceration or prolapse of iris. A choice between these incisions will depend on many factors, including the stability of the scleral bed in question. Use of the corneal incision carries with it a larger potential for corneal astigmatism persisting over the *sutures in* period, which can be neutralized with appropriate compensating compression sutures. Eventually, with through-and-through closing sutures removed, closure of the corneal incision induces minimal stable corneal astigmatism.

The 4.5 to 6 mm scleral tunnel incision has the least inherent tendency to induce early or delayed corneal astigmatism. By using horizontal suturing techniques and the T incision, with PMMA oval or round haptics, astigmatic neutrality can be achieved in as little as 1 week. No suture technique has been demonstrated to be feasible; biologic glues are the next logical step to enhance wound stability. The goal of astigmatically neutral cataract surgery with intraocular lens implantation without the necessity for a sutured incision is within the grasp of every modern cataract surgeon.

Chapter 13

Surgical Management of Congenital and Postcataract Astigmatism

Transverse incisions for high postcataract astigmatism have a long and colorful history. In 1869 Snellen described penetrating corneal incisions to reduce high postoperative cataract astigmatism, as Bates theorized for congenital astigmatism in 1891. Snellen was responding to the high *against the rule* astigmatism that often accompanied the unsutured cataract incisions of the day. Lack of good suture material, instruments, and knowledge prevented him from directly revising the wound dehiscence at the site of the cataract incision as we would have advised him to do with today's more advanced instrumentation. Moreover, the instruments for making repeatable corneal incisions were not nearly good enough, and these incisions were not performed on more than a very few patients. The first significant work using incisions for the control of astigmatism came with the arcuate relaxing incisions described by Troutman in the mid-70s. Although some cases were performed for idiopathic and postcataract astigmatism, the majority of these procedures were performed following penetrating keratoplasty.

The introduction of anterior radial keratotomy by Fyodorov generated great interest in the surgical manipulation of corneal shape (see Chapter 16). The *L* and *RL* procedures introduced by Fyodorov established the principle that radial incisions along a given axis can correct low to moderate amounts of astigmatism. The theory behind the *L* procedure was that corneal fibers would be *released* by the multiple radial incisions along that axis. Subsequent addition of transverse incisions resulted in significant astigmatic corrections at the cost of an even more instability of the cornea. In an attempt to harvest the effectiveness of the transverse incisions, a variety of operations were proposed. In particular, Ruiz introduced the trapezoidal keratotomy, which in its original form proved to be effective but unpredictable with significant long-term complications. We will examine these procedures in detail to gain a better understanding of the contribution of various shaped and oriented anterior corneal incisions as they relate to astigmatic correction.

TRAPEZOIDAL RELAXING INCISION

The original Ruiz procedure was introduced in 1983 (Plate 13–1,A) to quantify astigmatic correction for idiopathic and post-corneal transplant astigmatism with the operating parameters included in a computer program. It soon became obvious that the radial and transverse incision should not connect because the results of many incisions in a small area of the cornea coupled with connecting the incisions allowed *block lifts* of tissue with poor healing. The procedure was modified several times with changes in the length and orientation of both the radial and transverse incisions (Plate 13–1,B). Despite these modifications, the procedure was found to be unstable and unpredictable. A pathologic study by Deg and Binder (1987) showed nonhealing incisions that were present several years following the procedure. An initial theory that the semiradial incisions *blocked* the astigmatic coupling to the opposite meridian was shown to be inaccurate because strong coupling was observed, unfortunately in an unpredictable manner. In the later modifications of the procedure, an attempt was made to influence spherical equivalent using this coupling effect by changing the length of the transverse incisions, as reported by Buzard et al. (1987). Over time it became clear that incisions longer than 5 mm, when used with the Ruiz procedure, gave paradoxical effects that sometimes worsened the astigmatism. In addition, predictable control of spherical equivalent proved to be difficult or impossible, and this concept was abandoned.

In an attempt to isolate the important astigmatic features of the Ruiz procedure and to minimize complications, Lavery and Lindstrom (1985) performed a cadaver eye study that examined the effect of each incision of the Ruiz procedure starting with the paired transverse incisions, progressing to semiradial incisions, and finally examining the contribution of additional transverse incisions. These results help us to appreciate salient features of the effect of combination radial and transverse incisions on corneal curvature. First, transverse incisions appear to have a maximum effect at approximately a 5 mm optical zone with decreasing effect as the optical zone is made smaller or larger. Second, the radial incisions appear

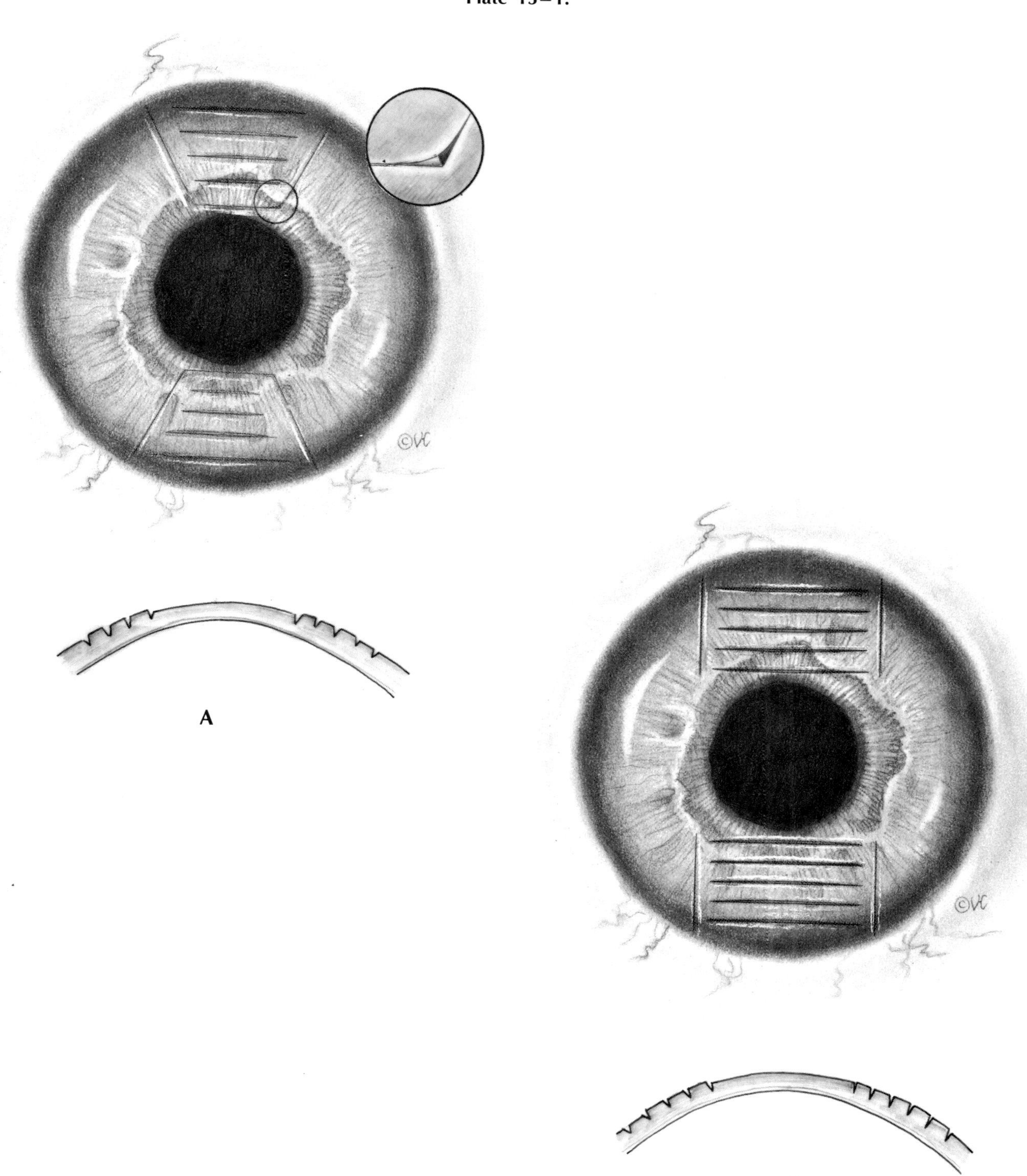

A, original Ruiz procedure with five transverse incisions flanked by semiradial incisions with connection of radial and transverse incisions leading to *block lift* of tissue below cross section. **B,** modified Ruiz procedure used unsuccessfully to attempt control of *coupling* by varying length of transverse incisions, leading to corneal instability with long transverse incisions below cross section.

Surgical Management of Congenital and Postcataract Astigmatism　　**319** to have an increasing effect as they approach the optical axis. Finally, the additional transverse incisions seem to have a small effect on the final procedure. This information made several adaptations of the full Ruiz procedure a reasonable consideration. First, a simple pair of transverse incisions appears to provide a considerable percentage of the effect of the full Ruiz procedure, as reported by Buzard and others (1987), and it seems that incisions closer to the optical axis, within a 5 mm optical zone, give no significant benefit. Second, it appears that removing some of the transverse incisions from the full Ruiz pattern gives almost the effect of a full Ruiz pattern.

Lindstrom developed the modified Ruiz procedure, which consists of only one pair of transverse incisions at 5 mm with semiradials on each side (Plate 13–2,A) and suggested adding an additional pair of transverse incisions later if an undercorrection was encountered (Plate 13–2,B). Today, the various forms of the trapezoidal keratotomy, including the modified Ruiz procedure, are used infrequently because they require a large number of incisions in the cornea, often lead to corneal instability, and are difficult to modify if an undercorrection is encountered. In general, these procedures should be used only in special situations, if at all.

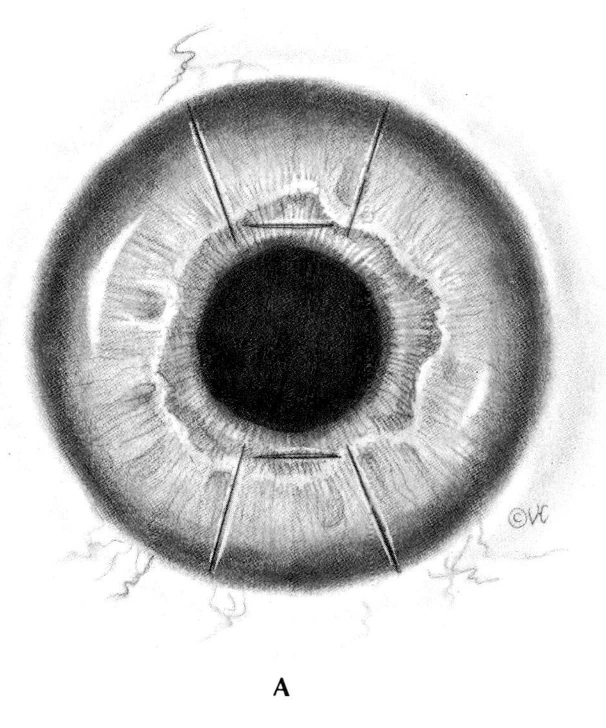

A

B

A, Lindstrom modification of Ruiz procedure, deleting all but one pair of transverse incisions. B, additional transverse incisions for enhanced astigmatic corrective effect.

STRAIGHT TRANSVERSE INCISIONS

Interest in the simple transverse incision (Plate 13–3,A) for correction of astigmatism began with radial keratotomy and was bolstered by the observations of Lavery and Lindstrom. The Fenzel flag incision, the Thornton *T* incision, the Hofmann *T* incision, and the Fyodorov *TR* incision patterns are all variations on the concept of using transverse incisions to correct post–radial keratotomy astigmatism.

Considerations of Symmetry

The issue of symmetric vs. asymmetric incisions is largely a matter of philosophy. As the maxim in architecture goes, form follows function. If the cornea being corrected is asymmetrical in terms of astigmatic error, the incisions should be correspondingly asymmetric. In the typical radial keratotomy patient, the astigmatism is symmetric because it is congenital in nature. Taking this into account, it is our belief that symmetric transverse incisions (Plate 13–3,B) should be performed instead of single asymmetric transverse incisions (Plate 13–3,A) to avoid the possibility of irregular astigmatism with correspondingly decreased, best-corrected visual acuity. It is true that a single incision placed under the upper lid has a better opportunity to heal and, in fact, in the small degree of astigmatism being corrected, probably induces little irregular astigmatism. This approach may be used in patients with dry eye or poor wound healing to avoid postoperative complications.

If an incision is short, that is, less than 3 mm, the degree of curvature with a 5- to 7-mm optical zone will be negligible over this length. However, for longer incisions, curvature can be a significant issue and straight incisions longer than 5 mm have a tendency to heal poorly and to produce progressive effects. Even in the smaller incisions, the issue of straight versus curved is significant from a theoretical standpoint. Anyone who has observed the elegant plots of corneal contours produced by the Topographic Modeling System will be struck by the basic circular symmetry of the eye.

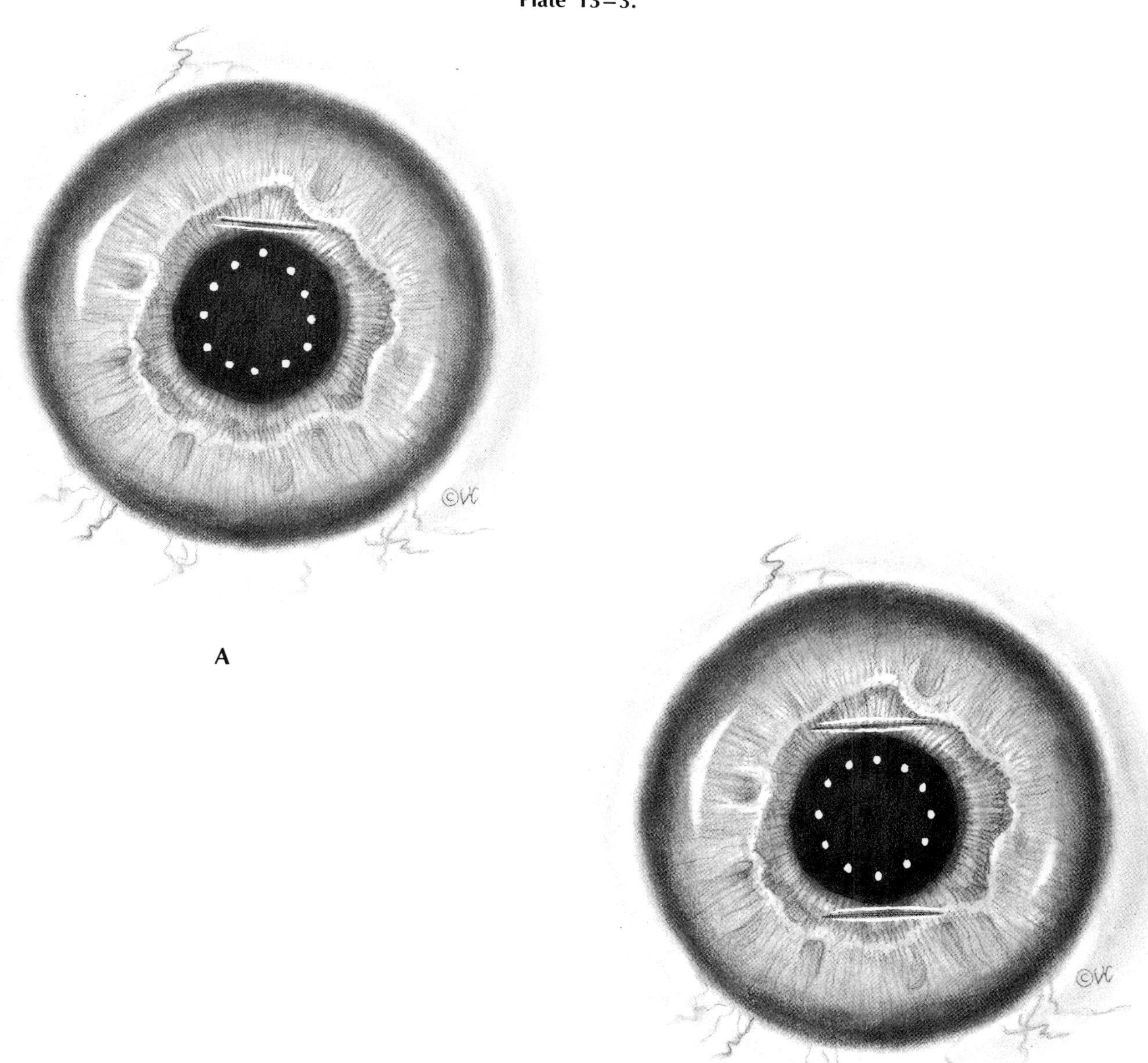

A, irregular *teardrop*-shaped reflex from operative keratometer after application of asymmetric short transverse relaxing incision. **B,** more regular-shaped reflex from operative keratometer after application of symmetric short transverse relaxing incisions.

We are often confronted with the Cartesian coordinate system, which uses straight lines oriented perpendicularly to measure and locate objects on a grid. This system is used in our cities and towns to create streets because these are usually linear straight objects. The eye is a round object, and the Cartesian coordinate system does not naturally adapt itself to round objects (Plate 13–4,A). A coordinate system that is perfectly adapted to describing round objects is the Polar coordinate system, which measures the location of objects in terms of their radius or distance from a central point (Plate 13–4,B) and angular displacement from a given radius (Plate 13–4,C). Thus, to respect the circular symmetry of the eye, we should think and describe objects or incisions on the cornea in terms of radius and angular displacement in degrees rather than using linear measurements, such as millimeters.

Straight transverse incisions, even short ones, are not circular and violate this basic symmetry leading to stresses that are not equal over the length of the incision. With this in mind, we believe an attempt should be made to create curved incisions of any length. For the short straight incisions that we are discussing here, in practice the curved incisions will undoubtedly look almost the same as straight incisions of the same length.

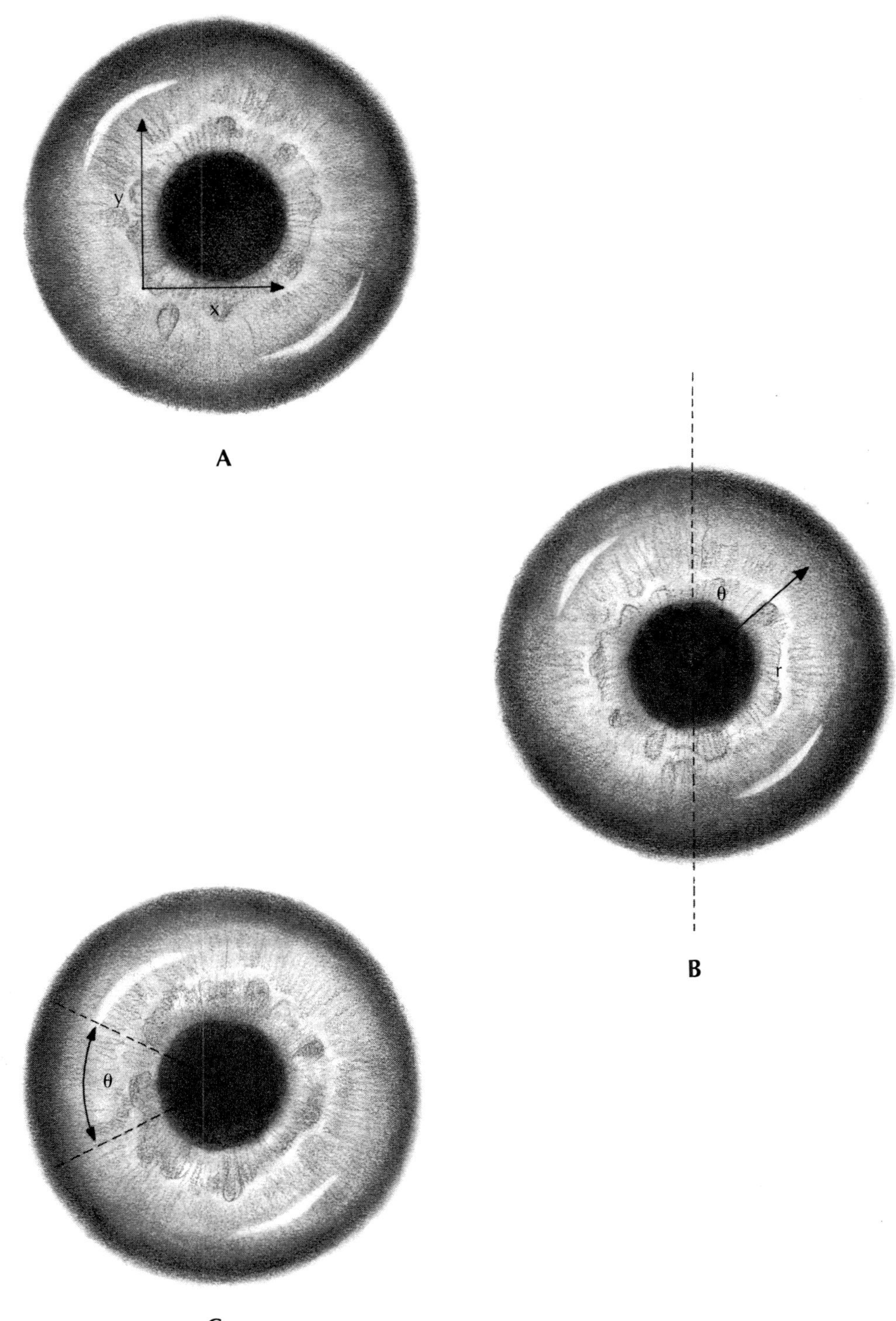

A, Cartesian coordinate system overlay on circular cornea demonstrating mismatch in symmetry. **B,** radial component of polar coordinate system measured from optical axis demonstrating matching symmetry with circular cornea. **C,** angular displacement component of polar coordinate system measured from optical axis demonstrating matching symmetry with circular cornea.

Considerations Relative to Astigmatic Meridian

If the transverse incisions are placed incorrectly relative to the patient's final astigmatic meridian, a cross-cylinder effect will come into play that will, in effect, give an astigmatic error at an entirely new axis (see Chapter 6). If the surgeon does not consider the cross-cylinder effect, an attempt to correct this astigmatism may be made with incisions along the new axis. This will not correct the problem but instead will lead to an even more complex cross-cylinder effect. In the past, this has led to a situation in which multiple transverse incisions were created around the cornea in an attempt to correct the patient's astigmatism, ultimately leading to an unstable cornea due to the multiplicity of incisions (Plate 13–5,A). The photokeratometry shows irregular astigmatism reflected by this patient's poor best-corrected visual acuity with spectacles (Plate 13–5,B).

If the situation of incisions along the incorrect axis occurs, the surgeon should suture the incorrect transverse incision, allow it to heal, and later perform incisions along the appropriate axis. In some cases, simply extending the transverse incision can allow proper centering on the patients astigmatic meridian, thus avoiding the cross-cylinder effect.

For astigmatic errors greater than 3 D, the Troutman operative keratometer can be used to verify the flat and the steep axis. For astigmatic errors of less than 3 D, this operative aid cannot be used, and the surgeon should mark the cornea as we describe in the operative techniques section.

Considerations Relative to Coupling

Throughout this book and in the literature, the importance of *coupling* has been emphasized as the way transverse incisions accomplish the reduction of astigmatic error. As we have discussed, flattening occurs along the axis of the transverse incision, whereas steepening occurs in the axis 90 degrees away as Troutman observed in 1970. The degree of coupling depends on the length and configuration (straight versus arcuate) of the incisions and, as a practical matter, does not seem to be consistent enough to predict accurately.

For simple transverse or arcuate incisions (less than 5 mm), coupling occurs in a way so that the spherical equivalent is preserved. The Ruiz procedure seems to approximately correct the minus cylinder spherical equivalent, which was believed to be due to the blocking effect of the radial incisions. Early in the development of these astigmatic procedures, it was hoped that the coupling effect could be used to predictably correct spherical error in addition to astigmatism by varying the length of the incision. Buzard, Haight, and Troutman investigated this theory with the Ruiz procedure and demonstrated erratic coupling combined with poor wound healing for the longer transverse incisions. This was one of many

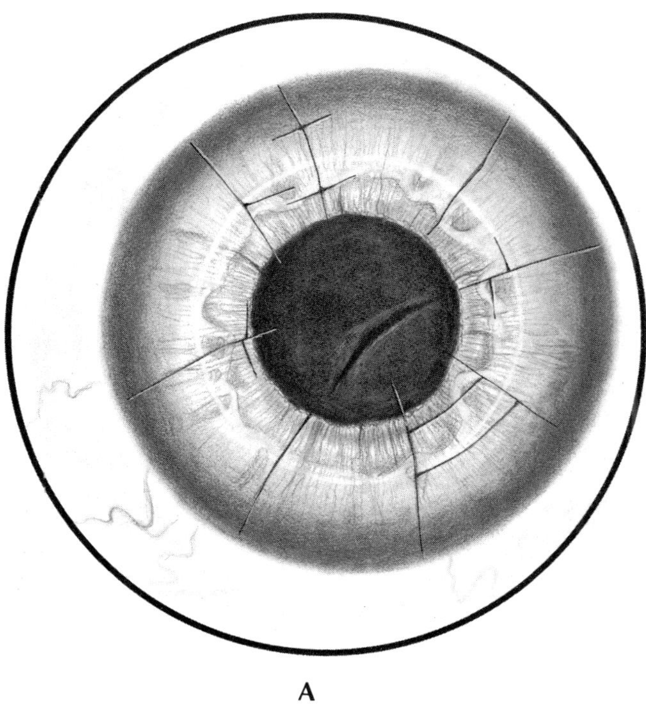

A

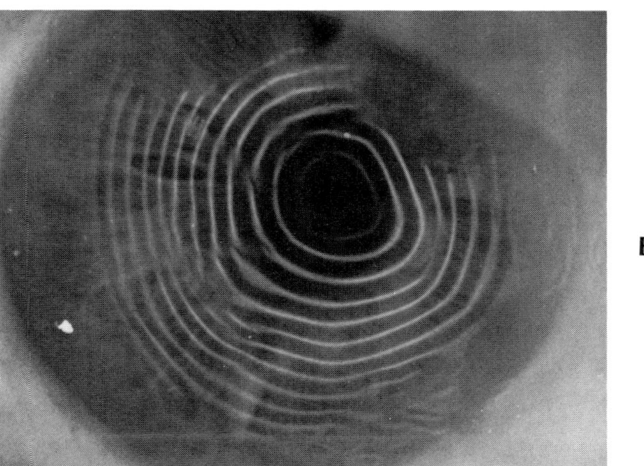

B

A, patient with excessive corneal incisions, resulting from attempt to correct cross-cylinder effect after Ruiz procedure along improper meridian. **B,** photokeratometry of the same cornea, showing severe irregular astigmatism leading to diminished best-corrected visual acuity.

reasons why the Ruiz procedure was abandoned in favor of more predictable and stable operations.

Investigations by Buzard of short simple paired transverse incisions have consistently indicated decreased coupling relative to the Ruiz procedure. For the simple transverse and arcuate incisions considered here, a rough estimate of coupling dictates that the spherical equivalent is conserved. For example, a patient with the refraction $-2.00 - 2.00 \times 90$ would have a refraction of -3.00 sphere after short, paired transverse relaxing incisions conserving the spherical equivalent. If a Ruiz procedure were performed, correcting minus cylinder astigmatic error, the final refraction would be -2.00 sphere. These considerations are less important here than when considered in conjunction with radial keratotomy, but they emphasize the important concept of *coupling*.

This discussion also highlights an important principal, *algebraic addition of corneal incisions*, that in effect states that the effect of incisions is additive, either at the time of surgery or in the situation in which incisions are created at separate times. Thus in the Ruiz procedure, the correction of minus cylinder sphere is a result of the coupling effect of the transverse incisions steepening the cornea at 90 degrees away. The flattening effect of radial incisions in the axis of the incision also occurs at 90 degrees away. Thus slightly more flattening is obtained, the additive effect resulting in a change in the coupling from spherical equivalent to the correction of minus cylinder astigmatic error. This subject is explored in more detail in Chapter 16. *We believe that isolated radial, transverse, or arcuate incisions are incapable of the true blocking effect so well demonstrated by the corneal optical ring or post-keratoplasty pseudo–optical ring.*

Independent Variables in Transverse Incisions

The pertinent variables to consider in varying the effect of the transverse incision are the depth, number, length, optical zone, and age of the patient. The depth is less critical than for radial keratotomy and should be between 80% and 90% of the cornea. In general, a setting of 0.6 mm for the diamond knife is appropriate if the practitioner does not own a pachymeter, although pachymetry is advised to obtain a more exact knife setting. Increasing the number of transverse incisions can actually have a diminished effect on astigmatic error by blunting the *breaking* effect of the cornea over the transverse incision(s), as shown by Buzard. Increased effect has been shown by Thornton, Lindstrom, and others, with multiple transverse incisions indicating a variable effect possibly related to incomplete wound healing. (Plate 13–6). If too many transverse incisions are made in a small area of the cornea, wound healing problems will be induced, resulting in a large astigmatic effect with long-term instability. The critical variables of length of incisions and optical zone are modified by

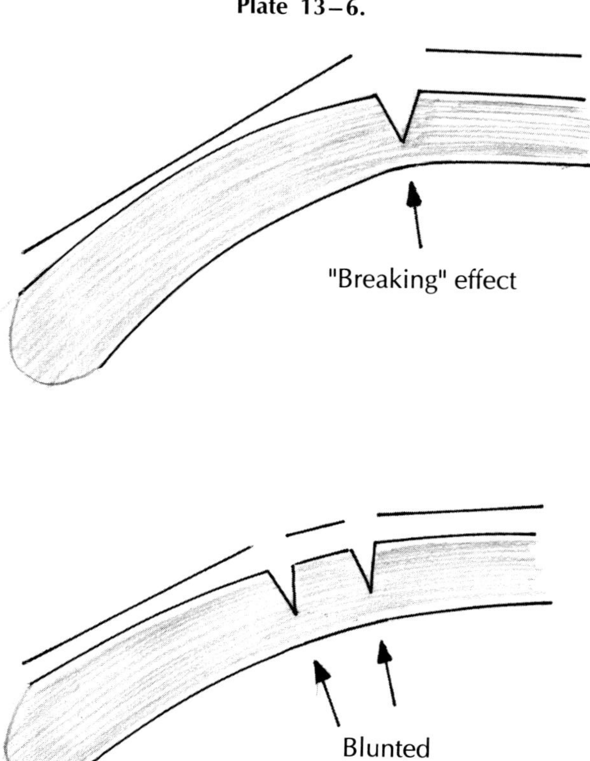

Breaking effect of transverse incisions on corneal curvature, showing blunting of *breaking* effect and possible diminished astigmatic correction with multiple incisions as compared with single incision, not increased central flattening with multiple transverse incisions.

age, although age is a less important modifier because of the relatively short incisions. Longer incisions, such those encountered in radial keratotomy, are more affected by age-related healing factors.

In the past, transverse incisions have been straight and short, in the range of 2 to 3 mm. A useful concept is the idea of segment length introduced by Thornton and defined as the distance between adjacent pairs of an eight-incision radial keratotomy. These can be easily defined geometrically to obtain the appropriate numerical values (Plate 13–7). Even if radial incisions are not present, the distances can be marked with a radial incision marker.

This concept of segment length is important because it places these incisions in the context of the circular symmetry of the eye. Angular displacement of individual incisions is another important concept and implies that a one-segment incision placed at 5 mm subtends the same angular displacement as a one-segment incision at 7 mm.

From previous work, we are aware that short incisions near the optical axis give similar astigmatic effects as longer incisions placed farther from the optical axis. A reasonable case can be made for the concept that the astigmatic effect is directly related to the angle subtended by the incision, independent of the optical zone, subject to certain limitations.

This concept, which has also been advanced by Rowsey, has not been conclusively proved in the laboratory. However, using the clinical results of various investigators, Rowsey has demonstrated a close approximation of this theory. This would certainly explain why separate investigators using various length incisions in different optical zones can obtain similar results. According to this theory, longer incisions in larger optical zones would give similar results as shorter incisions in smaller optical zones. The limitations of this approach would be the paradoxical effects seen with incisions of 5 mm or more and the difficulties of reproducing the length of the incision accurately. Straight incisions longer than 4 to 5 mm have been observed clinically to give erratic immediate postoperative results and unstable long-term results due to healing abnormalities. We believe that straight incisions of this length violate the circular symmetry of the eye and thus subject themselves to gaping and incomplete wound healing. Recent investigation in our laboratory (Sabates et al.) in eye bank eyes suggests that this linear theory of segment length is incorrect. We found that by using the same "segment length" significantly more effect is seen at 5 to 6 mm vs. 7 to 8 mm, because of increased coupling at the 5 to 6 mm optical zone.

One of the problems in comparing results of transverse incisions from one investigator to another is determining exactly how long and deep the incisions are. Short transverse incisions tend to be difficult to make, because the natural tendency of a knife inserted into virgin tissue is to come slowly to full depth as the knife is moved forward (see Chapter 8). By rocking a

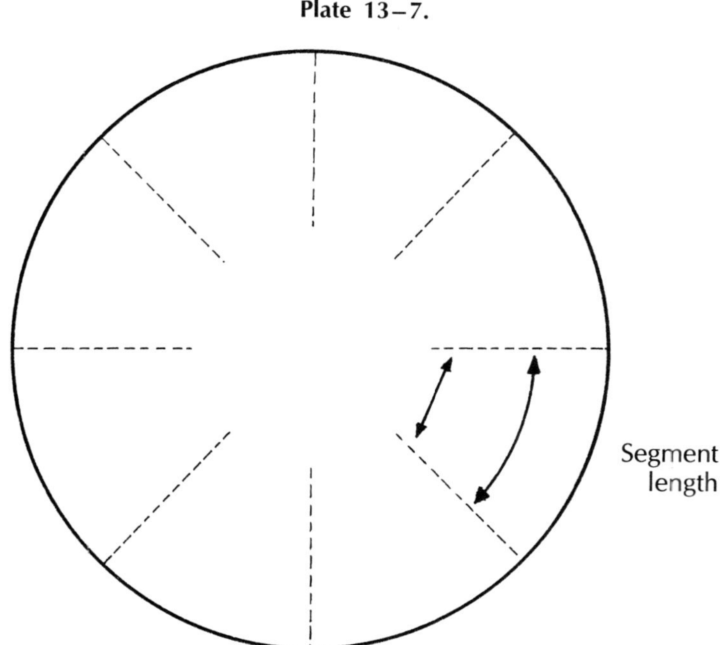

Incision Length at Varying Optical Zones

Length (mm)	Optical Zone (mm)			
	5	6	7	8
½ seg	1.1	1.3	1.5	1.7
⅔ seg	1.4	1.7	2.0	2.3
¾ seg	1.6	1.9	2.3	2.6
1 seg	2.1	2.5	3.0	3.4
1¼ seg	2.7	3.2	3.8	4.3
1½ seg	3.2	3.8	4.5	5.1

Segmental length and numerical values for various optical zones (taken from Thornton, courtesy of Spencer P. Thornton, M.D.).

double-cutting diamond knife back and forth in the very short incision and systematically reversing its orientation, a reproducibly deep incision can be made. Another approach involves the use of a square trifacet diamond knife that can be moved back and forth in the incision without reversing the orientation. The true length and depth of the incision thus will be quite variable, and perhaps this can explain the variation in individual results.

The authors feel that varying the optical zone is more predictable and simpler than varying the length of small transverse incisions, as advocated by Thornton. The effect is similar because by making a fixed-length incision of varying optical zone, we are changing the effective segment length of the incision. In addition, we believe that shorter (2–3 mm) incisions heal more predictably and thus transverse incisions in the 5 to 7 mm zone provide a better alternative than longer incisions in the periphery. The disadvantage of mid-peripheral distortion caused by incisions at the 5 mm optical zone has not been significant enough to warrant the risk of diminished wound healing encountered with longer incisions at larger optical zones for small (less than 3 diopters) astigmatic errors.

TROUTMAN RELAXING (ARCUATE) INCISIONS–COMPRESSION SUTURES

Long arcuate incisions (Plate 13–8,A), have been used extensively for the correction of postkeratoplasty astigmatic errors. The presence of a corneal transplant is not mandatory for the use of this technique to correct astigmatism. Indeed, shortly after introducing the technique, Troutman performed several cases for the correction of idiopathic congenital astigmatism, but these incisions were not used often, because of difficulty in creating reproducible incisions with the knives available at the time. A knife that is wide and thick will tend to cut in a linear fashion (see Chapter 8), and in fact provides an excellent means of obtaining straight incisions in radial keratotomy. To create arcuate incisions, the knife should be extremely thin and sharp, such as a double-cutting ultra-thin diamond knife, and the angle of attack should be narrow, that is, a 30-degree rather than a 45-degree angled knife. Knives such as this will adapt much more readily to the creation of curved incisions and make possible regular and reproducible arcuate incisions.

The first systematic use of Troutman relaxing (arcuate) incisions for the correction of congenital astigmatism was the work of Merlin, which demonstrates several important features of these incisions. Merlin investigated incisions ranging from 100 to 160 degrees and optical zones ranging from 5 to 7 mm. He found astigmatic correction increased from 100 to 120 degrees and diminished when incisions were made longer. He also found progressive diminished effect as the optical zone was shifted from 5 to 7 mm. The effect on spherical equivalent was null for 100-degree incisions and produced steadily larger hyperopic effects, implying steepening of the cornea, as the incision length increased to 160 degrees. Thus, coupling for long arcuate incisions of less than 90 to 100 degrees is essentially the same as for short transverse incisions, preserving spherical equivalent.

Rowsey and Tripoli have separately examined the effects of arcuate incisions as a function of angular displacement with photokeratometry and eye-bank eyes. They have shown evidence of wound instability as the incisions approach 120 degrees. For this reason, the authors suggest that arcuate incisions should be created with a maximum extent of 90 degrees, as originally suggested by Troutman. Rather than extending the incisions beyond 90 degrees to create larger astigmatic corrections (Plate 13–8,B),

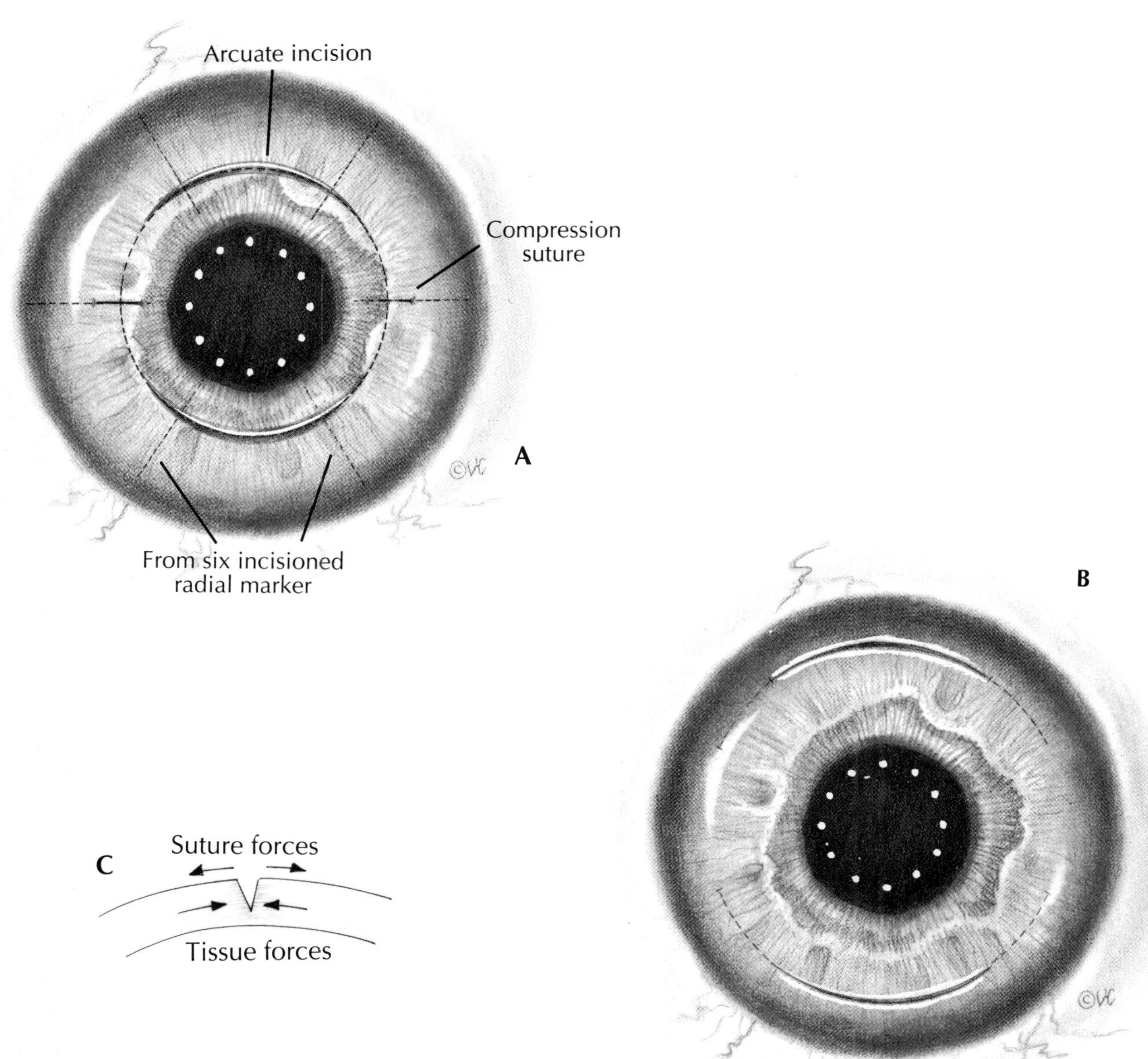

A, long Troutman relaxing (arcuate) incisions of 90 degrees at a 7-mm optical zone with compression sutures and overlay of six-cut radial incision marker demonstrating measurement of angular displacement. **B,** long arcuate incisions of 90 degrees at an 8-mm optical zone, showing possible extension of incisions to 120 degrees *(dotted lines),* which is not advised. **C,** balanced forces *gaping* arcuate incisions with Troutman compression sutures showing gaping forces by compression sutures opposed by wound closing forces of adjacent tissue.

the technique of compression sutures is used to augment the effect of the operation.

When arcuate incisions are used to correct postkeratoplasty astigmatism, the effect often is variable, and little effect is seen as the two 90-degree arcuate incisions are created. To solve this problem, Troutman introduced compression sutures to augment the gaping of arcuate incisions and to increase the corrective effect of the procedure (Plate 13–8,A). Because the incisions have a tendency to close, the compression sutures, in effect, create a temporary overcorrection by predictable and stable gaping of the incision during wound healing (Plate 13–8,C). This combination of incisions and compression sutures is less dependent on the vagaries of wound healing and tend to give more reproducible results. The sutures are removed consecutively as they loosen or as indicated by the astigmatic correction obtained. As much as 8 to 10 D of astigmatic error may be corrected with this technique.

The choice of the appropriate optical zone should be made in the context of ease of creation of incisions of the proper length and configuration and midperipheral distortion. Because these incisions have been performed in many patients at 7 to 8 mm optical zones, as a result of the usual size of a corneal graft, it is sensible to continue with an optical zone of at least 7 mm. Smaller optical zones make it difficult to easily create arcuate incisions, and the issue of mid-peripheral distortion becomes a factor. At an optical zone of 7 mm, the incisions create little distortion and the authors have been satisfied with the astigmatic results. Of interest is the fact that even Lindstrom has largely abandoned the modified Ruiz procedure (private communication) in favor of Troutman relaxing (arcuate) incisions for astigmatic correction above 3 D, and this approach seems to be the procedure of choice for moderate and high astigmatic errors at the present time.

Krumeich Procedure

An extension of the curved incision concept is a procedure described by Krumeich in which a Krumeich or Hanna corneal trephine is used to create a circular incision to 80% to 90% depth, which is then resutured using an antitorque suture pattern (Plate 13–9,A,B). Under observation with the operative keratometer, the running suture pattern is adjusted to nullify corneal astigmatism. The advantage is the production of an arcuate incision with minimum difficulty and the efficient redistribution of corneal forces due to the circumferential incision.

This incision can be useful in treating the patient with large (greater than 4–5 D) astigmatic errors and hyperopic spherical equivalent. Just as we have seen with the data presented by Merlin, the circular incision allows a slight steepening of the central cornea, which leads to reduction of

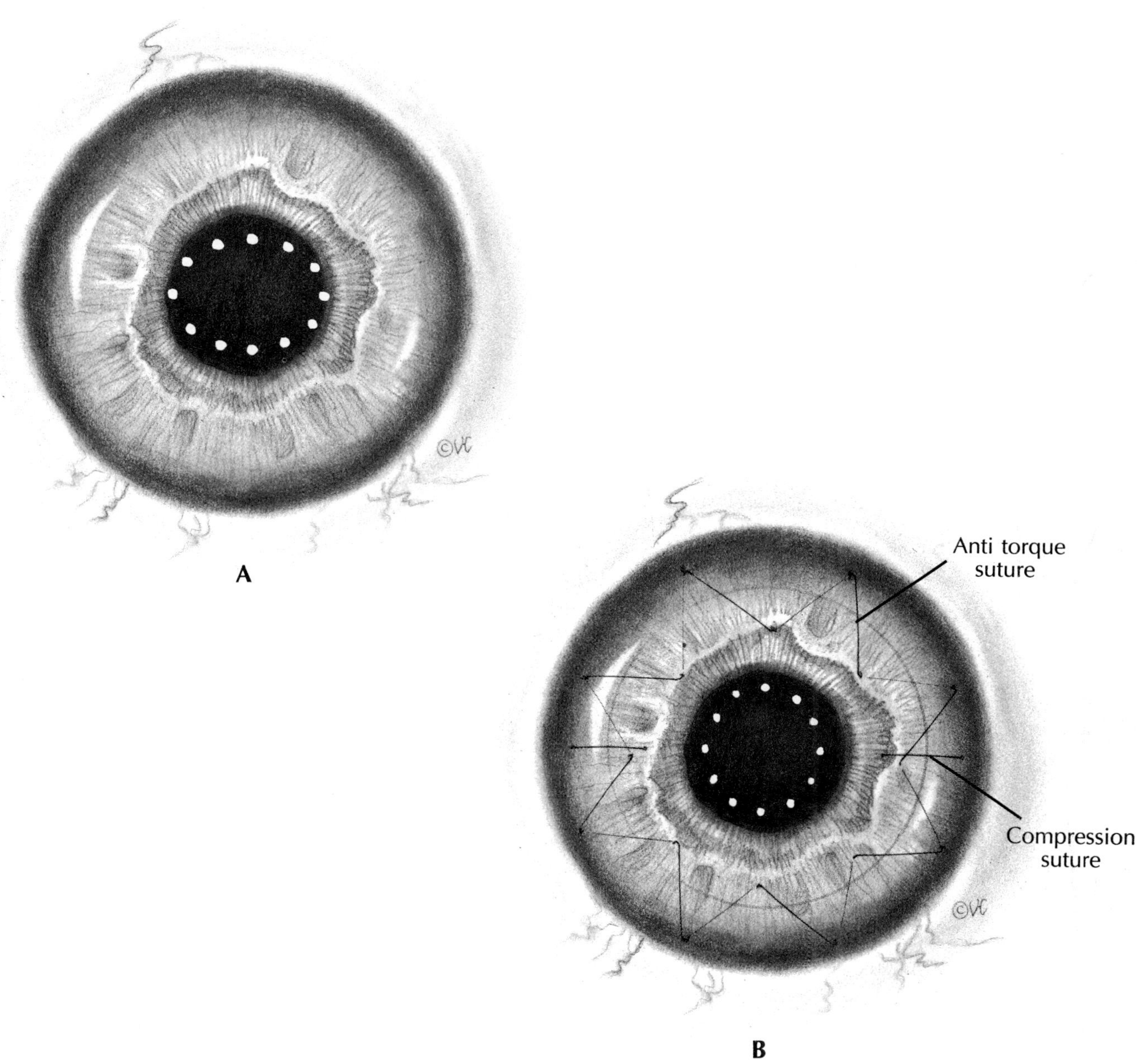

A, preoperative cornea with *with the rule* astigmatism. **B,** Krumeich procedure seen postoperatively showing partial penetrating circumferential incision at 8 mm, with antitorque suture and compression sutures at 180 degrees creating a slight overcorrection seen with the operative keratometer.

hyperopia depending on the suture pattern used to close the wound. Buzard has performed several of these procedures, and has found that the astigmatic correction reverses if only an antitorque closure is used to close the wound. The addition of interrupted compression sutures is required along the preoperatively flatter meridian to maintain a permanent correction (Plate 13–9,B). *In effect, this procedure works like Troutman relaxing incisions connected circumferentially, the differential healing being achieved by the interrupted sector compression sutures. The antitorque suture serves only to prevent dehiscence of the long arcuate (circumferential) incision.* Thus the running suture can be removed at 3 months, but the interrupted compression sutures are removed later as indicated by refraction or loosening of the suture(s).

This technique suffers from the problems of extended postoperative care due to healing of the long corneal wound with its attendant problems of diurnal variation of vision, irritation from sutures, and possible problems with infection and wound healing. It is a good policy to leave the cornea slightly overcorrected, as with Troutman relaxing incisions, removing interrupted sutures as needed in the postoperative period. In addition, many practitioners do not own the Krumeich or Hanna corneal trephine with which such an accurate fine arcuate incision can be produced, although the effect can be obtained with a diamond knife in combination with guarded trephines. Indications for this procedure are consequently somewhat limited, and for the majority of cases, paired arcuate relaxing incisions with compression sutures will serve almost the same purpose with fewer problems.

Bowtie Procedure

Another variation on the use of long arcuate incisions is the bowtie procedure in conjunction with radial incisions introduced by Tchah (1985). This procedure involves a four-incision radial keratotomy connected at the limbus by two arcuate incisions straddling the steep axis. The peripheral radial and arcuate incisions are connected, and the astigmatic corrective effect of the operation is determined by the length of the radial incisions (Plate 13–10).

Merlin investigated arcuate incisions adjacent to the limbus and concluded that the effect was excessively variable because of healing influences from the limbal vessels. In addition, the connection of radial and arcuate incisions represents an important error in refractive surgery, allowing block lifting of the tissue if prompt healing is not achieved. Buzard has performed a small number of such procedures in elderly postcataract patients, and has observed wound dehiscence and block lift in the area in which the radial and arcuate incisions connect, requiring suturing to correct the problem. This procedure is quite variable in its cor-

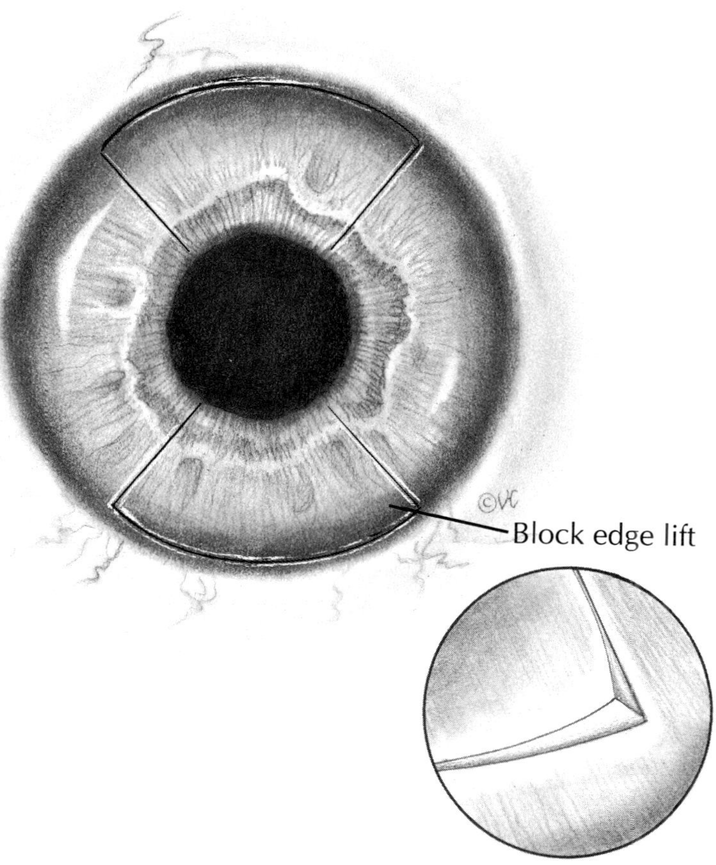

Bowtie procedure performed on patient with *with the rule* preoperative astigmatic error, showing arcuate incisions adjacent to limbus connecting with radial incisions.

rection of astigmatic error even in younger patients and should probably
be avoided.

PREOPERATIVE CONSIDERATIONS

The initial problem in refractive surgery for astigmatism is to identify
the visual (optical) axis, which is different from the geometric axis of the
eye, often not coinciding with the center of the cornea (Plate 13–11,A).
The visual or optical axis must be determined by asking the patient to observe a lighted object, and assuming the observation is along the same
line as the light (Plate 13–11,B). Localization of the optical axis on the cornea can be obtained by the location of the reflex of the lighted object
(Plate 13–11,C). The optical axis is generally slightly nasal to the geometric center of the cornea, and this is called a positive angle kappa, refer-
ring to the angle between the geometric and optical axes of the eye. It is
clear that if the observer is not directly in line with the optical axis, the
reflex seen on the cornea will not correspond to the location of the optical
axis on the cornea due to parallax between the observer and the light reflex.

Several pitfalls of refractive surgery are encountered at the time of determination of the optical axis on the cornea, and it is clear that an error
at this point will seriously jeopardize the remainder of the operation. In
the early days, determination of the optical axis was performed using the
reflex from the coaxial illumination of the microscope. The patient was
asked to look directly at the light. With the surgeon looking through his or
her right eye, a mark was created with a needle at the lower left-hand
corner of the reflex from the filament of the lamp. Two aspects of this
method led to problems. First, the coaxial illumination is excessively
bright, and the patient often failed to look directly at the light, leading to
an error in the determination of the optical axis. Second, marking the optical axis with a needle could leave a small scar directly in the visual axis,
leading to a decreased best-corrected visual acuity secondary to irregular
astigmatism.

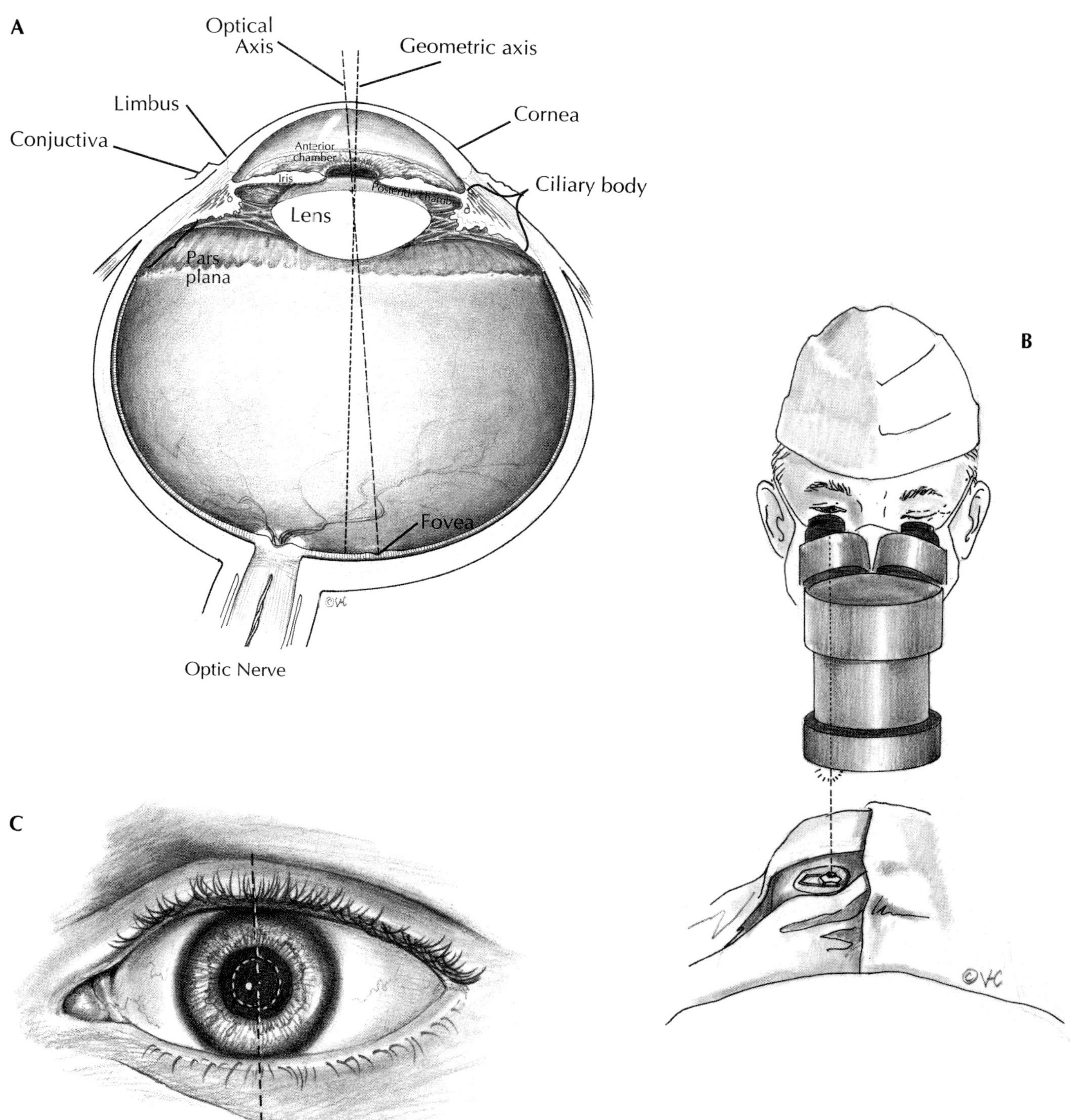

A, demonstration of *angle kappa* between geometric and optical axes of the eye and separation on corneal surface between central cornea and optical axis. **B,** demonstration of coincident axis of surgeon's right eye, fixation light, and optical axis. **C,** appearance of cornea from the surgeon's right eye, showing location of optical axis defined by specular reflection of fixation light and separation from geometric center of cornea.

In general, the optical zone should either be marked with a blunt instrument or not at all, using the cross hairs of the optical zone marker as a direct guide to the optical axis. Waring has shown that decentration of the optical axis in eccentric penetrating keratoplasty leads to induced astigmatism with the flat axis along the axis of decentration. In precisely the same manner, decentration of the optical axis creates a shifting of the *optical cap* or optical zone that can lead to development of regular astigmatism. If the optical axis is excessively decentered, actual irregular astigmatism can result from interference of the incisions with the optical clarity of the cornea. If, as is often the case, the optical zone is small, such as a 3-mm optical zone required in radial keratotomy for high myopia, even a small decentration of the proposed visual axis can lead to a significant percentage change in the visual axis relative to the 3-mm optical zone. For these reasons, it is advisable to avoid using the coaxial light to determine the visual axis and to use instead a dim light, such as an LED (Plate 13–12,A) or a filtered version of the coaxial light on which the patient can more comfortably focus. Creating a light source that is truly parallel to both the optical axis and the surgeon's eye was first addressed by Topcon (a second one is now available from Mastel) with a device that attaches to the operating microscope (Plate 13–12,B). This device has a fiberoptic cable that transfers a small portion of the light from the coaxial illuminator to a point directly opposing the surgeon's right eye (Plate 13–12,C). This places the fixation light along the line of sight of the surgeon's right eye, avoiding the problem of parallax. Even with these precautions, determination of the visual axis can be a significant problem because the distance of the light from the patient's eye is short enough and the light is lacking in detail sufficiently that fixating on the light itself may be next to impossible for the patient.

As a precaution, the pupil can be constricted with pilocarpine so that a secondary check of the gross location of the visual axis is available. However, occasions arise in which the visual axis does not lie within the constricted pupillary zone. If the light reflex is found along the edge of the pupil when constricted, it is likely that the patient has either an eccentric visual axis or an abnormality in pupillary constriction and should be rescheduled for another day without the use of pilocarpine.

The instruments used to mark the optical zone represent another important choice. Various means of delineating the center of the optical zone are available, including wire cross hairs, a single point, and bulls eye. We prefer the wire cross hairs for the best nonintrusive indication of the optical center. However, it should be noted the wires are very delicate and easily moved and should be checked periodically. In addition, the optical zone marker should have a reasonably sharp edge to mark the optical zone. One should check the diameter accuracy of the optical zones with a

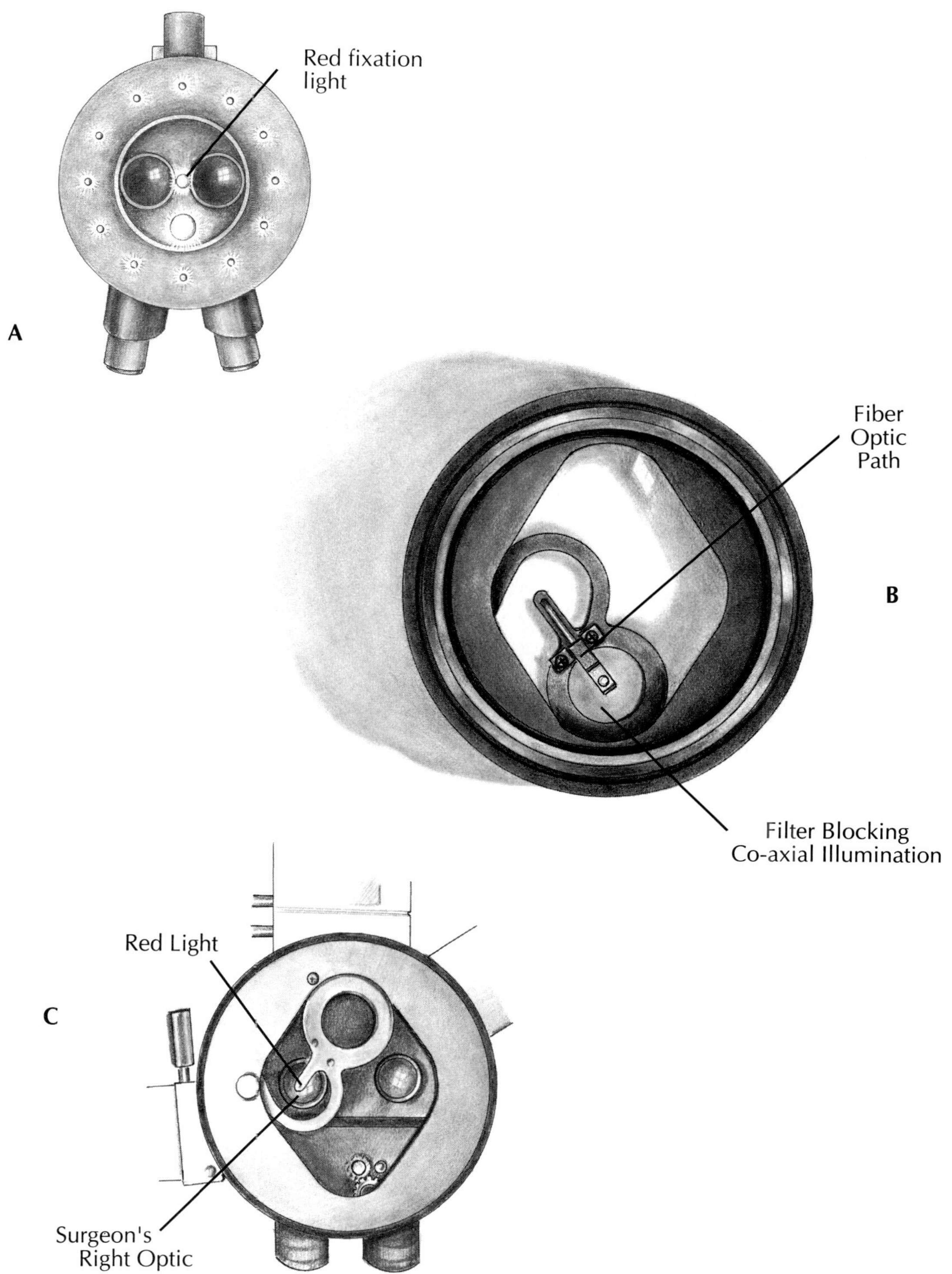

A, patient's view of operating microscope with Troutman keratometer and LED fixation device between optics of microscope. **B,** fixation device provided by Topcon for identification of optical axis. **C,** fixation device provided by Topcon for identification of optical axis on microscope showing fixation light central to right optic and thus, to surgeon's right eye.

device such as the Baribeau micronscope to determine whether the measurement is marked from the inside or outside diameter.

Various specialized markers have been developed to mark the length of the short transverse incisions, and their use will depend on the degree of convenience that is afforded by the instrument in question. Personally, we prefer to mark the cornea with instruments from our basic set (see Chapter 7) and thus to use an optical zone marker followed by spatula-style markers for the length of the incision. An alternative is to use a very small (2–3 mm) optical zone marker to indicate the length of the incision.

When long arcuate incisions are contemplated, the use of an optical zone marker combined with a 6 or 8 radial incision marker (used in radial keratotomy) can conveniently provide angular markings. Additionally, the appropriate location of the compression sutures, if needed, are indicated on the circumference of the optical zone.

The proper choice of the crystalline knife and appropriate preoperative calibration are discussed in Chapter 8. Pachymetry is performed in the appropriate location to obtain the proper setting for the knife. The knife should be set at 100% of the pachymetry. For short transverse incisions, a trifacet ultra-thin diamond knife set in an Osher-style handle has proved to be an effective means to cut a uniform depth along the entire incision, with excellent visualization. For long arcuate incisions, a 30-degree double-cutting ultra-thin diamond knife in the same Osher handle allows convenient visualization and facilitates the creation of curved incisions.

As discussed in Chapter 7, the most appropriate device to stabilize the globe for transverse and arcuate incisions is the ring-style fixation device. This provides excellent torsional stability, and in addition is the most comfortable for the patient. Anesthesia is accomplished by topical means that can be augmented throughout the procedure. Although these surgical interventions take little time, the cornea should be kept moist throughout the procedure to prevent thinning of the cornea by desiccation.

Prior to the procedure, the cooperative adult patient should be seated vertically and asked to fixate on a distant object. Using a needle, the vertical axis should be marked by means of a small scratch at the 6-o'clock position. This technique provides a simple reference when the surgery is in progress and provides a check on proper axis identification with a Mendez gauge. It is not uncommon to observe significant oblique muscle function resulting in eye torsion even if the patient is cooperating fully. The patient is often somewhat apprehensive concerning the surgery, and we have found it prudent to place a heparin cannula to administer 1 to 2 mg midazolam (Versed) prior to the procedure and augment it as necessary. Pilocarpine is used to constrict the pupil prior to surgery.

In the past, cataract removal has been associated with variable amounts of iatrogenically induced astigmatism (see Chapter 13). Today, with the advent of *small incision* cataract surgery involving phacoemulsification, scleral tunnel incisions, and horizontal or no suturing, astigmatically neutral cataract removal is the rule rather than the exception. If a cataract patient has a significant astigmatic error, the surgeon may consider performing an astigmatic procedure, such as relaxing incisions, at the time of the cataract removal. We discourage this approach for several practical reasons. First, the surgeon will not devote full attention to the astigmatic procedure, because the cataract removal is the primary operation. Second, determination of optical axis is complicated by dilation, the retrobulbar block, and the inability of the patient to actively participate. Finally, if the incisions are performed before the cataract removal, they may gape, limiting visualization of the cataract procedure. If performed after the cataract removal, the eye may be soft and incision depth suboptimal. Even if an appropriate astigmatic operation is performed, the possibility remains that the astigmatic axis or power may change after cataract surgery. For these reasons, we believe that astigmatic procedures should be performed only after successful cataract removal.

In the older patient wound healing often is suboptimal. Thus the first concern of the surgeon with a patient with excessive astigmatism after cataract removal should be evaluation of the healed wound with keratometry, photokeratometry, and slit-lamp examination. If *with the rule* astigmatism is identified, tight sutures may be cut or removed. If *against the rule* astigmatism is identified, the wound should be evaluated for dehiscence and possible wound repair. Only after these considerations have been fully explored should the surgeon consider incisional corrective procedures. In the older patient the minimal surgery having the least chance of overcorrection, should be performed. Thus linear transverse incisions should be kept short and lengthened only as necessary. Arcuate incisions should be kept at 60 degrees or less in patients 65 years and older, enhanced later, when required, with compression sutures and/or lengthening of the incisions. Buzard believes that, with few exceptions, patients older than 75 years should not undergo incisional astigmatic procedures but should have revision of the cataract wound.

The surgical techniques for correction of congenital and for iatrogenically induced astigmatism are essentially the same, and are discussed as one technique. The patient is prepared with a standard antibacterial preparation and draped with sterile towels. A locking lid speculum is used to maintain lid position. The Topcon fixation device (see Chapter 7) supplied with the microscope is most convenient. The optical zone is marked directly without marking the optical axis by means of optical zone markers with cross hairs. The location of the optical zone is verified by means of photokeratometry taken preoperatively and taped to the microscope. Preoperative keratometry and refraction are indicated on this same form to avoid confusion in the operating room (Plate 13–13). Using a graduated ring with the 90-degree axis placed against the mark left preoperatively on the cornea along the vertical meridian, the proper meridian of surgery is identified and marked. Currently, we do not use an axis marker as described in Chapter 7; however, this prevents errors and is a good practice for beginning surgeons. The axis of surgery is verified from the photokeratometry and keratometry sheet taped to the microscope (Plate 13–13).

For short transverse incisions, the length of the two incisions is marked with a spatula-style or an optical zone marker. For long arcuate incisions, we use a six-zone radial incision marker with one set of marks parallel to the flat axis, at the location of the compression sutures. This provides an indication for 60° arcuate incisions that can be lengthened or shortened depending on astigmatic error.

Incisions are created using a ring-type device for fixation of the globe and Osher-style knife handles fitted with appropriate diamond blades as previously discussed. The knife is gently rocked in the incision to assure *square* ends and proper depth. Generally, cutting is performed in the *front cutting* configuration of the knife to allow proper visualization and to achieve adequate depth. Irrigation of the incisions with a cannula allows verification of extent and depth of the incisions.

For the larger astigmatic errors (greater than 3 D) using arcuate incisions, constant attention to the operative keratometry reflex allows interactive control of the operation. If inadequate correction is achieved after the placement of the arcuate incisions, compression sutures should be placed along the flat axis to augment the effect. Each suture should be placed and tied temporarily with a slipknot to allow sequential adjustment of the suture tension prior to locking the knots. As always, the knots should be buried and a slight overcorrection should be seen on operative keratometry.

Postoperatively, the pupil is dilated using one drop of 10% phenylephrine (Neo-synephrine) and 1% cyclopentolate (Cyclogyl). In the older pa-

Plate 13–13.

DATE		SURGERY SCHEDULING		

NAME	ACCT
DATE OF BIRTH	AGE

DATE SCHEDULED	TIME	EYE

PREVIOUS RK IN EYE SCHEDULED	DATE	PREVIOUS CE IN EYE SCHEDULED	DATE

IF A PREVIOUS PK HAS BEEN DONE YOU ARE USING THE WRONG FORM
NO ANESTHESIOLOGIST / NO ASSISTANT / REGULAR CONSENT REQUIRED

PRE-SURGICAL TESTING

PHOTOKERATOMETRY	EYE	OD	OS	OU

KERATOMETRY	
OD	VA oc
OS	VA oc

MANIFEST	
OD	VA cc
OS	VA cc

CELL COUNT	
OD	OS

SURGERY

OPTICAL ZONE	Number of Cuts	BLADE DEPTH
PACHYMETRY		NOTES

Preoperative refractive workup sheet used by Buzard in operating room, showing preoperative photokeratometry, refraction, and keratometry.

tients, the eye is patched with an antibiotic ointment, and in the younger patients, a disposable contact lens is used with an antibiotic steroid drop and artificial tears hourly to control postoperative pain and accelerate visual rehabilitation. As we have previously discussed, the disposable soft contact lens provides relief of pain through separation of the action of the lid on the cornea and provides excellent appositional protection of the anterior corneal surface. For both of these reasons and for rapid visual rehabilitation, the use of these lenses can reduce patient apprehension concerning refractive surgical procedures.

NOMOGRAMS

Transverse and arcuate keratotomies are by their nature more variable in effect than radial incisions, as we have emphasized in this chapter. Nevertheless, rough guidelines are useful (Plate 13–14). These guidelines are formulated for the most frequent applications of the procedures, and although few nomograms exist for these procedures, both Thornton and Lindstrom have made their personal nomograms available through Chiron. In general, these nomograms agree with the numbers presented here, although differences appear in the age modifier, which we believe is smaller in good wound healing, and in terms of preferred operations. The surgeon should be aware of available nomograms but should choose only one to follow to avoid problems related to assumptions and techniques built into the particular nomogram. As the surgeon develops his or her technique with one of these nomograms, individual variability will demand a personalized nomogram.

We have chosen two primary age groups, 30 and 65 years old, with age modifiers of approximately 1.5% per year. Thus an operation that provides 2 D of effect in a 30-year-old patient will provide approximately 3 D of effect in a 65-year-old patient, assuming normal wound healing. The nomogram shows steps of 0.5 mm to the 6-mm optical zone, then steps to a 7-mm optical zone. The effect of incisions is greatest near the 5-mm optical zone, and falls nonlinearly past the 6-mm optical zone. Thus the appropriate next location at which to add incisions is the 7-mm optical zone (as indicated in the nomogram), not the 6.5-mm optical zone.

Short, transverse keratotomies are a practical procedure for less than 3 D of corneal astigmatism. For more than 3 D, long arcuate incisions should be the procedure of choice, again modified by considerations of age. For more than 4 D, Troutman compression sutures will allow even larger corrections with the interactive tightening of the compression sutures described previously. Incisions more than 60 degrees are used only in exceptional circumstances in older patients. We prefer to rely on compression sutures for additional effect. A majority of the cataract patients with astigmatism can be corrected with short transverse incisions because

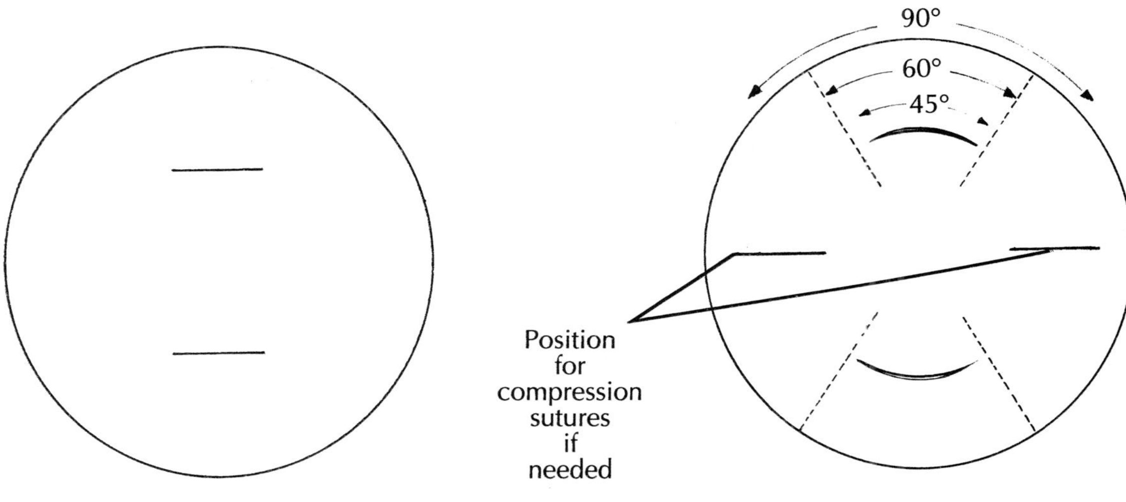

T-cuts		Arcuate Incisions	
	(All values approximate)		
Incision Length 2.0–2.5 mm		Optical Zone −7.0 mm	
30 Years Old		30 Years Old	
Optical Zone	Effect in Diopters	Incision Length	Effect in Diopters*
5.0 mm	2.0	45 Degrees	2.0
5.5 mm	1.5	60 Degrees	3.0
6.0 mm	1.0	90 Degrees	4.0
65 Years Old†		65 Years Old†	
Optical Zone	Effect in Diopters	Incision Length	Effect in Diopters*
5.0 mm	3.0	45 Degrees	3.0
5.5 mm	2.25	60 Degrees	4.5
6.0 mm	1.5	90 Degrees	6.0‡
7.0 mm	1.0		

*Add compression sutures for larger astigmatic corrections.
†Age modification factor approximately 1.5% per year calculated from 30-year-old parameters.
‡Not recommended.

Buzard nomogram for short transverse and long arcuate incisions.

we can obtain up to 3 D in this age group. For younger patients, only about 2 D of correction can be obtained with short transverse incisions, and long arcuate incisions are more common in this age group. Both short transverse and arcuate incisions can be lengthened or deepened if undercorrection occurs. For example, to obtain 2 D of astigmatic correction in a 65-year-old patient, perform T-cut incisions at a 6-mm optical zone. If undercorrection results, extend or deepen the incisions later. Radial keratotomy provides a situation in which slightly more effect can be obtained with the use of short transverse incisions, as we will discuss later.

Astigmatic errors above 3 D should always be viewed in the context of progressive corneal ectasias, such as keratoconus. Astigmatism correcting refractive procedures are *not* designed to be used in unstable corneas, and their inadvertent application in these situations can lead to long-term corneal instability as the corneal ectasia progresses. For large astigmatic errors, particularly in the presence of myopia, careful evaluation of corneal topography photokeratometry and keratometry in addition to pachymetry must be performed.

SUMMARY

Transverse and arcuate incisions for the treatment of postcataract and congenital astigmatism are a safe and effective means of treatment. They can reduce glare, distortion, and improve both corrected and uncorrected visual acuity. Although the techniques are simple, many factors enter into a safe and appropriate application. In this chapter, we have outlined many of these potential problems and have suggested our approach based on previous clinical experience and laboratory evaluations. Because congenital and post-cataract astigmatism in small to moderate amounts is a common problem, we believe they represent an excellent point to begin a refractive career. The operations described here are forgiving and can provide both the patient and surgeon with tremendous satisfaction. The same principles can be applied to other refractive procedures because the surgery will always involve determination of optical axis and optical zone and the precise surgical manipulation of the cornea.

Pathophysiology and Prevention of Astigmatism Secondary to Penetrating Keratoplasty

Before discussing the prevention of astigmatism resulting from penetrating keratoplasty, it is first necessary to understand the forces at work in the cornea. These tend to maintain its curvatures or resist or assist any attempt at their modification. Returning to the tenets and principles outlined in chapters 1 and 3, before attempting a primary or secondary intervention, the surgeon should carefully examine the cornea with particular attention to the integrity of the corneal optical ring. If this ring has been damaged by previous surgery, trauma, or disease, it will be necessary to compensate for the involved sector at primary surgery or to anticipate the necessity for secondary correction. The peripheral support zone internal to the optical ring must be similarly evaluated. A thinned, thickened, or vascular sector will tend to influence postoperative graft curvatures. If the anterior reflective surface is of good quality, clinical keratometry will quantify not only optical zone curvature but whether a corneal ametropia is present. Photokeratoscopy and, if available, computerized corneal topographic analysis will indicate peripheral distortions that may affect graft curvature. When such information is difficult to obtain from the pathologic eye and the fellow eye is normal, its measurement can indirectly indicate the probable optical state of the involved cornea prior to the onset of the pathology or trauma mandating the keratoplasty.

Some idea of relative corneal thickness can be obtained with the biomicroscope and more exactly with optical or ultrasonic pachymetry. Thinned sectors of the cornea tend to induce steepening in the affected meridian, whereas thicker wound profiles tend to better maintain normal curvatures or become flatter. In some instances when the pathologic cornea is flatter or steeper than the normal fellow cornea, a larger or smaller diameter corneal button may be indicated to better approximate the normal corneal curvature in the healed graft.

Whether the cornea is incised circumferentially or in sector, as the wound deepens, the anterior corneal edges tend to fall away from the knife edge as it forms an increasingly deep V shape. In a circumferential trephine incision, the internal cornea tends to bulge forward, steepening as the incision deepens, inducing undercutting of the recipient (see Plate 8–10,C). The optical corneal ring retains its diameter and circumference as does the secondary ring, formed at the level of the incision, as demonstrated by the guy wires at these two levels in the illustration. This is prevented when a suction trephine with an obturator, such as the Krumeich and Hanna instruments, is used, as this tends to maintain the central cornea in the same plane and curvature while the peripheral cut is completed. This undercutting routinely occurs with the Barron trephine or a manual trephine without an obturator and can induce astigmatism from the defective recipient wound profile.

Although it is important to measure corneal parameters preoperatively, because of the inherent limitations of our present mechanical surgical armamentarium, such observations are often only mental exercises. Attempts to predict, even qualitatively, the astigmatism that will be induced by keratoplasty, let alone to devise a means to compensate for it at the primary surgery, remain disappointing. Under these circumstances, the best approach is to use a standard primary technique that gives the least induced average astigmatism across a broad range of pathology. Essential to this technique is the creation of a full-thickness scar that, when necessary, can be modified predictably to effect correction of any residual astigmatic, spherical, or compound errors.

Therefore, in this chapter, the first emphasis will be on prevention, detailing a standard operative procedure, which, in our hands, meets the above criteria, is applicable to any penetrating keratoplasty, phakic or aphakic of whatever pathology, and assures a firm, full-thickness scar that can be manipulated predictably in the event an excessive astigmatic or spherical error should occur after an otherwise successful clear graft. In chapter 15, we present the several procedures that are used to secondarily correct the astigmatic and spherical residuals. It is as important for the surgeon to be familiar with these secondary techniques as it is for the patients who are to undergo penetrating keratoplasty to understand the limitations of the primary procedure and the probability that astigmatism may limit their optical result. The patients must also be aware that effective secondary procedures exist to correct the almost certain residual ametropia. The surgeon must avoid the mind-set that because these corrective procedures do not give uniform and perfect results, they should be avoided. The patient who is informed that secondary surgery is a probability will be better able to accept a less than perfect primary postoperative result and any indicated secondary corrective procedure. Although when these procedures were introduced it was our practice not to secondarily correct astigmatism of less than 5 D, the informed patient not only better accepts but also frequently requests secondary correction of 2 or 3 D of astigmatism. These are often our most satisfied patients, as they can be more accurately corrected and have more stable results than patients with higher degrees of astigmatism.

STANDARD PENETRATING KERATOPLASTY TECHNIQUE: DONOR AND RECIPIENT PREPARATION

To be useful, a standardized procedure should embody principles applicable to any number of individual approaches. No matter what standard technique is adopted, first and foremost, it must result in a firm full-thickness scar. This can be achieved only by close attention to vertical as well as horizontal apposition of well-formed graft to recipient edges.

Exposure and Fixation

Exposure of the eye should be effected in such a way that the arms of the speculum do not exert unequal pressure on the globe, which can affect the regularity of manual trephination. The Barraquer open light-wire speculum has been consistently effective in our hands. When manual trephination is to be used, a ring support of the globe should be used. The suture fixation of the ring must be balanced to prevent inducing a sector distortion. A 15 mm Pierse scleral strap fixated with a continuous 6-0 or 7-0 silk suture armed by a C-6 side-cutting spatula needle (Ethicon) provides excellent stabilization just distal to the corneal optical ring. The loosely tied continuous suture prevents ring collapse and sector corneal distortion during trephination.

When using a suction trephine such as the Krumeich or Hanna, placement of a corneal ring is difficult or impossible. When recipient trephination is complete, a stabilizing corneal ring is virtually unnecessary.

Trephination of Recipient

Before trephination of the donor or recipient is attempted with any technique, the trephine sizes to be used must be selected and the blade edges inspected under the surgical microscope. If there are any irregularities or edge defects, the trephine blade should be discarded.

Selection of Donor-Recipient Diameters

When manual trephination is being performed and the donor cornea is cut posteriorly by a punch set, an 8.0 mm trephine is used to cut the recipient, and an 8.2 or 8.25 mm trephine is used to prepare the donor button. When the recipient cornea is significantly flatter than the cornea of the normal fellow eye, a larger diameter donor button (0.5 mm to 1.0 mm) difference may be chosen. In normally curved corneas and in keratoconus, a 0.2 mm larger diameter donor button averages 43 D postoperatively in our hands. Corneas, on average, become flatter when donor and recipient of the same diameter are used. Donor buttons that are smaller than the recipient diameter can induce wound problems, irregular or excessive astigmatism, and glaucoma.

The major difficulty in using manual recipient trephination is that of maintaining verticality while avoiding distortion and undercutting from excessive pressure. This problem can be minimized by the use of a lightweight, narrow-diameter trephine holder that can be centered, unobscured by the handle, so that the corneal periphery can be observed outside the trephine blade. The trephine is supported by the index finger and twisted by the thumb and second finger. The only pressure exerted should be from the weight of the trephine, the index finger being used to steady and maintain centration and verticality of the trephine as the blade descends. The blade is rotated through at least 360 degrees before being reversed to cut more evenly around the circumference. The blade is advanced until fluid escapes around the edge of the blade. Any remaining posterior lamella is trimmed with fine curved Troutman keratoplasty scissors.

These scissors have blades of equal length. The lower blade cuts inside the curvature of the upper blade to minimize shelving of the posterior lip of the incision. The scissors must be held vertical to the iris plane, slightly overcorrected from the corneal plane to avoid undercutting the cornea or inducing a shelf. A shelf, particularly in a thinner recipient, displaces the donor button forward, inducing corneal myopia. If a shelf is inadvertently created, it should be excised. However, should trephination produce sloping or irregular cuts, these are usually better left alone. Although such cutting errors can be anticipated to induce a higher than average astigmatism, any attempt to rectify them by scissors excision may cause more severe irregularities. If the disparate edges are allowed to heal with firm full-thickness apposition, any residuals can be dealt with secondarily.

Parel (1988) has shown that manual trephination performed as we have described can produce graft and recipient edges almost as regular as some corneal suction cutting sets. An exception is the Barron suction trephine and its predecessor the Hessberg-Barron trephine (see Chapter 7). He has shown that this instrument can cause severe undercutting of the recipient cornea, making it virtually impossible to accurately align the shelved recipient edge to the vertical edge of a punch-cut donor button. When poor edge matching is combined with superficial suturing, the incidence of both spherical ametropia and astigmatism are increased and become more difficult to correct predictably at a second procedure.

Cutting Donor and Recipient With Suction Trephine Sets

Parel has shown that the best donor and recipient match is obtained when both donor and recipient have been cut with one of the suction fixated cutting sets designed for this purpose by Hanna and Krumeich (see Chapter 7). With the Krumeich set, both the donor and recipient corneas are cut from anteriorly using the same diameter trephine blade. The donor is cut using an artificial anterior chamber, and the recipient is cut using a specially designed suction unit, both allowing full penetration of the blade. Because scissors are not required to complete the cut, better matching edges are obtained.

With the Hanna system, the recipient is cut using a suction-fixated trephine that also permits full penetration (see Plates 14–4 and 14–5). The donor is cut with a piston punch unit that incorporates a suction in its base to fixate the donor cornea (see Plate 14–6). Hanna has introduced (1991) an artificial anterior chamber that allows his trephine unit to be used for cutting the donor (not illustrated). At this writing we have not had the opportunity to evaluate it. It does have the advantage that multiple blade diameters from 6 mm to 9.5 mm are available and can be used interchangeably.

Cutting Donor Cornea

The blade and obturator are fitted to the trephine assembly with the micrometric advancing screw fully retracted (see Plate 7–16). The screw and the obturator should never be coated with sodium hyaluronate (Healon), because it will harden and freeze the mechanism. The obturator is aligned to and pressed into the shaft of the trephine holder, concave side down, and seated flush. The 8 mm trephine blade, (standard manual type: Wick, Katina), having been carefully inspected for the quality of its edge, is slid onto the shaft of the trephine holder and pressed flush. Under microscopic control, using the micrometric adjusting screw, the blade edge is advanced to be level to the end of the shaft. The shaft assembly is inserted into the blade-shaft holder and the split ring expander is retracted to lock the assembly in the zero cutting position (see Plate 7–17).

The artificial anterior chamber is fitted with a three-way stopcock to which are also attached an IV set connected to a bottle of balanced salt solution (BSS) and a 5 mL syringe filled with BSS (see Plates 7–14, 7–15). With the IV bottle suspended 25 inches above the anterior chamber, the stopcock is opened to displace all air from the unit. The stopcock is then turned to the 5 mL syringe, blocking off the IV set. Any residual air is evacuated with the syringe. A donor cornea with an approximately 15 mm diameter rim is coated on its internal surface with sodium hyaluronate, held vertically to the anterior chamber, and then gradually allowed to seat itself over the center of the anterior chamber unit as the BSS-filled syringe displaces any air bubbles from behind it. When it is seated loosely, it is centered over the anterior chamber. Excess BSS is removed, and the primary fixating ring is seated over it, aligned by the two holes provided on either side of the face of the chamber. The threaded secondary fixation ring is then screwed down to fix the cornea to the anterior chamber base with a watertight seal. The stopcock is turned to open the IV set. When pressure equilibrium is reached the IV tube is clamped off with a mosquito clamp. *The progressive clamp supplied with the set should never be used to clamp off the set, because it will increase the pressure in the line as it is pushed down to squeeze the tube closed.* The previously assembled trephine is fitted into the dovetail on the top of the secondary fixation ring and locked in place. Occasionally the eye bank donor cornea scleral rim will be too wide to fit within the secondary fixation ring, and it can be trimmed to an exact diameter using the 15-mm trephine supplied with the Krumeich set (see Plate 7–20). If persistent leaking around a too small rim occurs, the piston punch set should be used alternatively.

The advancing screw of the trephine handle is advanced one mark, approximately 0.05 mm, and a complete turn of the trephine is made manually. This process is repeated successively until the trephine blade has been fully advanced. The trephine holder is released from the dovetail and the blade retracted. The completely cut-through button will be found resting against the obturator. Rarely, a lamella of Descemet's membrane may be present in a small sector, which can be readily cut with corneal scissors.

The Krumeich trephine has the advantage of using a disposable blade of standard manufacture. Occasionally, a blade will be slightly short and should be moved closer to the end of the trephine holder before advancing the screw to set the blade flush at zero. At this level the blade can be fully extended to cut through the donor cornea in every instance. This caution is true also when setting up the trephine to cut the recipient cornea. The same 8.0 mm blade used for the donor cornea may be used for the recipient after it has been inspected and zero set.

Cutting Recipient Cornea

The dovetailed recipient suction cup is screwed onto its handle firmly but without excessive torsion, because the joint fixing the screw to the suction cup can be fractured (see Plate 7–18). A rigid-walled flexible tube attaches the handle to a suction unit, which is adjusted to approximately 18 psi or 800 mbars. The suction head is then inserted between the lids. Sometimes, it may be difficult to insert this unit between a narrow lid aperture; however, once the suction is applied, the globe can be lifted forward between the lids without distorting the cornea (Plate 14–1). It is important not to press backward with the suction ring against the eye but always to lift it away between the lids. When the suction unit is in place on the wetted cornea, centered on the pupil, suction is applied using the foot control. Krumeich advises that the suction be activated by using the foot control while an assistant crimps the tube. When the ring is in position the tube is released, eliminating the delay before adhesion. The gauge of the suction unit should indicate 800 mbars. The eye, held firmly in the suction unit, is elevated between the lids to the position for the trephine cutting assembly to be locked in the dovetail.

It is important that the suction cup be carefully inspected before and cleaned immediately after each use. If fouled, suction will be incomplete and cutting errors will occur.

The trephine is placed in the suction dovetail, inserting the trephine dovetail proximal to the surgeon and then locking it in place against the lower end of the suction shaft (Plate 14–2,A,B). With the trephine in place, the micrometric screw is advanced successively one mark (0.05 mm) at a time and rotated a full 360 degrees until its limit of advancement is reached (Plate 14–3). Because the anterior chamber is retained, the

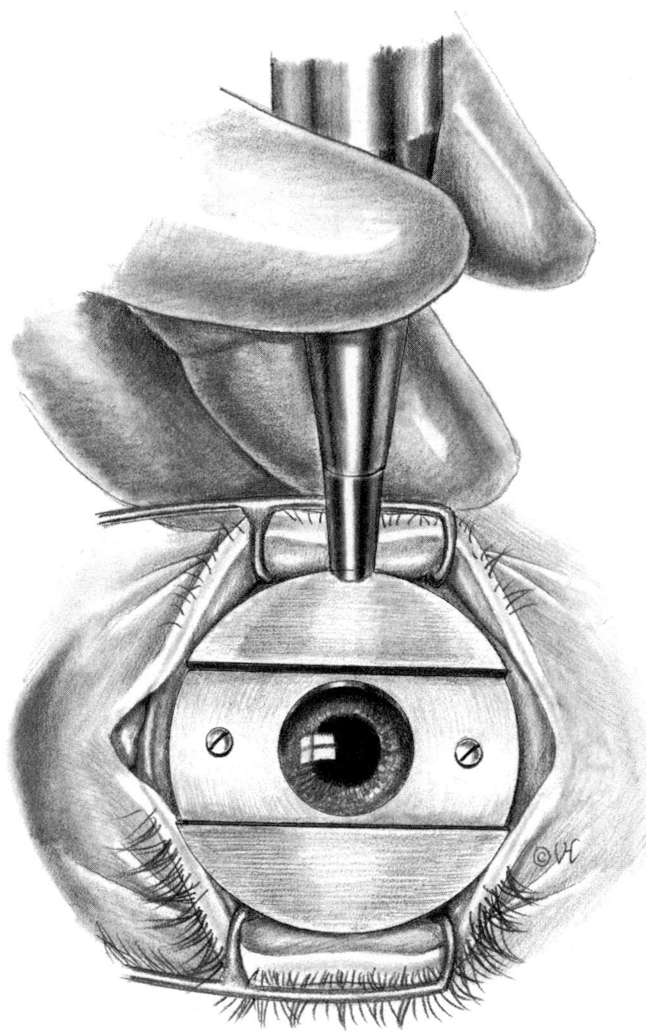

Krumeich recipient suction dovetail in place, elevated between lids for insertion of trephine.

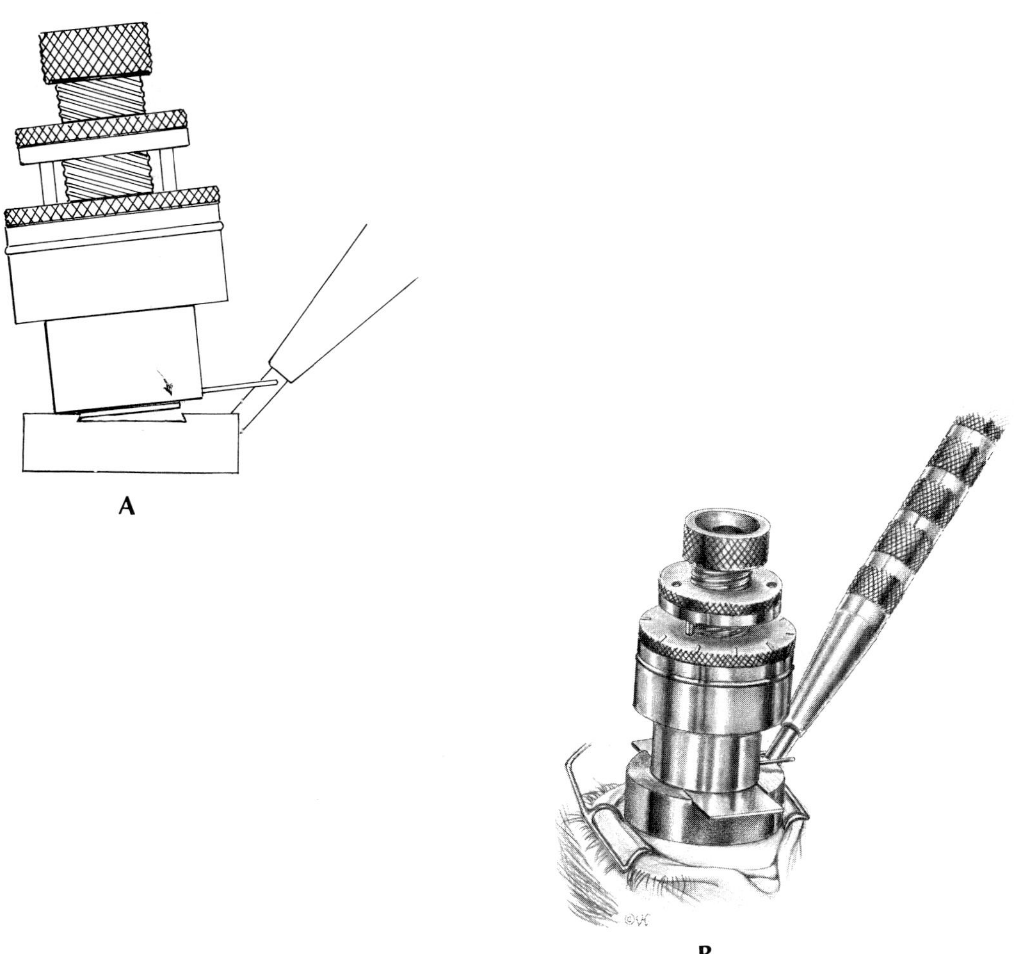

A, Krumeich trephine being snapped into place in recipient suction dovetail. **B,** trephine locked in suction dovetail on recipient cornea.

cornea can be cut in full thickness around its circumference. If, during cutting, aqueous humor is seen to leak into the internal shaft of the obturator, the suction must be released and the trephine suction cup assembly lifted away. In an aphakic or pseudophakic eye, the cornea should be only partially penetrated, not more than 10 marks, because the chamber seems to be more readily lost in these eyes. Especially with an anterior chamber lens, the implant haptic can displace, to cause premature loss of the anterior chamber.

When the trephine blade has achieved partial or full penetration, the suction is released and the pressure allowed to equalize. The entire assembly is then carefully removed from between the lids. When the cornea is fully penetrated, the button is retained in the barrel of the trephine. When partially penetrated and the cut is completed with scissors, care must be taken not to create shelving.

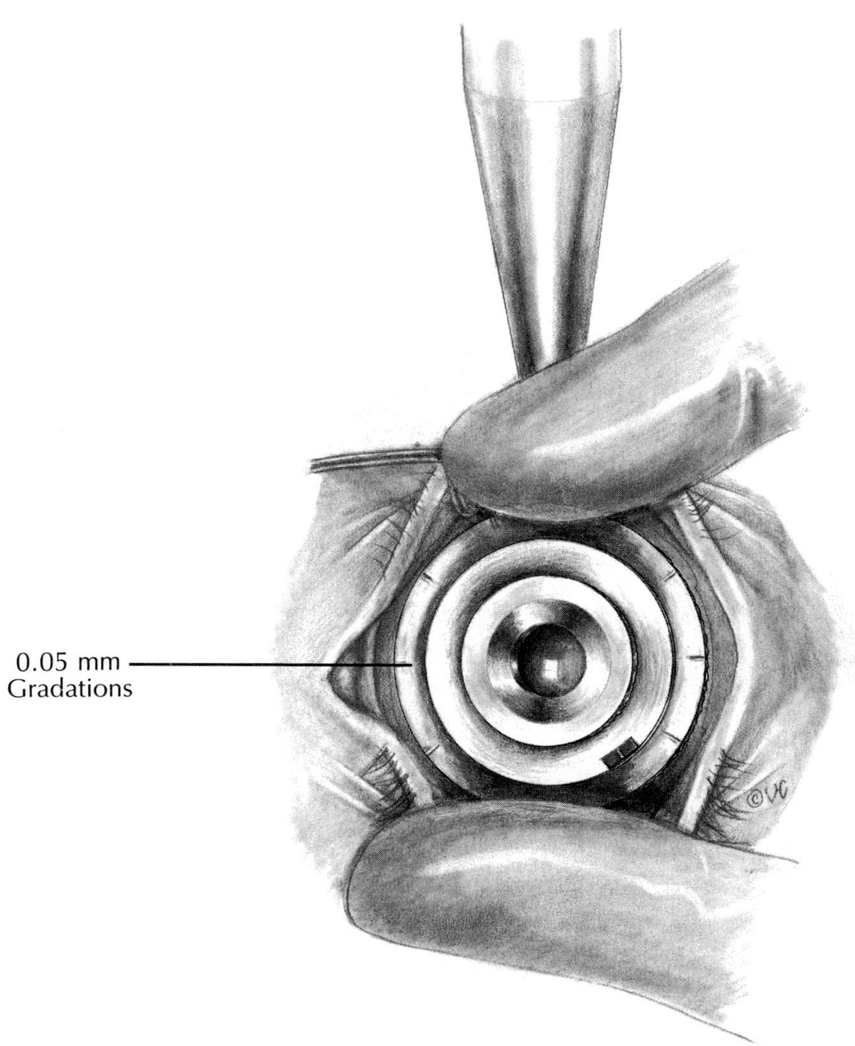

Surgeon's view of trephine showing micrometer adjusting screw, 0.05-mm gradations.

Pathophysiology and Prevention of Astigmatism Secondary to Penetrating Keratoplasty   **359**

USE OF HANNA SUCTION TREPHINE SET
Cutting Recipient Cornea

The Hanna trephine set also uses suction to permit circumferential penetration of the recipient (Plate 14–4). Its suction cone is fixed by a foot-controlled motor-driven suction device at 600 mm Hg (800 mbar). The cone is fitted internally with a trephine holding device that can be set to a preselected depth by means of an adjustable ratcheted ring. The trephine holder rotates within the suction cone. The blade is driven into the cornea by means of a knurled knob projecting from the top of the cone, angulated so that the surgeon can observe the progress of the trephination through the central internal cone-shaped opening in the trephine holder.

This instrument has the advantage to accept blades of different diameters from 6.0 to 9.5 mm, which also may be used if the corneal punch that is supplied with the unit is used for the preparation of the donor button. The precision-manufactured disposable blades are precisely fitted in a slotted holder at the base of the cutter and locked in place by a bezel, which turns to firmly fix the haptics, positioning the trephine blade in the cutting position. With the blade in the cutting position, the angled knurled knob is retracted to its stop, the zero position. It is then lifted slightly from its seated position and turned to rest at right angles to its slot. The depth selected for the particular trephination is then set with a special knurled tool in 12 0.1-mm increments. In practice, these increments approximate 0.05 mm. In the usual cornea full penetration can be achieved with a setting of 10, or 1.0 mm. The internal mechanism of the trephine is designed in such a way that the blade descends gradually to the preset depth and then continues to turn without further penetration to deepen the cut evenly to completion.

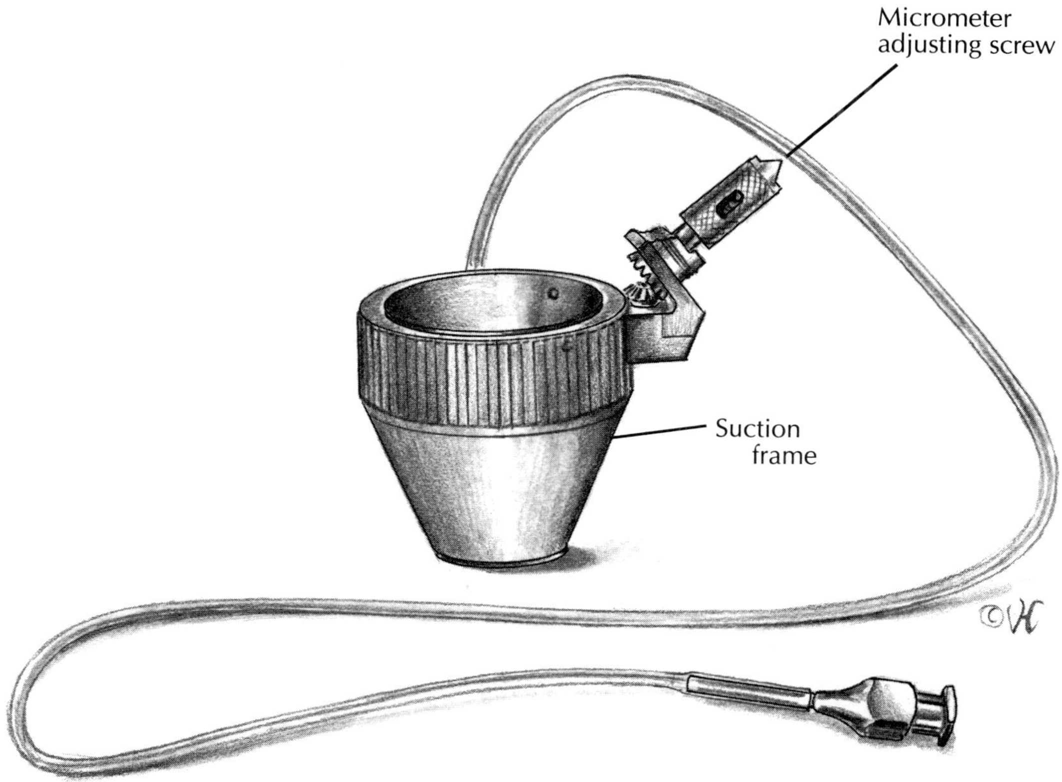

Plate 14–4.

Hanna suction trephine, micrometer adjusting screw, suction tube.

To use the trephine, the surgeon first marks the center of the cornea with a pointed instrument and a dye, for example, methylene blue. Then the trephine is centered with its sighting device on the wetted recipient cornea so that the central hole of its obturator coincides to the mark (Plate 14–5). Suction is applied through a polypropylene tubing to the suction cone. The surgeon then turns the knurled knob to full penetration, at which level a slight decrease in resistance will be felt. The cut may be completed at depth by turning the knob two or three 360-degree rotations. Should aqueous be seen, the suction is released and the cone removed. In most instances, the cornea will be completely cut through, but if a small tag of Descemet's membrane remains, it is cut with corneal scissors.

Suction is verified by lifting the assembly slightly, observing the corneal adhesion, and the suction reading is verified on the suction unit gauge. Suction can be applied by an on-off or a "dead man" foot switch; for safety, the latter is preferred. Although determination of anterior chamber depth is easier with the Hanna unit, it has a tendency to drift on the cornea, and centration must be maintained carefully.

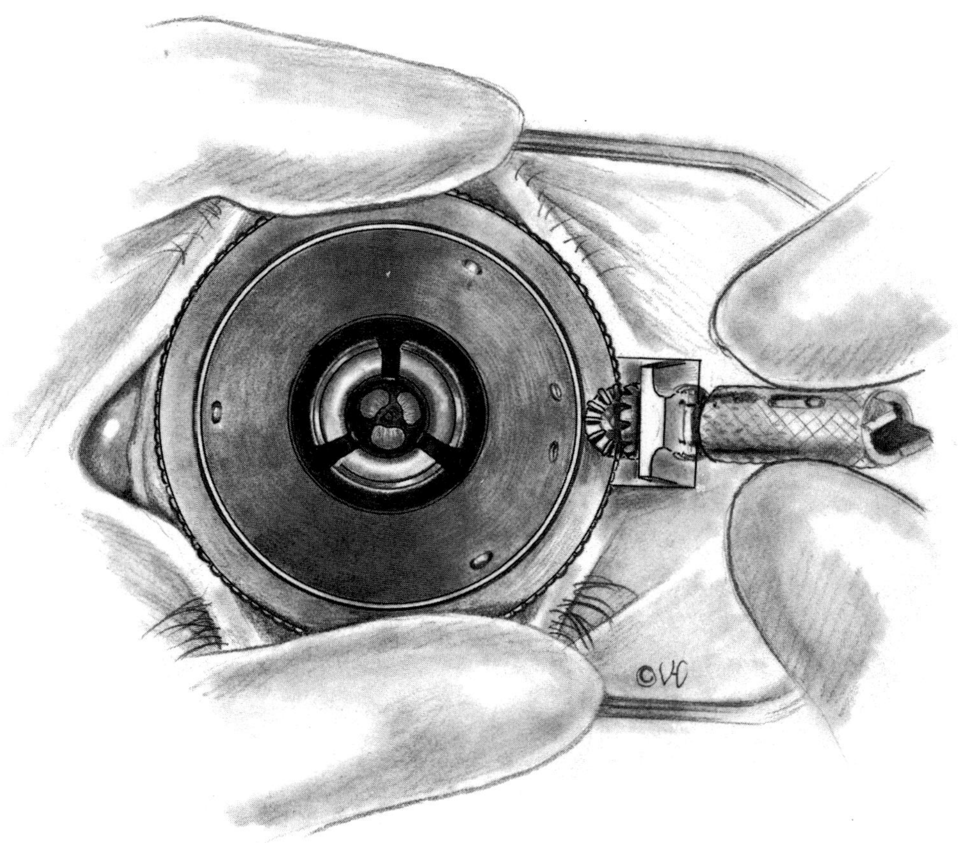

Surgeon's view: Sighting device centered on corneal mark, micrometer screw advanced to penetration.

Cutting Donor Cornea

With the original Hanna trephine set, the graft is cut from the donor cornea with a modified corneal punch (Plate 14–6). This corneal punch set has a cutting block with multiple tiny holes through which suction can be applied to the donor cornea to hold it securely in place during cutting. The cornea is placed convex side down on the cutting block, and suction is applied from either the suction unit or by a syringe through a polypropylene tube attached to the base. The external piston wall of the cutting unit is then screwed to the base, the central piston is inserted and allowed to rest on the cornea. Cutting pressure is applied to complete the cut. Parel (1988) has shown that this system produces superior donor buttons. This is probably as much due to the extremely sharp razor blade edge precision disposable trephines as to the suction system. Before the cut is performed, the blade of the selected diameter, usually 0.25 mm larger than that used for cutting the recipient, is fixed to a bezel at the base of the cutting piston that is identical to that used in the recipient cutting set. It is important before using either this unit or the recipient cutting set to carefully inspect the blade edge after it has been placed in the cutting frame because the delicate edge may have been damaged during manipulation.

Alternatively, Hanna (1991) has introduced an artificial anterior chamber that can be used in combination with the recipient trephine unit to cut the donor button. We have found this technique useful to prepare donor lamellar grafts, because of the wider range of available trephine diameters. We have not had sufficient experience at this writing to evaluate its use for penetrating keratoplasty.

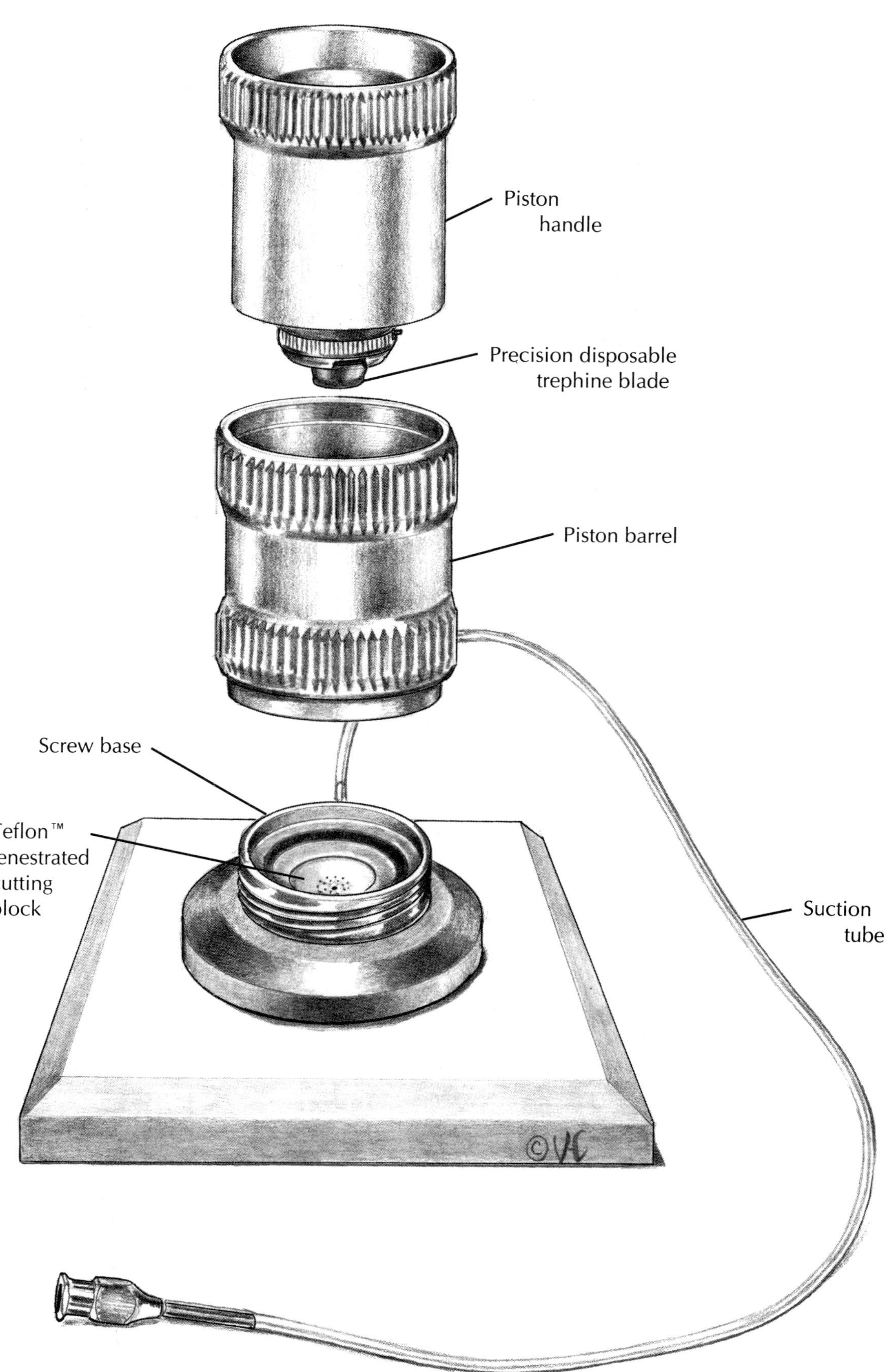

Hanna corneal punch: exploded view, note Teflon fenestrated cutting block and suction tube.

Cutting Recipient Cornea

This system has been recently redesigned and is now known only as the Barron trephine (Plate 14–7). It is essentially the same as its predecessor except for the addition of a marking device incorporated in the base. This marking device allows easier equidistant positioning of the interrupted or continuous suture bites preferred by the surgeon. Because this unit is disposable and relatively inexpensive, it has achieved a wide following among corneal surgeons, despite its well-known tendency to undercut the recipient cornea.

This device is simple to use. After it is removed from its sterile package, it is examined under the microscope and the spokes on the top of the blade assembly turned to align the edge of the blade with the inner wall of the vacuum chamber (zero position). The blade is then retracted three quarters of a revolution, which prevents loss of vacuum as it is set on the wetted corneal surface. One can observe the marking spokes of the new instrument as they surround the vacuum ring. The center of the cornea is marked with the gentian violet marking pen that is included with the set. The cross hairs of the unit are lined to the central mark, and the plunger of the suction syringe is pushed in as the trephine base is pressed against the cornea and released. After 30 seconds, the blade is lowered into the cornea by turning the spokes clockwise; each complete revolution equals 0.25 mm after the zero position is reached. *It is important not to penetrate the cornea with this set, because the iris may be damaged.* The incision is completed with a razor knife and keratoplasty scissors. At the completion of the trephine cut, the surface of the cornea is dried with a cellulose sponge and the radial impressions made by the trephine are marked with the pen provided in the set so that they may be used to position the suture placement from donor to recipient.

Cutting Donor Cornea

The donor cornea is cut with one of several donor piston cutting sets, for example, Troutman (1977) donor piston trephine set.

INTRAOCULAR LENS SURGERY AND PENETRATING KERATOPLASTY

One of the most frequently seen conditions requiring penetrating keratoplasty is pseudophakic keratopathy. Because this surgery is important to the refractive result, the technique for removal and replacement of the offending intraocular lens is important to the total surgery. The selection and technique for primary insertion of intraocular lenses is discussed in Chapter 12. Anterior chamber lenses, as in cataract surgery, should be

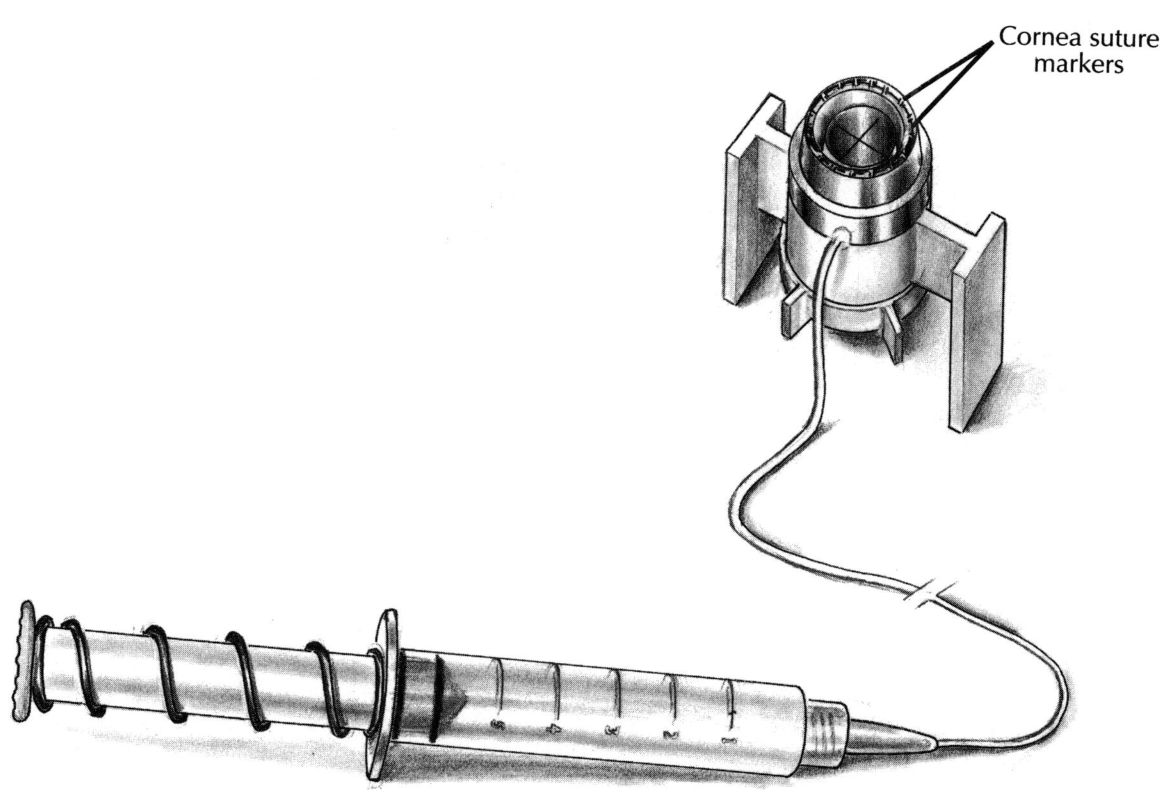

Barron trephine attached to spring-loaded suction trephine.

avoided when possible. With penetrating keratoplasty, though they may not always induce secondary pseudophakic keratopathy, they can be productive of postoperative astigmatism. Their stiff haptics distort the corneal ring, inducing flattening of the corneal curvature along the axis of the haptics as they impinge into the opposite angles. When an anterior chamber lens is present in an eye at the time of penetrating keratoplasty, it is particularly important to use the Krumeich or Hanna suction trephine to cut the recipient. Ovaling of the recipient from uncompensated haptic distortion is prevented because the suction holds the cornea in a block to minimize cutting distortions. An open loop posterior chamber lens fixated to the iris, or into the ciliary sulcus, does not induce astigmatism.

Removal of Offending Intraocular Lens

Several techniques are used for lens removal. The replacement technique depends on the presence or absence of capsular support. Prior to the surgical procedure, the surgeon needs to consider not only the surgical approach but the anticipated optical and functional vision result. Every attempt should be made to duplicate or normalize curvatures in the postoperative cornea. Using new and original A-scan data together with preoperative and postoperative refractive information, the power of the lens to be substituted intraoperatively can be calculated. The refractive calculation in the normal fellow eye, if present, can aid in this process. The range and standard deviation of the postoperative refractive result will not be as accurate as in a primary case, because the final corneal curvatures can differ from the curvature used in the lens calculations.

Removal of Closed Loop Lens

The no longer used closed loop anterior chamber lens now figures less prominently among the several types of anterior chamber lenses encountered during keratoplasty for pseudophakic keratopathy.

The closed loop single curved haptic lens, such as that of Leiske, is removed more readily than the several types with angular haptics or positioning holes. When the trephination is complete, the flexible haptics of these lenses will allow the optic to move into the recipient opening from posterior pressure, and vitreous may follow. Following anterior vitrectomy, fine sharp scissors, such as the Vaness type, are used to sever the polypropylene haptics at their four points of attachment to the optic, and the optic is removed (Plate 14–8,A). The haptics will almost always be found in a fibrovascular cocoon on one or both sides of the angle. Because they have a single curve, they are easily rotated out of the cocoon without disinserting the iris root (Plate 14–8,B). Use of two instruments—one to

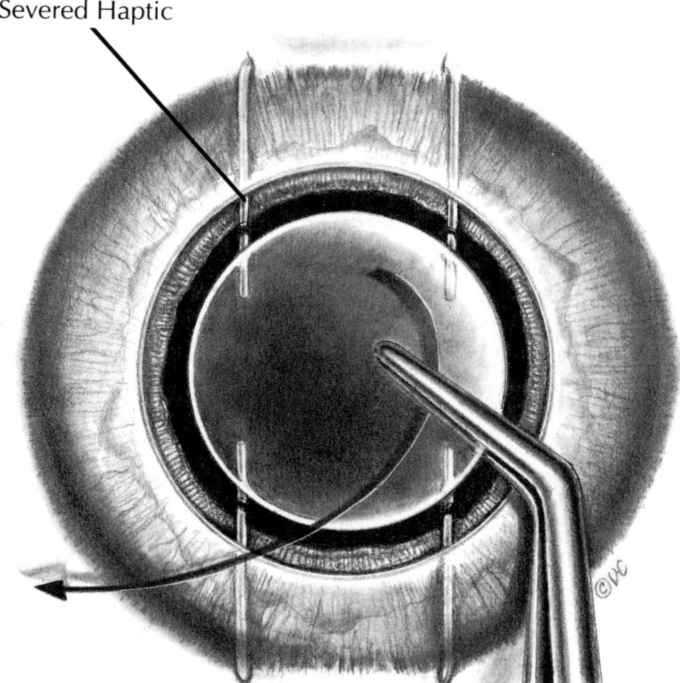

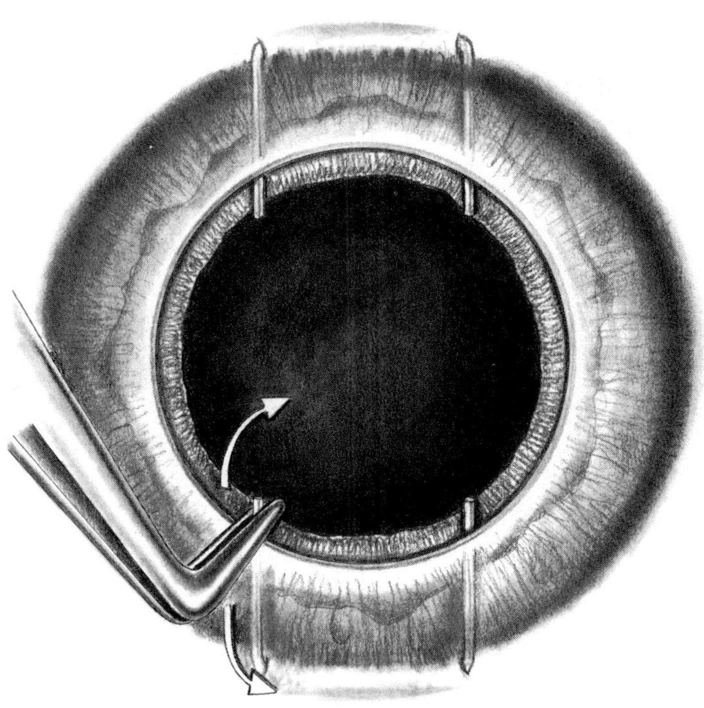

A, optic of closed loop intraocular lens removed after severing haptics. **B,** rotating haptic from fibrovascular cocoon.

stabilize and the other to manipulate—facilitates this maneuver. Occasionally, when the haptic has a projection or positioning hole, it may be necessary to leave a piece of haptic in the cocoon to avoid angle disinsertion and bleeding. When the haptics are made of methylmethacrylate, they tend to fragment as they are cut with the scissors. It is important to perform this maneuver under moderately high magnification so that any loose fragments can be visualized and removed.

Removal of Open Loop Lens

More commonly encountered is the Kelman-style open loop lens, which not only has multiple reversing curves but also dilations or holes in the ends of the haptics that firmly lock them in the angle. As with open loop lenses, the optic must be severed from the haptics before any attempt is made to remove them from the angle (Plate 14–9,A). When they are firmly fixated and cannot be removed without the probability of severe trauma, the visible haptic should be cut free and the portion trapped in the angle left in place (Plate 14–9,B). Often in these eyes one haptic will be fixed in the angle and the other free, and removal may be attempted by grasping the entire lens. This should be avoided. One should always resect the trapped haptic from the optic before attempting its removal of the trapped haptic(s). These lenses often create ovaling of the recipient opening caused by tension of the semirigid lens across the anterior segment, which distorts the optical corneal ring. On their removal, the optical ring will return to its normal circular shape if the recipient has been cut with either the Hanna or Krumeich trephine. Ovaling of the recipient may persist after the anterior chamber lens removal if manual trephination has been used, and excessive astigmatism may result.

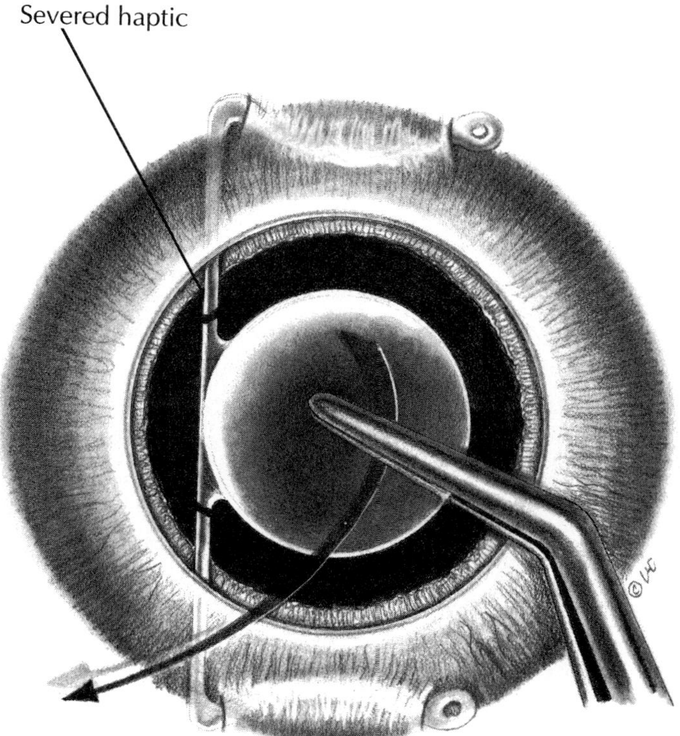

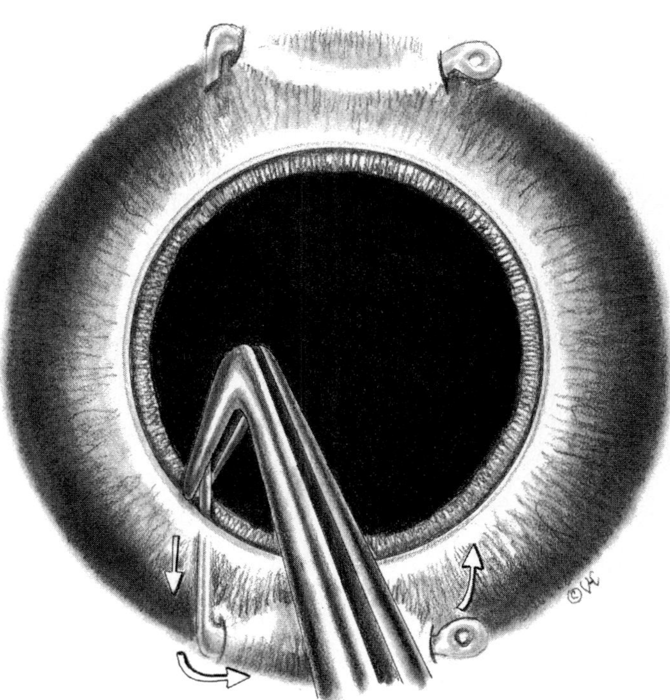

A, optic being removed after severing from angular haptics of Kelman-style intraocular lens. **B,** inverse removal of angular haptic. Second haptic left in place because of danger of hemorrhage.

Pathophysiology and Prevention of Astigmatism Secondary to Penetrating Keratoplasty **371**

Removal of Posterior Chamber Lens

Rarely, a posterior chamber lens will be malpositioned or of inappropriate power and needs to be removed at the time of keratoplasty. In these instances, the keratopathy is more likely to be from the primary surgical procedure rather than related directly to the implant. Nevertheless, it is better to remove and replace the offending lens, especially when of inappropriate power, than to try to reposition it because it is common for the lens to spring back into its eccentric position. To remove a posterior chamber lens, an attempt is made to rotate the severed haptics out of the capsular cocoons (Plate 14–10,A,B). If resistance is met, as usually is the case with capsulorhexis, the trapped haptics are left in place. Care must be taken not to dislocate the posterior capsule because it will be important for support of the replacement lens. If this threatens, the visible portion of the haptic is resected and the peripheral portion is allowed to remain embedded in the capsule.

Preparation for Insertion of Posterior Chamber Intraocular Lens

The surgeon's job is considerably simplified when the peripheral posterior capsule can be left intact for a sulcus fixation, and particularly if a posterior capsulotomy or a capsulectomy has not been performed. Often, however, the iris may be adherent to the posterior capsule, and to center the replacement lens, posterior synechiae must be carefully separated by spatulation, or better by severing them with fine scissors, for example, Galand scissors (see Chapter 8). The blade angle of the Galand scissors approximates the plane between the iris and the posterior capsule, facilitating such dissection. If vitreous is present, an anterior vitrectomy should be performed to allow the capsule to fall away from the iris as the synechiotomy is performed. An intraocular lens with narrower haptics (e.g., Shearing style) will better avoid residual synechiae as it is slid into the prepared tract and centered. In the face of extensive posterior synechiae, a smaller diameter lens or an oval-shaped lens should be used.

Insertion of Posterior Chamber Intraocular Lenses in Absence of Posterior Capsule

In the event of fragmentation or absence of the posterior capsule, an anterior vitrectomy should be performed with the vitrectomy extending toward the vitreous base in the meridian where the lens is to be inserted. As a rule, the lens is inserted obliquely to avoid the iris or long ciliary vessels, whether it is fixated to the iris or into the ciliary sulcus. For fixation of an intraocular lens in the absence of capsular support, iris fixation is technically less time-consuming than sulcus fixation and has been shown

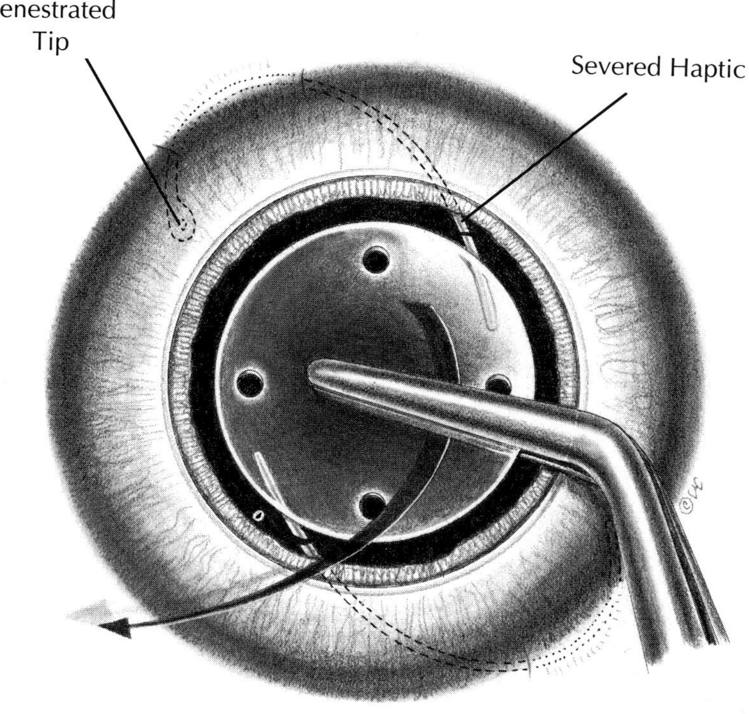

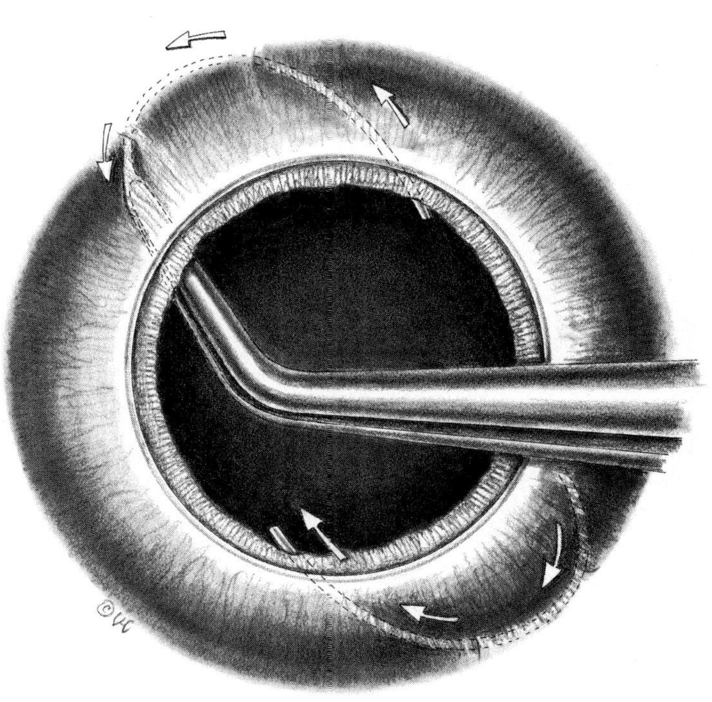

A, optic of posterior chamber intraocular lens severed from haptic and removed. **B,** inverse removal of fenestrated tip haptic.

to be as effective when appropriately used. Sulcus fixation must be used alternatively when the iris has been compromised to the point at which fixation to it is not possible. Several intraocular lenses have been designed with appropriately positioned suture fixation holes on their haptics that can be used for either technique (e.g., Troutman "lens for all reasons"; ORC) (Plates 14–11, 14–13, 14–14).

Iris Fixation

An anterior vitrectomy is performed to free a tract for the lens haptics so that they can reach and impinge the sulcus. BV100-4 needles double arming a 2-inch 10-0 polypropylene thread (Ethicon) are prefixed through the proximal hole in the haptic of an appropriately powered one-piece "lens for all reasons" (Plate 14–11,A). In the event that this type of lens is not available, the thread can be fixed with a cinch knot to the haptic of another one-piece lens style, approximately one third of the distance from the optic to the curve of the haptic. The paired suture needles, separated by approximately 2 mm, are passed through the mid-periphery of the iris from behind. The paired sutures are positioned to opposite sides of the pupil in the oblique meridian. Single slipknot ties are fashioned in the respective paired fixation sutures. Then one haptic is slid under the iris into the sulcus, followed by the second haptic to the opposite side. The slipknots are brought down, and the sutures are lifted to bring the haptics forward against the posterior iris and into the sulcus (Plate 14–11,B and C). When the optic is centered, the drawn-up slipknots are locked with square knots and the suture ends are cut, leaving approximately 1 mm suture ends. A drop of sodium hyaluronate is placed on the anterior lens surface, and the standard keratoplasty corneal closure proceeds.

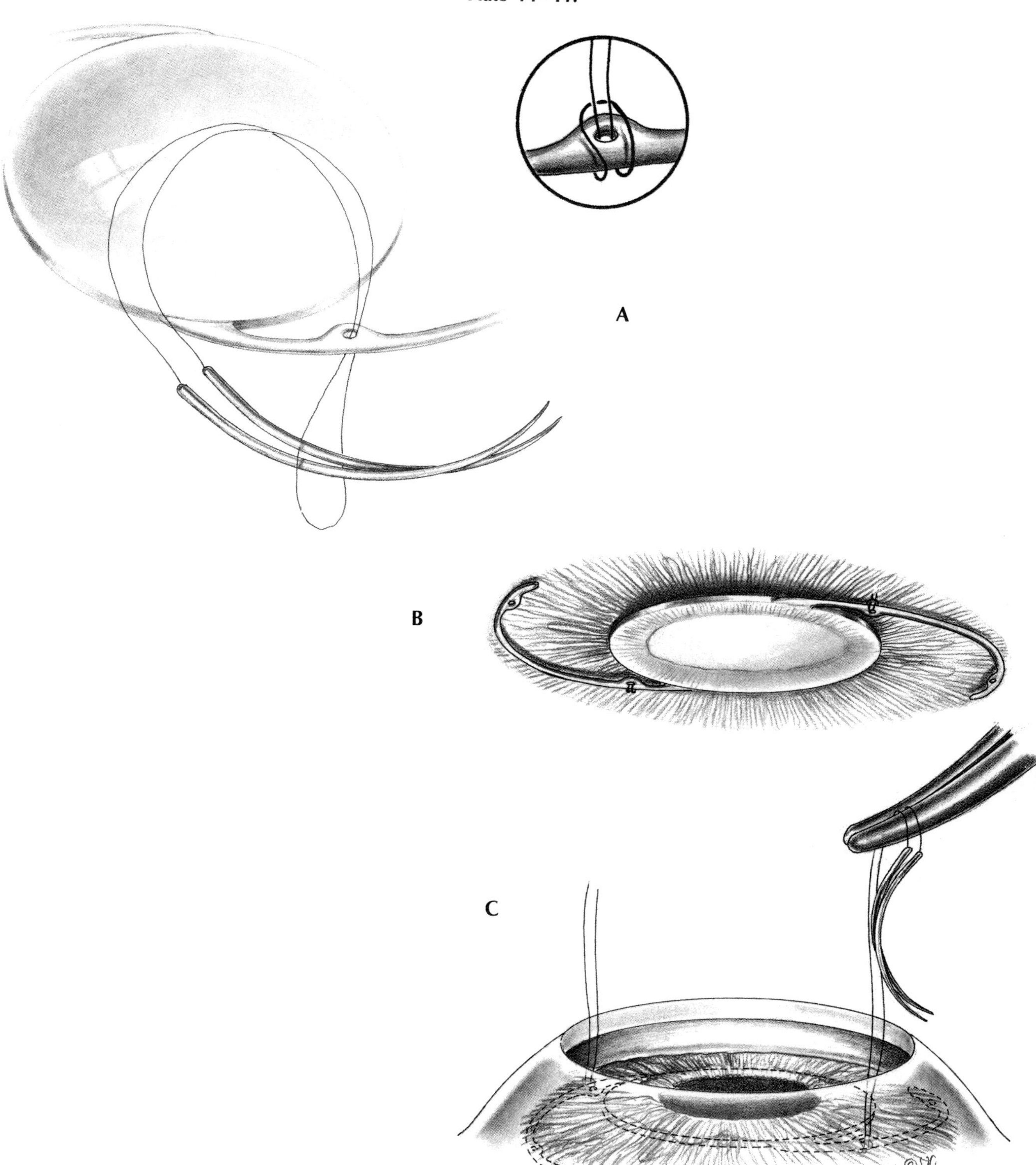

A, BV100–4 arming a 2-inch 10.0 polypropylene thread (Ethicon) looped through internal haptic fenestration of Troutman "lens for all reasons." *Inset,* cinch knot formed through haptic hole. **B,** posterior chamber intraocular lens sutured through intact iris, centered on pupil. **C,** anterior view.

Sulcus Fixation

Scleral fixation through the sulcus can be accomplished by one of several methods. Both techniques described begin prior to trephination with the preparation of episcleral flaps positioned to cover the externalized knots of the haptic fixation suture (Plate 14–12). These triangular flaps are placed obliquely, based at the limbus, with their apices toward the periphery at approximately the 1:30- and 7:30-o'clock positions in the left eye or the 10:30 and 4:30 positions in the right eye to provide the best access to the limbus area during suturing.

A technique has been developed by Lewis for fixation of a secondary posterior chamber lens without capsular support after cataract surgery, which we have modified for use when placing a posterior lens in aphakic or pseudophakic keratoplasty.

The trephination is performed and the offending anterior chamber lens, if present, is removed. When using a Krumeich or Hanna trephine, full penetration should be avoided because the preplaced needle holes (Plate 14–12) under the prepared scleral flaps may leak and the anterior chamber may be lost, with ensuing iris damage from a penetrating trephine blade. An anterior vitrectomy is performed, removing the vitreous to its base in the area internal to the external scleral flaps to allow unimpeded haptic insertion.

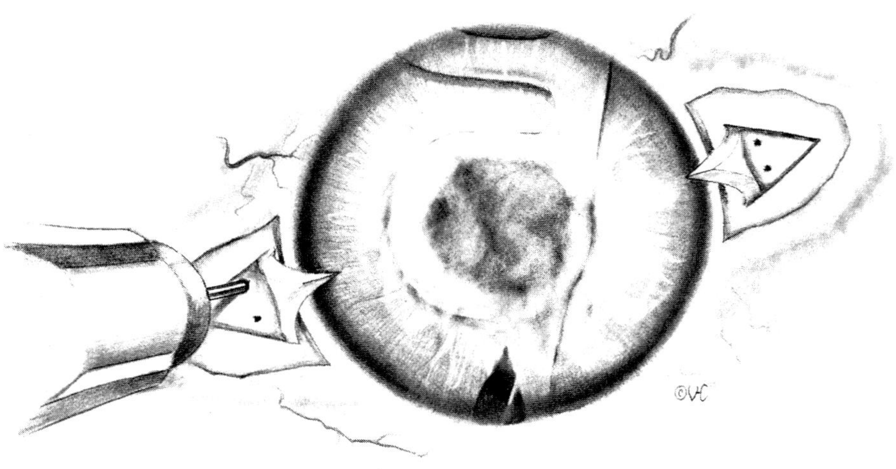

Position of episcleral flaps and preplaceing needle entrance holes in preparation for sulcus fixation of posterior chamber intraocular lens, by Lewis technique.

In this technique, a 27-gauge hypodermic needle, bent to avoid globe displacement, is passed through a preplaced needle hole under the scleral flap from externally at 1 mm distal to the limbus, until its tip, bevel up, is seen behind the pupil (Plates 14–12, 14–13,A). The needle tip is brought up through the pupil, and one arm of an ST-6 or a BV100-4 suture needle of a double-armed 2-inch 10-0 polypropylene thread (Ethicon) fixed to the lens haptic is inserted into the needle barrel (Plate 14–13,B). With the suture needle in the barrel, the 27-gauge needle is drawn back through its scleral entrance (Plate 14–13,C). A second thread is placed in the same fashion so that a mattress closure can be formed beneath the prepared scleral flap. A second pair of suture threads are passed to the opposite side.

When the lens has been appropriately placed and centered, the exteriorized suture ends are tied together with slipknots over the lamellarized scleral bed. When the centration of the lens is verified, these knots are locked with square knots. The protective scleral flaps are closed with a single interrupted suture at the tip of each triangular flap, and the fornix-based conjunctival flap is sutured or cautery fixated in place.

After a drop of sodium hyaluronate has been placed over the intraocular lens and on the back of the graft, the button is sutured in place, using the standard keratoplasty technique.

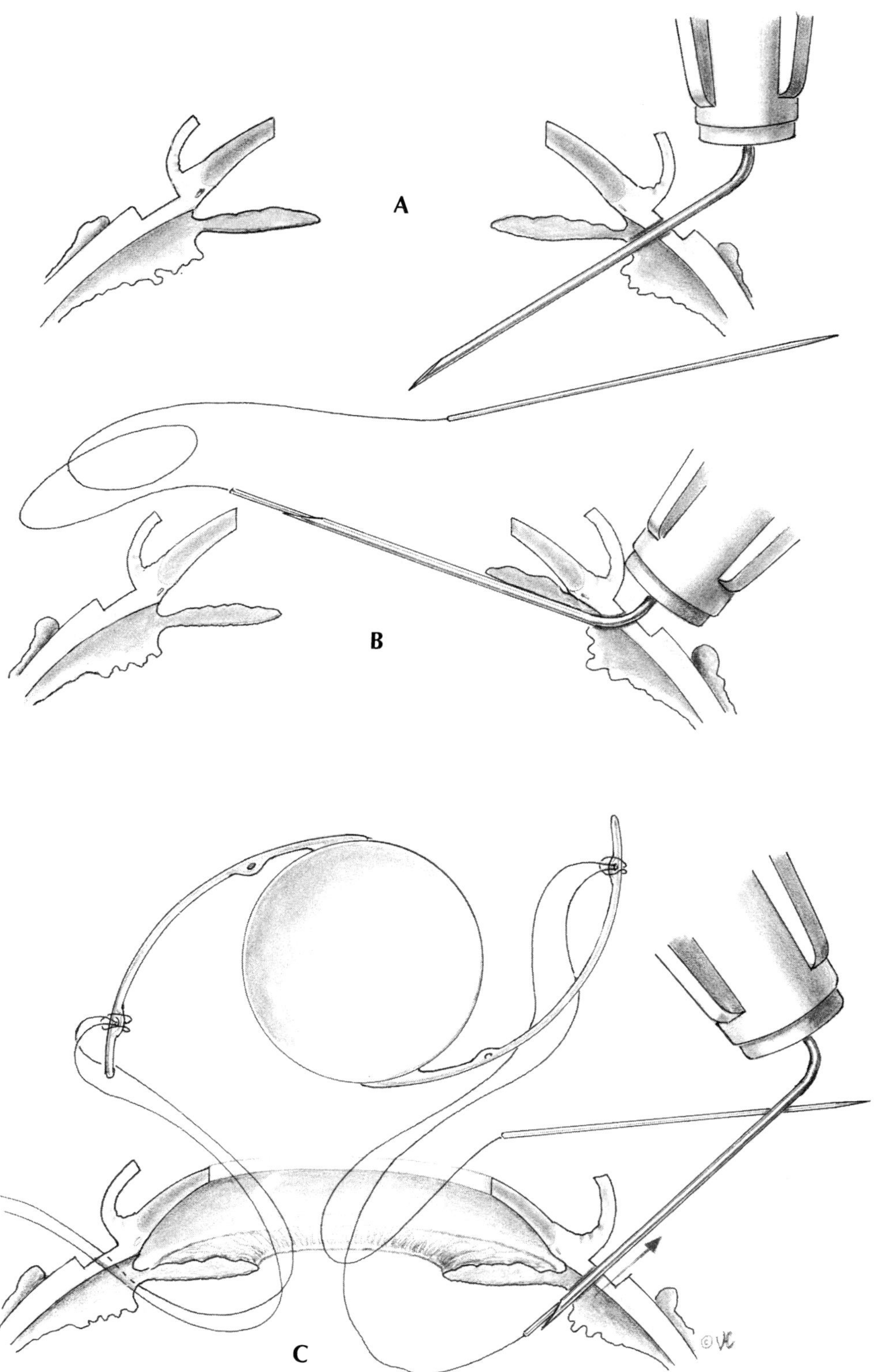

A, cross section of insertion of 25-gauge needle for Lewis technique. **B,** elevation of needle point to accept ST-6 or BV100 needle arming 2-inch 10-0 polypropylene thread (Ethicon). **C,** *right,* withdrawal of 25-gauge needle; *left,* double-armed suture in position in sulcus. Both sutures have been attached to distal fenestration of Troutman "lens for all reasons" in preparation for insertion.

Internal (Blind) Sulcus Fixation

A commonly used technique for sulcus fixation is the so-called blind technique. As with the previously described technique, two limbus-based triangular episcleral flaps are raised for oblique insertion of the lens (Plate 14–12). A 2-inch polypropylene thread double-armed with CIF-6, 10mm long, 30-degree curved cutting needles (Ethicon) is prefixed through the distal hole in the periphery of each haptic of an appropriately powered "lens for all reasons" (Plate 14–14). A vitrectomy is performed to prepare a tunnel to the sulcus for insertion of the lens. The paired needles are passed in turn beneath the iris to engage the internal sulcus. Slight pressure is applied to determine if the needle point is positioned at the appropriate area, 1mm distal to the base of the scleral flap. Using counterpressure from a slightly opened tying forceps, the first needle is exited between the blades but not withdrawn. The second needle then follows the path of the first, exiting beneath the flap for a mattress closure. The same technique is repeated on the opposite side (Plate 14–14). Each haptic in turn is slid beneath the iris and pulled into the sulcus with the externalized fixation threads. The threads are tied with slipknots to fixate the haptics into the sulcus. When the lens is verified to be centered and positioned, the ties are completed, the flaps closed, and a drop of sodium hyaluronate placed on the lens. The donor graft is then positioned and sutured into the recipient, using the standard keratoplasty closure technique.

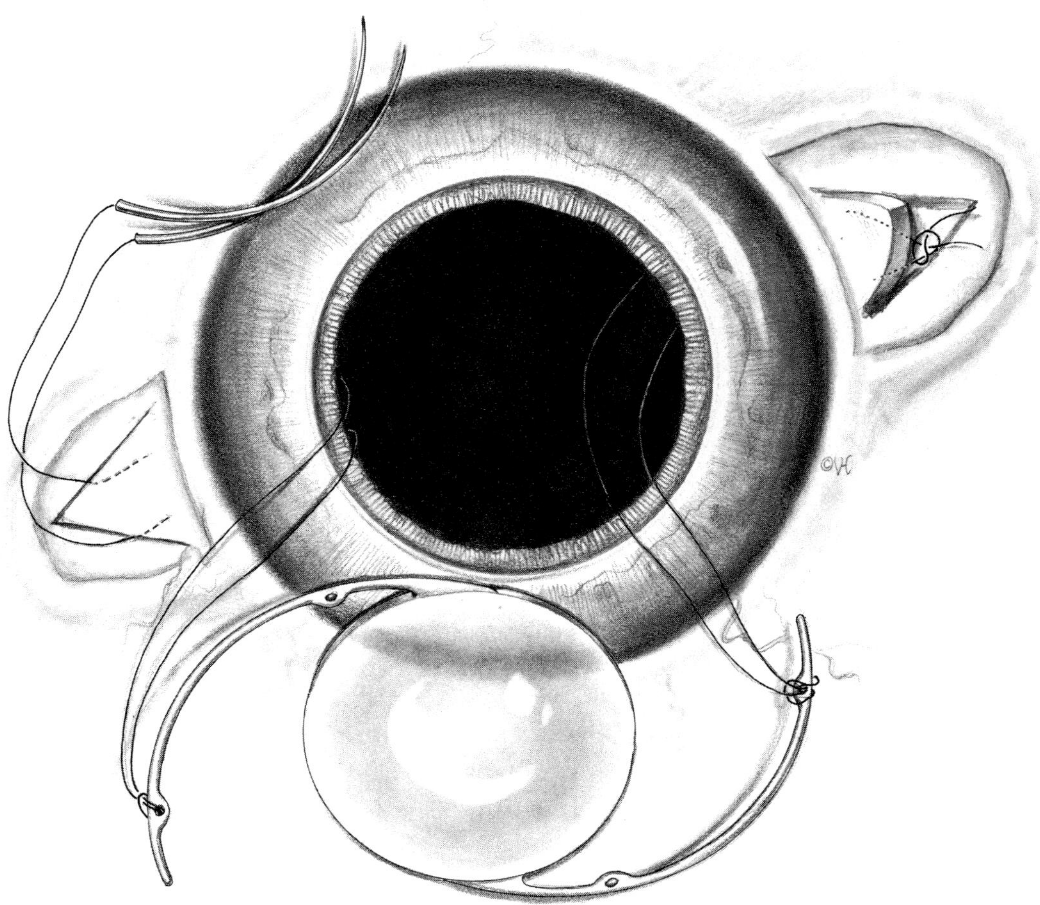

Blind sulcus fixation of posterior chamber intraocular "lens for all reasons," using CIF-6 needles arming 10-0 polypropylene thread (Ethicon).

In any sulcus fixation technique, there is always a possibility of intraocular hemorrhage from the penetration of one of the annular or long ciliary vessels. There is also the problem of the optimal position of the lens haptic in the sulcus. An oblique position approximately 1-mm behind the optical corneal ring not only better avoids long ciliary and annular vessel involvement but also reduces or eliminates potential astigmatic distortion resulting from displacement of the optical ring.

Triple Procedure: Extracapsular Lens Extraction

This discussion would not be complete without detailing one of the more frequent internal ocular procedures performed in conjunction with the standard keratoplasty technique. Endothelial corneal dystrophy is more frequently found in our aging population, and combining lens extraction with penetrating keratoplasty has made this procedure safer and less visually disabling than separate procedures.

The lens extraction requires a special technique because it is done *open sky* through the recipient cornea. Because phacoemulsification cannot be done in the open chamber, capsulorrhexis should not be done because the capsular bag may be torn as the nucleus is expressed. A square capsulectomy allows nucleus expression without significant lateral tearing and leaves visible flaps under which the lens haptics can be inserted. A large capsulorrhexis may permit nucleus expression but makes retention of the intraocular lens in the bag difficult. Four puncture capsulotomies are performed with a 25-gauge needle (Plate 14–15,A). The Galand scissors are used to incise the square of capsule, first outlined vertically and then horizontally (Plate 14–15,B). The lens nucleus is removed by hydrodissection and by counterpressure and rotation, taking care to separate it from the posterior capsule as it is delivered (Plate 14–15,C). The lens cortex is then removed with an infusion-aspiration cannula. Because the anterior chamber is absent, the technique is more time-consuming and the possibility of capsular rupture is increased. It is important that the aspiration line be kept free of air so that the cortex will be evacuated readily once engaged. As the cortex is approached, the tip of the cannula is tilted to the right or the left to avoid the capsular flap (Plate 14–15,D). *Stroking* must be avoided because the cannula is in contact with the bulging posterior capsule at all times. The Kuglin hook is useful for retracting the iris sphincter so that the lens cortex can be engaged under direct visualization, but it should not be used for capsule retraction. At the completion of the cortical evacuation, a viscoelastic is gently placed between the capsular leaves, and the distal haptic is inserted. As the optic is pressed back against the posterior capsule, the proximal haptic is placed in the bag. A

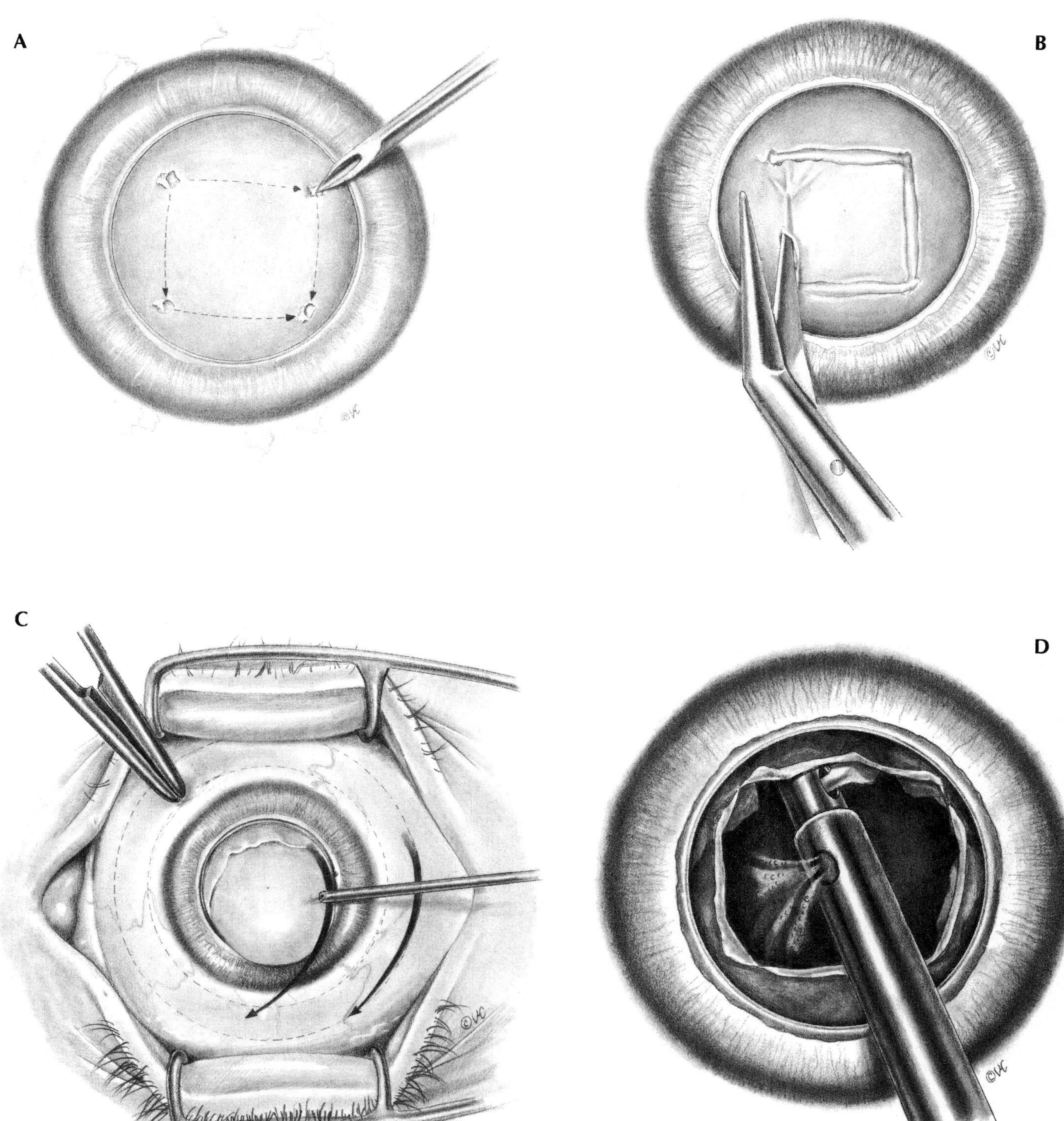

A, triple procedure, needle puncture capsulotomies. **B,** excising the capsule with Galand scissors. **C,** expressing the lens nucleus. **D,** aspiration of lens cortex; note aspiration aperture turned to right, away from capsular flap, irrigation ports horizontal.

Pathophysiology and Prevention of Astigmatism Secondary to Penetrating Keratoplasty   **383**

drop of viscoelastic is placed on the lens surface and on the back of the donor cornea that is to be inserted (Plate 14–16).

Coreoplasty—Iris Suture

Iris disease frequently coexists with corneal and anterior segment pathology in the eye that requires penetrating keratoplasty. As with penetrating keratoplasty, the iris is not only important as an anatomical structure but also optically. When possible, the anatomic structure of the iris should be restored to create a flat iris diaphragm to prevent anterior synechiae and to center a pupil of relatively normal dimensions behind the optical zone of the cornea. If a large coloboma is left behind a clear cornea graft, the image will be degraded whether or not an astigmatism is present.

To repair an iris defect, the iris first must be mobilized by separating it from adhesions to the lens, to the vitreous, to the cornea or an old incision, and to itself. This is best accomplished either by spatulation or by sharp scissors dissection, as required, with the Galand scissors. Once mobilized, an attempt should be made to close any colobomas by suturing with 10-0 monofilament polypropylene suture (see Chapter 10). One should not use a cutting needle for this purpose, because it may fragment the already diseased, damaged, fragile iris. The BV100-4 round blood vessel needle manufactured by Ethicon is ideal for this technique. The iris tissue apposed in the suture loop will eventually heal. Occasionally, it will be impossible to close a coloboma, in which case the thread is left across the residual opening to hold the iris diaphragm flat during corneal healing to prevent delayed formation of anterior synechiae. Although the restoration of the anatomic integrity of the iris diaphragm and pupil is probably more important to the eventual outcome of the penetrating keratoplasty procedure, the restoration of the stenopeic pupil will nevertheless be an important secondary benefit to restore visual function.

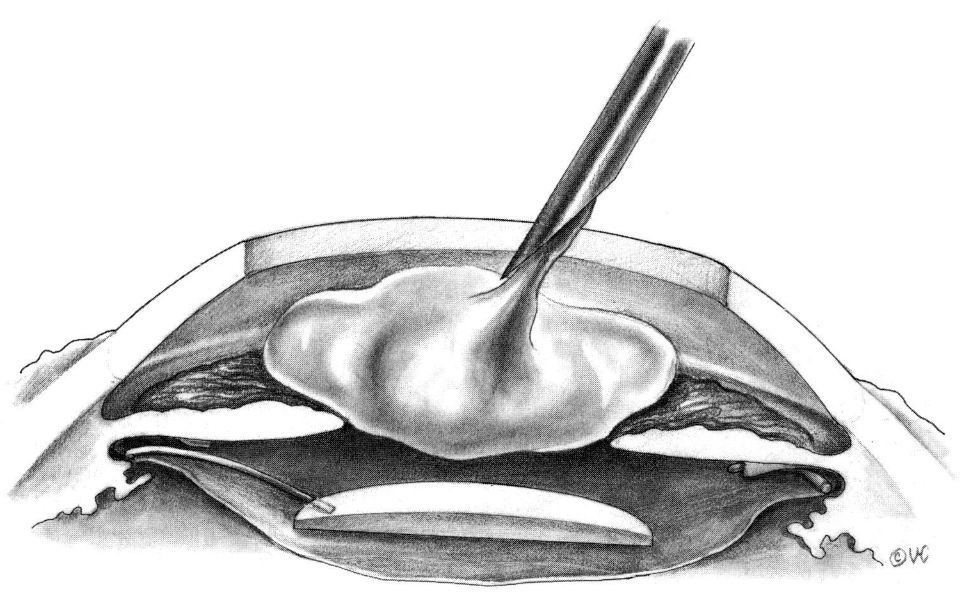

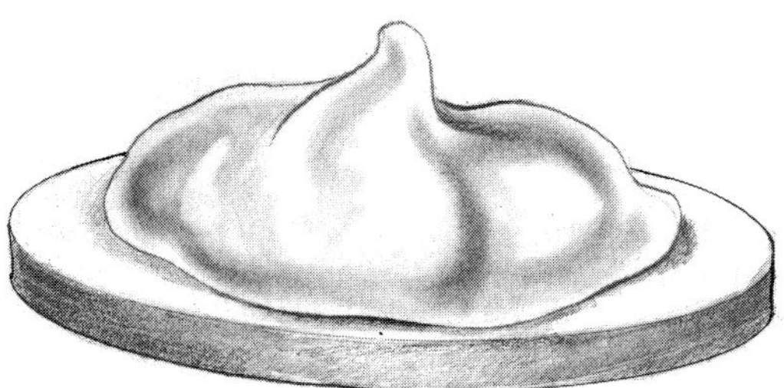

Intraocular lens "in the bag" viscoelastic over lens surface protecting graft endothelium. Avoid Healon in chamber angle.

STANDARD KERATOPLASTY TECHNIQUE: DONOR-RECIPIENT CLOSURE
Positioning and Fixating Donor to Recipient

As with preparation of the donor button and trephination of the recipient, positioning and suture fixation of the donor button to the recipient bed has been standardized to minimize suture-induced astigmatism as well as residual astigmatism after all sutures have been removed. As stated at the beginning of this chapter, both the incision and the closure are designed not only to create a regular spherical anterior corneal surface but also to produce a full-thickness graft to recipient scar. Then, should a secondary corrective procedure be required, it can be more accurately and more predictably performed. This technique takes into account the various problems that can be encountered in the recipient periphery, such as thickness variations (e.g., keratoconus), tissue alteration (e.g., trauma), and vascularization (e.g., disciform keratopathy). Continuous closure is preferred over interrupted suture fixation because it not only provides overall firmer wound apposition and better anterior support but also because the tension of individual suture loops can be more readily adjusted both intraoperatively, under surgical keratometer control, or postoperatively to correct excessive astigmatic bands.

Rotational Positioning of Graft—Antitorque Closure

When an appropriately sized donor button is inserted in the recipient area and the edges approximated, the surgical keratometer projection can indicate moderate to severe meridional distortion (Plate 14–17). This distortion can be compensated for by selective rotation of the donor button within the recipient opening until the reflection of the surgical keratometer indicates approximate sphericity, as presented by Belmont and Troutman (1985). It is important to level the donor edge to the recipient edge at each successive position to avoid a false reading from tilt. The keratometer projection is observed as the anterior surface of the cornea is leveled. With the Krumeich and Hanna suction trephine systems, the more regular matching of wound edges often does not necessitate rotation.

Once the graft is appropriately positioned, the suture pattern used for fixation of the graft to the recipient should maintain their relationship circumferentially and in depth. Troutman's double-opposing continuous suture (Plates 14–19 to 14–21) accomplishes these ends, combining the simplicity of continuous suture closure and the antitorque properties of the more time-consuming, less secure interrupted closure technique.

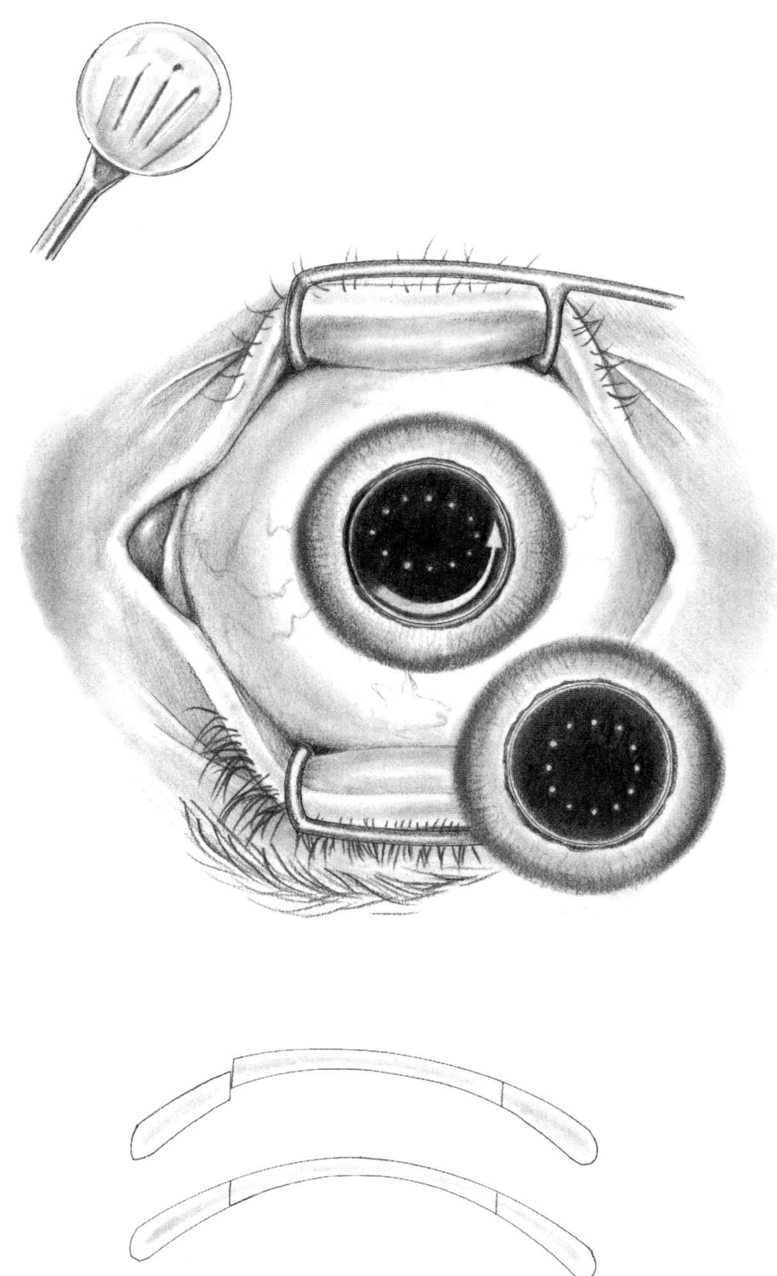

Rotational positioning of graft for best optical fit under surgical keratometer, top. Bottom, donor button should be leveled to recipient cornea.

Interrupted Fixation Sutures

With the donor button appropriately positioned, six equidistant interrupted through-and-through fixating suture loops are placed and tied, using adjustable slipknots to assure even apposition (Plate 14–18). The second suture, which determines the graft position, is the most important. If the six interrupted fixation sutures are accurately placed, the anterior chamber should readily re-form, making possible the use of the surgical keratometer to ascertain the initial relative sphericity of the donor button in preparation for the first, clockwise, continuous suture placement. The fixation suture loops are placed with short 0.5 mm through-and-through radial bites to assure firm anterior, posterior, and circumferential positioning of the graft to the recipient.

Length of Suture Bites

When the corneal periphery is softened by disease or is vascular, longer bites are taken in the softer or vascularized recipient sectors. Monofilament nylon suture rests postoperatively on top of an intact Bowman's layer, both on the donor and on the recipient. If the suture loop is placed over an area in which Bowman's layer is absent, the anterior loop cuts prematurely into stroma when the suture loop compresses the tissue. The suture loop loosens before it can work its way forward into the posterior stroma, and fistulization may lead to infection or epithelial downgrowth. Placing a longer bite to the periphery, in the case of a diseased or vascular cornea, better assures optimal tension on the appropriate suture loop until its internal aspect is retracted into posterior stroma.

Suturing Edges of Disparate Thickness

It is essential that through-and-through sutures be used to approximate a graft to a recipient of different thickness, especially when this is present in a sector rather than circumferentially. In this case, the anterior edges of both the donor and the recipient should be closed at the same level, and the vertically disparate edges of the posterior cornea should be apposed in full thickness to avoid posterior gaping and subsequent excessive astigmatism.

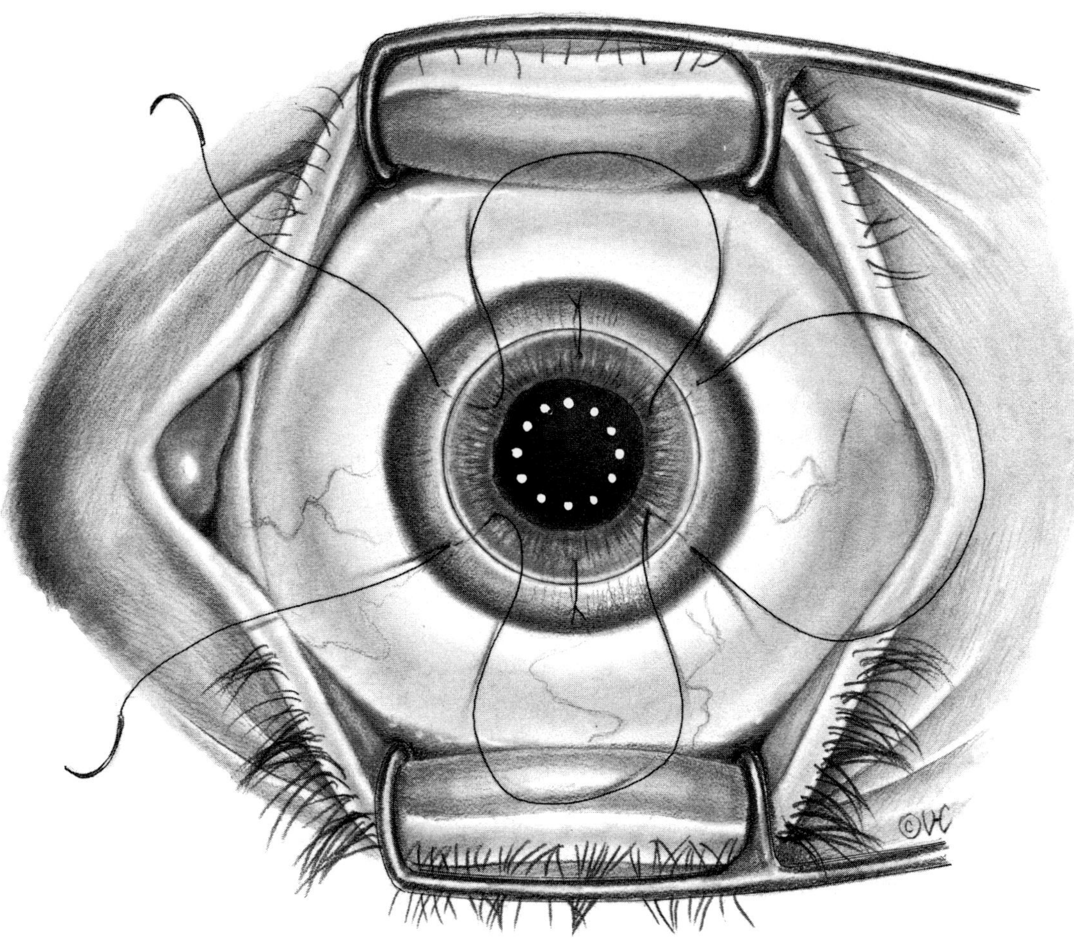

Two interrupted fixation sutures in place, additional four sutures in place before tying placed continuously to facilitate suturing.

DOUBLE OPPOSING CONTINUOUS SUTURE (ANTITORQUE)
Clockwise Continuous Suture

The first limb of the double opposing continuous suture is placed with through-and-through suture bites of appropriate length clockwise around the circumference of the rotationally positioned and fixated donor button. These suture bites are placed equidistant to each other in a radial direction without regard to the position of the fixating interrupted sutures. To insert the successive suture loops, the cornea is grasped with Pierse forceps and the compound curved needle driven through the corneal thickness, as described in chapter 9, to both sides of the incision. It is usually unnecessary to grasp the recipient cornea during needle insertion, but the corneal forceps is used to control needle passage. The number and length of bites taken in the first continuous suture depend not only on the disease process but also on the age and reliability of the patient. A minimum of 12 to a maximum of 18 bites are placed. The ends of the continuous suture are joined with a single slipknot for appositional tensioning; then the knot is completed for adjustment of suture loop tension, to reduce any meridional distortion detected by the Troutman operative keratometer (Plate 14–19).

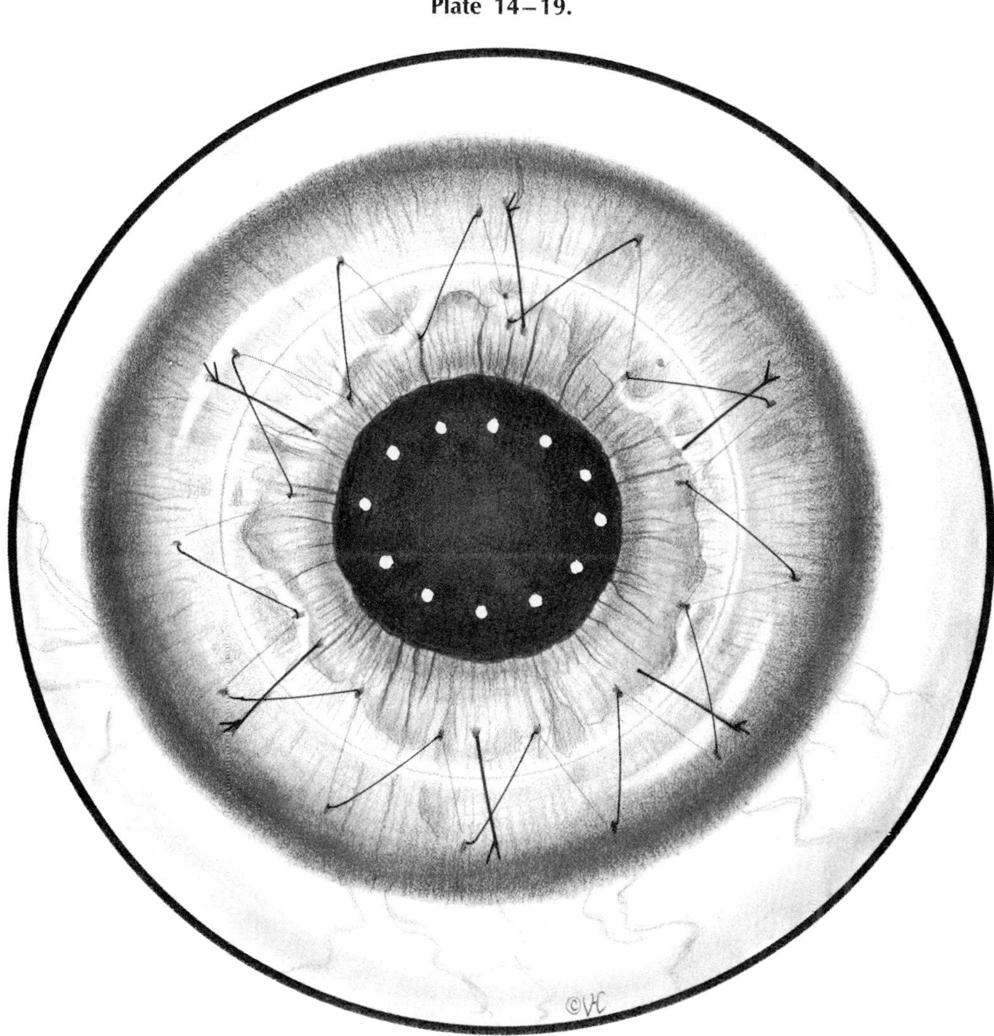

Clockwise continuous suture, inducing *with the rule* astigmatism. Before suture adjustment (note displacement of deep suture bites from torquing effect of single continuous suture).

Appositional tensioning is done in two stages. While holding the distal end of the continuous thread with the straight tying forceps, the closed curved tying forceps are inserted under the successive loops, lifted, and lightly tensioned around the circumference of the graft. A slipknot is formed and adjusted so that the knot is adjacent to the opening of the needle tract on the donor side of the cornea. This reduces the necessity to adjust the suture further after the second adjustment has been made. Then, holding the suture threads to avoid displacing the knot, each suture loop is grasped in turn and tensioned by pulling it in the direction of its overlying loop until the circle is again completed. Any slack created is drawn up by the slipknot, which is then locked down with a square knot and trimmed flush with the razor knife. The knot is buried in the suture tract in the donor cornea adjacent to it by slightly loosening the loop to either side of the tract and then pulling on the thread toward the recipient side while directing the knot into the tract from the donor side. Should difficulty be encountered in burying a knot, it can be lubricated with a drop of viscoelastic before it is pulled into the tract.

The suture loop tension then is adjusted to reduce meridional distortion while the cornea curvatures are being observed with a surgical keratometer until approximate sphericity is indicated. This is accomplished by successively tightening suture loops in the flatter meridian and loosening suture loops in the steeper meridian (Plate 14–20).

When the first suture has been completed, it will be noted that the formerly radially placed continuous suture bites are turned oblique clockwise (Plate 14–19). The interrupted suture bites will also be observed as turned to an oblique position and to be slightly loosened as well. This torquing effect of the successive overlying bites of the continuous suture causes the graft to rotate clockwise in relation to the recipient (see Plate 14–19). Troutman in 1967 proposed an antitorque "limited movement of force" suture to control this effect. A single continuous suture with obliquely placed suture bites was initially proposed as a means to prevent graft rotation. This suture was placed to form a series of isosceles triangles that tended to equalize rotational stresses around the graft circumference, blocking rotation. Because corneal needles at the time were difficult to pass obliquely, a second counterclockwise opposing radially placed continuous suture was used to equalize the torquing effect of the clockwise suture (Plate 14–21). The single antitorque continuous suture has been used primarily for lamellar keratoplasty and has been popularized by José Barraquer for antitorque suturing of keratophakia and keratomileusis lamellar buttons. In lamellar keratoplasty, fewer closing suture loops are required for apposition than with penetrating keratoplasty, where the incision is under continuous posterior displacement pressure. The advantage of the double opposing continuous suture pattern is its ver-

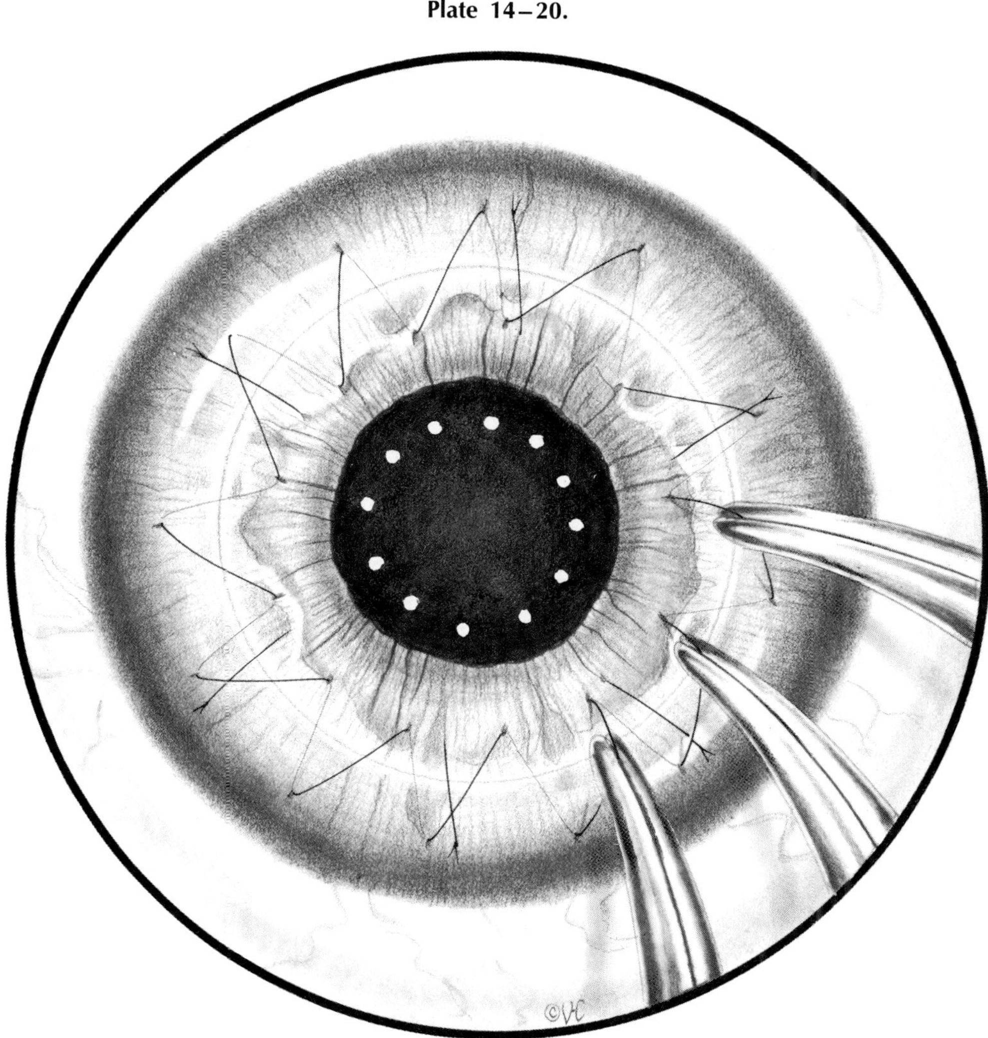

Astigmatism compensated by sequential suture loop adjustment, tightening flatter meridian.

tical and lateral stability, induced by the web of suture support it provides on the anterior surface of the cornea.

Counterclockwise Opposing Single Continuous Suture

To compensate for the now oblique, torqued position of the first continuous suture, a second opposing continuous suture is placed counterclockwise with the full-thickness bites *between and parallel to* the now obliquely displaced deep bites of the clockwise suture. Because the graft has now been firmly apposed to the recipient by the first suture, the compound curved needle can be passed obliquely through the full thickness of both the donor and the recipient cornea in a single movement without the necessity for forceps fixation. When the second circular suture has been completed, the two-step tightening, as described for the clockwise suture, is performed in the reverse direction to compensate for the torquing effect of the clockwise continuous suture. As the counterclockwise suture is tensioned, the intracorneal portion of the loops of the first continuous suture will again assume their radial direction. The interrupted sutures will also return to their previous radiality, becoming still further loosened as the second suture is tightened and tied.

When the knot of the second suture has been buried in the donor button, as described for the clockwise continuous suture, the surgical keratometer reflection is observed and the second continuous suture adjusted to achieve approximate sphericity (Plate 14–21). At this point, all of the loosened interrupted sutures are removed, taking care not to cut either one or both continuous sutures adjacent to their loops.

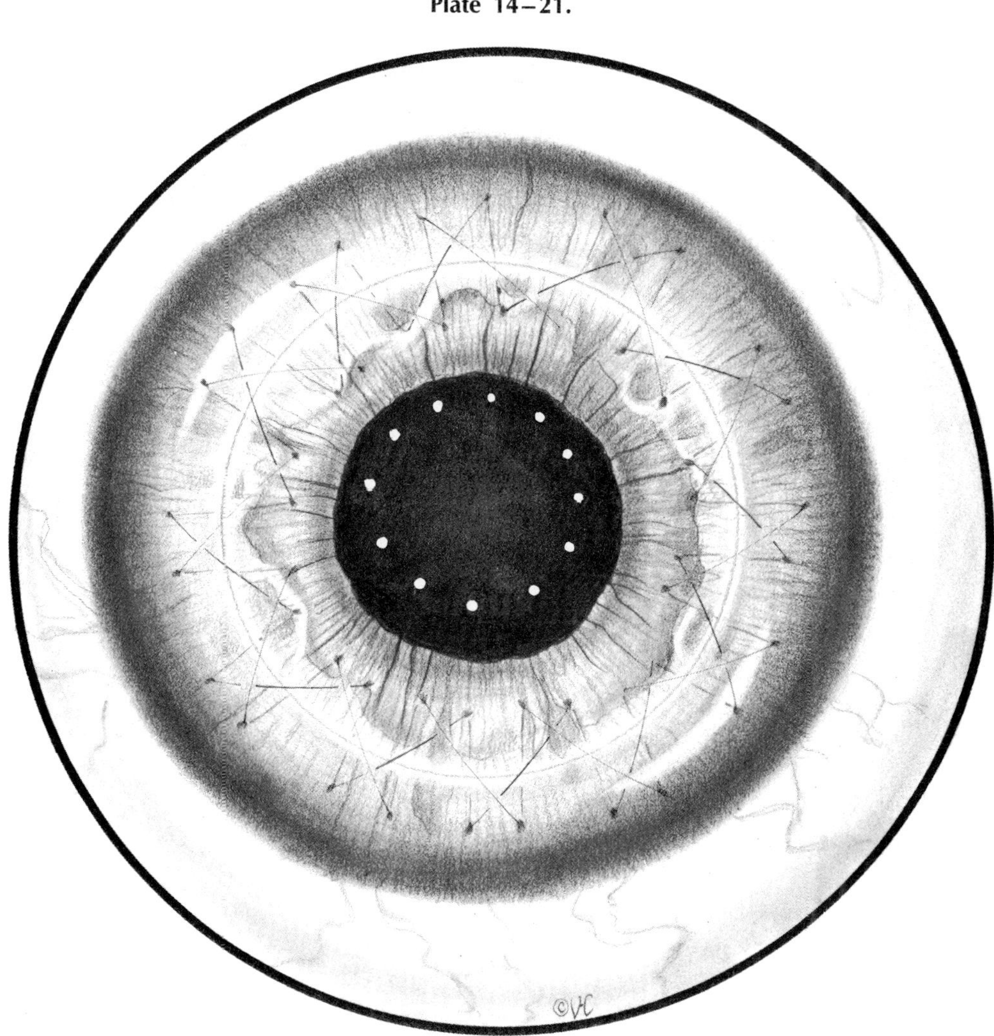

Counterclockwise opposing continuous suture in place and adjusted to compensate torque- and suture-induced astigmatism. (Note all deep bites are radial, indicating torquing effect of clockwise continuous suture compensated.)

Single Continuous Suture

In spite of its tendency to cause the donor button to rotate within the recipient opening, for simplicity a single continuous suture is preferred by many surgeons. As soon as a single continuous suture is tightened and tied, the radially placed bites rotate to assume a more or less oblique direction (Plate 14–19), depending on the number of bites taken around the circumference. If any single or several bites are not equidistant, not only will the angle of the closing suture loop change, but also the cornea will tend to flatten in the meridian of the more widely placed loop or loops (Plate 14–22,A). When this occurs, it is not often possible to accurately adjust the suture loops to compensate for the meridional distortion. An interrupted suture will have to be inserted to close the wound dehiscence that induces the astigmatism (Plate 14–22,B). If these microdehiscences are not compensated for at surgery, they will need to be compensated for during the postoperative course. Since suture adjustment or selective suture removal of interrupted sutures, if also in place, may either compound the problem or fail to relieve it, suture addition is the preferred alternative (see Chapter 4).

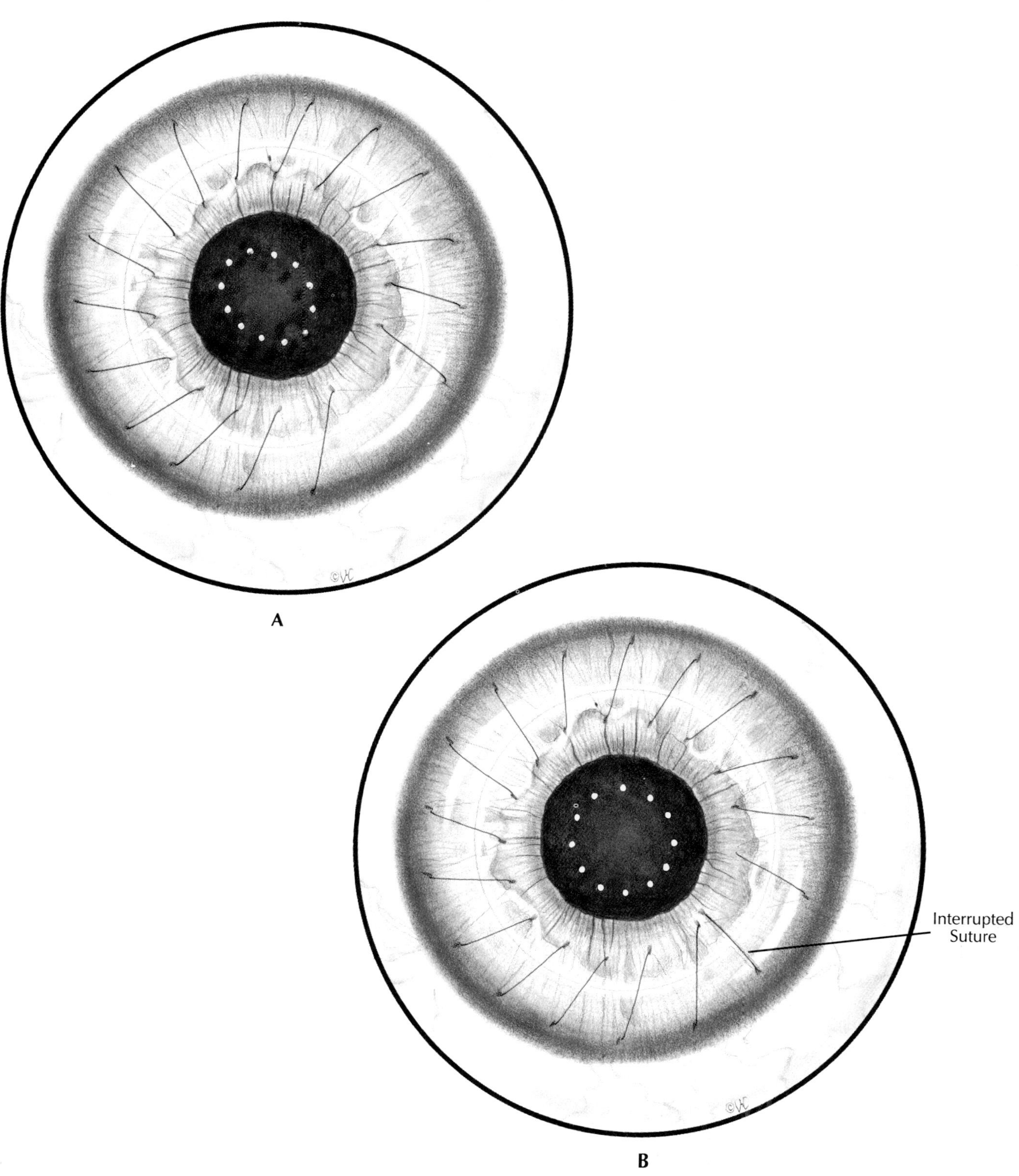

A, single continuous suture with unequally placed loops inducing oblique astigmatism. **B,** astigmatism corrected by placing interrupted suture across flatter meridian.

Pathophysiology and Prevention of Astigmatism Secondary to Penetrating Keratoplasty   **397**

Interrupted Sutures

Advocates of selective suture removal prefer interrupted sutures or continuous and interrupted sutures (belt and suspenders technique) because the interrupted sutures can be removed to compensate for astigmatism. Accurate placement of interrupted sutures at the primary procedure must be done to assure, if possible, that there will be no necessity to remove more than a few sutures to compensate for an astigmatic distortion before wound healing has taken place. When one or more sutures is tighter or looser, the suture(s) should be removed and replaced, adjusting the tension with slipknots while observing the astigmatic band with the surgical keratometer (Plate 14–23,A,B). Rather than weakening a stronger wound sector by removing a suture(s) in the steeper corneal meridian to balance a weaker flatter sector, we prefer suture addition or adjustment of a continuous suture, if also in place.

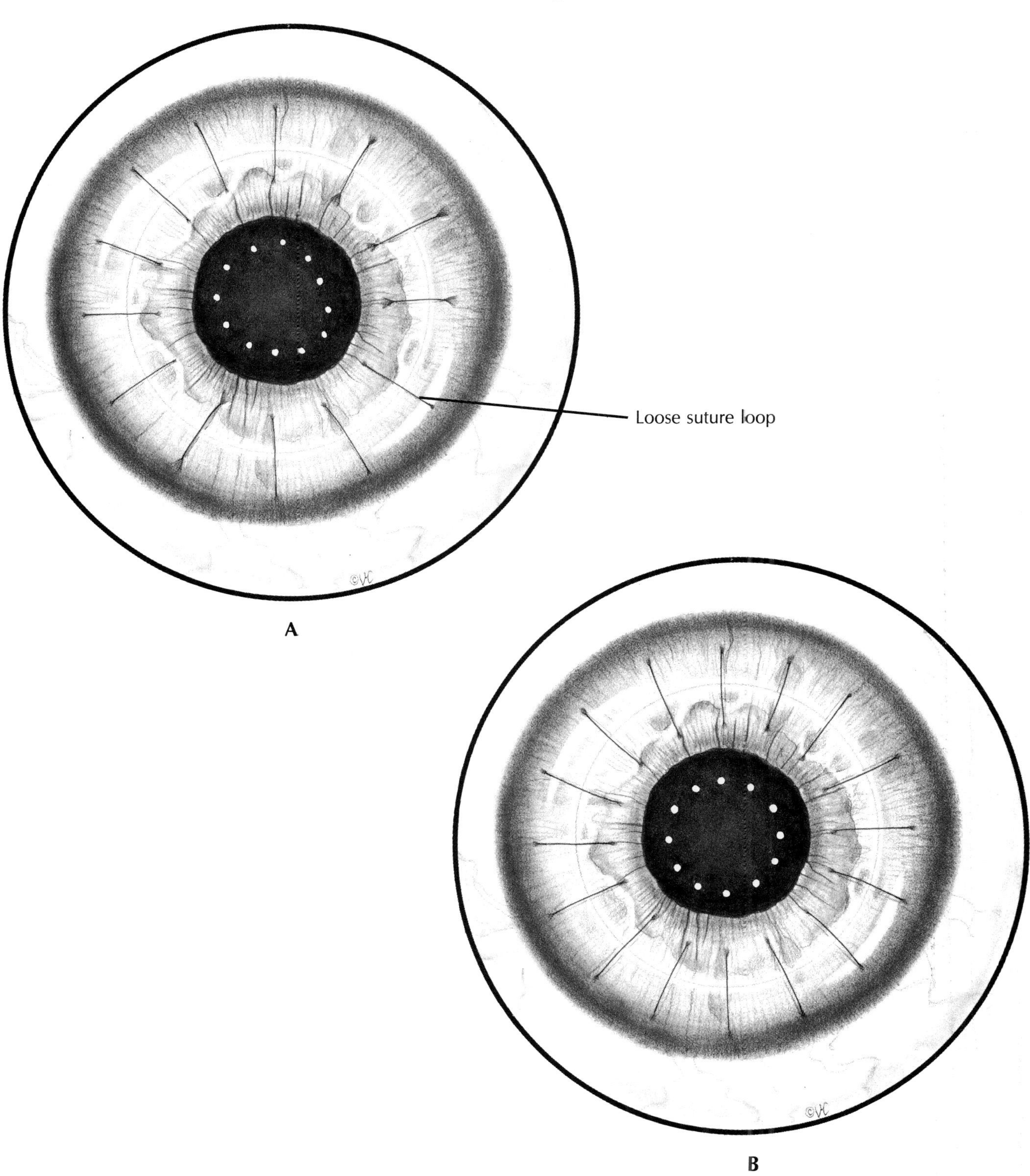

A, interrupted suture closure with unequal suture loop tension inducing oblique astigmatism. **B,** looser sutures removed and replaced to compensate for induced astigmatism.

Pathophysiology and Prevention of Astigmatism Secondary to Penetrating Keratoplasty   **399**

Double Continuous Sutures: 10-0 and 11-0 (Torque Inducing)

Another popular suture pattern is to place two clockwise continuous sutures of different diameters with alternating bites (Plate 14–24). The 10-0 suture is removed at 3 months postoperatively, and the second 11-0 suture is left in place indefinitely. Four or more interrupted sutures may be placed for sequential removal to control postoperative astigmatism. This suture does not compensate for graft rotation because both sutures are placed in the same direction, inducing and maintaining torquing of the graft in relation to the recipient. The 11-0 suture, being more elastic, allows some stretching of the wound, and the graft tends to be steeper and more myopic when all sutures biodegrade or are removed. Astigmatism can also be more difficult to correct because of the thinner wound resulting from early removal of the stronger thread.

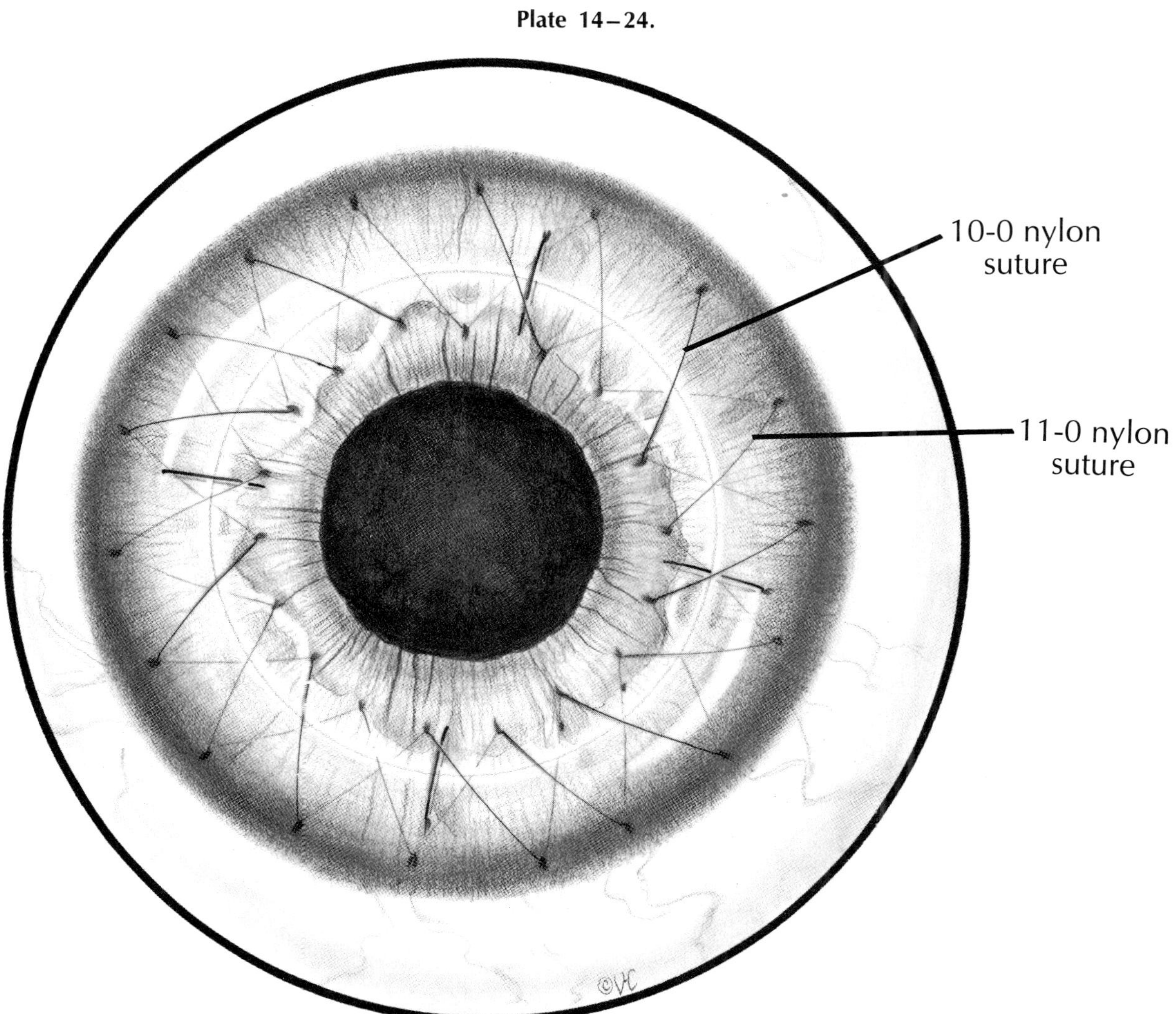

Double continuous sutures, 10-0 and 11-0, with interrupted sutures. (Note torqued position of continuous threads.)

Stromal Overgrowth

Other than iatrogenic appositional errors, monofilament thread causes few complications. In some cases, however, corneal stroma will extrude from the suture points, usually from the donor side of the wound, and spread under the epithelium around the wound. If this occurs only in a sector, that sector will become flattened. If it occurs circumferentially, the entire cornea will flatten, becoming more hyperopic (Plate 14–25). The meridional distortion or corneal flattening can be relieved by removing the stroma from Bowman's layer. Under slitlamp magnification, an edge is elevated until it can be mobilized and gripped with a smooth forceps. Usually the whole stromal sheet can be stripped from Bowman's layer. Care should be taken not to dissect near suture points or a suture may be prematurely released.

Maintaining Anterior Chamber

With any suture technique, it is essential that the anterior chamber be maintained at approximately normal intraocular pressure during suture placement, particularly when adjusting suture tension under surgical keratometer control. As detailed in chapter 9, with through-and-through passage of suture needles, especially when the peripheral cornea is opaque or vascularized, care must be taken to avoid including the iris or other adjacent internal ocular structures in a suture loop. With careful technique the anterior chamber should not require frequent refilling during suturing. Any iris inclusion should be released before proceeding to the next suture loop. At the close of the procedure, the wound should be free of adhesions and the anterior chamber fully re-formed. If any questionable area is seen, a drop of fluorescein dye on the cornea will detect a wound dehiscence. Usually adjustment of the continuous sutures will close a leak. Occasionally one or several interrupted sutures may be required.

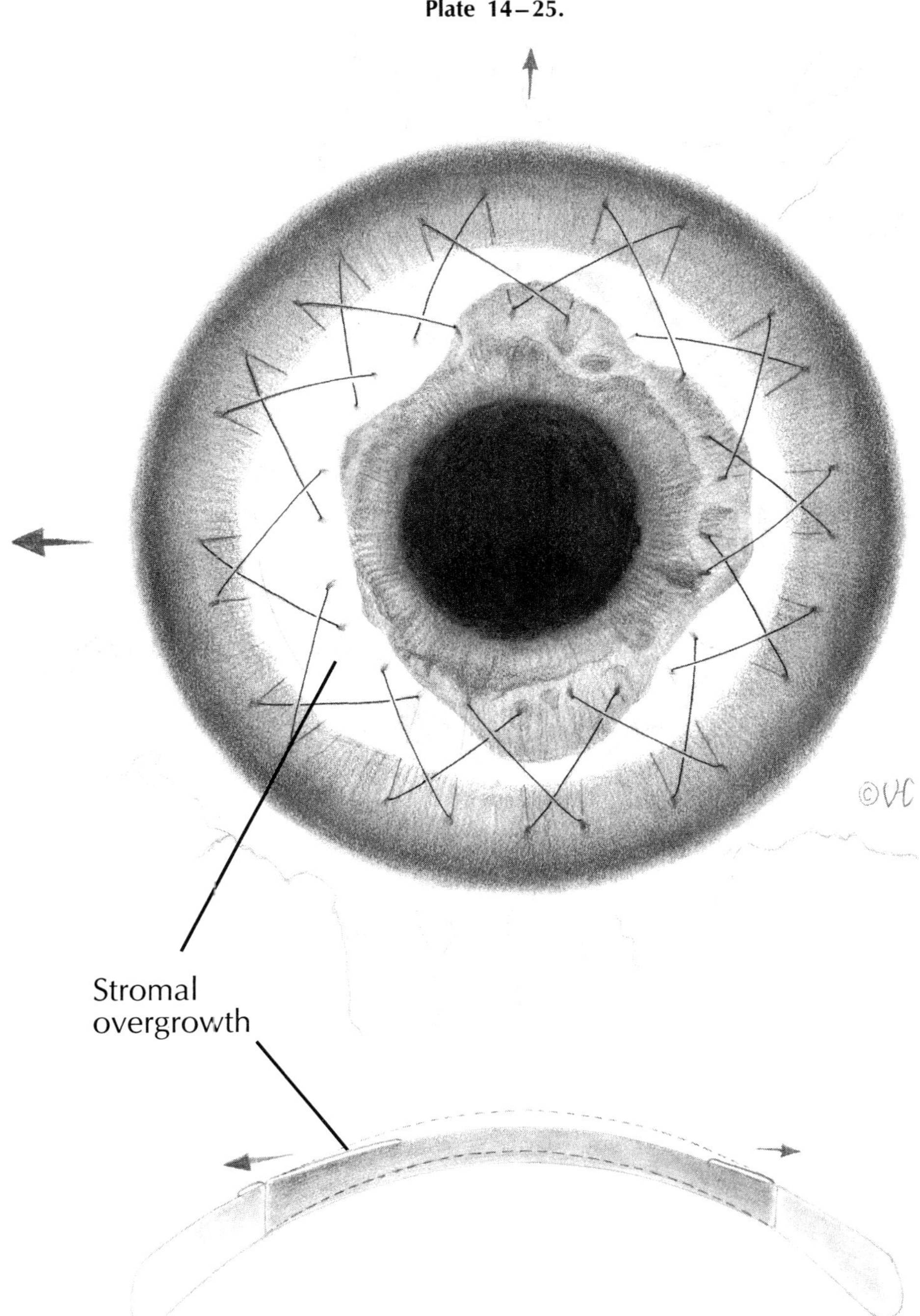

Stromal overgrowth. *Top,* frontal view; *bottom,* induced flattening of cornea.

SUMMARY

Penetrating keratoplasty is productive of excessive astigmatism more than any other ophthalmic surgical procedure and has defied our efforts to correct it primarily and, until relatively recently, secondarily as well. In this chapter, a standard penetrating keratoplasty technique is proposed and described as a partial solution to this surgical dilemma. Only by cutting the donor button and recipient opening as accurately as possible can we hope to achieve a precise fit of the donor to the recipient. Sutures need to be placed not only to close the incisional edges anteriorly and posteriorly but also to prevent rotation of the appropriately positioned graft. To accomplish this a technique using through-and-through suturing and double continuous antitorque closure is described. If we do not achieve full-thickness circumferential healing, then correction of any residual astigmatic defects becomes less predictable.

We have described recent advances in the cutting instruments that are used to prepare the donor and recipient, which in our hands have achieved significant improvement in graft recipient matching and apposition that, in turn, have resulted in reduced astigmatism both with through-and-through sutures in place and after their removal.

Recently, the excimer laser has been used (Lang et al., 1990) for cutting both the donor and the recipient, using oval donor and recipient shapes. Even if the laser should provide more accurate cutting of these shapes than we have been able to accomplish mechanically, we can still anticipate residual astigmatism unless and until the relatively crude suture closure techniques currently in use can be replaced by new technologies such as laser welding and enzymes that would promote more accurate, rapid wound healing.

The final functional result of corneal surgery depends not only on a clear, optically regular cornea but also on the power of the lens or of a substitute. We have therefore described intraocular lens replacement procedures used in conjunction with keratoplasty. In addition, we have emphasized the importance of the restoration of the lens iris diaphragm and stenopeic pupil. The combined goal of these modalities is the improved function of the postkeratoplasty eye, avoiding if possible the necessity for secondary optical corrective surgery.

Chapter 15

Surgical Management of Post–Penetrating Keratoplasty Astigmatism

Success in penetrating keratoplasty can no longer be measured only in terms of the anatomical result and the clarity of the graft. All too often, the functional result of an otherwise successful surgical intervention suffers as a result of moderate to marked corneal ametropia, particularly astigmatism. Excessive residual astigmatism has become the most common complication of penetrating keratoplasty. Corneal surgeons will commonly accept residual astigmatism that they would consider unacceptable after any other anterior segment surgery. Now the patients are becoming more intolerant of such surgical residuals, expecting, as in modern cataract surgery, that they will require little or no optical correction to achieve a perfect functional result. Consequently, the corneal surgeon is now obliged not only to correct excessive astigmatism but also to correct more moderate meridional errors. In addition, we have come to expect that these corneas may be modified to correct surgically or pathologically induced corneal spherical ametropias, as we have done with radial keratotomy and, recently, with excimer laser photoablation techniques. This chapter will address the current means to correct such visually debilitating errors that have yet to be controlled at primary penetrating keratoplasty.

MANAGEMENT OF POST–PENETRATING KERATOPLASTY ASTIGMATISM WITH "SUTURES IN"

Following successful penetrating keratoplasty, while interrupted, torque-inducing single or double continuous, or antitorque single or double opposing continuous sutures are in place, the patient should be able to enjoy some degree of functional acuity through the optically clear cornea graft. Serial keratometer measurements combined with subjective refraction will determine when the central corneal curvatures are stable enough to permit optical correction. In most instances, when intraoperative keratometry has been used to adjust the curvatures of the graft, appropriate spherocylindrical correction will permit the patient to use the vision potential of the recently operated eye. When continuous suture closure has been used and an excessive uncorrected astigmatism persists, one of several methods may be used for its reduction.

Suture Addition Technique

Buzard is of the opinion that excessive *sutures-in* postoperative astigmatism can be induced by small dehiscences of the wound between a loop or loops of a double continuous suture. These *microdehiscences* can be identified at about 6 to 12 weeks postoperatively. At this time the graft is usually optically stable and clear enough to permit functional vision, but prevented from optimal acuity by an excessive meridional error. Photokeratometry or topographic corneal mapping will demonstrate the relatively flatter or steeper corneal meridians. The flatter meridians, identified by the topography, are carefully examined with the slitlamp. Small elevations of the wound edge or an apparent loosening of a suture loop just opposite to the excessively flatter meridian will usually be seen. In an outpatient surgical operating facility, one of several interrupted sutures are inserted across each of the microdehiscences on the flatter meridian. They are tied and tensioned with slipknots, then locked with square knots when the surgical keratometer indicates approximate sphericity. Several days subsequent to the interrupted suture placement the corneal topography is again mapped, and if some astigmatism is still present, either additional sutures are placed or the continuous sutures are adjusted to reduce the residual astigmatic error.

Buzard (1991) has shown that circumferential additional sutures can be used to reduce myopia-inducing corneal steepening during the *sutures in* phase of penetrating keratoplasty. These circumferential interrupted additional sutures must be added within 3 months of the original penetrating keratoplasty to obtain permanent flattening of the cornea.

Continuous Suture Adjustment

When faced with an excessive postoperative astigmatism in the absence of or after closing microdehiscences, adjustment of one or both double opposing continuous sutures is used to regularize corneal curvatures. The double opposing continuous suture technique has the advantage that only one continuous suture may have to be adjusted to correct the surgically induced error. Before doing the adjustment, topographic mapping of the cornea is performed, and the flatter and steeper meridians are identified. Under the slitlamp, which is fitted with a modified surgical keratometer for real-time monitoring of the adjustment effect, the tighter suture loops are located and adjusted under topical anesthesia. A suture handling forceps, or alternatively a fine blunt hook, such as a Sinsky hook, is used to elevate and tighten successive loops across the flatter meridian, transferring the slack toward the steeper corneal meridian (see Plate 14–20). When possible, a quantitative keratometer should be used intermittently to refine the correction. After several days, the topography is reevaluated and, if required, adjustment of the second continuous suture may be performed. The first suture acts in its turn as a safety net should the second suture be ruptured during adjustment.

Other authors (Lin et al., 1990) have described the adjustment of a single continuous suture combined with opening of the healing incision. This ostensibly allows rotation of the graft to a position of less astigmatism as the tension on individual loops is adjusted. *Opening of the healing incision is not necessary when double opposing antitorque sutures are adjusted, because the graft position within the circumference of the recipient bed is not altered by the adjustment.*

Sequential Removal of Interrupted Sutures

One of the means, popularized by Binder, used to control corneal astigmatism with the sutures in place is the selective sequential removal of interrupted suture loops, sometimes protected by a continuous 10-0 or 11-0 suture. In this technique, beginning 6 weeks to 3 months after surgery, the corneal topography is analyzed, using the photokeratometer or a corneal mapping system, and the tighter sutures in the indicated steeper corneal meridian are removed successively. When postremoval topographic corneal mapping and refraction indicate the necessity, additional suture loops are removed. Unlike selective suture addition at microdehiscences or continuous suture adjustment, or both, in which the weaker part of the incision is strengthened, in this technique, it is the stronger part of the incision that is weakened. This may explain the tendency for corneas managed by this technique to have a steeper overall corneal curvature when all sutures are removed. This technique may succeed until the protecting continuous suture is removed, only to have a severe astigmatism appear in the non-suture-compensated cornea.

MANAGEMENT OF POST–PENETRATING KERATOPLASTY ASTIGMATISM WITH "SUTURES OUT"

Following any of the these techniques, remaining sutures eventually must be removed or they will become weakened, loosened, or biodegrade. The residual astigmatism that they have compensated for then will become manifest and surgical correction often will be indicated.

Earlier suture removal from the full-thickness healed wound is possible when double opposing antitorque continuous sutures with through-and-through wound apposition have been used at the primary surgery. In the case of keratoconus and hereditary dystrophies, sutures are routinely removed 6 months after surgery. In softer corneas, for example, pseudophakic keratopathy, they are usually not left more than 1 year. When sutures are left for longer periods of time, not only is visual rehabilitation delayed, but there is a greater tendency toward irregular astigmatism. It has been our experience that prolonged suture apposition, more than 1 year, does not significantly reduce the astigmatism, which becomes manifest when all sutures are eventually removed. When the wound is closed with through-and-through sutures, earlier full-thickness wound healing is achieved. The resulting stable regular corneal curvature makes possible earlier and more accurate secondary correction.

Mechanism of "Sutures-Out" Corneal Astigmatism

When all sutures have been removed and the wound has stabilized and the corneal astigmatism is determined by refraction, keratometry, and topographic mapping, not only its presence but its mechanism will be important to the selection of the appropriate secondary correcting procedure. In the case of a severe residual astigmatism, the mechanism is usually from sector wound slippage from a poorly healed wound, commonly seen following penetrating keratoplasty for keratoconus in which a sector of the cornea, usually inferior, is thinned and sutured to a normal-thickness donor button (Plate 15–1,A). With the closing sutures in place, the unequal forces around the periphery of the graft may be compensated. However, when the sutures are removed, although the circumference of the peripheral corneal optical ring remains constant, a sector of the more central pseudo-optical ring stretches forward, inducing flattening as indicated by a distortion of the surgical keratometer projection (Plate 15–1,B,C). This is seen after rotational grafts (Plate 15–1, D and E), be-

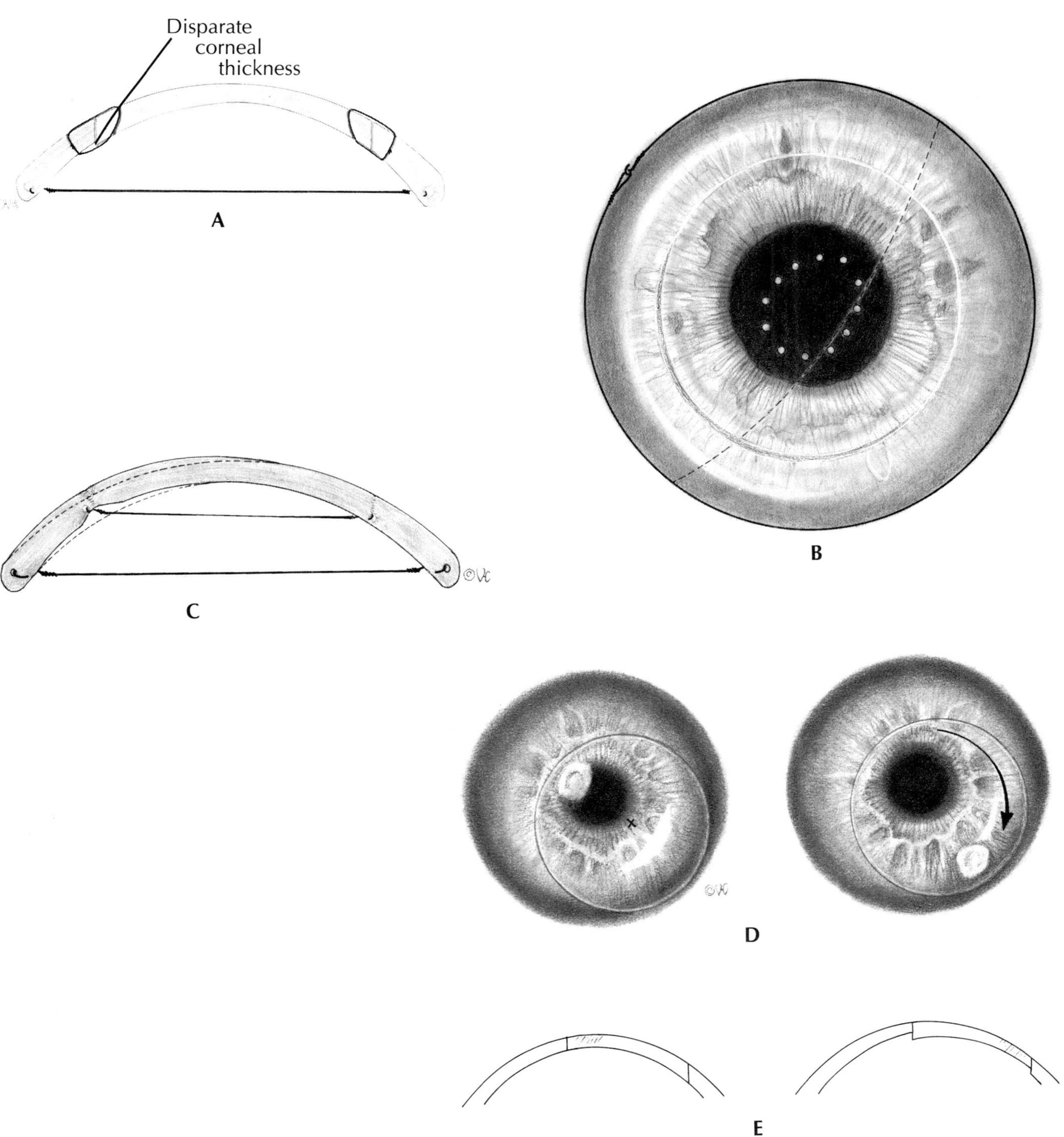

A, normal thickness corneal graft sutured to thinner recipient area, astigmatism controlled with sutures in. **B,** after sutures are removed, keratometer projection indicates flattening of meridian of thinner scar. **C,** cross section showing flattening effect on meridian of thinned scar. **D,** rotational graft, central scar rotated to periphery. **E,** disparate central thicknesses of graft and recipient inducing astigmatism.

cause the thicker peripheral cornea is rotated centrally to displace a central scar. Moderate to severe astigmatism can occur, but when an autograft is indicated it is correctable, whereas graft failure may not be. In these instances, because the astigmatism is induced by a thinner sector of the wound, its correction would be best effected by excision of the defective wound and suture, using the Troutman corneal wedge (block) resection (Plate 15–2,A,B).

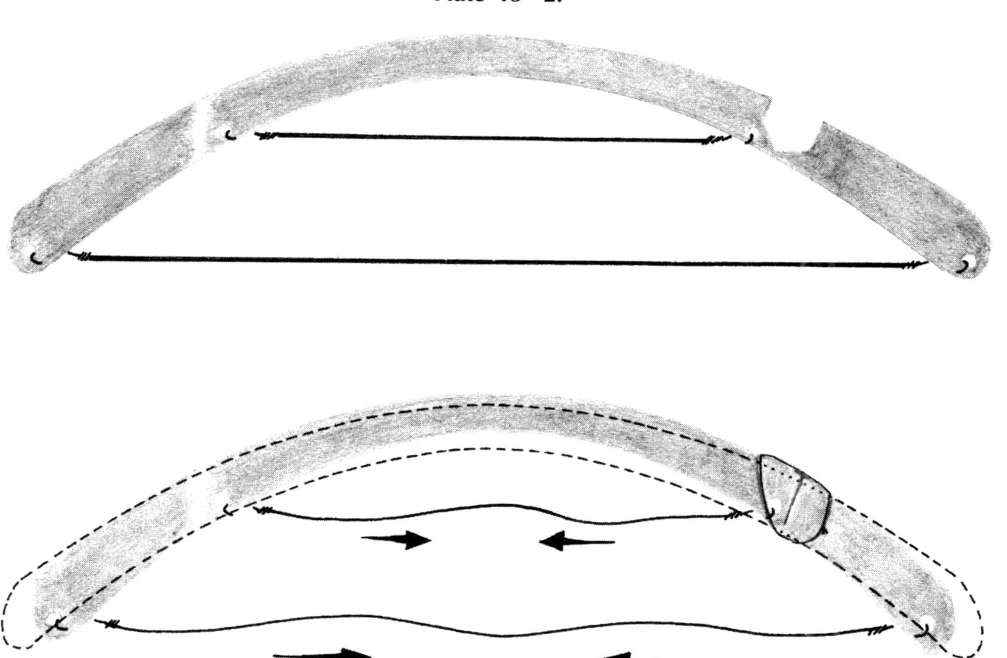

A, block excision of thinned scar sector to steepen flatter corneal meridian. **B,** block excision closed steepening flatter corneal meridian, temporary overcorrection induced.

In a corneal distortion in which the wound is well healed in full thickness around its periphery, both the peripheral corneal optical ring and the pseudo optical ring are stable. In this instance, there will be more symmetry, usually a smaller degree of astigmatism, and a full-thickness scar around the graft circumference (Plate 15–3,A). Correction of these errors is better accomplished by Troutman corneal relaxing incisions, enhanced by compression sutures (Plate 15–3,B).

Astigmatism in eyes with marked differences in peripheral corneal thickness around their circumferences tends to be markedly asymmetric; wedge resection alone does not often fully compensate for the astigmatic error and an undercorrection can result. This phenomenon has recently been demonstrated by topographic corneal mapping and has led to combining corneal wedge resection with corneal relaxing incisions (see Plates 15–20 and 15–21). A better circumferential balance of forces has been achieved as well as a more accurate stable correction.

SECONDARY CORRECTION OF POST-KERATOPLASTY ASTIGMATISM

When keratometry and refraction indicate relative stability of the central corneal curvatures, careful clinical evaluation of the wound combined with topographic corneal mapping is performed to determine the mechanism as well as the amount of postoperative astigmatism. Depending on the amount of the astigmatism and the evaluation of the mechanism, the appropriate corrective procedure is selected. When there is an obvious sector wound defect, a corneal wedge (block) resection or combined with corneal relaxing incisions will be the procedure of choice. If it is determined that the scar is uniform, corneal relaxing incisions with compression sutures will be performed. The topographic map is used to identify the appropriate meridians for the selected procedure, in the case of corneal relaxing incisions across the steeper corneal meridian, and in the case of a corneal block resection, or a combination of both procedures, first across the flatter corneal meridian.

Correction of Residual Astigmatic Error: 1 to 5 D

Originally it was considered appropriate to correct only corneal astigmatic errors in excess of 5 D because of the limited accuracy of early corrective techniques. Smaller degrees of astigmatism are now routinely corrected, and patients, who were formerly satisfied with the improvement of vision even with higher astigmatic residuals, are more willing to have secondary corrective procedures. Smaller corrections are more indicated because we have been able to obtain improved symmetry of the graft, using a standard penetrating keratoplasty procedure aided by one of the new suction trephine sets. This range of errors, as with the correction of

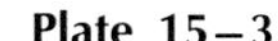

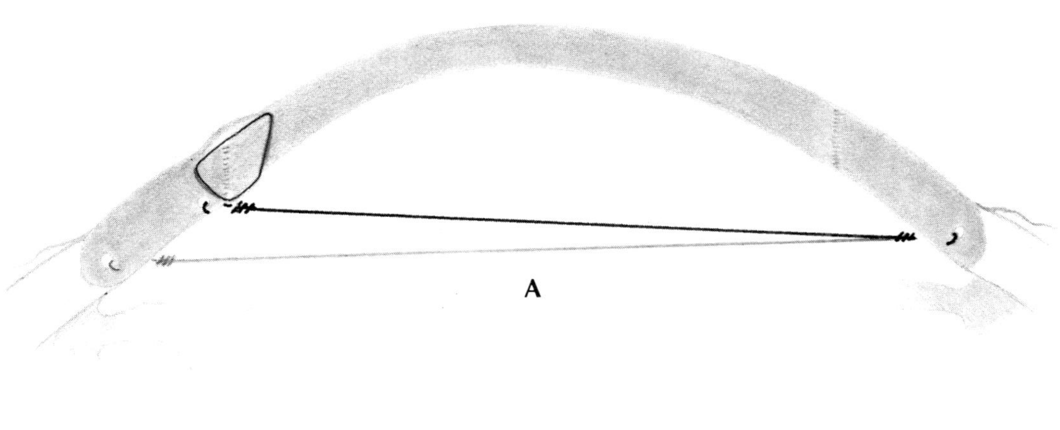

A

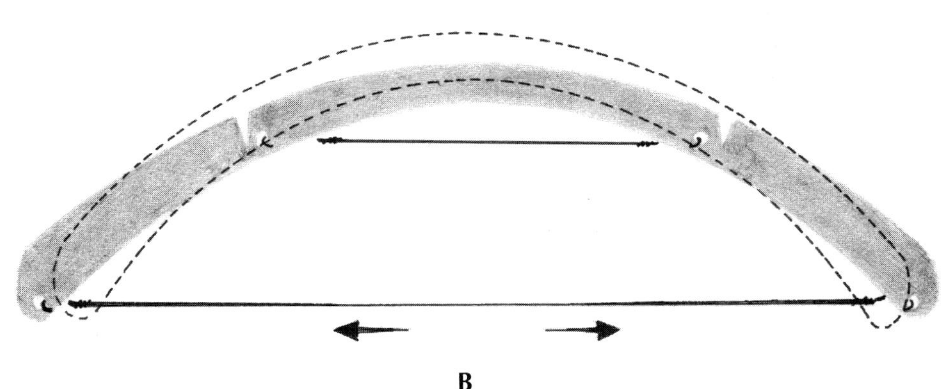

B

A, astigmatism induced in cornea with uniform circumferential healed full-thickness scar. **B,** relaxing incisions correcting steeper corneal meridian (enhanced by compression sutures).

the lower degrees of spherical myopia, is now considered appropriate for secondary correction. Often, such corrections can be effected more accurately with greater reliability and subsequent patient satisfaction than can higher degrees of astigmatism.

Errors under 5 D are best corrected by Troutman corneal relaxing incisions alone or in combination with compression sutures. Not only are relaxing incisions less difficult to perform than a Troutman corneal block resection, but they give more immediate results. Although corneal relaxing incisions can sometimes be performed as an office procedure, it is more appropriate to perform relaxing incisions with compression sutures in an outpatient surgery setting, as with corneal block resection and combined techniques. In either setting, these procedures should be performed only after diagnostic corneal topography, monitored by a surgical keratometer to assure accurate placement of the incisions and compression sutures. This is especially important when using a corneal topographical map because it is now evident that the astigmatic corneal meridians are almost never exactly symmetrical either in their axis or in the lateral extent of the sector involvement at the graft-host junction.

Technique of Corneal Relaxing Incisions: Asymmetric

Although the procedure can be performed under topical anesthesia, peribulbar or retrobulbar anesthesia provides better patient comfort. The computerized topographic corneal map is taken to the operating room and used to delineate the incision and compression suture parameters. *To avoid error the map should be inverted to correspond to the surgeons view, from above, as opposed to the photo from the clinical instrument view from below.* The surgical keratometer is used to verify the approximate axis of the astigmatic band. Using a trephine of the approximate diameter of the graft scar, a mark is made around the circumference of the graft and colored with a dye marker (Plate 15–4,A,B). Using a ring axis marker (see

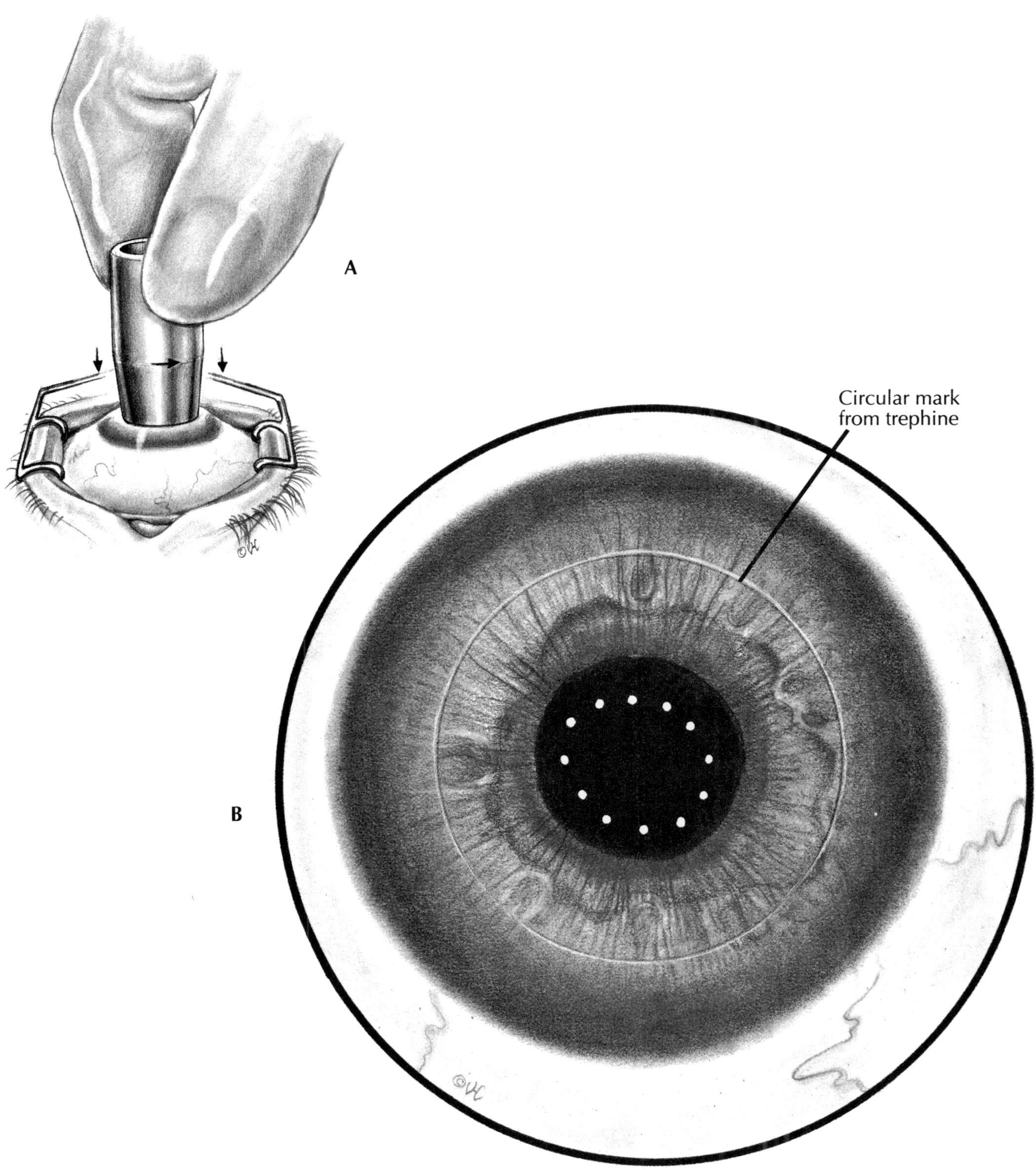

A, trephine being used to mark incision line for relaxing incisions or corneal wedge resection. **B,** marked cornea showing steeper oblique vertical meridian prior to relaxing incisions.

Surgical Management of Post-Penetrating Keratoplasty Astigmatism **415**

chapter 7, Plate 7–27), the appropriate incisional arcs corresponding to the steeper meridians indicated by the topographic map are marked by light radial cuts with a diamond knife. These are dye marked (Plate 15–5). With the Topographic Modeling System, the length of the incision in the graft scar is determined by the width of the red band at the graft junction, varying from 40 degrees up to 90 degrees. The opposing incisional meridians are usually asymmetric, both in their axes and extent.

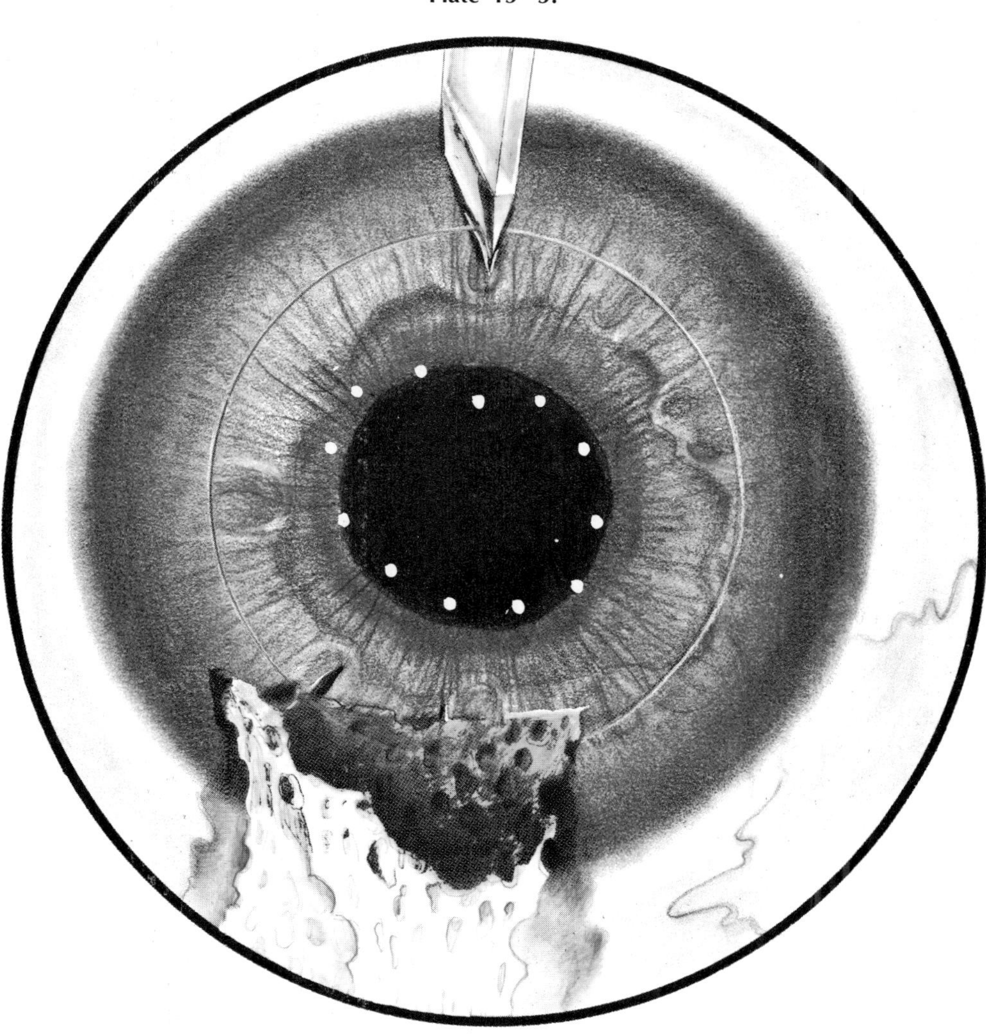

Dye marking incision parameters across steeper corneal meridian indicated by topographic mapping.

A micrometer diamond knife is adjusted to extend its front cutting blade 0.5 mm for an approximate 80% depth cut as determined by ultrasonic pachymetry. The eye is fixated, using ring fixation rather than point fixation, and the incisions are made into the graft scar, following the curvilinear outline mark of the trephine (Plate 15–6). In a longer incision, it is helpful to use the multiple punch technique of Buzard to maintain the symmetry of the incision line. In this technique, the blade first makes multiple unconnected puncture points along the line of the incision, in effect, hyphenating the incision. Then the knife is used to sever the intermediate uncut zones at depth completing the curvilinear cut.

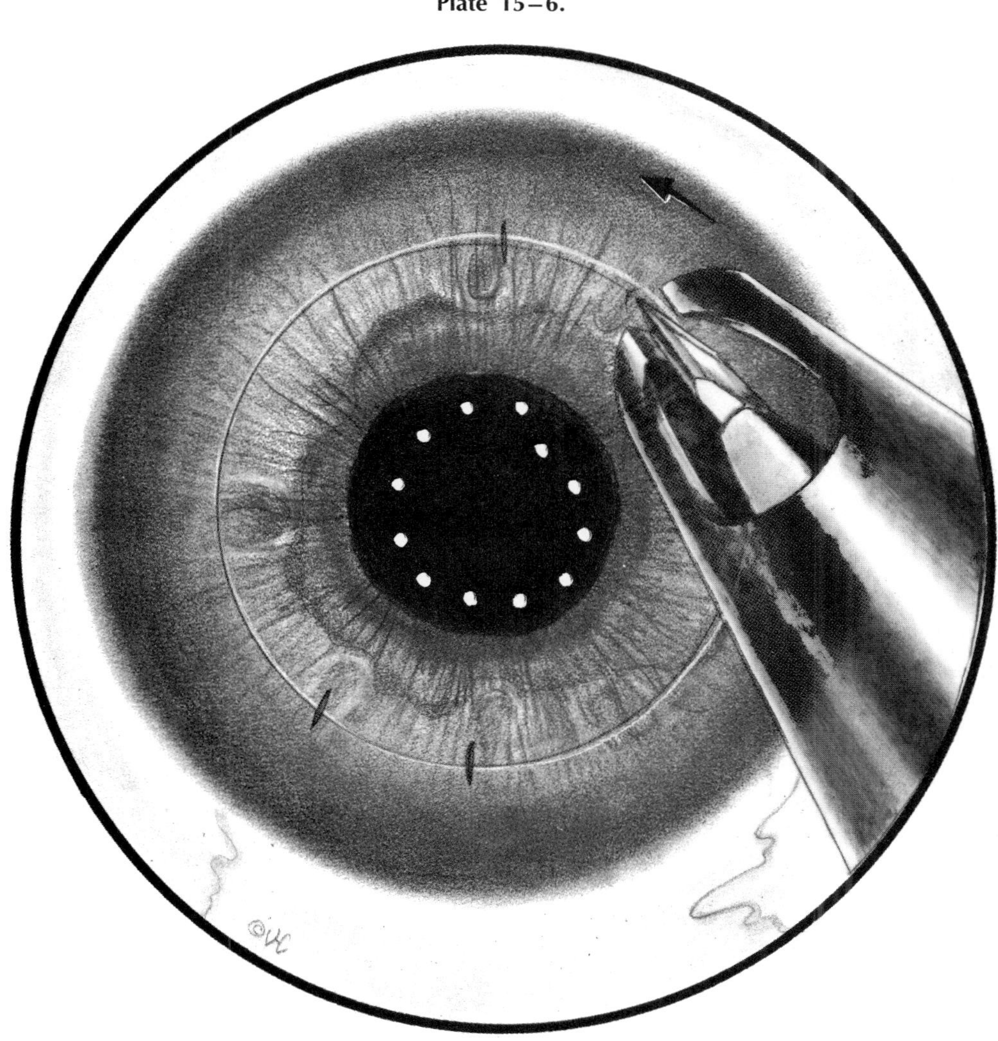

Making relaxing incisions in the graft scar to 80% corneal thickness with micrometer diamond knife.

After the incisions have been completed, the surgical keratometer projection, which had been used initially to confirm the approximate cylinder axis, is used to evaluate their effect. The effects of the relaxing incisions are not always immediately evident. However, some correction will usually be noted. If an overcorrection is not indicated, the surgical keratometer indicating no astigmatism or a slight undercorrection, compression sutures will be added (Plate 15–7). An undercorrection or overcorrection

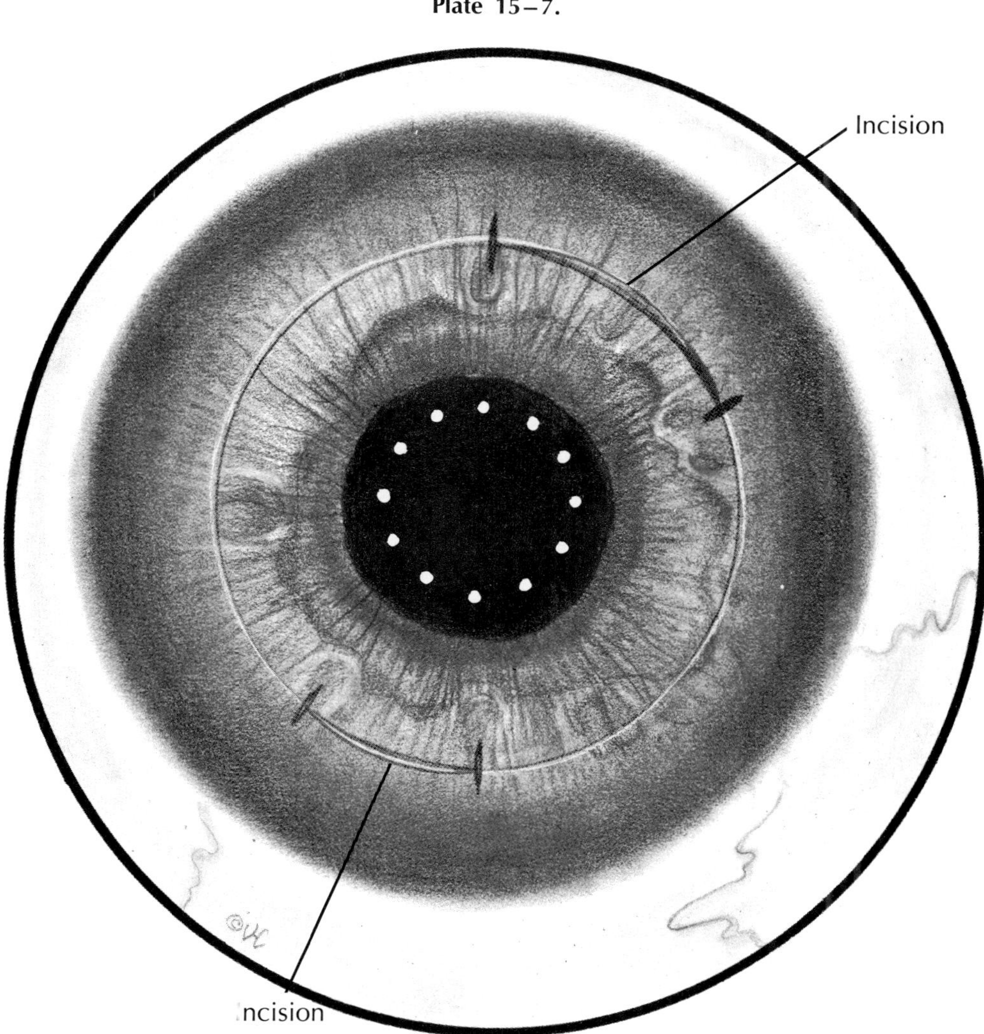

Completed incisions showing partial correction effect.

may be due to unrelieved pressure of the speculum, the relative ocular rigidity, or other factors. Thus, it is not appropriate to rely on surgical keratometer measurements alone to determine a final result. In our opinion, compression sutures should always be used. Their position, indicated by the color-coded topographic map, is centered on the blue, flatter corneal meridian to either side of the incisional meridian, usually at approximately right angles, or 90 degrees (Plate 15–8).

The compression sutures are closed with single slipknots that are adjusted to induce steepening of the preoperatively flatter meridian for an overcorrection of approximately 50% of the preoperative amount. If a flatter zone on one side of the meridian is wider, two compression sutures should be placed. In this instance, usually only one suture will be required on the narrower opposite side of the compression meridian.

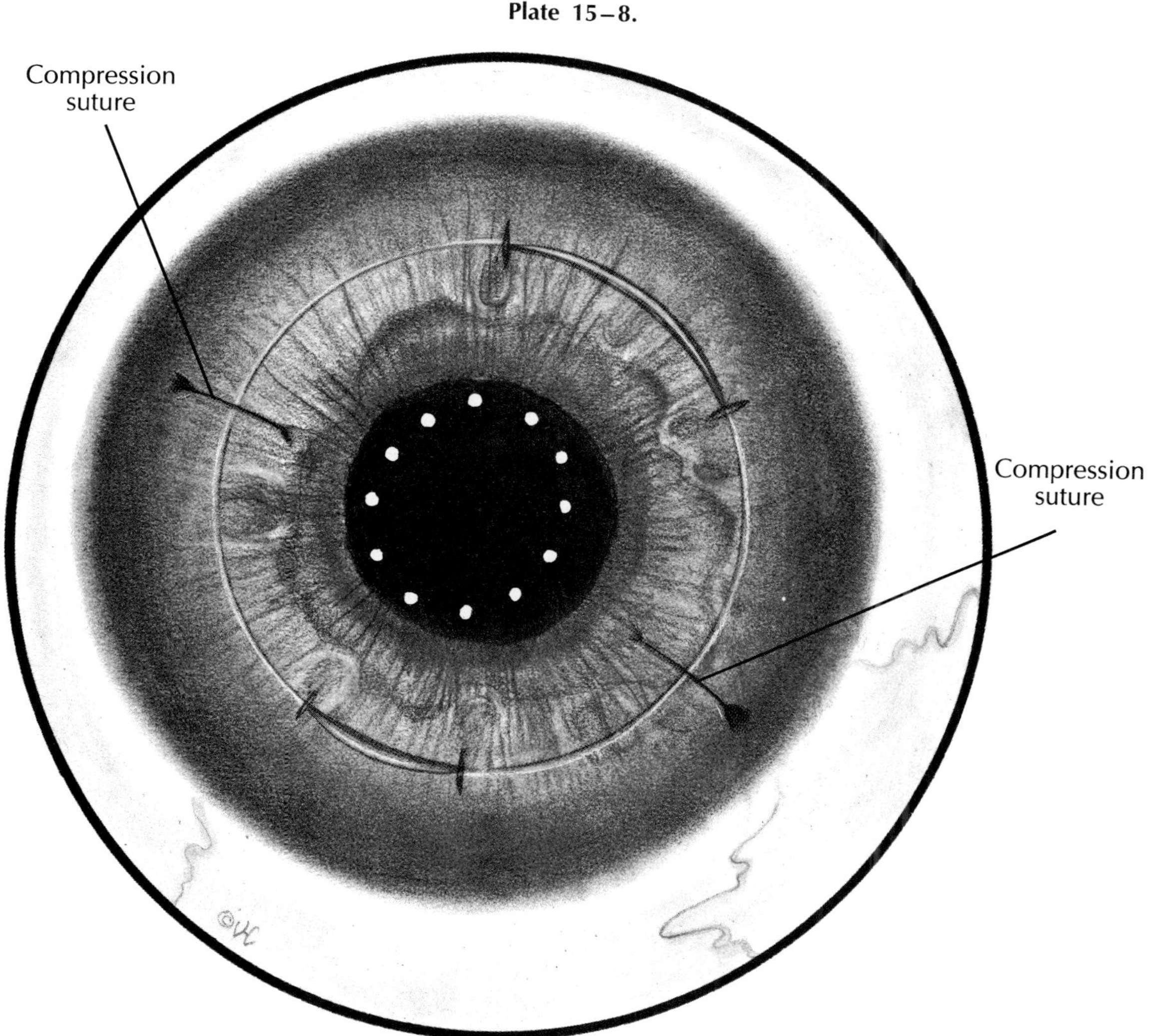

Compression sutures inserted across flatter meridian to induce overcorrection.

Relaxing Incisions: Symmetric

When a corneal topographical mapping system is not available, symmetric relaxing incisions, based on clinical keratometer measurements confirmed in the operating room by the surgical keratometer, are performed (Plate 15–9). Marking of the arcs of the incisions and positioning of compression sutures are facilitated by use of the six-incision radial keratotomy marker (see Chapter 7). Then marking with the trephine is followed by symmetric paired arcuate incisions centered on the axis of the steeper corneal meridian, as indicated by the surgical keratometer and

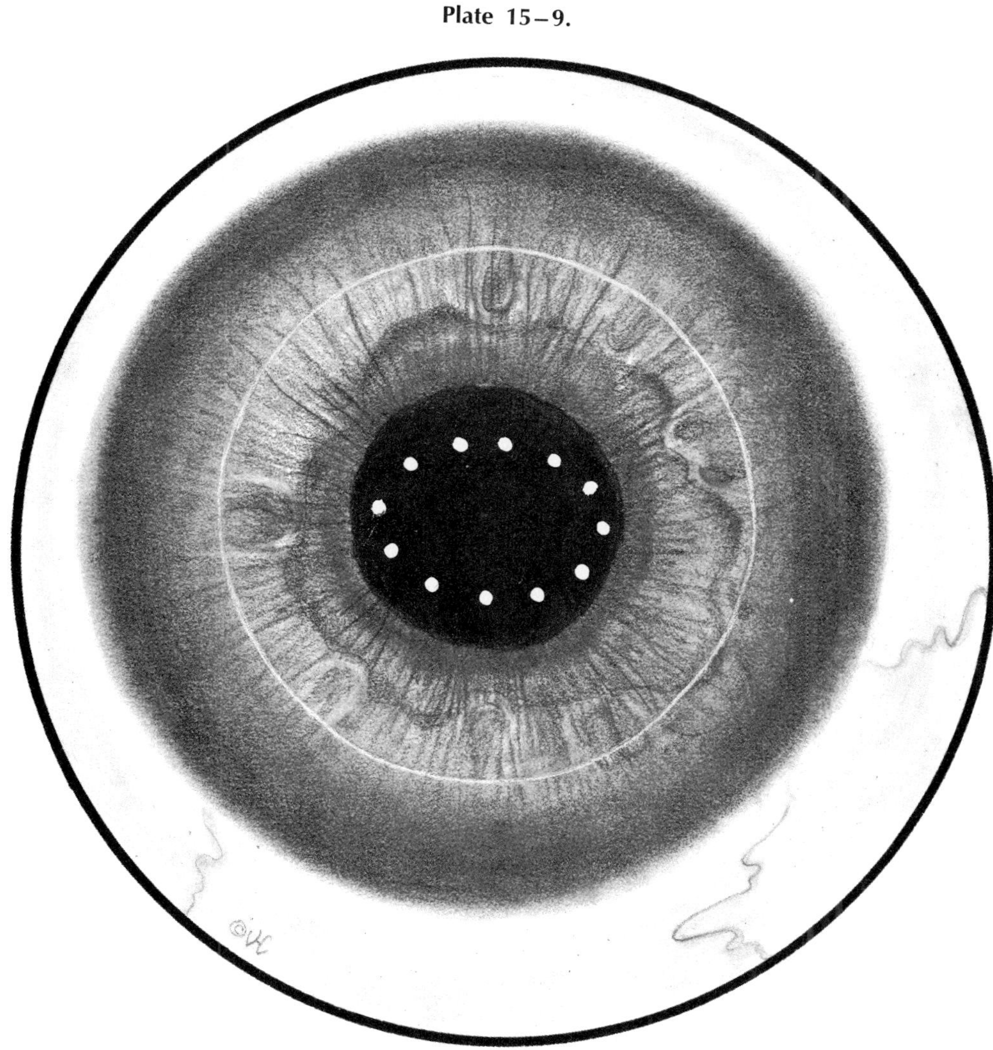

Steeper vertical meridian, incision periphery marked with trephine blade and radial keratotomy marker in preparation for symmetrical relaxing incisions.

the marks (Plate 15–10,A). These are made with a guarded-blade diamond knife, as described earlier, or they can be made with less accuracy by a single-blade diamond knife or a razor blade. As in the previous technique, incisions are made in the corneal scar. The multiple puncture technique can be useful to assure accurate curvalinear incisions.

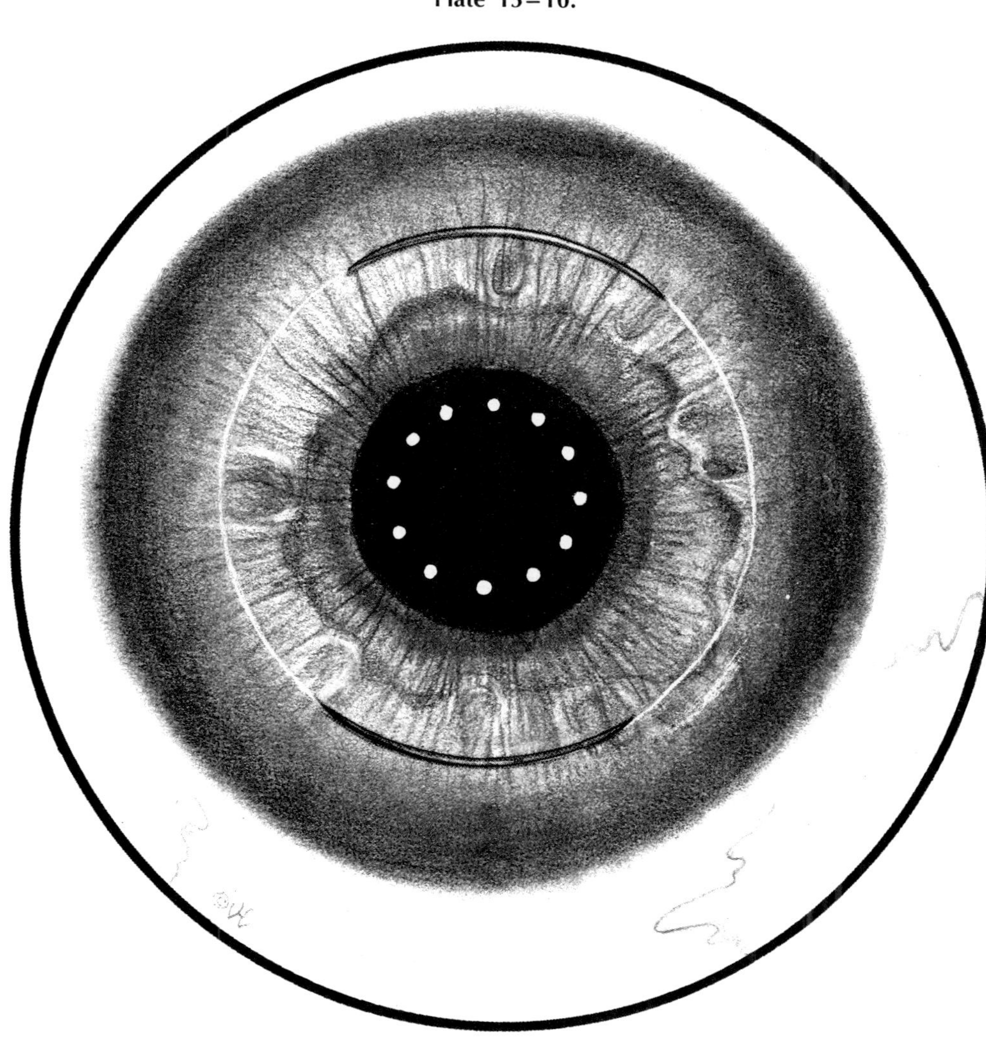

A, relaxing incisions performed across steeper corneal meridian. Partial correction achieved before compression sutures. *Continued.*

Compression sutures are placed at 90 degrees to the axis of the incisional meridian along the preplaced marks and adjusted with slipknots for an approximate 50% overcorrection (Plate 15–10,B).

The effect of relaxing incisions is to induce flattening of a steeper meridian within the pseudo optical ring, the peripheral optical ring remaining constant in diameter and circumference (Plate 15–10,C).

Postoperative Care

For relaxing incisions to be effective, there should be an overcorrection of at least 50% from the preoperative level of astigmatism. The compression sutures are removed sequentially, beginning at 6 weeks.

If an *undercorrection* occurs, a further correction can often be achieved by using the *tickle* technique of Buzard to reopen and deepen or lengthen the incision.

If an *overcorrection* occurs, it will be necessary to place one or several interrupted sutures across the most gaping portion of a relaxing incision under keratometric control, aiming for a slight undercorrection. This suture should be left in place for 3 months or longer until the wound edges heal and the correction is maintained.

The patient should always be informed in advance of surgery that, as with all refractive surgery, some undercorrection and overcorrection not only can but will occur and that one or more minor adjustments may be necessary to achieve an optimal result.

Relaxing incisions give less consistent results for over 5 D of astigmatism, much as the accuracy of radial keratotomy diminishes above 5 D of myopia.

Troutman first proposed this procedure in 1975, adding compression sutures in 1980 and asymmetric incisions in 1988. The technique was originally always done to coincide with the graft scar, and this was the technique used by Krachman and Fenzl (1981), who were the first to confirm his findings. Krachman later proposed the term "augmentation sutures" for compression sutures. Several surgeons have advocated making the cuts internal to the graft scar; however, this does not seem to significantly improve the results and can result in irregular astigmatism.

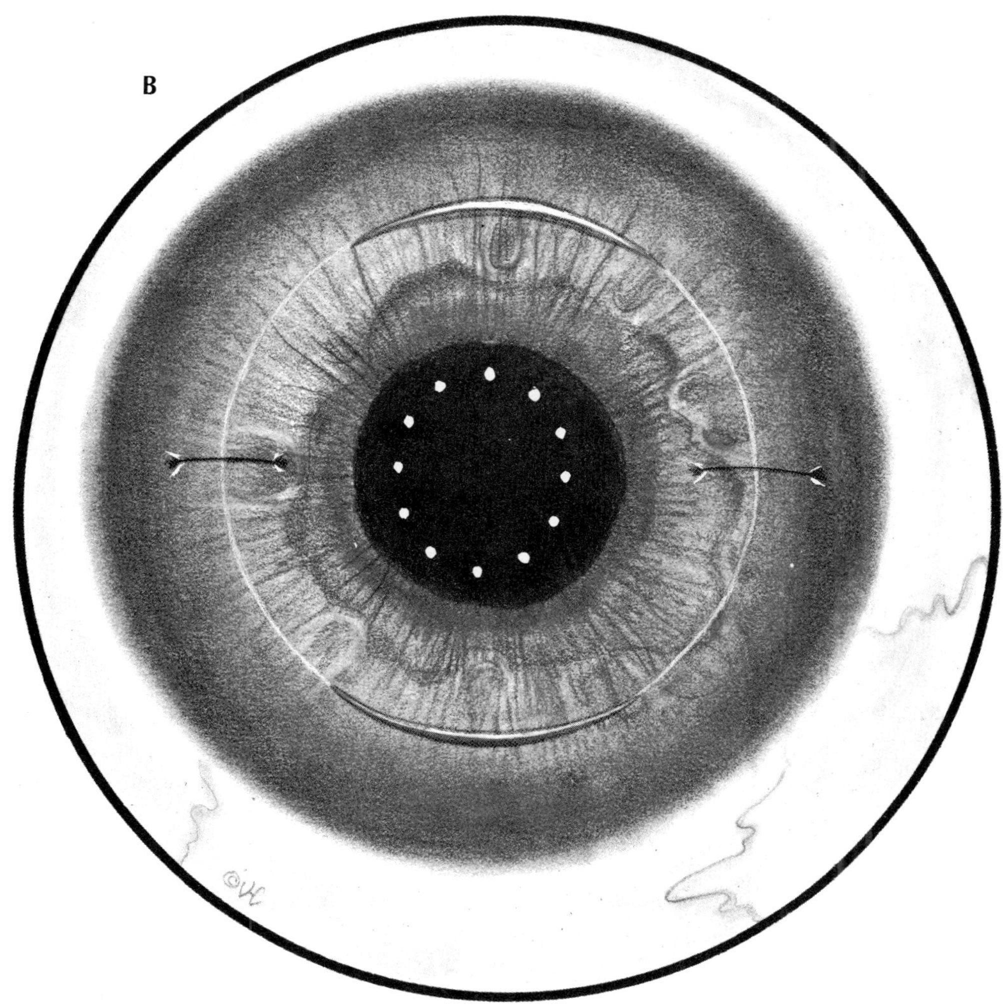

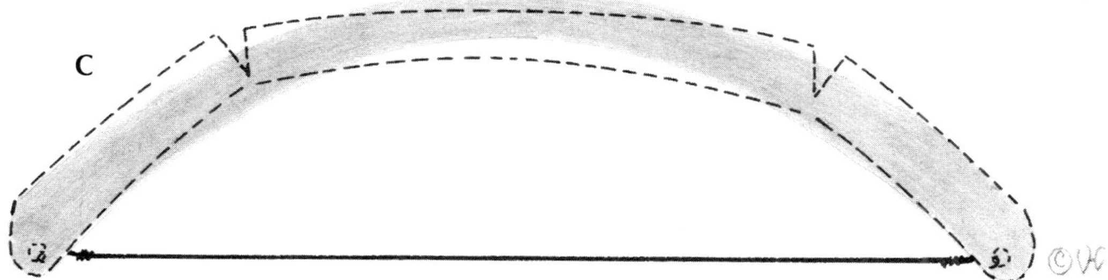

B, corneal flattening induced by relaxing incisions combined with compression sutures. **C,** effect seen in cross section.

Surgical Management of Post-Penetrating Keratoplasty Astigmatism   **429**

CORNEAL WEDGE (BLOCK) RESECTION FOR EXCESSIVE CORNEAL ASTIGMATISM 5.0 D AND GREATER

In point of fact, the term "wedge resection," proposed in 1970 when Troutman originated the technique, should no longer be used generically because we now resect the area as a rectangular block rather than as a triangle or wedge shape. This is not only performed more accurately with improved instruments, but it also serves to reduce the anterior width of resection necessary to achieve a given correction. As a result, when the edges of the block resection are firmly apposed to induce the mandatory overcorrection, there is less tendency toward irregular astigmatism. When combined with compression-compensating sutures, added to the technique in 1980 by Troutman, early rehabilitation of vision and a more comfortable patient are better assured during the sometimes prolonged sutures-in postoperative course.

Corneal Block Resection Technique

The corneal topographic map or a photokeratometry picture is inverted to correspond to the surgeons view, which helps to avoid any positional error when identifying the area to be resected. The flatter resection meridian will usually be seen to be asymmetric, in both extent and axis. For wedge (block) resection, the flatter sector of the wound, invariably the one with the most extensive thinned scar or elevated wound edge, is on the side of the meridian selected for the resection.

With the lid speculum placed to avoid deforming the globe, the surgical keratometer identifies the approximate axis of the flatter corneal meridian, which is then marked with a pen in the area selected for the resection (Plate 15–11). Using the Mendez gauge (protractor ring; see Chapter 7, Plate 7–24), the length for the resection is then marked to correspond to the width of the periphery of the blue, flatter meridian as indicated by the topographic map (see frontispiece for color maps). A trephine blade of appropriate diameter is used to make a light circumferential mark over the scar (see Plate 15–4). The marking cuts are colored with a marking pen. The gimbaled fixation ring is placed around the cornea (see Plate 7–21). The double-bladed block resection knife (see Plate 7–11,A) is set to the selected resection width, not less than 0.5 mm or more than 1 mm, de-

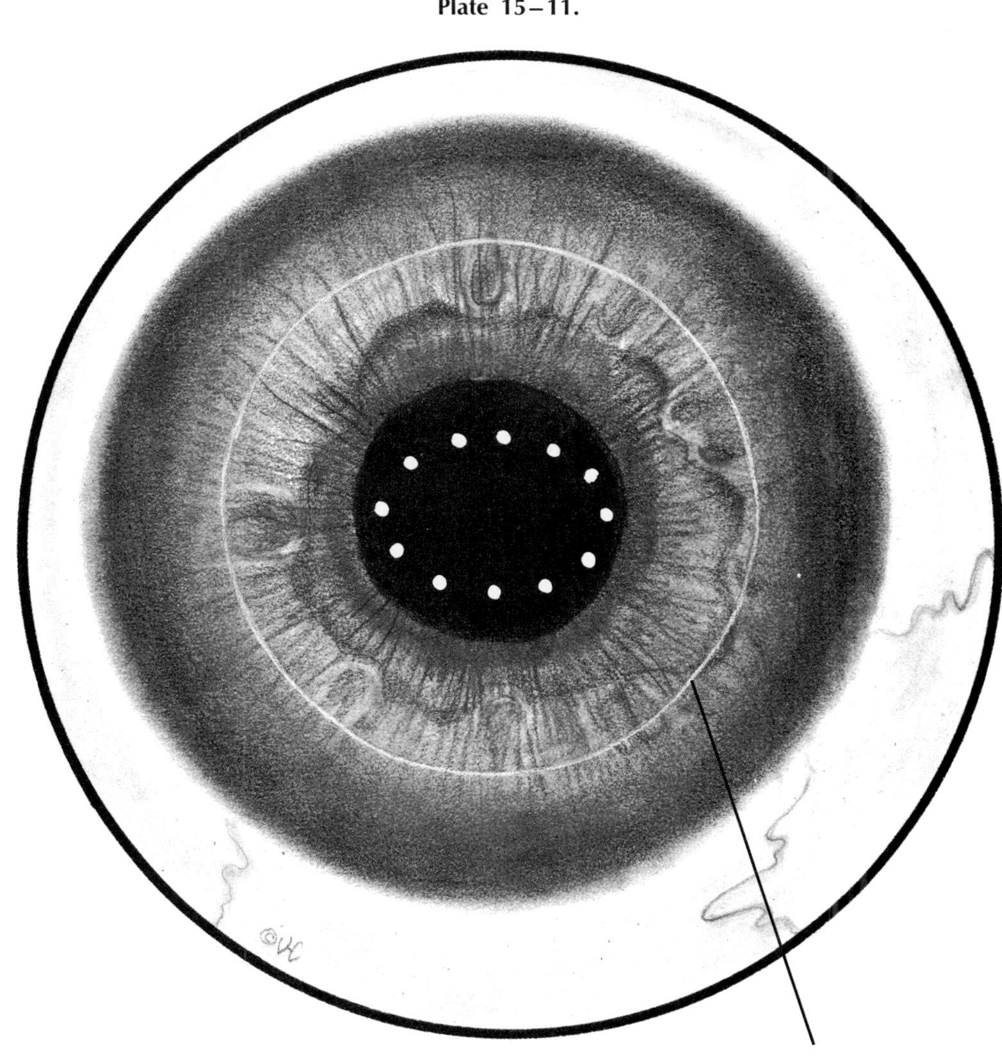

Cornea with flatter meridian at 180° with trephine mark and wedge resection sector as indicated by corneal topographical map. (Confirmed with surgical keratometer.)

pending on the width of the scar and the length of the area to be resected. The shorter the area to be resected, the wider the resection should be to effect the same correction. A longer resection requires less resection width because the same amount of more corneal tissue is being removed. The double-blade knife is placed to straddle the dye-marked graft incision (Plate 15–12,A). Buzard prefers resecting the block completely within the donor cornea, rather than straddling the wound, to maintain an even host contour should regrafting be required. Both techniques are effective. Troutman prefers removing the defective stretched scar inducing flattening of the meridian. Double, partial penetrating, half-thickness incisions are made along the marked resection zone from one end to the other. With a single-blade knife, the external ends of the wounds are extended to meet approximately 1-mm peripheral to the marked area, creating a point for better closure at each end of the incision. The incisions are deepened with another pass of the double-blade knife and the depth of the cuts confirmed. Using the single-blade diamond knife, the block outline is completed to the level of Descemet's membrane (Plate 15–12,B). The block is resected with the Vaness scissors, tensioning the block as it is being resected, to facilitate deep, even resection (Plate 15–13). With the

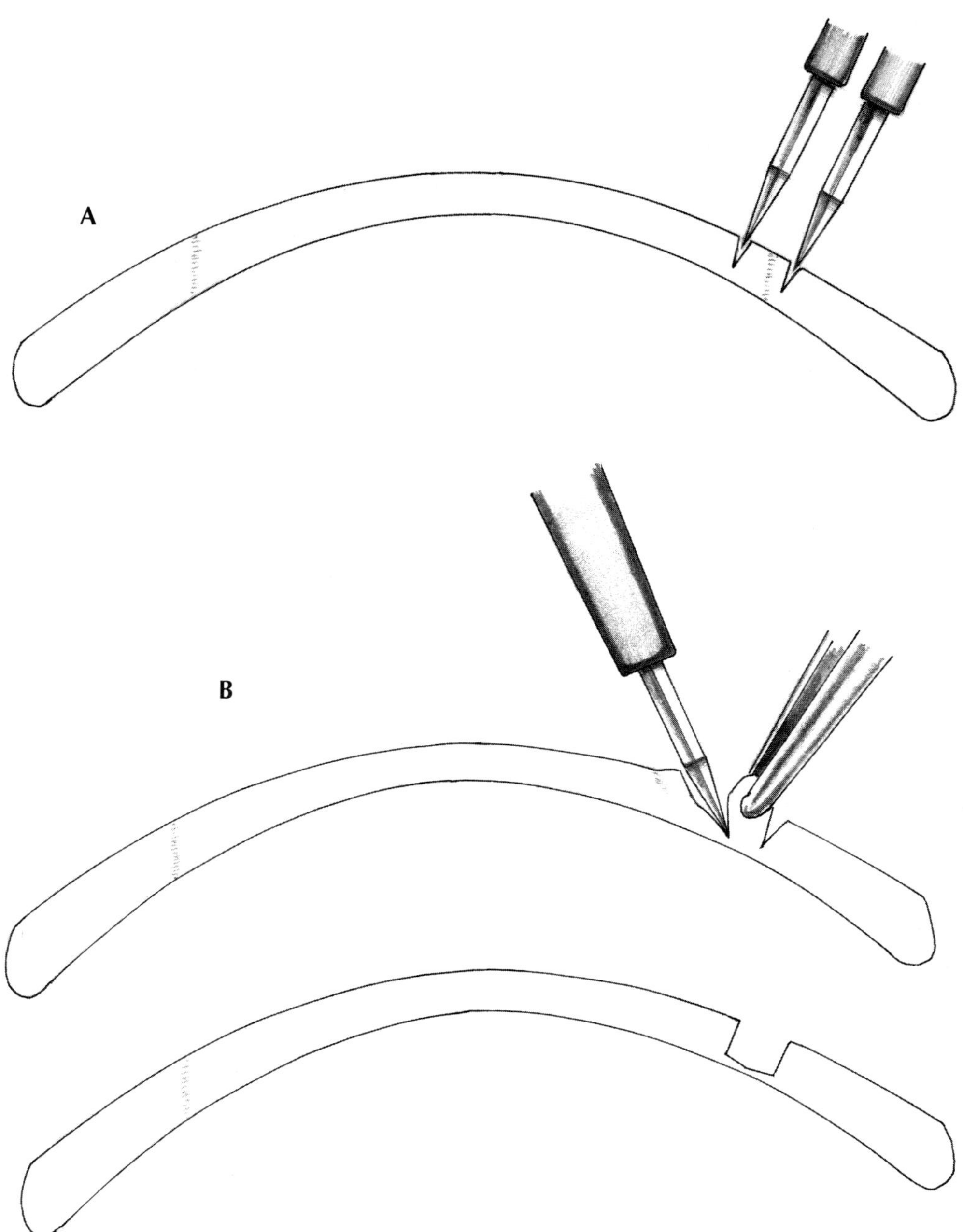

A, double-blade diamond knife outlining block resection. **B,** completing dissection block with single blade diamond knife.

block removed, the donor and recipient edges are lamellarized at the depth of the excision 1 mm from the wound edges to allow some sliding of the wound edges and easier suture apposition (Plate 15–14). A paracentesis may be made to release some aqueous humor so the edges of the wound can be approximated.

Plate 15–13.

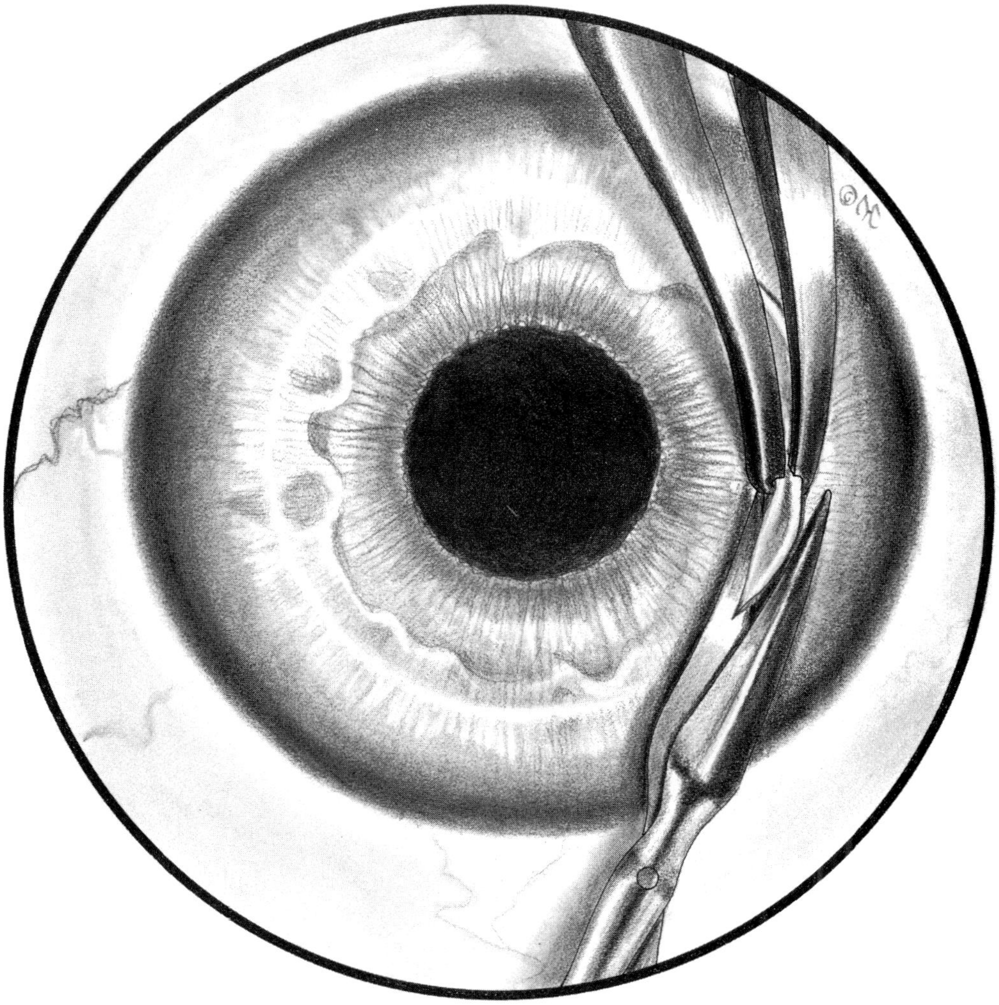

Resection of block at base with Vaness scissors.

Using the compound curved needle, a through-and-through suture loop is placed to approximate the donor to the recipient edge across the center of the excision, entering and exiting about 0.5 mm from the edges. Short, deep bites are essential to prevent central distortion and irregular astigmatism. This loop is completed with a double slipknot and drawn up to approximate the edges, but it is not locked. Two additional full-thickness suture loops are placed between the central suture and the ends of the incision and similarly completed with double slipknots. Using the surgical keratometer as a guide, the slipknots are adjusted to effect both a secure apposition of the tissue edges and the reversal of the preoperative

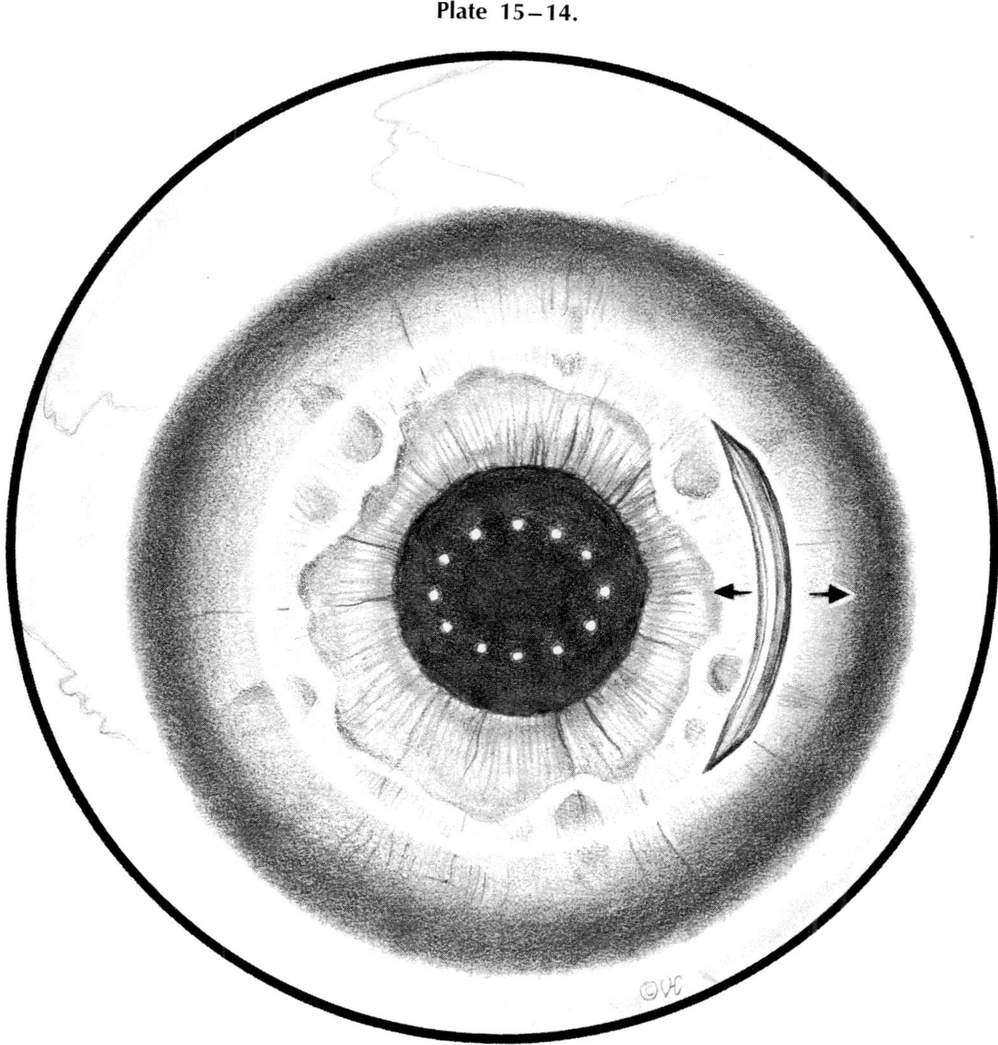

Plate 15–14.

Lamellarized block resection area after paracentesis to facilitate closure.

astigmatic band. If the wound margins are tightly apposed and there is still an incomplete reversal of the astigmatic band, then insufficient resection has been done and a small additional resection is performed. It may be necessary to replace some or all of the three initial sutures. These sutures are locked with square knots, and four or more additional sutures are placed between and peripheral to them to effect the final closure (Plate 15–15). All suture loops should encompass the full thickness of the cornea to effect full-thickness apposition of the opposing edges. When the suturing is complete, the knots are buried on the donor side of the wound. They should not be buried on the recipient side because they may stimulate vascularization and will be more difficult to remove. The knots *must* be buried because these sutures may have to remain in place for up to 1 year postoperatively.

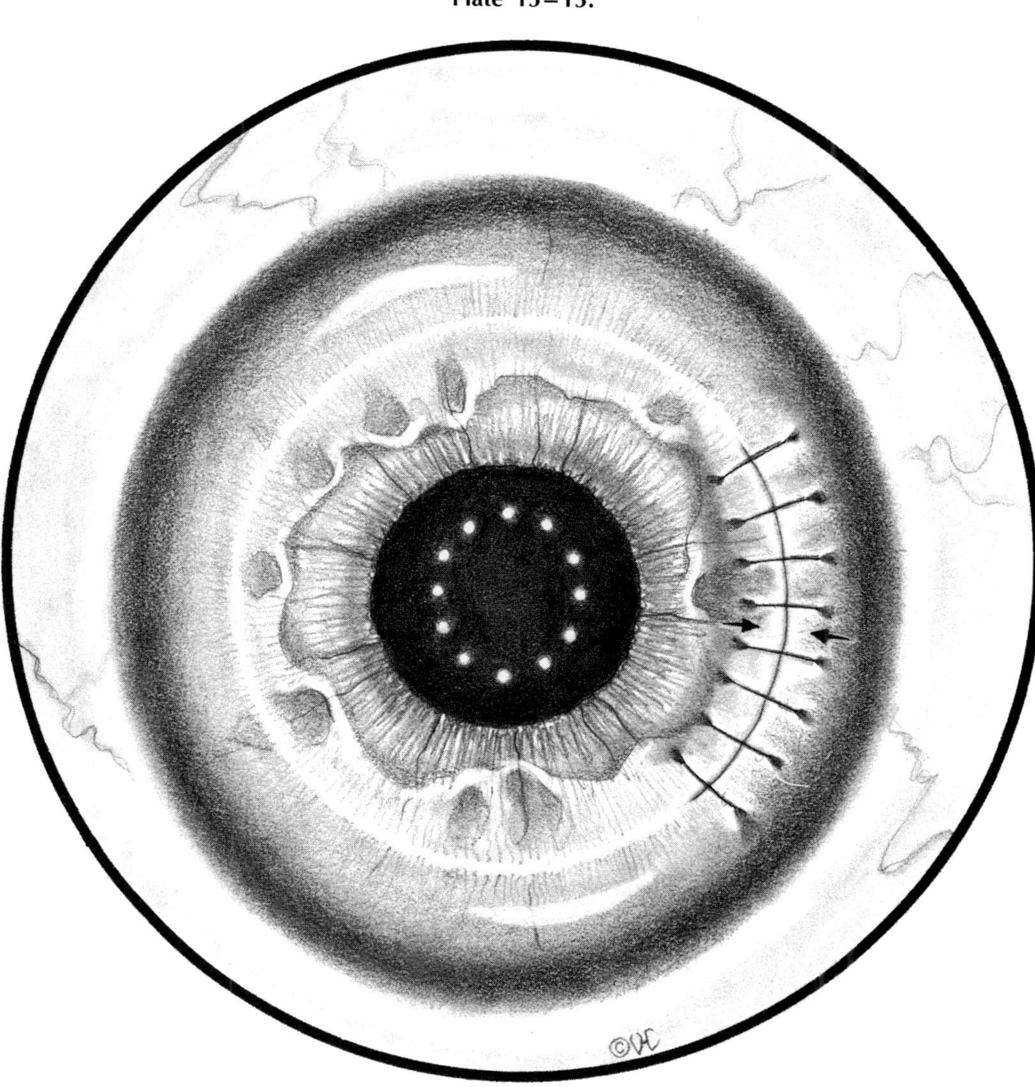

Wedge resection area closed with multiple interrupted through-and-through sutures, note overcorrection.

Compensating Compression Sutures

The overcorrected meridian is identified with the surgical keratometer, and two or more full-thickness interrupted loops are placed across the graft incision at approximately 90 degrees distal to the ends of the block resection. These are completed with single slipknots. With the eye normotensive, the loops are adjusted until the projection of the surgical keratometer indicates sphericity (Plate 15–16). They are locked down and the

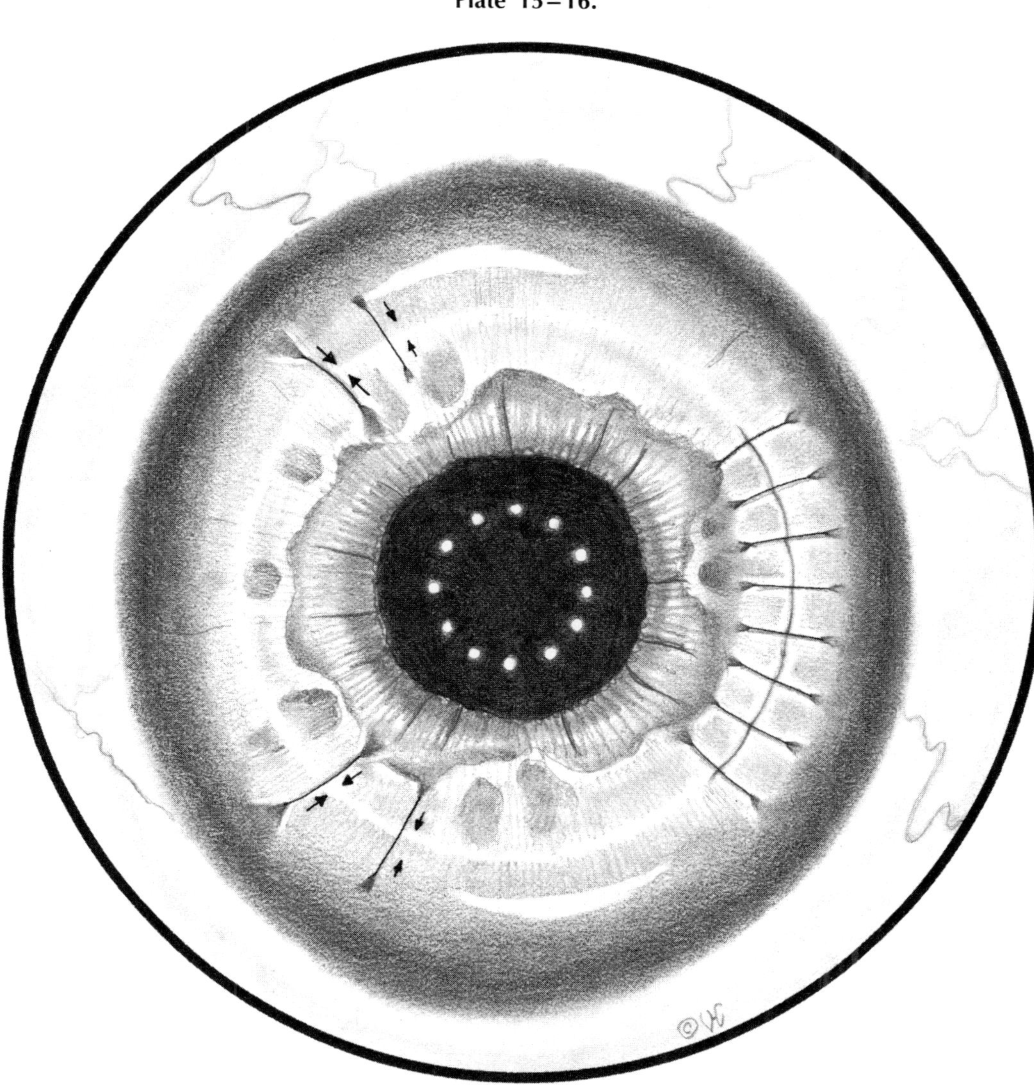

Compression-compensating sutures inserted to compensate for overcorrection and to reinforce the graft incision opposite to resection area.

knots are buried in the donor, not the recipient, cornea. The position of these two or more sutures should be such that they provide, in addition to their optical correcting function, support to the graft wound opposite to the resection meridian (Plate 15–17,A,B,C). It has been observed in some cases, especially when wedge resection may have been done relatively soon after suture removal, that the wound opposite can stretch from the tension of the resection, partially nullifying its effect. To prevent this occurrence, reinforcement should be done even if the surgeon feels that the compensating compression sutures are unnecessary.

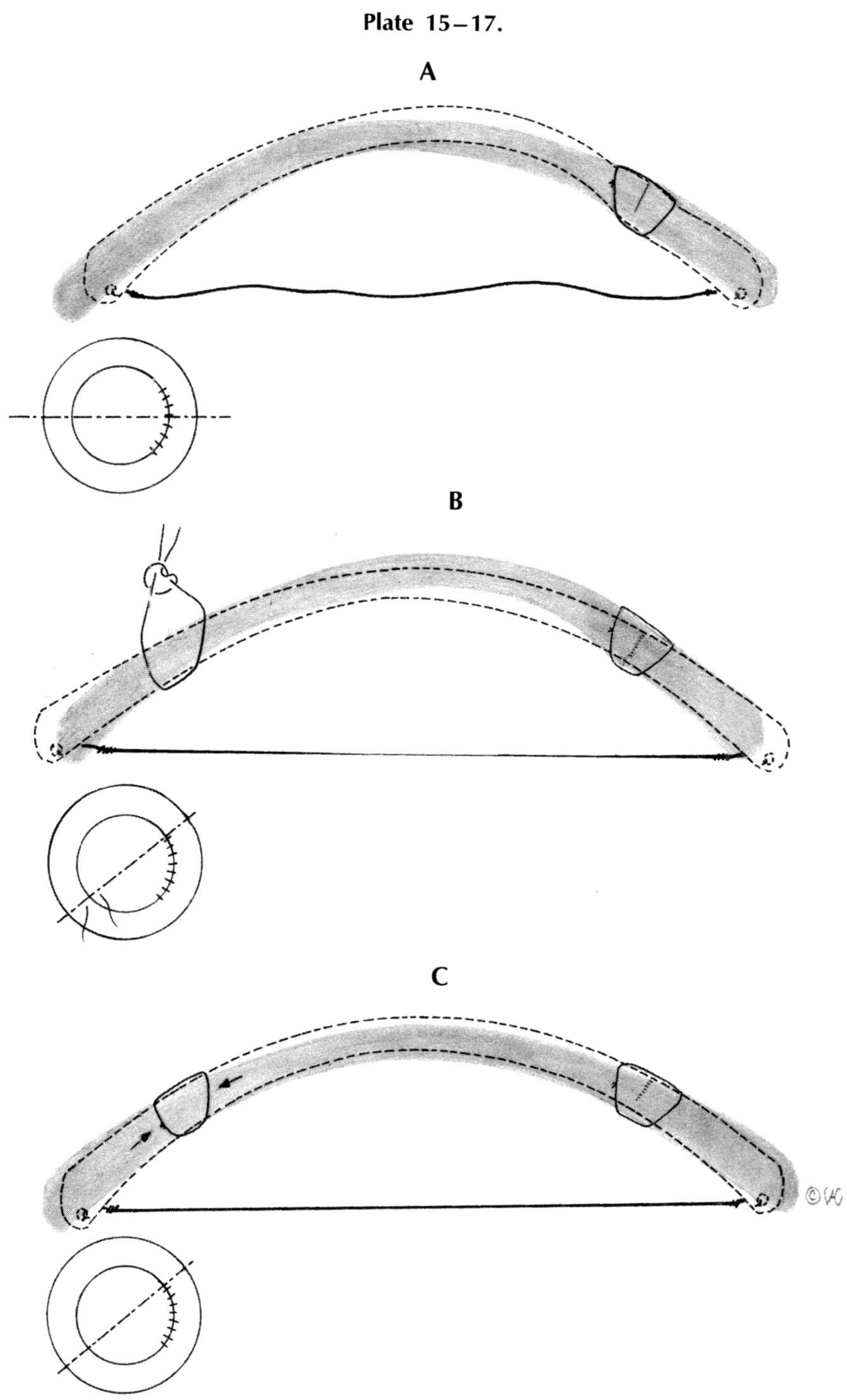

A, steepening effect of wedge-resecting closing sutures on preoperatively flatter corneal meridian. B, positioning of compensating compression suture loop across healed keratoplasty wound. C, compensation of overcorrected meridian by completed compression suture loop.

The corneal relaxing incisions technique is summarized in Plate 15–18, and the corneal wedge resection technique in Plate 15–19.

Postoperative Care

It is important that no sutures be removed from a corneal wedge resection for a minimum of 3 months after surgery, no matter what the optical state. The wound will dehisce in whole or in part, and any temporary correction achieved will be lost. The one exception is if a suture should become loosened, then it should be removed to prevent irritation and possible infection.

At 3 months the compressed cornea at the wound will begin to release and an overcorrection in the orthogonal meridian may appear, at which point one or more compression compensating sutures can be removed sequentially. Then if an overcorrection occurs in the resection meridian, the tightest sutures, as observed by the slitlamp and confirmed by computerized topographic analysis, should be removed leaving the less tight sutures in place. If an undercorrection is present, only loosened sutures should be removed and all apposing sutures should remain in place for an additional 3 months. One can begin to remove the sutures at 6 months at intervals of 2 to 4 weeks, until all have been removed and the final correction achieved.

It is important for the patient to understand both the inexact nature of the wedge (block) resection procedure and the variability that can be anticipated in the result. The patient should be advised that, in addition to sequential suture removal, one or several touch-up procedures may be required to achieve the optimum correction. Corneal graft rejection, which may or may not be related, has been reported. To avoid this possibility, it is necessary to remove a loosened suture or sutures immediately.

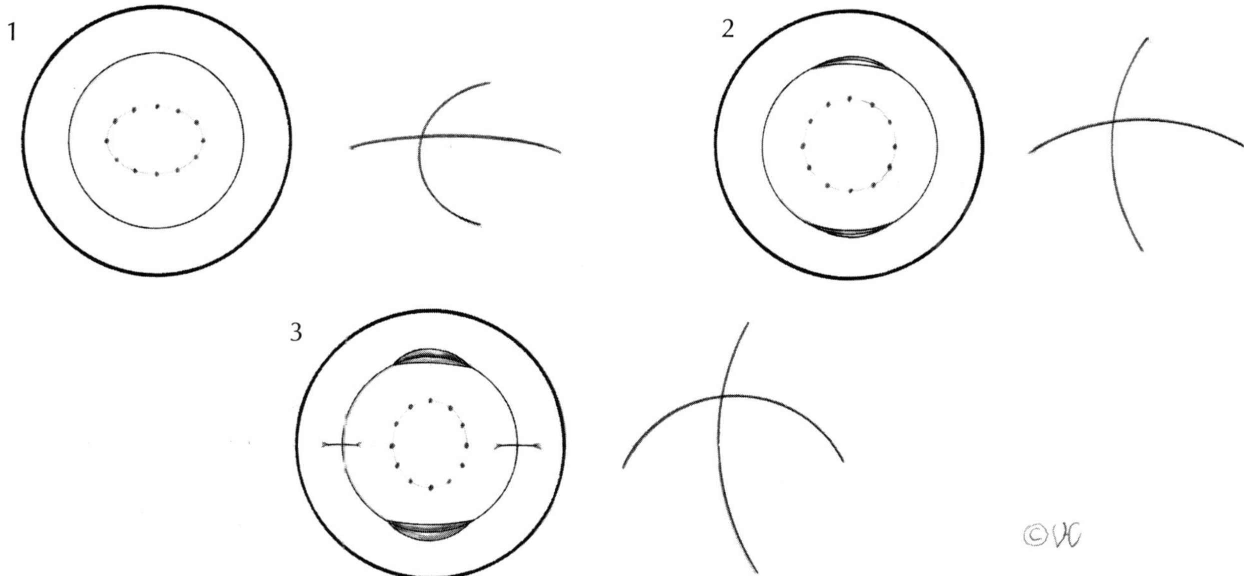

Summary of corneal relaxing incisions technique: **(1)** Steeper vertical corneal meridian. **(2)** Relaxing incisions partially correcting steeper corneal meridian. **(3)** Overcorrecting compensating sutures.

Plate 15–19.

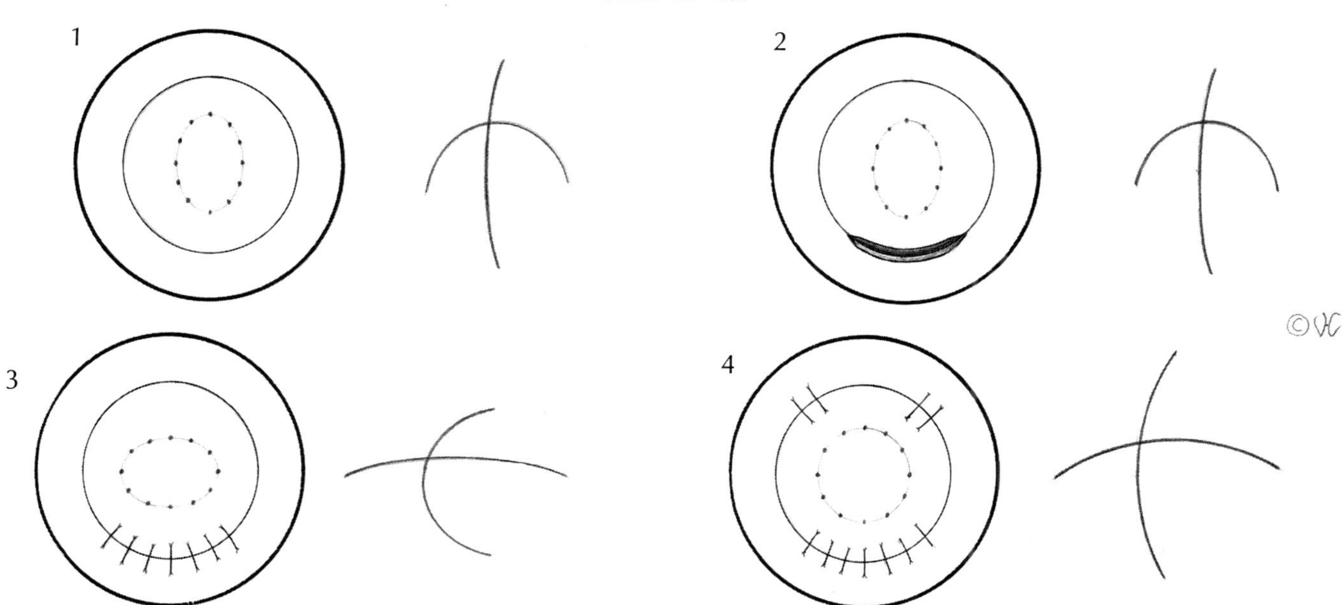

Summary of corneal wedge resection technique: **(1)** Flatter vertical corneal meridian. **(2)** Block resection of thinned corneal scar across flatter meridian. **(3)** Overcorrecting closing sutures. **(4)** Compression-compensating sutures correcting induced astigmatism and reinforcing wound opposite to resection.

COMBINED CORNEAL WEDGE RESECTION AND CORNEAL RELAXING INCISIONS FOR ASTIGMATIC ERRORS GREATER THAN 10 D

In the past, errors greater than 10 D have been difficult to correct fully and with reasonable accuracy by corneal wedge resection or corneal relaxing incisions, alone. Corneal topographic mapping, by indicating to us the irregularity and asymmetry of the flat and steep sectors of the peripheral cornea, has led us to attempt combined procedures. We perform relaxing incisions, forcing the overcorrection with a corneal block resection in place of one or more compression sutures, or, after corneal block resection, corneal relaxing incisions to enhance the effect.

In both cases, we use compression-compensating sutures to partially close one or both relaxing incisions to provide a temporary spherical postoperative result. Sutures are left in place for a minimum of 3 months up to a maximum of 1 year before being removed.

Corneal block combined with corneal relaxing incisions is shown in Plate 15–20, and corneal relaxing incisions combined with corneal block resection in Plate 15–21.

The combined procedure brings home even more clearly the fact that this technique is an art and not a science. It is only with the knowledge of corneal optics gained from photokeratometry and more recently from corneal topographic mapping, for example, the CMS and TMS and the surgical keratometer, that incisions and excisions can be made that can balance the unequal forces created by the keratoplasty scar. In most primary cases, we have performed the procedure by doing the relaxing incisions first and then, if these are not effective, adding the wedge (block) resection secondarily. Only when the wedge (block) resection does not overcorrect at the procedure do we add relaxing incisions to induce a greater correction.

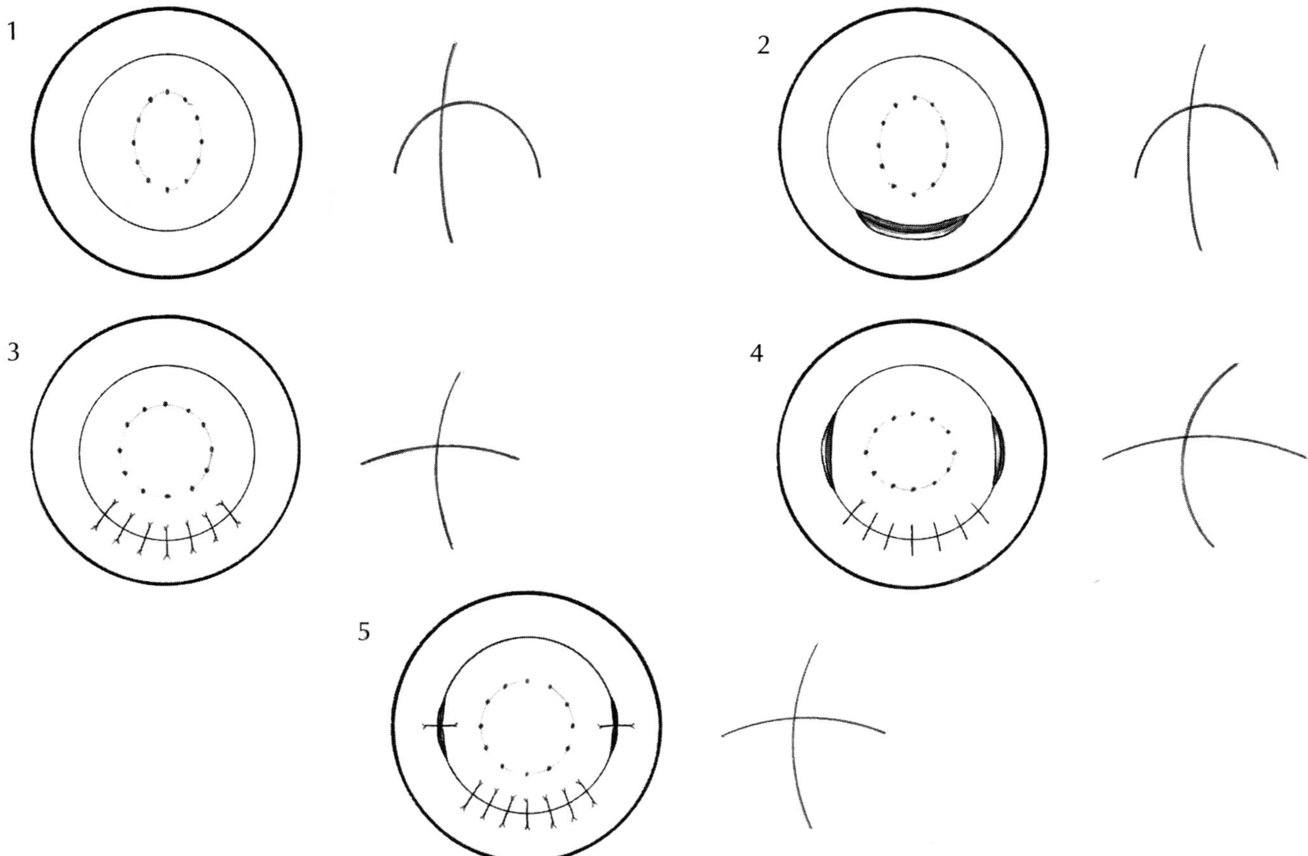

Summary of corneal block resection combined with relaxing incisions: **(1)** Flatter vertical corneal meridian. **(2)** Block resection of thinned cornea. **(3)** Apparent undercorrection. **(4)** Addition of paired relaxing incisions. **(5)** Compression-compensating sutures across paired relaxing incisions.

Postoperative Care

As with corneal wedge resection alone, sutures are left in place for at least 3 months before any are removed. First the compression compensating sutures and then the interrupted sutures closing the block resection are removed sequentially at intervals of 2 to 4 weeks until approximate sphericity has been achieved. The remainder are left in for up to 1 year. According to preoperative and postoperative corneal topographic maps, this procedure gives us not only better corrections but also a more regular periphery.

MANAGEMENT OF SPHERICAL AMETROPIAS IN COMBINATION WITH POST-KERATOPLASTY ASTIGMATISM

The management of these compound errors often requires multiple procedures individually or in combination. Simple correction of astigmatism by corneal block resection, relaxing incisions, or a combination, has a minimal effect on average corneal curvature, approximating the spherical equivalent of the astigmatism; in the case of corneal wedge resection becoming slightly flatter, in the case of corneal relaxing incisions becoming slightly steeper.

On occasion an otherwise successful penetrating keratoplasty will result in an excessively steep cornea. Troutman performed a circumferential wedge resection in 1976 in a single traumatic case, correcting 12 D of induced myopia. Buzard has performed several circumferential and hemicircumferential wedge resections, with reduction of myopia of 5 to 10 D. This technique flattens the cornea analogous to undersizing penetrating donor buttons to flatten the cornea and reduce corneal power. This may become technically more feasible with a "double trephine" blade being constructed by Moria for the Hanna trephine, or the excimer laser may better perform this function.

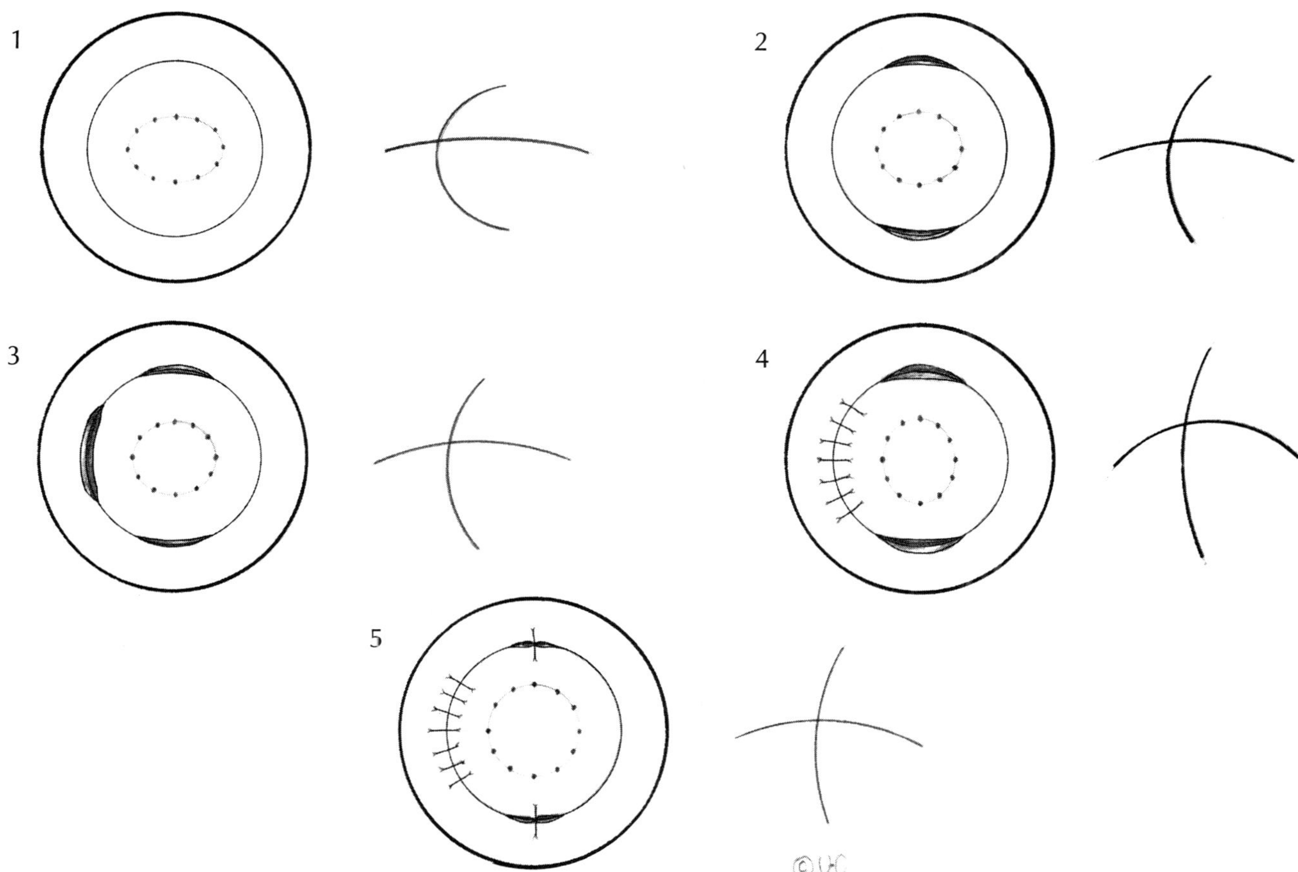

Summary of corneal relaxing incisions combined with block resection: (1) Steeper vertical corneal meridian. (2) Paired relaxing incisions with apparent undercorrection. (3) Addition of corneal block resection. (4) Overcorrection accomplished. (5) Compression-compensating sutures across paired relaxing incisions.

SUMMARY

In this chapter we have outlined the correction of astigmatism resulting from penetrating keratoplasty. As we have seen in Chapter 14, prevention is the obvious choice. However, with current surgical mechanical instrumentation, routine achievement of this goal is not possible. Not only is prevention important, but also the character of the scar resulting from the keratoplasty. A full-thickness healing can be achieved only with full-thickness antitorque wound closure. When significant post-keratoplasty astigmatism occurs, a full-thickness scar can be manipulated more accurately with more predictable results than one resulting from a wound that was closed superficially and that has marked thickness irregularity in the scar, inducing the astigmatism.

When astigmatism of less than 5 D occurs, then corneal relaxing incisions with compression sutures are the procedure of choice, giving the most accurate corrections and the greatest patient satisfaction. Between 5 and 10 D, a corneal block resection has been used primarily. More recently, and especially with astigmatism above 10 D, combined procedures with corneal relaxing incisions followed by corneal block resection, or the reverse, have been performed.

The simultaneous correction of spherical ametropias from the graft may or may not be possible, depending on the severity and cause, but can be performed as a tertiary procedure in severe cases.

Chapter 16

Pathophysiology and Surgical Management of Post–Radial Keratotomy Astigmatism

Anterior radial keratotomy as introduced by Fyodorov in the late 1970s has been an operation in constant evolution. Almost immediately, Fyodorov recognized that the original operation of 32 radial incisions gave nearly the same effect as 16 incisions and recommended reducing the number of incisions to simplify the operation. The original radial keratotomy gave far less effect than its modern counterpart. For instance, 16 incisions in 546 patients gave only 2.77 D of myopic effect, whereas 32 incisions performed in 22 patients gave 2.79 D of myopic effect. This relatively small reduction in myopia, despite the large number of incisions, was a result of several factors. The incisions were planned to be at only 75% depth, and with the metal blades available at that time, the depth of the incisions was often considerably less. The introduction of crystalline knives and improved surgical technology in general led to the realization that fewer incisions could give significant reductions in myopia. It was soon recognized that with incisions of 90% depth or more, 16 incisions resulted in only 10% more effect than eight-incision radial keratotomy. Even more interesting was the observation that four incisions provided 60% of the effect of an eight-incision radial keratotomy.

As the number of incisions decreased, the relative importance of each incision became more prominent. Variations in configuration and depth often led to situations in which an irregular astigmatism or an astigmatism that was considerably changed from the original error became manifest during the postoperative period. At the present time the use of variable depth radial incisions to correct astigmatism has not been exploited. A poorly performed radial keratotomy varying in terms of depth of incisions or orientation of those incisions may lead to circumstances in which correction of induced astigmatism may be quite difficult. Therefore, any discussion concerning the correction of astigmatism in radial keratotomy must, by its nature, be preceded by a careful description of radial keratotomy as performed at the current level of technology. The goal of this discussion will be to identify those areas of greatest variability and difficulty and to describe the current approaches to avoid problems. Certainly in its optimal configuration, the radial keratotomy operation should be centered squarely on the visual axis with symmetrical incisions of equal depth.

RADIAL KERATOTOMY

Prevention of astigmatic error with radial keratotomy is largely a matter of proper placement and performance of radial incisions. Radial keratotomy is a forgiving procedure, but only in a limited sense, and small details can often lead to significant problems that can only be resolved with a much more difficult surgical procedure. Planning and forethought are essential to avoid serious errors such as poor positioning of the optical axis and incision pattern.

If we consider our model of the cornea with a limbal *guy wire*, we can appreciate the fact that a *pseudo optical ring* is created along the optical zone on which the eight radial incisions abut. For an eight-incision radial keratotomy the orientation of the *pseudo optical ring* is dependent on the symmetrical and equal movement of the cornea in each of eight directions (Plate 16–1). The situation is similar to a table with eight legs. If one leg is short or long, the table will not be level. Similarly, if one incision produces less effect, as seen in a shallow incision, or more effect, as seen in a microperforation, the curvature will be asymmetric, resulting in regular or irregular astigmatism. These problems assume even greater significance when dealing with a four- and six-incision radial keratotomy. Displacement of the optical zone causes similar displacement of the *pseudo optical ring,* which can itself lead to astigmatic error, as shown in penetrating keratoplasty by Van Rij (1985).

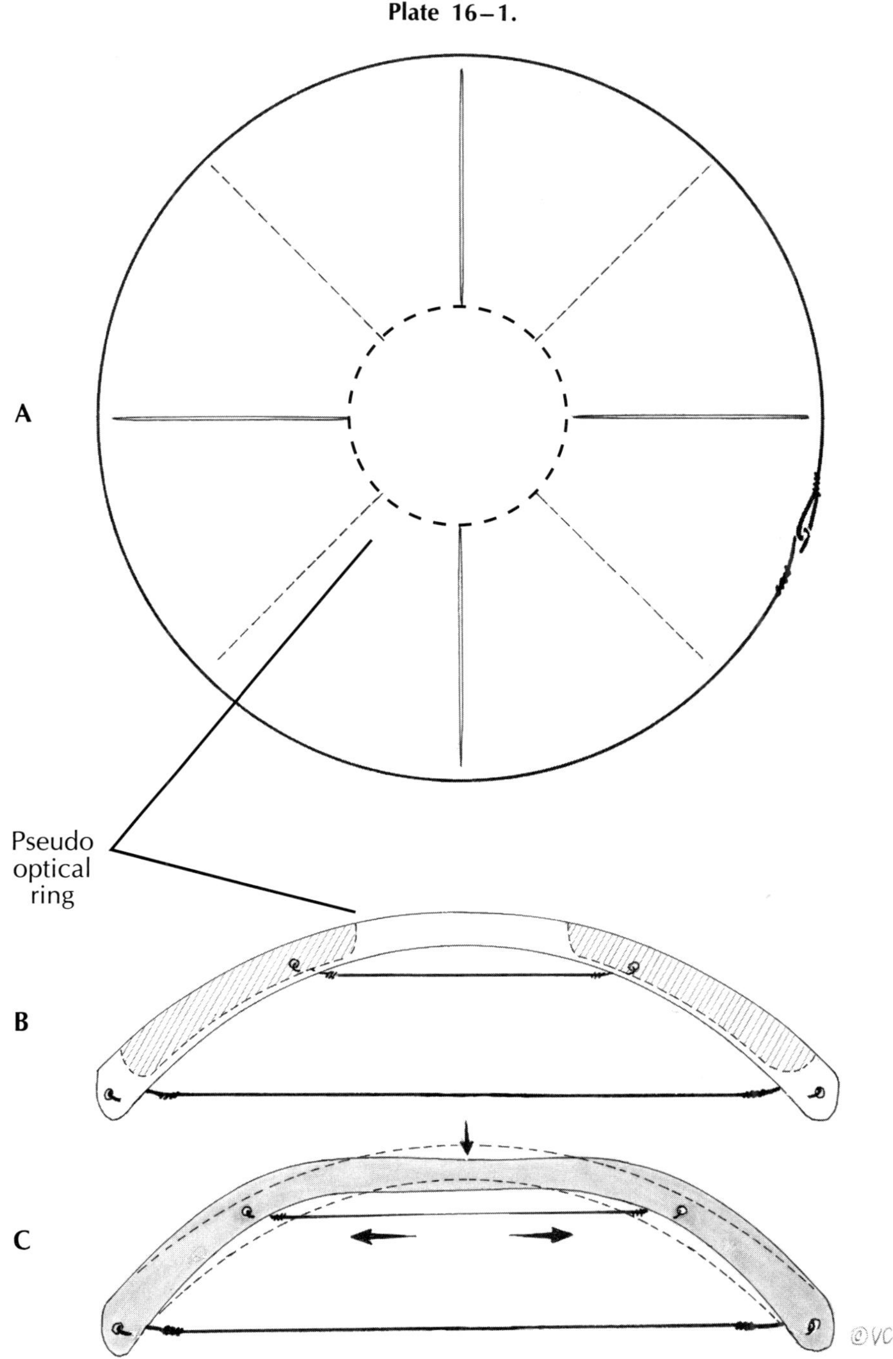

Action of radial keratotomy with development of *pseudo optical ring*. **A,** frontal view of cornea after radial keratotomy, showing creation of pseudo-optical ring. **B,** cross section of cornea before radial keratotomy, showing proposed radial incisions and guy wires. **C,** cross section of cornea after radial keratotomy, showing central flattening and mid-peripheral ectasia induced by radial incisions, resulting in stretching of mid-peripheral guy wire.

Optical Axis and Zone

We have discussed identification of the optical axis and marking of the optical zone in detail in chapter 13. The same approach is used in radial keratotomy, although even more care is required due to the smaller optical zones. As a precaution, the pupil is usually constricted with pilocarpine for verification of the gross location of the visual axis. However, occasions arise in which the visual axis does not lie within the constricted pupillary zone. If the light reflex is found along the edge of the pupil when constricted, it is likely that the patient has either an eccentric visual axis or an abnormality in pupillary constriction and should be rescheduled for another day without the use of pilocarpine.

The instruments used to mark the optical zone represent another important choice. The wire cross hair is preferred for the best nonintrusive indication of optical center (see Plate 7–19,A). The very delicate wires are easily moved, and their alignment should be checked periodically. To mark the optical zone, the optical zone marker should have a reasonably sharp edge. One should check the accuracy and edge of the optical zone markers with a device such as the Baribeau Micronscope to determine whether the measurement is calibrated to an inside or outside diameter. Every effort should be made when performing the radial keratotomy to create a perfectly round, central optical zone with the incisions abutting on the mark created with the optical zone marker. Early experiments using an oval optical zone showed that small amounts of astigmatism can be induced if the incisions do not converge to form a circle. Irregular astigmatism with decreased best-corrected visual acuity also is a possibility if a single incision is left short.

Marking and Creating Symmetric Radial Incisions

A truly perfect radial keratotomy should be symmetric. It is clear from our understanding of the function of radial incisions, which is felt to be a flattening along the axis defined by the incision, that incisions that are placed too close to one another will overly flatten that area and lead to astigmatism in this meridian. An extreme example of this phenomenon would be the *L* procedure of Fyodorov or the fan-shaped Binder procedure in which multiple radial incisions are placed along the steep axis of the cornea. Although small variations from perfect symmetry will cause little effect, the individual eye can show more significant effect if the deviation is large. Thus the positions of the incisions should be marked with a suitable marking device. A radial keratotomy marker, such as the Grandon marker from Katina (see Plate 7–20), is quite useful with respect to correction of astigmatism because the steep axis of astigmatism can be straddled by the marks, whereas it is difficult to do so when judging the position of the incisions without a marker.

Eye Fixation and Hand Orientation Technique

The method used to stabilize the eye during the incisions may make a significant difference in the final configuration of incisions. An early technique that is still used by many practitioners consists of a bimanual movement in which the eye is grasped with a forceps and both the eye and the knife are moved in opposite directions to create the incision. This technique tends to create straight incisions, but the incisions often are not radial. In addition, it is more difficult to follow a preset mark than it would be if the eye were held stable and the hand holding the knife used exclusively to trace along a preset mark. For this technique a ring-type holder (see Plate 7–18,D) better stabilizes the eye in terms of both torsional and radial forces and is more accurate for creating radial incisions along preset marks. Another technique that can be used to produce straight radial incisions along the preset marks involves moving the knife in the space above the planned path of the incision several times just prior to actually incising the cornea. This technique allows the surgeon to orient the hand and wrist to a position in which the movement will be natural and undue lateral forces will be avoided.

Pachymetry and Knife Calibration

Measurement of the true thickness of the cornea by pachymetry is perhaps one of the greatest potential sources of error in radial keratotomy. Optical pachymetry has, for the most part, been superseded by handheld ultrasonic pachymetry. Errors in this procedure include inappropriate measurement location, tilting of the instrument, undue pressure, and inappropriate drying or wetting of the cornea. Although it is true that the cornea varies in thickness circumferentially around the optical axis and the most appropriate procedure would be to set the diamond knife separately for each incision, the time involved to do so would allow the cornea to either dehydrate or become overly hydrated if additional fluids were added. Therefore, as a practical matter, the knife-depth setting is usually determined on the lowest paracentral reading taken prior to surgery and not changed in the course of surgery. In addition, depending on whether the surgeon performs the incisions from the optical zone outward or from the limbus inward, the knife is usually set at 110% or 100%, respectively, of the actual reading to account for the malleability of the cornea as the knife is applied to it (see Chapter 8).

The choice of the appropriate knife is again a matter of great importance. As discussed in Chapter 8, the goal of the radial keratotomy incision is to produce an incision of repeatable depth that is straight and in the proper location. We have found that double-cutting knives tend to produce incisions that are reproducible in terms of depth but often have a tendency to create incisions that are not straight. Conversely, a single-cutting knife sharpened on the diagonal tends to produce very straight incisions, but they are often shallow. A compromise can be reached if the incisions are first created with a single cutting knife sharpened on the diagonal edge, cutting from the optical zone to the limbus, and then completed using a double-cutting knife, cutting with its vertical edge from the limbus to the optical zone. This provides both a straight incision and an incision of repeatable depth with a *square edge* at the end of the incision at the optical zone.

The use of a microscope such as the Micronscope to properly set the knife prior to its use is an essential part of repeatable depth radial keratotomy incisions. In the past, blocks of various configurations were used to visualize proper depth setting of the knife, but these have been found to be quite inaccurate. In addition, the micrometers that are provided with the knives are subjected to significant variations in temperature, which with normal use may gradually drift to the point of being out of range.

Number and Length of Incisions

The length of the incisions is an area of further concern. Usually the optical center of the cornea is eccentric, resulting in a fairly long incision temporally and a short incision nasally. Some authors have advocated making incisions of the same length both nasally and temporally, although experimental efficacy of this technique has been lacking. Certainly the available evidence and theoretical considerations indicate that the incisions should not extend through the optical corneal ring (limbus), because it represents a major structural support of corneal optical integrity, and blood vessels that are present in this location may tend to grow through the incision, creating asymmetrical wound healing. It is therefore advisable to discontinue the incision somewhat short of the surgical limbus to avoid these complications. When performing a four-incision radial keratotomy (Plate 16–2,A), one often finds the development of spurious astigmatism following the procedure. This may be traced to the rather poor approximation of a circle with four points. If one examines the photokeratometry or corneal topology of a four-incision radial keratotomy (Plate 16–2,B) versus an eight-incision radial keratotomy (Plate 16–2,C), one can observe a slightly square appearance of the four-incision radial keratotomy in the mid-periphery versus the reasonably round appearance of the photokeratometry with an eight-incision radial keratotomy. This has led to the suggestion that an additional four very short incisions be created in the mid-periphery between the original four long incisions to *regularize* the cornea in four-incision radial keratotomy.

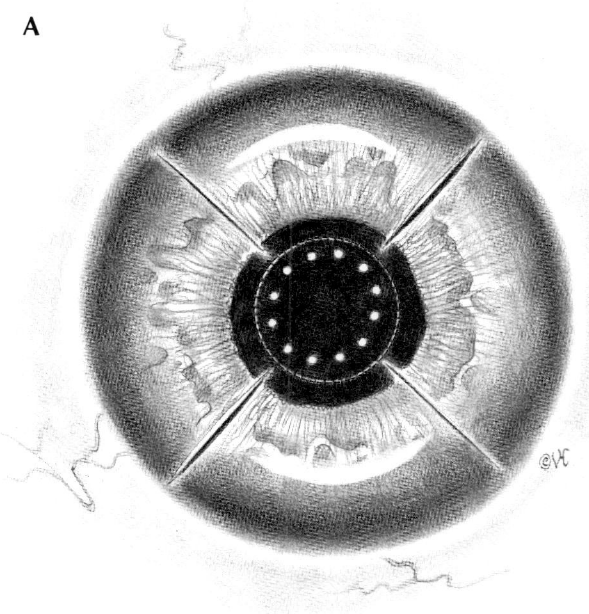

A

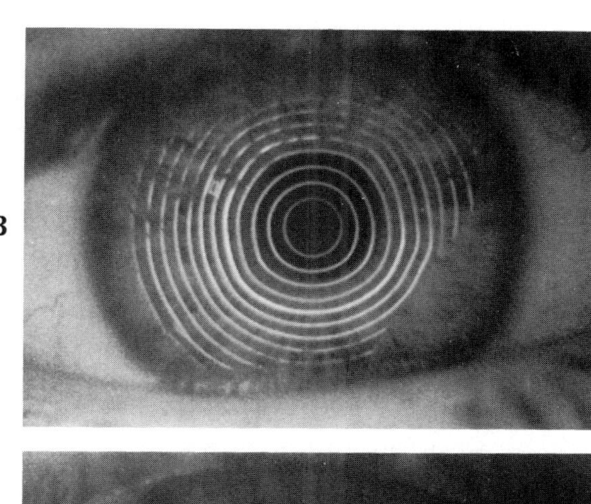

B

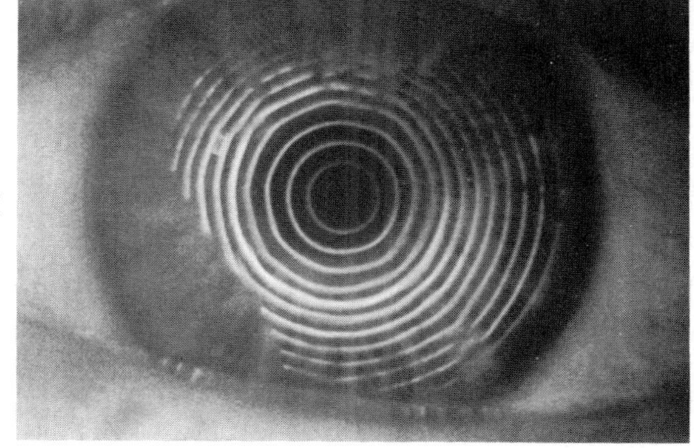

C

A, four-incision radial keratotomy. **B,** photokeratometry after four-incision radial keratotomy showing *square* appearance of mires from photokeratometer, indicating mild irregular astigmatism. **C,** photokeratometry after eight-incision radial keratotomy showing better approximation to *round* mires from photokeratometry.

Cleanup and Postoperative Care

At the conclusion of surgery, the incisions are customarily irrigated both to remove surgical debris and to recheck the depth of the incisions. The precise location of the proximal end of each incision should be checked by moving the irrigation cannula to this location, and if variation is noted among the incisions relative to the optical zone mark, this should be corrected by extending the affected incision(s) before the surgery is completed. The customary postoperative care for radial keratotomy involves the use of a patch for the first night postoperatively. We believe that a therapeutic contact lens better provides an appositional surface to hold the anterior cornea to provide good wound apposition during this time. Moreover, postoperative pain is virtually eliminated and the patient is afforded the opportunity for very rapid visual rehabilitation. For patients with wound healing abnormalities, the contact lens is an excellent means to provide even wound healing and to avoid differential wound healing relative to lid exposure.

POSTOPERATIVE RADIAL KERATOTOMY

The PERK (Prospective Evaluation of Radial Keratotomy) Study and others have documented a significant spread of the effect of radial keratotomy in terms of both sphere and astigmatism after long follow-up. As in other forms of corneal surgery, such as penetrating keratoplasty, these variations can be traced either to irregularities occurring at the time of surgery, as outlined earlier, or to variations in wound healing.

Nonsurgical Manipulation of Wound Healing

The management of wound healing in the postoperative corneal patient, regardless of the surgery, is an important matter deserving of attention, as discussed in Chapter 4. Wound healing generally decreases with age and is slowed to some extent with topical steroids. Conversely, wound healing can be enhanced with use of topical pilocarpine 4% four times daily and possibly with timolol (Timoptic) and acetazolamide (Diamox), reducing intraocular pressure and presumably increasing wound healing by this mechanism. Dietz reports teaching a Valsalva-like maneuver to patients to increase myopic correction. Neumann has reported anecdotal cases in which patching at night for 1 month has produced an additional 1 D of effect possibly due to additional flattening caused by the pressure patch. Therapeutic plano contact lenses have been used by Buzard, who theorizes that wound healing is delayed by the induction of mild corneal edema, thus slowing corneal wound healing. The mechanism appears to be quite different from the patching method of Neumann. The contact lens method usually does not have a permanent effect, but may be used as a temporary measure to improve vision and patient confidence while awaiting further surgery.

Surgical Manipulation of Wound Healing to Increase Incisional Effect

Surgical means of increasing incisional effect centers on two basic manipulations, breaking the incision open or deepening it with the tickle procedure. Simple opening of the incision should be performed on all incisions simultaneously and has a relatively small effect, 0.50 to 0.75 D. Generally, undercorrection or induction of astigmatism in radial keratotomy is a result of shallow incisions that need to be deepened.

If corneal astigmatism is present with the steep axis adjacent to a shallow incision, as seen on slitlamp evaluation, a reasonable first step would be to deepen this incision(s). This procedure can be performed at the slitlamp and has been termed the *tickle procedure* by Buzard (1991). In most instances, not more than 1 D of astigmatic effect will result from this maneuver, but prior to creating any further secondary astigmatism correcting incisions in the cornea, an attempt should be made to optimize the underlying radial keratotomy.

Slitlamp visualization of incisions involves placing the beam to a fine focus and observing the paracentral depth of each incision next to the optical zone. If the incisions are of proper depth, they will appear to be nearly 100% of the depth of the cornea (Plate 16–3).

The tickle procedure is performed with the patient seated at the slitlamp, after having been anesthetized with topical anesthetic. The incision(s) to be opened are observed. A blunt hook, such as a Sinsky hook, is used to break open the incision. This process is successful only in the first few months after surgery, after which a knife must be used to open the incision. An Osher-style double-cutting diamond knife, at the same depth setting as used for the original surgery, is then placed in the incision and used in a front-cutting manner to deepen the incision and square the end nearest the optical center. Postoperative procedure is the same as for the original radial keratotomy, with the use of a disposable soft contact lenses if appropriate. If the incision remains shallow, the tickle can be performed again with extension of the blade of the knife. Although this procedure can be performed in the operating room, the lack of good visualization and expense make the procedure better suited to the slitlamp. Complications, such as unintended excursions into the optical zone, are no more frequent than in the operating room.

A useful maneuver prior to performing any additional astigmatic surgery should be an evaluation of the photokeratometry. If significant *breaking* of the mires over the incisions is present 1 month after the surgery (see Plate 4–10,B), the surgeon should carefully consider the various options for increasing wound healing because it is clear that wound healing is progressing at an abnormally slow rate. Such breaking of the mires often accompanies incomplete wound healing with induced astigmatic error and usually occurs only in the first few weeks after surgery. This finding represents localized corneal edema surrounding the radial incision. If such edema is present, it is evidence of a break in Bowman's layer, which is most likely incompletely closed with a possible epithelial plug. If additional radial or transverse incisions are placed in such a cornea, one can expect long-term instability with a possibility of an overcorrection as the cornea continues to change. Additional incisions should be placed in a recipient cornea only if corneal stability can be demonstrated both in subjective terms of manifest refraction and visual acuity and in objective terms such as keratometry, photokeratometry, and corneal topology.

Surgical Manipulation of Wound Healing to Decrease Incisional Effect

If medical means to improve wound healing are inadequate, the incisions may be sutured individually or collectively using a circular suture. The principle involves increased tension across the wound, allowing resumption of normal wound healing. The technique involves the use of an

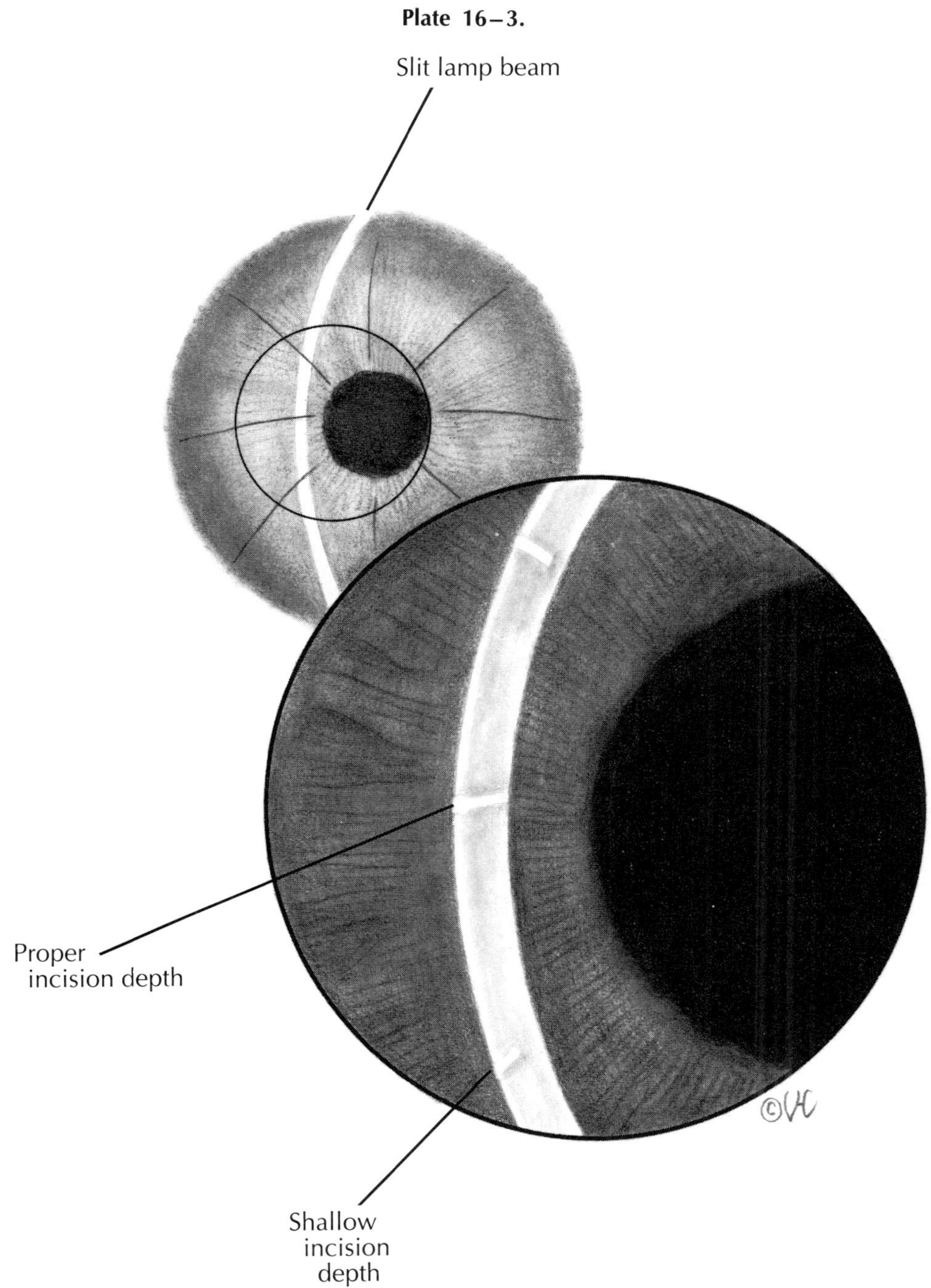

Estimation of incision depth at slitlamp, showing appearance of deep incisions extending 100% of corneal thickness and shallow incisions extending less than 100% of corneal thickness.

inextensible suture material, such as 10-0 dacron, placed approximately across the middle of each incision in the intermediate cornea.

The circular suture is placed to create a new pseudo-optical zone of approximately 7 mm by opening the incisions along this circumference (Plate 16–4,A) and entering and leaving the mid-cornea with the suture needle through these incisions around the circumference (Plate 16–4,B). The suture is then tied with a slipknot (Plate 16–4,C) and tightened until a slight depression occurs in the mid-corneal surface (Plate 16–4,D). The suture is locked and buried, at which time a circular suture extending at 50% corneal depth around the cornea at the new 7 mm optical zone. This tends to correct astigmatism as well as the spherical error. A problem with the circular suture technique is the development of small inflammatory foci at the intersection of the suture and incisions. These resolve eventually, and do not seem to cause a permanent problem.

Circular sutures work well for eight-incision or more radial keratotomies, because suturing individual incisions is considerably more difficult. For four-incision radial keratotomies, interrupted 10-0 nylon sutures are more appropriate because the interrupted dacron loops loosen too quickly. The interrupted sutures are placed along a 7-mm optical zone. Suturing improves the healing strength of any incision with delayed wound healing and can also be used to correct overcorrections in transverse and arcuate incisions.

The efficacy of removing the epithelial plug in delayed wound healing is debatable. We have found opening and scraping of the incisions to be a destabilizing procedure on the cornea, and we feel that the epithelial plug will extrude during the course of normal wound healing if sufficient tension across the wound is established. If these techniques fail, a lamellar keratectomy and homoplastic keratomileusis using the BKS microkeratome will restore anterior corneal curvature (see Plate 10–12, A).

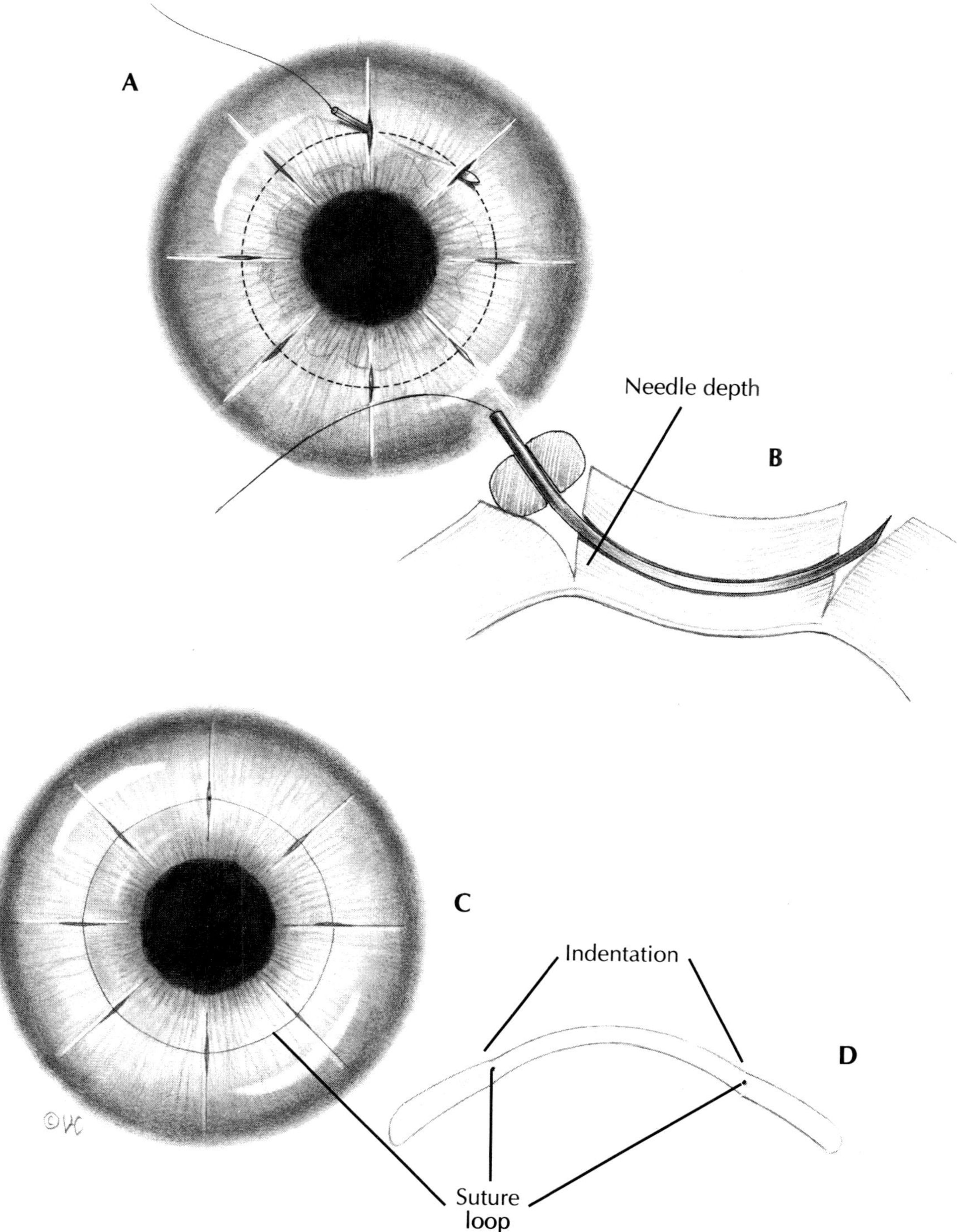

A, eight-incision overcorrected radial keratotomy marked with 7-mm optical zone with radial incisions opened along optical zone. **B,** path of needle between incisions showing 50% depth of needle. **C,** completed circular suture with knot buried in incision. **D,** appearance of cornea in cross section showing 50% depth of 10-0 dacron suture and depression in corneal surface indicating proper suture tension.

Pathophysiology and Surgical Management of Post-Radial Keratotomy Astigmatism   **463**

The issue of whether to perform additional surgery directed at the astigmatic component of the patient's refraction at the time of radial keratotomy is a subject of some debate. Originally, there was some hope that simply modifying the original surgery by means of producing an oval optical zone might correct a significant degree of astigmatism. This was found to be inadequate to correct more than a very small amount of astigmatism, and animal studies by Yau (1985) have confirmed this clinical observation.

The effect of radial incisions is to flatten the cornea in the meridian of the incision and 90 degrees away. This observation was made by Fyodorov early in his investigations of radial keratotomy and resulted in the *L* (for astigmatic correction alone) (Plate 16–5,A) and the *RL* (in combination with radial keratotomy for astigmatic and myopic correction) procedures. The multiple radial incisions centered on the steep axis of astigmatism certainly corrected large amounts of astigmatism but left the patient with an unstable result. The close proximity of the radial incisions led to block lifts of tissue, and the crossed incisions of the *L* and the *RL* procedures only made the situation worse. Binder attempted a modification of the *L* procedure by spreading the incisions in a fan shape (Plate 16–5,B). This technique, although simpler to perform and better avoiding the tendency to slide into adjacent incisions, still had a tendency to create instability over the long run.

A

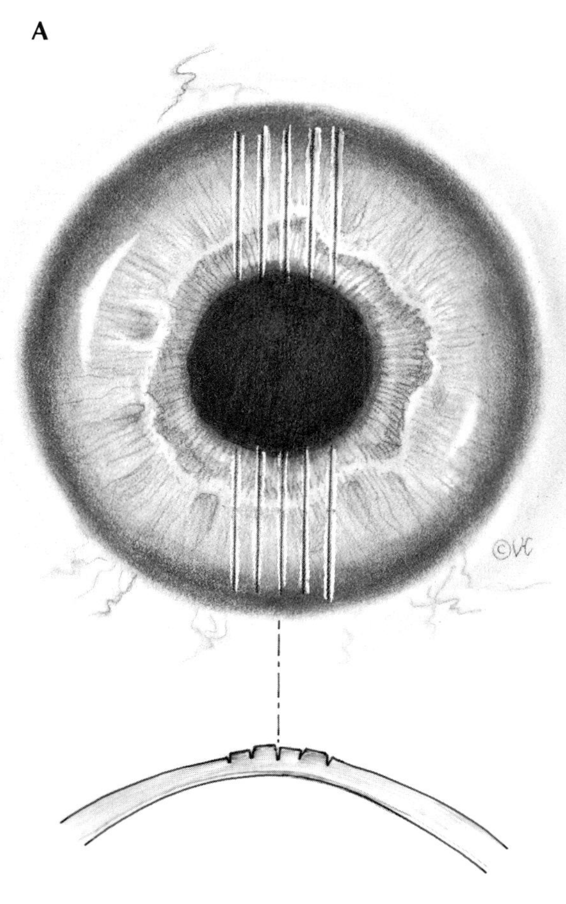

B

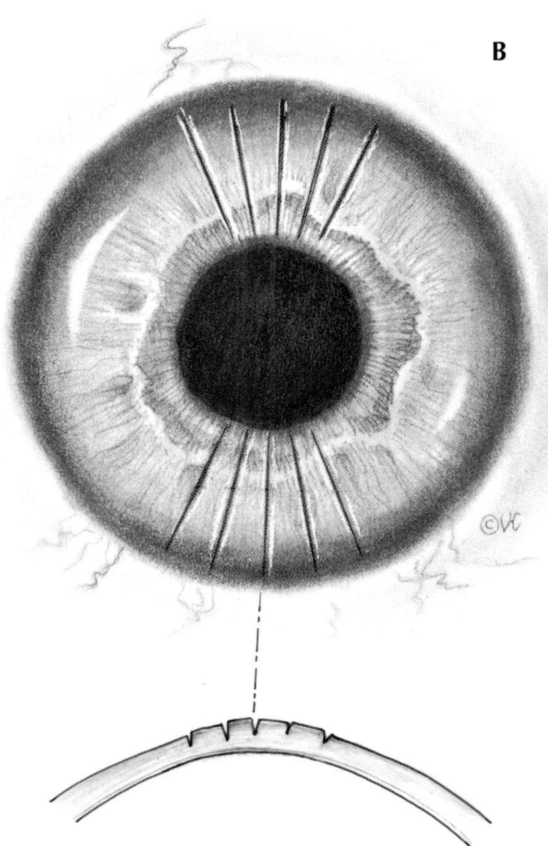

A, Fyodorov *L* procedure showing *block* lifting of tissue (below cross section) between incisions. **B,** Binder procedure showing continued problems with *block* lifting of tissue (below cross section) between incisions.

Continued.

The addition of one (Plate 16–5,C) or two (Plate 16–5,D) transverse incisions in the *TR* procedure was soon recognized to have powerful astigmatic properties, and it is this component that has survived in a variety of forms as the predominant method of treating the astigmatism with and following radial keratotomy. However, crossing radial and transverse incisions soon became a source of corneal instability that was made even worse when the number of transverse incisions was raised from a single pair to a pair of double incisions, particularly in the double *TL* procedure in which the crosshatched pattern resulted in severe instability (Plate 16–5,E).

By necessity, the issue of how to combine a transverse incision or incisions with the radial keratotomy incisions must center on the issue of stability. The grave instability produced by the *TL* procedure made surgeons very aware of the concept of block lift of destabilized corneal tissue. As experience grew, it became clear that even the crossing of a single radial and transverse incision could create instability in the area of crossing.

Even if a radial incision is allowed to heal and a transverse incision crossing a radial incision is placed 2 to 3 years after the original radial keratotomy, progressive instability can be observed in the area of crossing, including development of dot-map-fingerprint dystrophy in the area of the crossing often a deposition of calcium at the exact point of crossing (see Plate 4–7,C). This can lead to a progressive overcorrection, which can be seen on corneal topology or photokeratometry even before it affects the central cornea and best-corrected visual acuity. This important complication has led to several improved operations that place transverse and radial incisions in close proximity to but not actually crossing radial incisions.

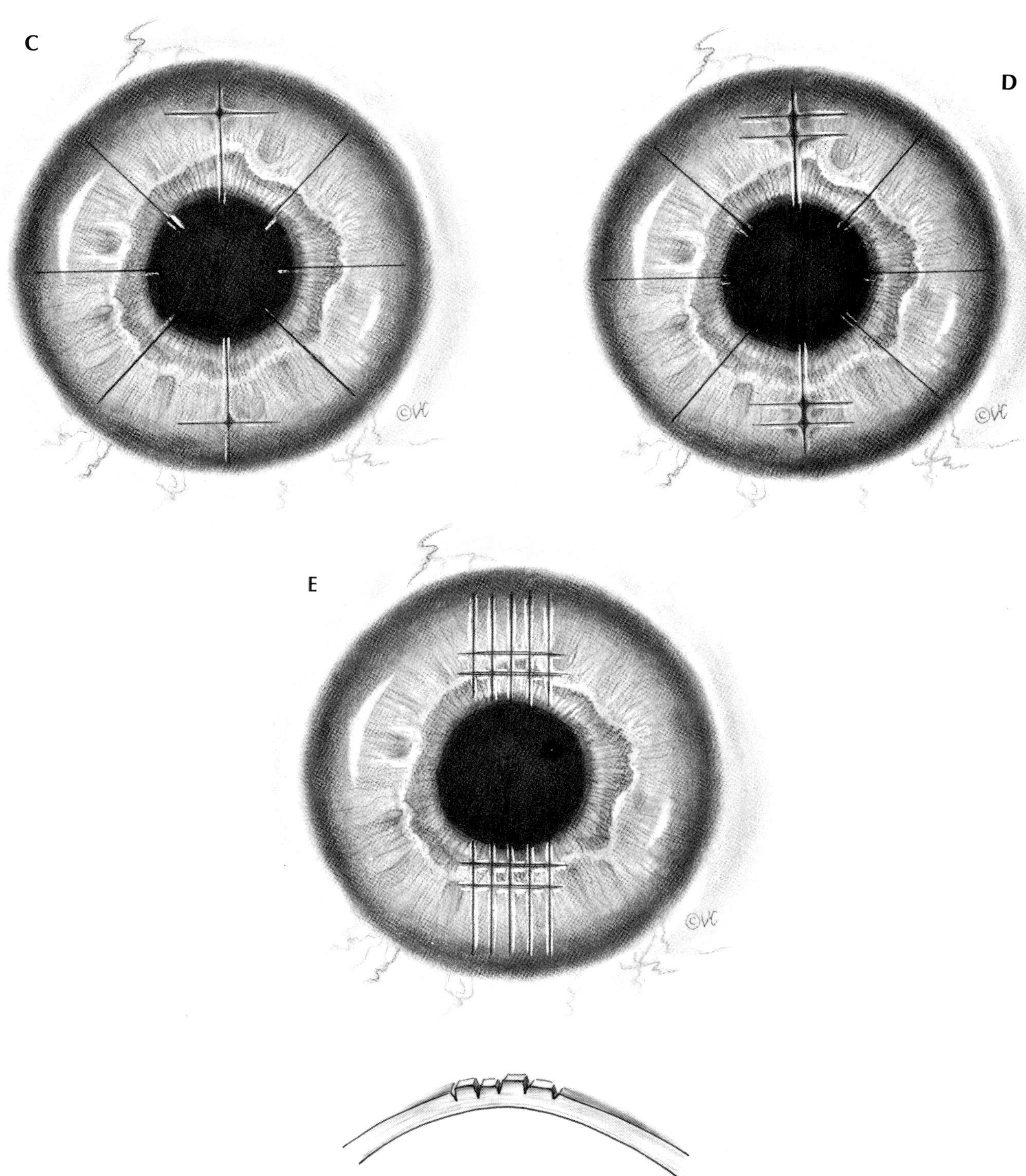

C, Fyodorov *TR* procedure with crossed radial and transverse incisions showing instability at area of crossing. D, Fyodorov double *TR* procedure showing two transverse incisions with severe *block* lifting of crosshatched incisional pattern. E, Fyodorov double *TL* procedure showing *block* lifting and instability in area of crossed incisions.

Pathophysiology and Surgical Management of Post-Radial Keratotomy Astigmatism   **467**

The Hofmann *T/I* is one example (Plate 16–6,A), as is the Thornton *T* incision (Plate 16–6,B), and these two procedures form the foundation for the current surgical correction of astigmatism in conjunction with radial keratotomy. In each method, the transverse incision is created so that the transverse incision does not intersect with a radial incision. This does not solve the problem of instability completely. Buzard compared transverse incisions created with and without radial incisions (not crossing), which demonstrate, over a period of several months, a small 0.5 D additional astigmatic shift can be observed only when the transverse incisions are combined with radial incisions. However, the debilitating wound dehiscence from crossing the incisions is avoided, and with a single incision the cornea usually stabilizes. This concept of relative stabilization should be kept in mind when performing astigmatic incisions in the presence of radial incisions to avoid corneal instability in an elderly patient or in patients with known compromised wound healing.

The addition of transverse incisions to radial keratotomy creates, in effect, a modified Ruiz procedure. Thus slightly more astigmatic effect is obtained in a patient of a given age and optical zone than would be obtained in a cornea without radial keratotomy. This is reflected in the nomogram presented on page 477.

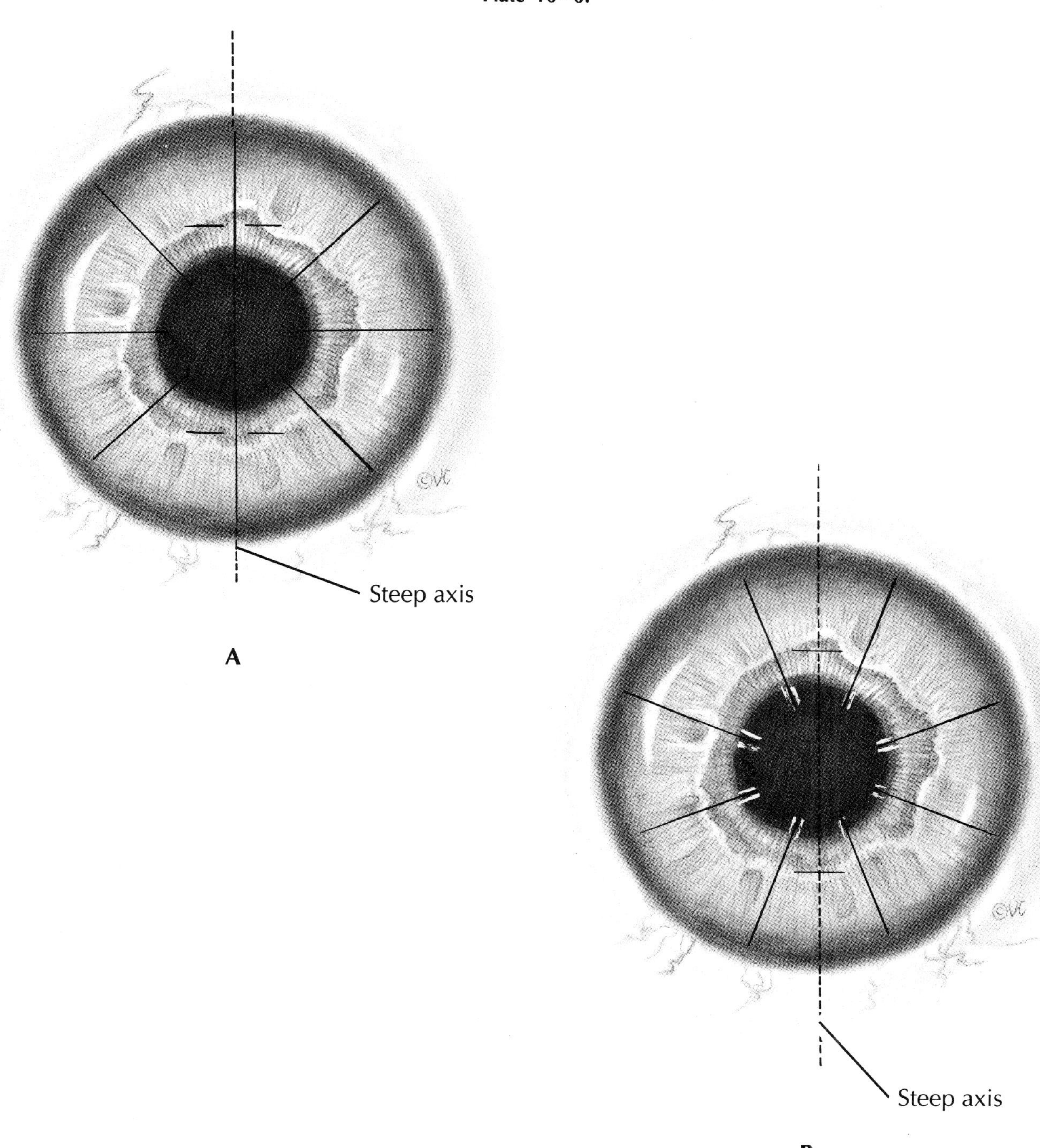

A, Hofmann *T/I* procedure showing *jumping* of transverse incisions to avoid intersection with radial incisions. **B,** Thornton *T* procedure showing placement of transverse incisions between radial incisions avoiding the necessity for *jumping* radial incisions.

TRANSVERSE INCISIONS AND RADIAL KERATOTOMY

The decision to perform transverse incisions in conjunction with radial keratotomy must depend in part on the amount of astigmatism involved. If the astigmatic error is small (<1 D), the patient often does well without additional astigmatic surgery, and in fact, depending on the means of measurement, the astigmatism actually may be eliminated by means of the radial keratotomy. This has been demonstrated in the PERK Study and elsewhere.

Timing of Additional Incisions

Studies by Buzard and others of transverse incisions made at the same time as the radial incisions and later, after healing of the radial incisions, show that virtually the same effect is created, regardless of the timing of the transverse incision. Thus, little advantage with respect to astigmatic effect is gathered by performing the astigmatic surgery at the time of the original radial keratotomy. A significant disadvantage in performing astigmatic surgery in conjunction with radial keratotomy is encountered both from the standpoint of actually performing the transverse incision and from the realization that the astigmatic error can change both in direction and amount after the radial keratotomy.

The concept of *algebraic addition for keratotomy incisions* is the basis for stepwise procedures for astigmatism (extending or adding incisions) (Plate 16–7,A) and for radial keratotomy (proceeding from four to eight radial incisions if the four-incision operation leaves the patient undercorrected) (Plate 16–7,B). Whenever possible, the surgeon should attempt to perform the fewest number of incisions at the primary procedure, returning at a later time to add or lengthen incisions if necessary. This will minimize overcorrections and prevent unpleasant surprises. This approach for staged astigmatic correction is similar to the approach advocated by Salz et al. (1986), suggesting four-incision radial keratotomy for low and moderate myopic correction followed by additional radial incisions, if needed.

Plate 16–7.

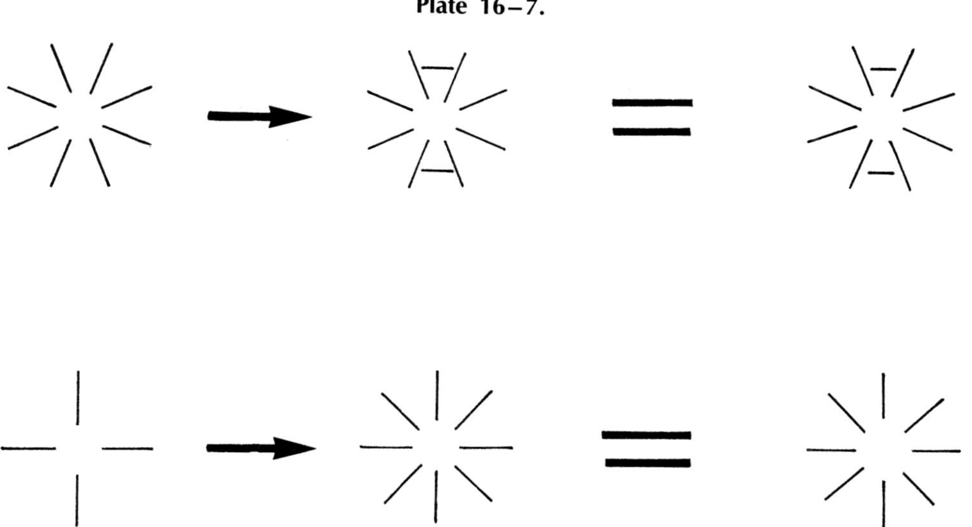

A, *algebraic addition of corneal incisions showing* the effect of radial and transverse incisions created at different times is equivalent to performing these incisions at the same time. **B,** *algebraic addition of corneal incisions* showing the effect of performing four-incision radial keratotomy with the addition of four incisions at a later time is equivalent to the effect of an eight-incision radial keratotomy.

When a transverse incision is done immediately after radial keratotomy incisions there is a tendency for the cornea to shift laterally *en bloc* because the lateral structural rigidity of the cornea is compromised (Plate 16–8,A). This can lead to a tendency both to intersect the radial incisions and to create shallow transverse incisions. These problems can be overcome to some extent by the use of multiple puncture wounds along the path of the transverse incision, but even this method can lead to shallow incisions in the presence of a *fresh* radial keratotomy (Plate 16–8,B). Given these considerations and the only possible positive benefit to the patient being to avoid a trip to the operating room, it appears most prudent to perform the transverse incisions, if they are required, at a later time for low to moderate astigmatic errors.

Considerations Relative to Astigmatic Meridian

If the transverse incision is placed incorrectly relative to the post–radial keratotomy astigmatic meridian, a cross-cylinder effect will come into play, which will, in effect, give an astigmatic error at an entirely new axis, as we have discussed in Chapter 13.

Given the choice of creating a transverse incision between radial incisions as in the Thornton *T* (Plate 16–6,B) or *jumping* over a radial incision as in the Hofmann *T/I* (Plate 16–6,A), it is clearly easier to orient the radial keratotomy pattern so that an opening between radial incisions occurs along the steep axis where transverse incisions will be placed. Even if transverse incisions are not anticipated at the primary procedure, the pattern should be rotated so that if transverse incisions are needed later, jumping the radial incisions may be avoided. The effect of transverse incisions between radial incisions and jumping radial incisions is approximately the same given the same length and position, although no formal studies on this issue have been performed. Additionally, approximately the same effect is obtained if the surgeon jumps the transverse rather than the radial incision, as has been demonstrated by Lipschitz (1990). The use of a radial incision marker, such as the Grandon marker, that can be rotated to vary the position and orientation of the radial keratotomy pattern is essential because it is quite difficult to create these incisions freehand.

Independent Variables in Transverse Incisions

The concept of angular displacement of incisions allows the surgeon to establish essentially similar astigmatic corrections with incisions of varying optical zone and length as long as *segment length* remains constant (see Chapter 13). Because of the inconvenience of jumping incisions, virtually all astigmatic corrections in radial keratotomy are accomplished with short transverse incisions rather than long arcuate incisions, although

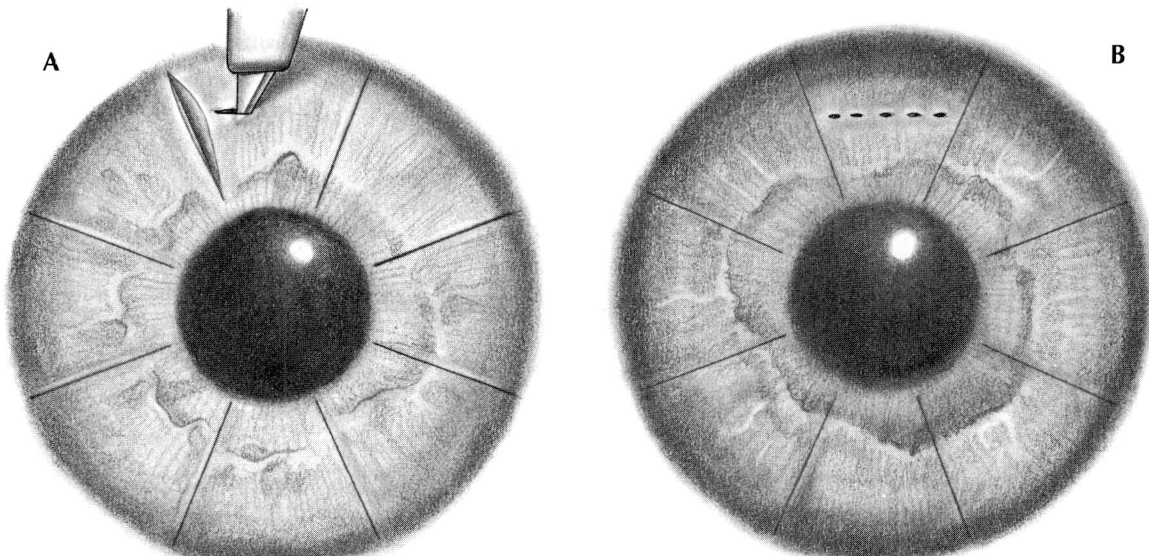

A, *block* movement of interincisional corneal tissue when transverse keratotomy is performed at the time of radial keratotomy. B, multiple puncture technique to achieve proper depth transverse incisions when transverse keratotomy is performed at the time of radial keratotomy. The incision is completed by cutting intermediate tissue in successively deeper connecting passes of the diamond knife.

even the short incisions are created in an arcuate manner. For practical purposes, short transverse and short arcuate incisions occupy the same segment length. Over a 2 to 3 mm incision, the degree of curvature is not terribly noticeable; however, wound healing and symmetry considerations dictate an attempt to curve the incisions.

The technique of short transverse or arcuate incisions will correct astigmatism in the vast majority of patients requesting radial keratotomy. If a patient presents with more than 3 D of astigmatic error and significant myopia, particular attention should be applied to examination of photokeratometry, keratometry, and corneal topography for the diagnosis of corneal ectasias (in particular, keratoconus; Plate 16–9). Because more incisions are created for the patient who receives radial keratotomy in addition to astigmatic surgery, the potential for corneal instability is greater. Also, corneal thickness can vary significantly in corneal ectasias, increasing the possibility of microperforation. Certainly, stability of the refraction should be verified with old records, and if any question concerning keratoconus exists, the surgery should be cancelled. If more than 3 D of astigmatic correction is required with radial keratotomy, long arcuate incisions (90 degrees) can be used, jumping the radial incisions.

PREOPERATIVE CONSIDERATIONS

The preparations and considerations discussed in Chapter 13 with regard to astigmatic correction of congenital and postcataract astigmatism are equally valid for radial keratotomy. Additional considerations, particularly for radial keratotomy, concern the issue of astigmatic meridian as it relates to the pattern of radial keratotomy incisions.

The astigmatic meridian and amount should be determined using a combination of photokeratometry, keratometry, corneal topology, and manifest

Plate 16–9.

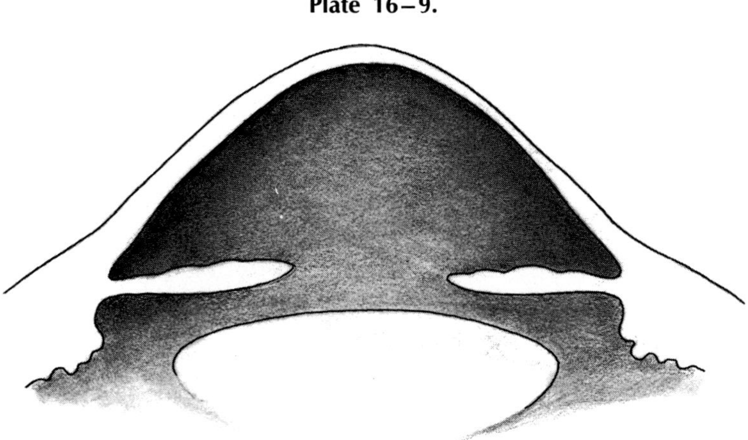

Cross-sectional appearance of the cornea in keratoconus showing significant corneal thinning. Radial and transverse keratotomy are contraindicated.

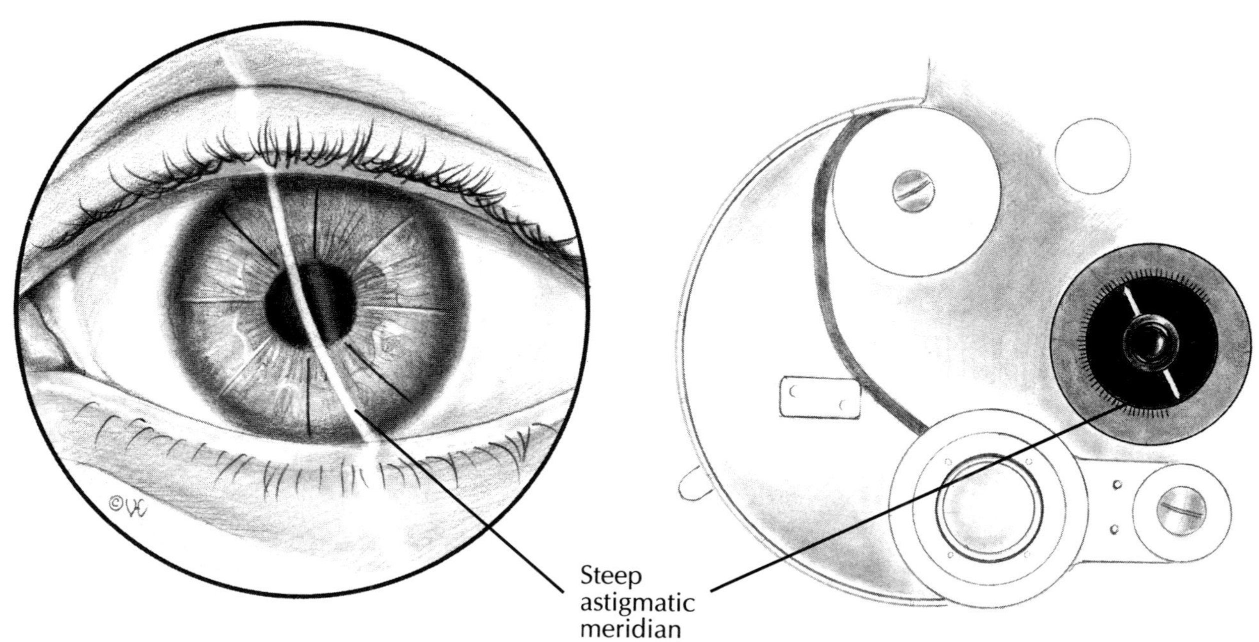

Preoperative technique to identify astigmatic meridian relative to radial incisions using the axis indicator on the phoropter placed near the patient's eye and marking adjacent radial incisions with a blunt needle

refraction. Following radial keratotomy, the standard measures of astigmatic error can be distorted by the surgery, and it is often difficult to determine the appropriate refractive error. After the astigmatic meridian is established, it should be placed in the phoropter next to the patient's head and compared with a thin slit beam directed along the same axis on the patient's cornea (Plate 16–10). This technique allows accurate determination of astigmatic meridian at the slitlamp. The configuration of radial incisions should be observed relative to the astigmatic meridian. If possible, the additional transverse incisions should be placed equidistant over or between incisions. Asymmetric placement of the transverse incisions relative to the radial incisions can result in disturbing anomalies, although minor variance from the astigmatic meridian will not usually cause significant problems.

Prior to surgery, the radial incisions bounding the astigmatic meridian should be marked with a blunt needle and stained with fluorescein dye. Visualization at the operating microscope is often suboptimal, and both realignment of the new optical zone to the optical zone used for the original radial keratotomy and avoidance of intersecting incisions can be accomplished with this technique. Additionally, these marked incisions provide landmarks that avoid confusion in the operating room.

Prior to bringing the patient to the operating room, the adjacent radial incisions are marked as noted, and constriction of the pupil with pilocarpine is performed to aid in identification of the visual axis and to lessen light sensitivity from the side illumination used during surgery. A heparin cannula is placed for administration of 1 to 2 mg of midazolam (Versed) to sedate the patient. The patient is prepped and draped with sterile towels, and lid closure is prevented with a locking lid speculum. Methylene blue is placed on the cornea to illuminate the marking of the radial incisions, and the appropriate optical zone marker is placed concentric with the optical zone of the radial incisions and the optical axis. A sheet with preoperative photokeratometry, keratometry, corneal topology, and manifest refraction is placed on the microscope to verify operative parameters and the optical axis, as discussed in Chapter 13 (see Plate 13–13). The length of the transverse incisions is marked with a spatula-style marker or small optical zone marker.

Using an Osher-style double-cutting diamond knife, the incisions are created in a front cutting manner. The knife is carefully rocked in the incision to assure proper depth and square ends. The orientation of the knife is reversed to square both ends of the incisions. The incisions are irrigated with balanced saline and checked for depth and length.

The patient is dilated and a disposable soft contact lens is used for comfort, if appropriate, and otherwise patched. If the contact lens is used, the patient is given antibiotic-steroid drops four times a day and artificial tears every hour while awake.

NOMOGRAM

As we have discussed, the measurement of astigmatism after incisional keratotomy is problematic at best because the usual keratometry measurements are confused by mid-peripheral distortion caused by the incisions. Additionally, the usual spherical subjective cues of visual blurring are not always present with astigmatic refractive errors. Instead, the patient may complain of glare, distortion, or vague symptoms of diminished visual quality. Despite these problems of postoperative measurement, the surgeon must have a general guide to perform these procedures. We present a guide based on Buzard's clinical experience. The nomogram presented here (Plate 16–11) is a starting point and may be modified by the surgeon's own technique, patient variables, and surgical results. Ultimately, each surgeon must create his or her own guide to any surgical procedure.

Short transverse incisions in the presence of radial keratotomy have slightly more effect for a given aged patient, and in a general sense, act as

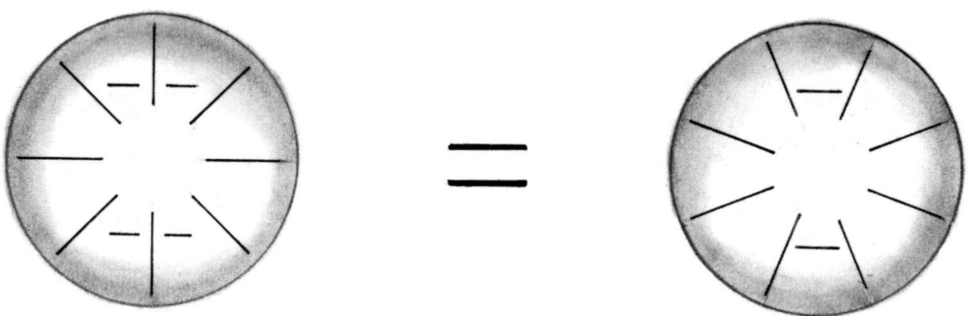

Buzard nomogram as a guide to short transverse keratotomy after radial keratotomy.

Length 2–2.5 mm (both incisions)	
30 Year Old	
Optical Zone	Effect in D*
5.0	3
5.5	2
6.0	1
55 Year Old†	
Optical Zone	Effect in D*
5.0	4
5.5	3
6.0	2
7.0	1

*Approximate values.
†Age modification factor approximately 1.5% per year calculated form 30-year-old parameters.

an age modifier, increasing the effective age of the cornea. For instance, a 30-year-old patient with paired short transverse incisions will obtain approximately 2 D of astigmatic effect without radial incisions and approximately 3 D of astigmatic effect in the presence of radial incisions. The radial incisions combined with the short transverse incisions create, in effect, a modified Ruiz procedure that develops an additional 0.5 D of astigmatic correction during the first 3 months. If incisions do not cross, the cornea can be expected to stabilize and heal. The nomogram shows steps of 0.5 mm to the 6-mm optical zone, then steps to a 7-mm optical zone. The effect of incisions is greatest near the 5-mm optical zone, and falls nonlinearly past the 6-mm optical zone, as shown by Salvates et al. (1991). Thus the appropriate next location at which to add incisions is the 7-mm optical zone, as indicated in the nomogram, and not the 6.5-mm optical zone.

If an undercorrection is encountered, the depth of the transverse incisions should be examined, and if shallow, they should be deepened and lengthened using the tickle technique, described previously. If necessary, after healing for 6 to 12 months, an additional pair of short transverse incisions may be added at the 7-mm optical zone to obtain approximately 1 D more astigmatic effect. This should not be considered until it is clear that the initial transverse incisions are appropriately deep. It is our experience that additional transverse incisions performed at the primary astigmatic surgery actually may diminish astigmatic correction (see Chapter 3).

If an overcorrection is encountered, photokeratometry should be consulted for evidence of a *microdehiscence* or delayed wound healing. In most situations this problem will resolve spontaneously, although older patients may have wound-healing problems leading to this situation. This problem can also be seen with intersecting transverse and radial incisions. Interrupted 10-0 nylon sutures can be applied under keratometric control to increase tension across the wound and resume normal wound healing. If intersecting incisions are observed, the *pursestring* suture closure described in chapter 10 for stellate lacerations can resolve wound-healing problems and reduce the overcorrection. Radial keratotomy, with or without astigmatic correction, should be performed with extreme caution in patients older than 55 years of age. Any nomogram will provide only relative predictability in these patients. In patients older than 55 years the surgeon always should begin with a four-incision keratotomy, adding radial incisions later if necessary.

SUMMARY

Radial keratotomy is an operation that reflects one of the basic tenets of life. It is both conceptually simple and yet full of contradictory decisions, whether made consciously or subconsciously, which have an impact on the final result. In this chapter we have attempted to outline some of these decisions. We have based these discussions on the common sense approach that the eye represents an object of circular symmetry revolving around the optical axis. Determination of the optical axis, and subsequent planning and execution of the operation, should always keep symmetry in mind. Deviations from circular symmetry, in areas such as wound depth, shape, and position, around the optical axis will inevitably result in various degrees of astigmatic refractive error or, worse, actual corneal instability. Adherence to these simple principles will save the practitioner many hours of agonizing planning and surgery to correct deviations from centration and circular symmetry that on the surface might appear inconsequential but that after they have been violated may prove to be exceedingly complex to repair.

Selected Bibliography

Ashton N, Cook C: Effect of cortisone on healing of corneal wounds. *Br J Ophthalmol* 1951; 35:708–717.

Barraquer JI: Queratomileusis y queratofaquia, Bogota, Columbia, 1980.

Barraquer JI: *Compilation of Reprints*. Vol 1: *Refractive Keratoplasty*. Bogota, Colombia, Instituto Barraquer de America, 1970.

Barraquer JI: *Compilation of Reprints*, vol 2: *Refractive Keratoplasty*. Bogota, Colombia, Instituto Barraquer de America, 1975.

Barraquer JI, Rutllan J: *Surgery of the Anterior Segment of the Eye*, vol 2: *Corneal Surgery*. Barcelona, Instituto Barraquer, 1971.

Barraquer JI, Rutllan J, Troutman RC: *Surgery of the Anterior Segment of the Eye*. Vol 1: *General considerations and intracapsular cataract extraction*. New York, McGraw-Hill, 1964.

Bates WH: A suggestion of an operation to correct astigmatism. *Arch Ophthalmol* 1894; 23:9–13.

Baum JL, Silbert AM: Aspects of corneal wound healing in health and disease. *Trans Ophthalmol Soc UK* 1978; 98:348.

Belin MW, Litoff D, Winn SS, et al: The Par Technology Corneal Topography System. Presented at the 3rd International Congress on Laser Surgery of the Cornea, Atlanta, 1990.

Belmont SC, Troutman RC: Compensating compression sutures in wedge resection. *J Refract Surg* 1985; 1:104–107.

Belmont SC, Troutman RC, Buzard KA: Control of astigmatism aided by intraoperative keratotomy. *Cornea*, accepted for publication.

Binder PS: Evaluation of through-and-through corneal sutures. *Arch Ophthalmol* 1978; 96:1886.

Binkhorst RD: The cause of excessive astigmatism with intraocular lens inplants. *Ophthalmology* 1979; 86:672–674.

Brightbill FS: *Corneal Surgery: Theory, Technique, and Tissue*. St Louis, CV Mosby, 1986.

Buzard KA: Paired relaxing incisions for the control of astigmatism. *Cornea* 1991; 10:38–43.

Buzard KA: Deepening of incisions after radial keratotomy using the "tickle" technique. *Refract Corneal Surg* 1991; 7:348–355.

Buzard KA: Use of immunosuppressive agents in uveitis. *Ophthalmic Pract* 1990; 8:250–255.

Buzard KA: Repair of the "microdehiscence" to correct postkeratoplasty astigmatism. *Ophthalmic Surg* 1989; 20:876–882.

Buzard KA: Compression sutures and penetrating corneal trauma, submitted for publication.

Buzard KA, Haight D, Troutman RC: Ruiz procedure for post-keratoplasty astigmatism. *J Refract Surg* 1987; 3:40–45.

Buzard KA, Hoeltzel DH: Biomechanics of the cornea. Progress in biomedical optics. *Proceedings of Ophthalmic Technologies.* 1991; 1423:70–77.

Buzard KA, Troutman RC: Keratophakia, in Schwab I (ed): *Refractive Keratoplasty.* New York, Churchill Livingstone, 1987, pp 69–94.

Buzard KA, Shearing SP: A comparison of postoperative astigmatism with incisions of varying length closed with horizontal sutures and without sutures, *J Cataract Refract Surg* 1991; 17(suppl):734–739.

Buzard KA, Shearing SP, Relyea R: Incidence of astigmatism in a cataract practice. *J Refract Surg* 1988; 4:173–178.

Castroviejo R: Atlas of keratectomy and keratoplasty. Philadelphia, WB Saunders, 1966.

Cohen SS: Isolation of a mouse sub-maxillary gland protein accelerating incison eruption and eyelid opening in the newborn animal. *J Biol Chem* 1962; 237:1555.

Crisp WH: A new cross cylinder test for astigmatic axis, without use of test type. *Trans Am Ophthalmol Soc* 1942; 40:54.

Daniele S, Frati L, Fiore C, et al: The effect of the epidermal growth factor (EGF) on the corneal epithelium in humans. *Albrecht von Graefes Arch Klin Exp Ophthalmol* 1979; 210:159–165.

Deg JK, Binder PS: Wound healing after astigmatic keratotomy in human eyes. *Ophthalmology* 1987; 94:1290–1298.

Denham DB, Barraquer E, Loertscher H, et al: Evaluation of manual, motorized, and laser trephines by shadow photogrammetric analysis. Presented at Association for Research in Vision and Ophthalmology (ARVO), May 1988.

Duane TD: *Clinical Ophthalmology,* vol 1. New York, Harper & Row, 1986.

Egan JA: A resume of cross cylinder application and theory. *Surv Ophthalmol* 1956; 1:513.

Eisner G: *Eye Surgery: An Introduction to Operative* technique. New York, Springer-Verlag 1980.

Friedlander MH, Mulet M, Buzard KA, et al: Holographic interferometry of the corneal surface. Progress in biomedical optics. *Proceedings of Ophthalmic Technologies* 1991; 1423:62–69.

Friedlander MH, Mulet M, Buzard KA, et al: Holographic interferometry of the corneal surface. Holographic Interferometry and Optical Pattern Recognition in Biomedicine. *Proceedings of Ophthalmic Technologies* 1991; 1429:36–43.

Friedlander P, Zinny ML: Effects of soft contacts of differing thickness on corneal wound healing in rabbits. *Invest Ophthalmol Vis Sci* 1989; 30:2138–2147.

Friedman B: The Jackson crossed cylinder. *Arch Ophthalmol* 1940; 24:4909.

Gallar J, Pozo MA, Rebollo I, et al: Effects of capsaicin on corneal wound healing. *Invest Ophthalmol Visual Sci* 1990; 31:1968–1973.

Heller MD, Irvine SR, Straatsma BR, et al: Wound healing after cataract extraction and position of the vitreous in aphakic eyes as studies postmortem. *Trans Am Ophthalmol Soc* 1971; 69:245–262.

Helmholtz H: *Treatise on Physiological Optics*, vol 1. New York, Dover, 1924.

Hessburg PC, Barron M: A disposable corneal trephine. *Ophthalm Surg* 1980; 11:730.

Ibrahim O, Tripoli N, Coggins JM, et al: Pattern analysis of color coded topographic maps and power arrays from corneas after penetrating keratoplasty, submitted for publication.

Jackson E: A trial set of small lenses and a modified trial size frame. *Trans Am Ophthalmol Soc* 1887; 4:595.

Jampel HD, Thompson JR, Backer CC, et al: A computerized analysis of astigmatism after cataract surgery. *Ophthal Surg* 1986; 17:786–790.

Kandarakis AS, Page C, Kaufman HE: The effect of epidermal growth factor on epithelial healing after penetrating keratoplasty in human eyes. *Am J Ophthalmol* 1984; 98:411–415.

Kervick GN, Simon G, Parel JM: The optical power of the epithelium. *Invest Ophthmol* 1991; 32:845.

Kratchmer JH, Fenzl RE: Surgical correction of high post keratoplasty astigmatism: Relaxing incisions versus wedge resection. *Arch Ophthalmol* 1980; 98:1400–1402.

Kratchmer JH, Ching SST: Relaxing incisions for high postkeratoplasty astigmatism. *Int Ophthalmol Clin* 1983; 23:153–159.

Lakshminarayanan V, Enoch JM, Rassch T: Refractive changes induced by intraocular lens tilt and longitudinal displacement. *Arch Ophthalmol* 1986; 104:90–92.

Lang GK, Naumann OH, Koch JW: A new elliptical excision for corneal transplantation using an excimer laser. *Arch Ophthalmol* July 1990; p 914.

Lavery GW, Lindstrom RL: Trapezoidal astigmatic keratotomy in human cadaver eyes. *J Refract Surg* 1985; 1:18–24.

Lin DTC, Wilson SE, Reidy JJ, et al: An adjustable single running suture technique to reduce postkeratoplasty astigmatism. *Ophthalmology* 1990; 97:934–938.

Lindquist TD, Rubenstein JB, Hofmann RF, et al: Astigmatic keratotomy, radial keratotomy. *Surg Tech* 1986; 6:117–129.

Lundergan MK, Rowsey JJ: Relaxing incisions: Corneal topography. *Ophthalmology* 1985; 92:1226–1236.

Mackensen G, Troutman RC, Roper-Hall MJ, et al: Microsurgery in glaucoma. Second Symposium of the Ophthalmic Microsurgery Study Group. Burgenstock, Switzerland, vol 22, 1968.

Maguire LJ, Singer DE, Klyce SD: Graphic presentation of computer analyzed keratotoscope photographs. Arch Ophthalmol 1987; 105:223.

Maltzman BA, Cinotti DJ, Horon CA, et al: Posterior chamber implants and postoperative refractive astigmatism. *CLAO J* 1983; 9:229–231.

Matsuda H, Smelser GK: Electron microscopy of corneal wound healing. *Grp Eye Res* 1973; 16:427–442.

Merlin U: Curved keratotomy procedure for congenital astigmatism. *J Refract Surg* 1987; 3:92–97.

Moore JG: Intraocular implants: The postoperative astigmatism. *Br J Ophthalmol* 1980; 64:318–321.

Morrison JC, Swan KC: Descemet's membrane in penetrating keratoplasties of the human eye. *Arch Ophthalmol* 1983; 101:1927–1929.

Morrison JC, Swan KC: Bowman's layer in penetrating keratoplasties of the human eye. *Arch Ophthalmol* 1982; 100:1835–1838.

Moses RA: *Adler's Physiology of the Eye: Clinical Application.* St Louis, CV Mosby, 1981.

Phan TM, Foster SC, Zagachin LM, et al: Role of fibronectin in the healing of superficial keratectomies in vitro. *Invest Ophthalmol Vis Sci* 1989; 30:386–391.

Robb RM: Refractive errors associated with hemangiomas of the orbit in infancy. *Am J Ophthalmol* 1977; 82:52.

Rowsey JJ: Review: Current concepts in astigmatism surgery. *J Refract Surg* 1986; 2:85–94.

Salz JJ, Villaseñor RA, Elander R, et al: Four-incision radial keratotomy for low to moderate myopia. *Ophthalmology* 1986; 93:727–738.

Sanders DR, Hofmann RF, Salz JJ: *Refractive Corneal Surgery* Thorofare, New Jersey; pp 243–288, 1986.

Sato T, Akiyama K, Shibata H: A new surgical approach to myopia. *Am J Ophthalmol* 1953; 36:823–829.

Shaw EL: A modified technique for conjunctival transplant, *CLAO J*, in press.

Shepherd JR; Induced astigmatism in small incision cataract surgery. *J Cataract Refract Surg* 1989; 15:85–88.

Simon G, Parel JM, Lee W, et al: Gel injection adjustable keratoplasty. *Graefes Arch Clin Exp Ophthalmol* 1991; 229:418.

Smith RS, Smith LA, Rich L, et al: Effects of growth factors on corneal wound healing. *Invest Ophthalmol Visual Sci* 1991; 20:222–229.

Stern D, Wei-Zhu L, Puliafito CA, et al: Femtosecond optical ranging of corneal incision depth. *Invest Ophthalmol Vis Sci* 1989; 30:99–104.

Storch RL, Troutman RC, Draga AE, et al: Postkeratoplasty (PK) astigmatism analysis comparing Krumeich guided trephine system (GTS) to manual trephination. Presented at American Academy of Ophthalmology (AAO) Annual Meeting, Sept 1990.

Tchah H. Hofmann R, Duffy R, et al: Delimited peripheral arcuate keratotomy for astigmatism: "Bow tie" configuration. *J Refract Surg* 1988; 5:183–190.

Thoft RA: Indications for conjuctival transplantation. *Ophthalmology* 1982; 89:335.

Tschering M: Etude sur la position du cristallin de l'oeil humain, in Javal E (ed): *Memoires d'Ophthalmometrie.* Paris, Masson Publishers, 1890.

Tripathi BJ, Kwait PS, Tripathi RC: Corneal growth factors: A new generation of ophthalmic pharmaceuticals. *Cornea* 1990; 9:2–9.

Tripoli NK, Cohen KL, Holman RE: Corneal topographic response to circumferential keratotomies. *J Refract Surg* 1987; 3:129–136.

Troutman RC: *Microsurgery of the Anterior Segment of the Eye,* vol 2. St Louis, CV Mosby, 1977.

Troutman RC: *Microsurgery of the Anterior Segment of the Eye,* vol 1. St Louis, CV Mosby, 1974.

Troutman RC: Microsurgery of keratoconus. *Proceedings of the Centennial Symposium, Manhattan Eye, Ear and Throat Hospital.* St Louis, CV Mosby, 1969, pp 242–253.

Troutman RC: Primary astigmatism control using the Troutman surgical keratometer, in Emery JM, Jacobson AC (eds): *Current Concepts in Cataract Surgery.* St Louis, CV Mosby, 1980, pp 241–243.

Troutman RC, Haight DH: Suture materials and techniques, in Brightbill FS (ed): *Corneal Surgery.* St Louis, CV Mosby, 1986; pp 265–268.

Troutman RC, Swinger C: Relaxing incision for control of postoperative astigmatism following keratoplasty. *Ophthalm Surg* 1980; 11:117.

Tuft SJ, Zabel RW, Marshall J: Corneal repair following keratectomy. *Invest Ophthalmol Visual Sci* 1989; 30:1769–1777.

Tuyet-Mai M, Foster CS, Zagachin LM, et al: Role of fibronectin in the healing of superficial keratectomies in vitro. *Invest Ophthalmol Vis Sci* 1989; 30:386–391.

Van Rij G, Cornell Fm, Waring GO, et al: Postoperative astigmatism after central vs. eccentric penetrating keratoplasties. *Am J Ophthalmol* 1985; 99:317.

Wagoner MD, Kenyon KR, Gipson IK, et al: Polymorphonuclear neutrophils delay corneal epithelial wound healing in vitro. *Invest Ophthalmol Visual Sci* 1984; 25:1217–1220.

Waring GO, Lynn MJ, Fielding B, et al: Results of the Prospective Evaluation of Radial Keratotomy (PERK) study 4 years after surgery for myopia. *JAMA* 1990; 263:1083–1091.

Waring GO, Lynn MJ, Gelender H, et al: Results of the Prospective Evaluation of Radial Keratotomy (PERK) Study one year after surgery. *Ophthalmology* 1985; 91:177–198.

Waring GO, Steinbert EB, Wilson LA: Slit-lamp microscopic appearance of corneal wound healing after radial keratotomy. *Am J Ophthalmol* 1985; 100:218–224.

Wilson G, Bell C, Chotai S: The effect of lifting the lids on corneal astigmatism. *Am J Optom Physiol Opt* 1982; 59:670.

Wunsh SE: The Cross cylinder, in Duane TD (ed): *Clinical Opthalmology.* New York, Harper & Row, 1982, pp 1–10.

Yau CW, Busin M, McDonald MB, et al: The effect of different radial keratotomy patterns on astigmatism in rabbits. *J Refract Surg* 1985; 1:201–205.

Glossary

absolute color scale   Used in computerized topographic corneal analysis as a predetermined scale of dioptric power, useful when large changes in corneal power are displayed.

additional suture technique   Method of astigmatic reduction in the sutures-in post–penetrating keratoplasty patient in which additional sutures are used to repair "microdehiscence" along the graft wound.

against the rule astigmatism   Less common form of regular astigmatism, seen in infants and older patients, in which the steep meridian is at 180 degrees and the flat meridian is at 90 degrees.

algebraic addition of corneal incisions   Theory that states that the effect of multiple corneal incisions will be the same if they are performed together or at different times.

American-style cutting   Radial incision that begins at the optical zone and proceeds to the limbus, using the diagonal cutting edge knife. Synonymous with back cutting or centrifugal cutting.

angulation of mires   Sign of irregular astigmatism in which the mires of the keratometer intersect at an angle.

arcuate incision   Curved transverse incision used for correcting astigmatism, for example, in the Troutman relaxing incisions procedure.

astigmatic coupling   Property of the cornea in which operations performed in one astigmatic meridian affect the meridian 90 degrees away.

astigmatically neutral cataract closure   Any closure technique that returns the cornea to the preoperative astigmatic error within 1 to 2 weeks after cataract surgery.

asymmetric corneal relaxing incisions   Technique that identifies asymmetric astigmatic bands with computed topology and corrects these areas proportionate to their occurrence on the cornea.

axis   Absolute measure reflected on the cornea related to the orientation of the cornea relative to the face and lids.

back cutting   Radial incision that begins at the optical zone and proceeds to the limbus, made with the diagonal cutting edge of the knife; synonymous with American-style cutting and centripetal cutting.

basement membrane   Substance secreted by the epithelium; mediates epithelial adhesion to Bowman's layer.

Bell's phenomenon   Tendency of a normal eye to roll upward with lid closure.

beveled lacerations   Lacerations angled relative to the corneal surface; closed with penetration of the needle through the tip of the bevel.

block lift   Wound healing abnormality seen when a block of corneal tissue loses adjacent support as a result of crossing incisions or incisions placed too close together.

blocking of radial incisions   Incorrect theory that postulates that the coupling of transverse incisions is blocked by the addition of flanking radial and semiradial incisions.

Bowman's layer   Anterior acellular envelope of the cornea beneath the epithelium, which does not regenerate.

bowtie procedure   Combination of radial and arcuate corneal incisions used to correct moderate to large degrees of astigmatism, but not recommended because of connection of incisions.

breaking of mires   Indication of incomplete wound healing; seen on photokeratometry by a break in the path of the mire over the incision.

capsaicin   Neurotoxin that blocks the action of nerves in corneal healing.

central corneal optical zone   Central 4 mm of the cornea, which provides the most important optical functions of the cornea and which is roughly spherical, with parallel anterior and posterior surfaces.

centrifugal cutting   Radial incision that begins at the optical zone and proceeds to the limbus, using the diagonal cutting edge of the knife. Synonymous with American-style cutting or back cutting.

centripetal cutting   Radial incision that begins at the limbus and proceeds to the optical zone, using the vertical cutting edge of the knife. Synonymous with front cutting or Russian-style cutting.

circle of least confusion   Area of greatest convergence of light rays from an astigmatic lens located between the principal foci.

circular corneal suture   Therapeutic maneuver used after radial keratotomy to compress the radial incision in the mid-periphery and to diminish overcorrections.

collagen fibrils   Long thick chains of collagen arranged in layers of differing orientation; provide strength to the corneal stroma.

compound astigmatism   Regular astigmatism in which both foci fall either behind or in front of the retina.

compound curved needle   Modification of a circular curved needle that allows short, deep corneal suture placement.*

conjunctival transdifferentiation   Process of the transformation of conjunctival cells to epithelial cells occurring at the limbus.

conoid of Sturm   Area between the principal foci of an astigmatic lens; roughly forms a cone-shaped figure.

continuous suture adjustment for astigmatism   Method of astigmatic reduction in the early post–penetrating keratoplasty patient in which the running suture pattern is adjusted to redistribute forces around the wound, usually at the slit lamp.

coreoplasty   Repair of iris abnormalities; also reestablishes iris tension and prevents anterior synechiae.

cornea splitter   Knife that is slightly dull; used for manual dissection of the lamellar keratoplasty bed.

corneal cataract incision   Located in clear cornea approximately 1–2 mm anterior to the surgical limbus.

corneal edge lift   Seen on biomicroscopy as an elevation of corneal tissue and evidence of poor wound apposition, with probable associated astigmatic error.

corneal endothelium   Monolayer of active cells that do not regenerate; responsible for the active water balance of the cornea.

corneal epithelium   Most anterior of the five layers of the cornea; responsible for production of basement membrane and regular stabilization of tear film.

Corneal Modeling System (CMS)   Computerized topographic corneal mapping system using computer analysis of specularly reflected rings, with provision for measurement of corneal thickness.

corneal optical zone   Central 4 mm of the cornea, that provides the most important optical functions of the cornea and is roughly spherical with parallel anterior and posterior surfaces.

*Dr. Troutman holds jointly with Walter McGregor of Ethicon Inc. of Somerville, New Jersey, the U.S. and foreign patents on the "compound curve" surgical needle concept and receives royalty compensation therefrom.

corneal stroma   Middle layer of the cornea, comprising 99% of its thickness and much of its anatomic strength.

corneal tear film   Actual anterior refracting surface of the eye; composed of the lipid, aqueous, and mucous layers.

cytotoxic medication   Nonsteroidal class of medications used to control inflammatory response, e.g., azathioprine (Imuran), cyclophosphamide (Cytoxan), and methotrexate.

Descemet's membrane   Posterior limiting membrane of the cornea, secreted by endothelial cells consisting largely of type IV collagen.

diurnal variation   Variation of visual acuity possibly related to incomplete wound healing by disturbance in corneal water balance.

double continuous suture pattern (10-0, 11-0)   Closure technique for penetrating keratoplasty that allows rotation of the donor disk, because of the inadequate apposing forces created by the 11-0 suture.

double-cutting diamond   Diamond with sharpened edges along both the diagonal and vertical edges, which is thus capable of cutting in two directions.

double slipknot   Technique that allows a sliding knot, which is capable of withstanding higher intraocular pressure than a single slipknot.

epikeratophakia   Thickness volume technique that involves placement of additional corneal tissue above Bowman's layer to effect hyperopic and myopic spherical correction.

epithelial growth factor (EGF)   Polypeptide found in mouse submaxillary glands and human urine; stimulates growth of epidermal cells.

epithelial plug   Indication of an early stage of wound healing on histopathologic study; can represent delayed wound healing if noted late in the course of healing.

excimer laser surface ablation   Surface modification technique involving controlled removal of surface corneal tissue by means of the unique ability of low ultraviolet radiation to ablate tissue.

EyeSys System   Computerized topographic corneal mapping system using computer analysis of specularly reflected rings.

Fenzel flag incisions   Touching transverse and radial incisions, which are stepped, can lead to corneal instability.

fibrin plug   Immediate response of tissue to injury that fills the wound, and is subsequently displaced as healing progresses.

fibroblast   Active cell derived from keratocytes in stromal wound healing; among other duties, elaborates collagen fibrils and proteoglycans.

fibronectin   Large glycoprotein that binds to collagen, fibrin, and extracellular matrix, and provides temporary epithelial adhesion in normal healing.

fogging   Method of astigmatic refraction that depends on collapsing the conoid of Sturm.

free conjunctival flap   Technique used after pterygium removal and other conjunctival surgery to replace the conjunctival covering of sclera.

front cutting   Radial incision that begins at the limbus and proceeds to the optical zone, made with the vertical cutting edge of the knife; synonymous with **centripetal cutting** and **Russian-style cutting**.

Fyodorov TR incisions   Crossing radial and transverse incisions; implicated in corneal instability.

Gauss' law of total curvature of toric surface   If a perfectly flexible and inextensible surface is bent in a given meridian, the total curvature remains constant as the second main radius changes in the opposite way. The total curvature is defined as the product of the inverse of the radius of each meridian.

glycosaminoglycans (GAG)   Proteoglycans responsible for the tendency of corneal tissue to swell; surround the collagen fibrils in corneal stroma.

Hanna trephine   Suction trephine system that adheres to the eye through corneal suction; capable of creating fine vertical incisions.

Hessberg-Barron trephine   Suction trephine system without an obturator that adheres to the eye through corneal suction but often creates beveled incisions.

Histoacryl glue   Form of cyanoacrylate glue that can be used to close small corneal perforations.

Hofmann T/I incisions   Short transverse incisions jumping radial keratotomy incisions.

holographic interferometry   Technique of measuring corneal topology in which interference of light is used to determine changes in corneal elevation.

hyperopia   Condition of spherical ametropia in which the focus is behind the retina.

incisional staining   Uptake of fluorescein dye over corneal incisions, indicating delayed or incomplete wound healing.

infinity cataract closure   Horizontal suturing technique that provides two horizontal bites for closure of larger scleral tunnel incisions.

intracorneal annular ring   Polymethylmethacrylate (PMMA) ring inserted in the periphery of the cornea to flatten or steepen the central cornea; also reduces central astigmatism by producing a regular peripheral optical ring.

irregular astigmatism   Astigmatic error that cannot be completely corrected with spectacle lenses, or a condition in which the astigmatic meridians are not symmetric.

irregular irregular astigmatism   Astigmatic error in which the surface is rough, preventing regular refraction of light, which also prevents full correction with spectacle lenses; often corrected with soft contact lenses, or in more severe cases with hard contact lenses.

Jackson cross cylinder   Combination of a plus and a minus cylindrical lens oriented at 90 degrees; used to determine astigmatic axis and degree.

jumped incisions   Technique of creating radial and transverse incisions in proximity in which one of the incisions is broken prior to contact with the other incision, thus preventing crossed incisions and subsequent corneal instability.

jumping of mires   Sign of irregular astigmatism in which the mires of the keratometer cannot be aligned.

keratoconus   Corneal ectasia resulting in distortion of the corneal surface and irregular astigmatism.

keratocyte   Cellular component of the stroma; participates in corneal wound healing.

keratometer   Device that measures, either subjectively or objectively, the curvature of the cornea.

keratometric astigmatic refraction   Method of astigmatic refraction that relies on keratometer readings as the initial determination of astigmatic error.

keratomileusis   Thickness volume technique that involves lathing central (myopic keratomileusis) or peripheral (hyperopic keratomileusis) corneal stromal tissue to achieve correction of spherical ametropias.

keratophakia   Thickness volume technique that involves the introduction of a disk of corneal stromal tissue to effect large hyperopic corrections in aphakia.

Krebs cycle   Aerobic cycle responsible for the production of adenosine triphosphate from glucose and oxygen.

Krumeich procedure   Astigmatic corneal technique that involves creation of a circumferential partial penetrating corneal incision, which is closed with a running suture and adjusted to remove corneal astigmatism.

Krumeich trephine   Suction trephine system that adheres to the eye through scleral suction; capable of creating fine vertical incisions.

L astigmatic procedure   Multiple semiradial incisions along a given meridian; used to correct moderate to large degrees of astigmatism; capable of creating corneal instability.

lambda-shaped wound profile   Corneal wound in which closure is not full thickness and the resulting wound spreads posteriorly, leading to wound weakness and loss of endothelial cells.

lamellar keratoplasty   Transplantation of corneal material to a host cornea without performing full-thickness penetration of the host.

limbal corneal cataract incision   Located in the transition zone between cornea and sclera; not recommended, because of problems with postoperative stability.

limbal guy wire   Artistic representation of the fixed circumference of the intact limbus.

linear guy wire   Artistic representation of the appropriate corneal diameter used to illustrate coupling effects in the cornea.

map-dot–fingerprint dystrophy   Abnormality of epithelial adhesion, usually due to defects in the basement membrane and resulting in recurrent erosions and poor wound healing.

meridian   Variable measure relating to the position of steep and flat positions on the cornea and referred to by their position relative to the absolute axis of the cornea.

mesodermal growth factor (MGF)   Naturally elaborated substance that accelerates wound healing.

microdehiscence   Abnormality seen on photokeratometry and computed corneal topography in which the mires display a characteristic V pattern pointing to an area of wound weakness.

microkeratome   Mechanical device used to create lamellar resection of corneal tissue; originally introduced by Barraquer.

mid-peripheral corneal distortion   Problem often seen after refractive surgery, in which distortions in the mid-cornea prevent accurate keratometry.

minification of mires   Sign of a steep cornea; may also indicate irregular astigmatism, as in keratoconus.

minus cylindrical lens   Astigmatic lens in which the axis of the correcting lens lies along the flat astigmatic meridian of the cornea.

mire   Specular reflection of a lighted object from the cornea; used to determine corneal curvature.

mixed astigmatism Regular astigmatism in which the focus of one meridian is in front of the retina and the other behind it.

modified Ruiz procedure Single pair of tranverse incisions flanked by semiradial incisions; exhibits less instability than a classic Ruiz procedure.

multiple puncture technique Means of creating two corneal incisions in close proximity by outlining the incisions with multiple punctures, which are then connected.

myopia Condition of spherical ametropia in which the focus is in front of the retina.

obturator Central device in a corneal trephine that prevents sliding of corneal tissue centrally.

optical ring Mechanical effect of the limbus that isolates the cornea from forces and operations in the sclera and participates in the process of astigmatic coupling.

paralimbal incision Any incision placed in proximity to the surgical limbus.

peripheral corneal support zone Area of the cornea outside the central 4 mm optical zone; varies in thickness with a complex curvature, which affects the regularity and astigmatic properties of the central optical zone by virtue of mechanical support.

photokeratometer Device with multiple lighted rings, camera, and chin rest that provides permanent documentation of subjective corneal topology.

physics of incompressible fluids Property that states that the volume of a structure filled with incompressible fluid is constant at all times; thus compression along one meridian requires extension along the meridian 90 degrees away.

placido disk Handheld device with multiple lighted rings; forerunner to the photokeratometer.

plus cylindrical lens Astigmatic lens in which the axis of the correcting lens lies along the steep astigmatic meridian of the cornea.

Poisson ratio Ratio of longitudinal extension to tangential extension for homogeneous materials, with a value of 0.5 for homogeneous biologic materials comprised mostly of water, due to the physics of incompressible fluids.

principle of least energy Law of thermodynamics that states that all physical systems will seek a configuration that minimizes their potential energy.

proteolytic enzyme   Substance secreted by inflammatory cells, such as polymorphonucleocytes, that causes melting and absorption of dead and sometimes living tissue.

pseudo-optical ring   Effect produced by a corneal transplantation or circular suture scar that isolates the central cornea from the peripheral cornea, preventing operations outside the pseudo-optical ring from achieving full astigmatic effect.

pursestring suture   Technique of closing stellate and crossing lacerations by closing circumferentially and drawing the tissue together.

radial keratotomy   Surface area modification technique that induces corneal flattening along both corneal meridians by addition of radial wedges of scar tissue, adding surface area to both corneal meridians.

Raster stereography   Device used to measure corneal topology by projecting a grid on the cornea and measuring its distortions.

regular astigmatism   Astigmatic error that can be corrected with spectacle lenses, in theory, with astigmatic meridians 90 degrees from one another.

regular irregular astigmatism   Astigmatic error in which the surface is smooth enough to regularly refract light but in which the power varies along the meridian, such as in keratoconus, thus preventing correction with spectacle lenses; usually corrected with hard contact lenses.

relative color scale   Used in computerized topographic corneal analysis as a scale determined by the range of dioptric power on a particular cornea; useful to display subtle corneal detail.

retrocorneal membrane   Fibrous tissue with fibroblast-like cells located on the posterior aspect of the penetrating corneal wound; often associated with poor wound closure.

RL astigmatic procedure   Multiple semiradial incisions along a given meridian combined with radial keratotomy; used to correct moderate to large degrees of astigmatism; has been found to create corneal instability.

running interrupted suture pattern   Closure technique for penetrating keratoplasty using single running and interrupted sutures, which are removed sequentially in an attempt to reduce postoperative astigmatism.

Russian-style cutting   Radial incision that begins at the limbus and proceeds to the optical zone, using the vertical cutting edge of the knife. Synonymous with centripetal cutting or front cutting.

Schirmer test   Test of aqueous tear function in which filter paper is used to quantitatively assess the production of aqueous; normal value ≥15 mm.

scleral tunnel cataract incision   Exterior incision located 1–2 mm scleral to the surgical limbus; the interior entrance to the eye usually is in clear cornea.

segment length   Term introduced by Thornton that indicates that an incision that occupies a 45-degree angle measured from the optical axis will have essentially the same refractive effect, independent of optical zone, recently shown to be incorrect.

sequential removal of sutures   Method of astigmatic reduction in the sutures-in post–penetrating keratoplasty patient in which tight interrupted sutures are identified on photokeratotometry and removed.

simple astigmatism   Regular astigmatism in which the focus of one meridian falls on the retina, the other in front of the retina (hyperopic astigmatism) or behind the retina (myopic astigmatism).

single-cutting diamond   Diamond with a sharpened edge along only the vertical or diagonal edge.

slipknot   Means of predictably controlling suture tension while tying.

small incision cataract surgery   Originally a term synonymous with the use of flexible intraocular lenses; now used with scleral tunnel incisions <5 mm long.

stellate lacerations   Lacerations that coincide at a central area of penetration; best closed with circumferential suturing.

stenopeic slit   Device that isolates an astigmatic meridian, allowing light rays to focus and serving the same purpose in astigmatism as the pinhole for spherical ametropias.

stromal overgrowth   Proliferation of fibroblasts above Bowman's layer and beneath the epithelium after corneal incisional procedures.

subepithelial fibrosis   Fibrous tissue located between epithelium and Bowman's layer; often associated with poor wound closure.

T cataract incision technique   Method of splitting the bed of the scleral tunnel to allow the intraocular lens to be introduced in a smaller incision.

T cut   Small linear transverse incision that acts to flatten the corneal meridian of the procedure and steepen the meridian 90 degrees away; used for correcting small degrees of astigmatism.

tachykinan neuropeptides   Mediators of neurogenic inflammation that promote both epithelial and stromal healing.

tangential or horizontal cataract closure   Suturing technique that minimizes radial forces on the scleral tunnel incision and results in little induced astigmatism.

tear breakup time   Test of the stability of the tear film; normal value ≥10 seconds.

tectonic lamellar keratoplasty   Graft performed primarily for structural support, usually done in the periphery rather than centrally, secondarily for optical improvement of vision.

tensor   Mathematical entity that must be described by a matrix of numbers of two or more dimensions.

Thornton T incisions   Short transverse incisions created between radial keratotomy incisions.

tickle procedure   Mechanical opening or deepening of refractive incisions to enhance refractive effect.

tickle technique   Means of creating corneal incisions using two diamond knives to achieve both straight and deep incisions.

time of flight ranging   Method of measuring distance in which sound or light is reflected from a given point and the time, and hence the distance, is determined.

Topographic Modeling System (TMS)   Upgraded version of the Corneal Modeling System, without provision for measurement of corneal thickness.

torque-antitorque suture pattern   Closure technique for penetrating keratoplasty of Troutman that prevents donor rotation and creates radial closure forces across the wound.

trapezoidal keratotomy   Introduced by Ruiz; uses a combination of T cuts and semiradial incisions for correction of astigmatism; not recommended, because of induction of corneal instability.

trifacet diamond   "Square" diamond with sharpened edges along all three edges; used for astigmatic incisions and capable of cutting in both directions.

Troutman operative keratometer   Surgical microscope mounted ring of lights projected on the cornea during surgery to objectively assess the astigmatic consequences of surgical technique.

Troutman relaxing incisions   Surface area modification technique that induces corneal flattening along the meridian of the procedure by addition of a wedge of scar tissue, adding surface area and steepening the meridian 90 degrees away.

Troutman wedge (block) resection   Surface area modification technique that induces corneal steepening along the meridian of the procedure by removal of a wedge or block of corneal tissue and suturing; flattens the meridian 90 degrees away.

vector   Mathematical entity that must be described by two or more numbers (e.g., an arrow, which is described by length and direction) or a one-dimensional matrix.

vortex epitheliopathy   Swirling visualization of epithelial migration seen with some drugs and sutures, sometimes resulting in irregular astigmatism.

with the rule astigmatism   Common form of regular astigmatism, seen in younger patients and in patients who have undergone cataract surgery, in which the steep meridian is at 90 degrees and the flat meridian is at 180 degrees.

Index